Novel Biomarkers in Alzheimer's Disease

Novel Biomarkers in Alzheimer's Disease

Editor: Lisa Scott

MURPHY & MOORE
www.murphy-moorepublishing.com

www.murphy-moorepublishing.com

MURPHY & MOORE

Cataloging-in-Publication Data

Novel biomarkers in alzheimer's disease / edited by Lisa Scott.
p. cm.
Includes bibliographical references and index.
ISBN 978-1-63987-400-2
1. Alzheimer's disease. 2. Biochemical markers. 3. Neurology. I. Scott, Lisa.
RC523 .N68 2022
616.831--dc23

Murphy & Moore Publishing,
1 Rockefeller Plaza,
New York City, NY 10020, USA

ISBN 978-1-63987-400-2 (Hardback)

Contents

Preface

Every book is initially just a concept; it takes months of research and hard work to give it the final shape in which the readers receive it. In its early stages, this book also went through rigorous reviewing. The notable contributions made by experts from across the globe were first molded into patterned chapters and then arranged in a sensibly sequential manner to bring out the best results.

The neurochemical indicators which help in the assessment of risk or the presence of Alzheimer's disease are known as Alzheimer's disease biomarkers. They help in an early diagnosis as well as tracking the progress of the disease in a reliable manner. The analysis of biomarkers becomes vital to the management of this disease since the neuropathologic changes occur years before the symptoms are seen. The most important biomarker used for the detection of Alzheimer's disease is amyloid beta. One of the novel approaches towards research on Alzheimer's disease is the usage of autoantibody. These can be used as both biomarkers and for future treatment. This book elucidates the concepts and innovative models around prospective developments with respect to novel biomarkers in Alzheimer's disease. It will also provide interesting topics for research which interested readers can take up. Researchers and students in this field will be assisted by this book.

It has been my immense pleasure to be a part of this project and to contribute my years of learning in such a meaningful form. I would like to take this opportunity to thank all the people who have been associated with the completion of this book at any step.

Editor

1

The potential of pathological protein fragmentation in blood-based biomarker development for dementia – with emphasis on Alzheimer's disease

*Dilek Inekci [1,2], Ditte Svendsen Jonesco [1], Sophie Kennard [1], Morten Asser Karsdal [1] and Kim Henriksen [1]**

[1] Nordic Bioscience, Biomarkers and Research, Herlev, Denmark, [2] Systems Biology, Technical University of Denmark, Lyngby, Denmark

Edited by:
Charlotte Elisabeth Teunissen, VU University Medical Center Amsterdam, Netherlands

Reviewed by:
Alison Louise Baird, University of Oxford, UK
Fabrizio Piazza, University of Milano Bicocca, Italy
Andreas Jeromin, Quanterix, USA

***Correspondence:**
Kim Henriksen, Nordic Bioscience A/S, Herlev Hovedgade 207, Herlev DK 2730, Denmark kh@nordicbioscience.com

The diagnosis of dementia is challenging and early stages are rarely detected limiting the possibilities for early intervention. Another challenge is the overlap in the clinical features across the different dementia types leading to difficulties in the differential diagnosis. Identifying biomarkers that can detect the pre-dementia stage and allow differential diagnosis could provide an opportunity for timely and optimal intervention strategies. Also, such biomarkers could help in selection and inclusion of the right patients in clinical trials of both Alzheimer's disease and other dementia treatment candidates. The cerebrospinal fluid (CSF) has been the most investigated source of biomarkers and several candidate proteins have been identified. However, looking solely at protein levels is too simplistic to provide enough detailed information to differentiate between dementias, as there is a significant crossover between the proteins involved in the different types of dementia. Additionally, CSF sampling makes these biomarkers challenging for presymptomatic identification. We need to focus on disease-specific protein fragmentation to find a fragment pattern unique for each separate dementia type – a form of protein fragmentology. Targeting protein fragments generated by disease-specific combinations of proteins and proteases opposed to detecting the intact protein could reduce the overlap between diagnostic groups as the extent of processing as well as which proteins and proteases constitute the major hallmark of each dementia type differ. In addition, the fragments could be detectable in blood as they may be able to cross the blood–brain barrier due to their smaller size. In this review, the potential of the fragment-based biomarker discovery for dementia diagnosis and prognosis is discussed, especially highlighting how the knowledge from CSF protein biomarkers can be used to guide blood-based biomarker development.

Keywords: dementia, Alzheimer's disease, biomarkers, blood, post-translational modifications

Introduction

Dementias are brain disorders that cause a progressive decline in mental function. In 2009, it was estimated that 35.6 million people were suffering from dementia worldwide and this number is expected to be 65.7 million by 2030 and 115.4 by 2050 (1). Alzheimer's disease (AD) is the most common cause of dementia, and accounts for 60–70% of all cases. Other common causes of dementia are dementia with Lewy bodies (DLB), vascular dementia (VaD), frontotemporal lobar degeneration (FTLD), and corticobasal degeneration (CBD). In addition to this, mixed dementias are also commonly seen (2–4).

The major risk factor for developing dementia is age, with increasing prevalence after age 65, followed by family history, environmental factors, and mutations (4). Cognitive and neuropsychiatric symptoms are the key clinical features of dementia (5).

The diagnosis of dementia is challenging and early and moderate stages of dementia are rarely detected thereby limiting the potential for early intervention. Additionally, a high number of dementia cases are left without a diagnosis (6).

It is generally accepted that there is a need for early diagnosis of dementia and many efforts have been made to develop early biomarkers with the ability to identify the pre-dementia stage of the disease before the onset of cognitive decline and brain degeneration (7, 8).

Another challenge is the differential diagnosis of dementia, as there is an overlap in the clinical features across the different dementia types (9–11). There is currently no single marker available that can differentiate between AD and other dementia types. Hence, there is a need for biomarkers that can distinguish between the dementias.

Additionally, successful development of disease-modifying drugs and prevention therapies require biomarkers that can recognize neuropathological changes in the pre-dementia stage and allow differential diagnosis. This would allow inclusion of the right patients in the clinical trials, monitoring of the treatment efficacy, and exclusion of patients that have already reached a point-of-no-return and would not have any beneficial effect of a given intervention (12, 13).

Unfortunately, the biomarker development has been hampered by the fact that tracking molecular pathological changes in the brain is a huge challenge due to the inaccessible nature of the brain. Currently imaging and CSF biomarkers provide the best method for diagnosing, staging, as well as predicting clinical progression of AD and related dementias. However their use is limited by cost, availability and by the fact that repeated brain scans and withdrawal of CSF by lumbar punctures are not advisable (14, 15). These aspects all underline the need for novel biomarkers which are easily obtainable.

The Proteopathy of Dementia

Most dementias can be designated as proteopathies characterized by aberrant processing of neuronal proteins such as fragmentations, aggregations and other post-translational modifications (PTMs) (**Table 1**) (3, 16).

The potential of these proteins as diagnostic and prognostic biomarkers has been extensively studied at the protein level. However, these investigations have been limited by the fact that the role of each of these pathological changes throughout the development of dementia is unresolved. This is due to the intrinsic difficulty of detecting the disease before patients display symptoms, which may be 20 years before the earliest cognitive changes are detected (28). Another complicating factor in diagnosing and determining progression of dementia is the significant crossover between the proteins involved in the different types of dementia. Thus, looking solely at protein levels is too simplistic to provide enough detailed information to differentiate between different dementia types. An alternative to this is the application of PTMs as biomarkers for AD. This is not a new approach, since it has already been investigated in the development of CSF-derived AD biomarkers $A\beta_{1-42}$ and phosphorylated tau (p-tau). This presents an excellent example of how understanding the molecular pathology inflicts certain protein fingerprints on key proteins, provides insight not only to central disease mechanisms, but also provides an opportunity to improve the protein's usage in terms of diagnostic and prognostic value for a specific dementia or even a subtype of dementia.

TABLE 1 | Common types of dementia and proteins affected.

Dementia type	Proteins affected	Reference
Alzheimer's disease (AD)	tau, Aβ, ApoE, α-synuclein	(17–19)
Vascular dementia (VaD)	tau	(20, 21)
Corticobasal degeneration (CBD)	tau	(22)
Dementia with Lewy Bodies (DLB)	α-synuclein	(19)
Parkinson's disease dementia	α-synuclein	(23)
Frontotemporal lobar dementia (FTLD)		
• FTLD-tau	Tau	(20, 22)
• FTLD-TDP43	TDP43	(24, 25)
• FTLD-FUS	FUS	(26, 27)

As we have previously proposed, AD pathology and other dementias may give rise to blood circulating fragments of key neuronal proteins, thereby allowing detection of disease specific post-translationally truncated fragments in the blood (29). This would allow easier and more frequent sampling and analysis and provide earlier diagnosis and prognosis of dementia.

The present review will focus on addressing the potential of disease-specific protein fragmentation for dementia diagnosis and prognosis and how these fragments can be utilized as biomarkers to segregate between the different types of dementia, especially highlighting how the knowledge from CSF protein biomarkers can be applied to investigate blood-based biomarkers.

Status of CSF Biomarkers

The pathological alterations in the brain at the molecular level are directly reflected in the CSF, therefore this fluid has been the most investigated source for development of biomarkers for AD and related dementias. $A\beta_{42}$, t-tau (total tau), p-tau, and α-synuclein are the most studied CSF biomarkers and their performance has been evaluated in several studies (30). Other biomarkers that will be described in this review are apolipoprotein E (ApoE), TAR DNA-binding protein 43 (TDP-43), fused in Sarcoma protein (FUS), and glial fibrillary acidic protein (GFAP).

$A\beta_{42}$ is the main component in the extracellular amyloid plaques of AD and is a marker of amyloid precursor protein (APP) processing and plaque load. In AD, a decrease in CSF $A\beta_{42}$ has been found, which is probably due to deposition in plaques (17, 31). Generation of $A\beta_{42}$ is an early event in AD, hence measuring CSF $A\beta_{42}$ is a very relevant strategy in prodromal AD to screen for early cases as well as monitoring disease progression. However as it is today the strategy of measuring CSF $A\beta_{42}$ only provides a supplementary test to support the diagnosis once cognitive dysfunction is apparent, and it gives little information on the disease progression as this biomarker has already found a steady-state of abnormality early in the disease progression (32, 33). CSF $A\beta_{42}$ is able to discriminate between AD and non-demented controls with a sensitivity of 59–96% and a specificity of 77–89% (17, 34–36). A change in $A\beta_{42}$ levels has also been studied for other types of dementia and shows a slight decrease in FTLD, DLB, and VaD (32). CSF $A\beta_{42}$ has been shown to predict the rate of cognitive decline in patients with very mild dementia and predict AD in subjects with mild cognitive impairment (MCI) (37, 38).

Cerebrospinal fluid t-tau is a biomarker of neuronal damage and neuronal and axonal degeneration and several studies have shown an increased level in AD patients compared with controls with a sensitivity and specificity of 70–83% and 81–92%, respectively (17, 34–36). However, CSF t-tau is not specific for AD and is also increased in other dementias such as Creutzfeldt–Jakob disease (CJD) patients and in a significant number of patients with DLB, FTLD, VaD, and CBD (20, 32).

Cerebrospinal fluid p-tau reflects aberrant phosphorylation and neurofibrillary tangle (NFT) burden. A strong increase in p-tau has been found in AD using ELISA methods that detect different phosphorylated epitopes such as p-tau(181) or p-tau(231). CSF p-tau differentiates between AD patients and controls with a sensitivity of 68–86% and a specificity of 61–73% (35, 36). A moderate increase in p-tau has also been found in CJD and DLB (17, 20). It has been reported that the use of p-tau instead of t-tau may improve the diagnostic sensitivity and differential diagnosis of AD versus DLB and FTD, respectively (34). Both t-tau and p-tau have been found to predict progression from MCI to AD (32, 39).

The combination of CSF biomarkers (t-tau/$A\beta_{1-42}$ and p-tau/$A\beta_{1-42}$) has been found to increase the sensitivity and specificity when compared to the single markers. The t-tau/$A\beta_{1-42}$ ratio shows a potential as a preclinical biomarker since it discriminates between MCI patients that progress to AD and those that do not progress, although the CSF sampling makes it virtually useless for this purpose (36, 40, 41). Furthermore, the ratio shows promise in prediction of dementia in cognitively normal older individuals (42).

Another interesting CSF biomarker is α-synuclein. Compared to tau and $A\beta_{1-42}$, little research has been done with respect to CSF levels of α-synuclein, which is the main component of Lewy bodies of DLB patients. Studies have demonstrated decreased CSF levels of α-synuclein in DLB and Parkinson's disease (PD) when compared to controls indicating a potential diagnostic use (43, 44). In contrast to this other research groups have shown no difference in CSF levels in DLB and PD patients compared with controls and other dementias (45–47).

In both PD and DLB patients, the level of α-synuclein oligomers is increased compared to healthy patients and other types of dementias (23, 48). In PD, the ratio of oligomers of α-synuclein to total α-synuclein is also significant. There is an increase in the ratio of oligomeric/total α-synuclein when compared to other dementias (49). Recent studies have also shown significantly elevated CSF levels of α-synuclein in AD patients (50) suggesting that α-synuclein may not be specific to DLB and PD, or again indicating that mixed pathologies are common.

Although, several CSF biomarkers show a promising diagnostic and prognostic potential, there are still important drawbacks limiting their clinical utility (**Table 2**). An important limitation is the lack of assay standardization and global cut-off values for biomarker concentrations. The handling of CSF and use of different technological platforms and antibodies are the major reasons for significant differences in biomarker concentrations between studies (51). Fortunately, international standardization initiatives have been initiated to reduce the large variations between studies and within laboratories (52). Another limitation of CSF biomarkers is the overlap between the protein profile of different types of dementia (20). Lastly, the clinical utility of CSF biomarkers is still hampered by sample collection, which requires a lumbar puncture. Despite the fact that there is minor complications related to lumbar puncture the procedure is still regarded as invasive in the general population and repeated follow-up measurement is challenging (14, 15), and hence they are not consistently applied in clinical trials. On the other hand, the CSF proteins described here all have a pathological link to the diseases of interest, and as such are of quite some interest for the development of blood-based biomarkers.

Status of Blood-Based Biomarkers

The use of blood as a source of dementia biomarkers is still under investigation. Blood is a more feasible biomarker source when compared to CSF due to its wide availability, low cost, time effectiveness, and easier sampling. Several different approaches for identification of blood biomarkers are available and these include biomarkers of the amyloid and tau pathology, biomarkers of inflammation, oxidative stress, mitochondrial dysfunction, neuronal and microvascular injury, and biomarker panels (15, 53). So far, the research has been hampered by two major challenges. The first is the complexity of blood and the large variation in samples and variation between studies. The difference in preanalytical and analytical methods is an important reason for this variation and these have been reviewed elsewhere (15). The second challenge is the fact that blood is not in direct contact with the brain. This limits the understanding of how the pathological alterations in the brain are reflected in blood analytes, as well as the absolute level of the analyte of interest in the blood. Additionally, the prevalent presence of non-specific proteins in the blood is an obstacle toward identification of disease-specific biomarkers. To overcome these limitations, the experience from the well-characterized CSF

TABLE 2 | Advantages and drawbacks of CSF biomarkers.

Advantages	Drawbacks
Diagnosis	Sampling
Prognosis	Standardization
	Diagnostic cut-off values
	False positive – false negative rates
	Overlap with other dementias

biomarkers, which in some cases are based on brain-specific pathological alterations, i.e., p-tau, may be a starting point for blood biomarker analysis. Pathological alterations in CSF proteins may be reflected in blood as a consequence of absorption of CSF into blood, by penetration due to barrier impairment in dementia or simply by diffusion (54–58). Whether a brain-derived protein can serve as a biomarker to be measured in blood will depend on the concentration, the change in concentration during disease, the molecular size and the half life in blood (57). Hence, exploring the dynamic range of brain proteins in the peripheral blood is of great interest.

The CSF biomarker tau is a brain-specific protein that can become a relevant biomarker to be measured in blood. So far, little is known about tau levels in blood and most studies have been hindered by the low abundance of the protein in blood (59). Zetterberg et al. (59) found that there was no correlation between CSF tau levels and plasma tau indicating that the clearance of tau is differently regulated (59). In healthy blood-donors tau protein concentration is in the range <10 and >100 pg/mL and the ratio between CSF:serum tau is 10:1 (57). Methods for determining tau in serum/plasma are under investigation. Few studies have reported elevated plasma tau levels in patients with AD (59, 60). The results from these studies are encouraging but highly sensitive detection methods are necessary. An ultrasensitive immunoassay for detection of plasma tau has been introduced and similar methods would be highly relevant (61).

Another CSF biomarker with potential to be a blood biomarker is Aβ. Plasma Aβ species have been examined by numerous studies but the results are contradictory. Some of these studies report high $A\beta_{42}$ or $A\beta_{40}$ whereas others show a decrease in AD. The overlap between patients with AD and healthy controls is also substantial. Importantly, Aβ is not brain-specific but is also expressed by other cells, and as such there is an interference of the peripheral Aβ species with the brain-derived species. Additionally, the binding of Aβ to plasma proteins and formation of Aβ oligomers may disturb the quantification by immunoassays (62, 63).

Finally, several studies have quantified plasma α-synuclein and α-synuclein oligomers in PD and DLB. However, additional studies are needed to evaluate blood α-synuclein as a valid biomarker and the high levels of α-synuclein present in red blood cells must be considered when quantifying the protein (64).

Plasma levels of ApoE, TDP-43, and GFAP have also been reported and the main results from these studies will be reviewed in the next sections.

Altogether, the inconsistent findings from plasma analyses illustrate the need for a pathology specific combination of protein and modification of this protein in order to enhance the possibility of generating a disease-specific biomarker, even more so in blood specimens than CSF.

Status of Protein Fragmentation Blood-Based Biomarkers

As mentioned identification and detection of brain-specific proteins in blood is restricted by the blood–brain-barrier, the substantial presence of non-specific proteins, and proteins from co-morbidities in the circulation. The use of post-translationally truncated protein fragments containing specific neo-epitopes as biomarkers of dementias may overcome these complexities (29, 65). Targeting protein fragments generated by disease-specific combinations of proteins and proteases opposed to detecting the intact protein could diminish the overlap between diagnostic groups. Proteolytic fragmentation of proteins is a post-translational process and several cleavage products have been identified in relation to AD and other dementias. $A\beta_{42}$, $A\beta_{40}$, and several other N- or C-terminally truncated Aβ peptides all represent examples of proteolytically cleaved protein fragments. Cleavage of tau, ApoE, α-synuclein, TDP-43, and GFAP has also been reported (66–70).

Although, several of the described protein fragments have been described in the literature and detected in CSF most of these have not been studied in blood. Targeting protein fragmentation by specific proteases may provide novel biomarkers for dementia and create a specific profile of each disorder based on the fragments and proteases that are involved in the pathology. Another advantage of using fragments as blood biomarkers opposed to the intact proteins may be the eased release from the central nervous system (CNS) into the periphery. The fragments may easier pass the blood-brain barrier due to their small size and be easier to detect (71–75) (**Figure 1**).

In addition to applying disease-specific protein fragmentation to identify new biomarkers for dementia, it is important to define and validate the ability of each novel biomarker. The BIPED classification system (Burden of Disease, Investigative, Prognostic, Efficacy of Intervention and Diagnostic) is a nomenclature first used for osteoarthritis and offers categorization of biomarkers in order to improve the development and validation of biomarkers (15). The use of BIPED classification in dementia would aid in the biomarker development process from target identification to validation in clinical trials.

In the following sections, neuronal proteins involved in the proteopathy of dementias will be reviewed with emphasis on proteolytic fragmentations (**Figure 2**).

Amyloid Precursor Protein

Derivatives from the full-length APP are the main components of the extracellular amyloid plaques. APPs are type 1 transmembrane

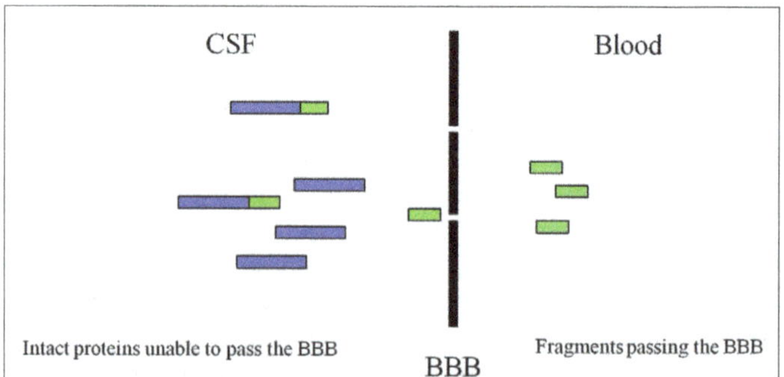

FIGURE 1 | Illustration of how the protein fragments may be able to cross the blood–brain barrier. Protein fragments may have the advantage of crossing the barrier as these breakdown products have a smaller size when compared to the intact protein. Modified from Ref. (29).

Protein	Proteases	Fragments
APP	ADAMs, BACE-1 and 2, Cathepsin B, γ-secretase	$A\beta_{42}$, $A\beta_{40}$, Aβn-42 (n=2-11), Aβ1-n (n=13-20), Aβ1-28, Aβ1-33, Aβ1-34, Aβ1-n (n=37-39), Aβ1-n (n=14-17)
Tau	Caspases, Calpains, thrombin, cathepsins and puromycin-sensitive aminopeptidase	Fragments cleaved at D13, E391 and D421, a 17 kDa fragment
ApoE	?	A 22 kDa N-terminally fragment, C-terminally truncated fragments
α-synculein	MMPs, Calpains, Cathepsins	N- and C-terminally truncated fragments
GFAP	Caspases	Fragments generated by cleavage at $VELD^{225}$ and $DLTD^{266}$
TDP-43	Caspases	Fragments of 25 and 35 kDa
FUS	?	?

FIGURE 2 | Key neuronal proteins involved in the proteopathy of different types of dementia, proteases involved in their truncation and fragments known from the literature. References can be found in the text.

proteins and exist in three isoforms in humans, APP695, APP751, and APP770. The APP695 is the main isoform in neurons and is the only isoform containing the sequence encoding Aβ (76, 77). In normal cells, APP is involved in kinase-based signaling, growth regulation, neurite outgrowth, formation of synapses and cell adhesion (33, 78). APP is cleaved by secretases and caspases at specific sites and this leads to the formation and release of several protein fragments (76, 78). The proteolytic processing of APP can follow the amyloidogenic or the non-amyloidogenic pathway. The major component of senile plaques, Aβ, is generated in the amyloidogenic pathway by sequential cleavage of APP by β-secretase and γ-secretase to generate $A\beta_{40}$ and $A\beta_{42}$. BACE1 (β-site APP-cleaving enzyme 1), BACE2 (β-site APP-cleaving enzyme 2), and cathepsin B have been identified as β-secretase responsible for production of Aβ. The γ-secretase activity belongs to a membrane-bound protease complex (presenilin 1, presenilin 2, nicastrin, Aph-1, and Pen-2) (76, 78). In the non-amyloidogenic processing, APP is cleaved by α-secretase which binds to and cleaves APP within the Aβ region and prevents formation of Aβ. All the identified α-secretases are from the family of disintegrin and metalloproteases (ADAMs).

The accumulation of Aβ is an early process in neurodegeneration leading to formation of oligomers, fibrils, and eventually extracellular plaques. CSF $A\beta_{42}$ levels become abnormal 5–10 years or more before the diagnosis (79, 80). The concentration of CSF $A\beta_{42}$ begins to increase abnormally followed by a drastic decrease. In mutation carriers (i.e., in the APP genes, presenilin 1, or presenilin 2), CSF $A\beta_{42}$ levels become abnormal up to 25 years before disease onset (28). Intracellular levels of Aβ initiate synaptic dysfunction, formation of NFTs and loss of neurons. The $A\beta_{42}$ is the main toxic form of Aβ, whereas $A\beta_{40}$ has been shown to have neuroprotective functions (78, 81).

$A\beta_{42}$ and $A\beta_{40}$ have also been detected in patients with cerebral amyloid angiopathy (CAA), which can be a co-occurring disorder with AD or a separate finding. CSF levels of $A\beta_{42}$ and $A\beta_{40}$ are lower in patients with CAA and CAA-related inflammation (CAA-ri) than controls (82–84). Furthermore, the level of CSF anti-Aβ autoantibodies is increased in CAA-ri which shares similarities with the amyloid-related imaging abnormalities detected in AD immunization clinical trials (84). It has been suggested that the CSF anti-Aβ autoantibody concentration can be used as a biomarker during immunization clinical trials in AD (84, 85).

The Aβ peptide is subjected to further truncations by different proteases and forms peptides of various lengths. The peptides are generated by N- or C-terminal truncation of Aβ and several of these have been identified in CSF, e.g., $A\beta_{n-42}$ ($n = 2$–11), $A\beta_{1-n}$ ($n = 13$–20), $A\beta_{1-28}$, $A\beta_{1-33}$, $A\beta_{1-34}$, and $A\beta_{1-n}$ ($n = 37$–39). These peptides have been found to be elevated in CSF of AD patients but only few are involved in plaque formation (86–89).

Recently, it was reported that some of the identified Aβ peptides in CSF are generated by an alternative APP processing pathway (90). In this pathway, APP is cleaved by α- and β-secretase without the involvement of γ-secretase. Many of the peptides derived from this pathway are elevated in CSF from AD suggesting an up-regulation of this pathway in AD as a response to the increase of the amyloidogenic pathway (90). The identified products of the alternative pathway are $A\beta_{1-14}$, $A\beta_{1-15}$, and $A\beta_{1-16}$. Eleven other truncated peptides with C-terminal at residue 15 in the Aβ sequence and start at the N-terminal end of the β-secretase site have been identified in CSF. The peptides contain a part of the Aβ sequence but are not degradation products of Aβ because they start upstream of the β-secretase cleavage site. Several of these were found to be elevated in AD and may also be generated in the alternative processing pathway (91).

Plasma levels of $A\beta_{42}$, $A\beta_{40}$, and the ratio $A\beta_{42}/A\beta_{40}$ have been examined in several cross-sectional studies with AD, MCI patients, and healthy controls. The results have shown a substantial overlap between diagnostic groups and the results between studies have been contradictory (92). $A\beta_{42}$ and $A\beta_{40}$ have also been studied in longitudinal studies to assess their association with disease progression. Although the results are not clear between individual studies the data show that a decreased baseline level of $A\beta_{42}$ predicts a greater risk of AD (92). A recent study has quantified $A\beta_{1-17}$ levels in plasma and has shown significant associations with the clinical diagnosis of AD, indicating the potential of the Aβ fragments (93). The plasma levels of the remaining Aβ cleavage products have only been examined in few studies. Highly specific antibodies and robust immunoassays must be developed and used for detection of these cleavage products of different size.

Tau

Tau is the basic component of the intracellular insoluble filamentous structures, also referred to as NFTs. The tau protein belongs to the family of microtubule-associated proteins and binds to, stabilizes, and promotes the assembly of microtubules. Tau is also involved in signaling pathways and cytoskeletal organization (94).

Tau is mainly expressed in the central and peripheral nervous system and most abundant in axons. There are six isoforms in the adult human brain, which vary in size and have either three or four microtubules-binding domains. The six forms each show functional differences (95, 96). The ratio between tau containing three and four domains is 1:1 in normal human brain but this ratio is altered in the different tauopathies. Additionally, different isoforms of tau are involved in the different tauopathies and affect distinct brain regions, hence it has been suggested that the isoform profiles can be used to classify the different tauopathies (97, 98). Besides AD, the tauopathies include FTLD, progressive supranuclear palsy (PSP), CBD, and prion diseases (20, 98).

In AD, the concentration of CSF t-tau and p-tau become abnormal after $A\beta_{42}$ and their levels increase progressively up to the time of diagnosis. Thus, tau levels are higher in MCI patients with an early conversion compared with late converters (79, 80). Increased CSF levels of tau are increased 15 years before symptoms in mutation carriers (28).

The conversion of soluble tau protein to insoluble inclusions is a central event in AD and other tauopathies. Formation of inclusions is mediated by protein aggregation and misfolding. The aggregates have been shown to be self-propagating and spread from one neuron to another (99). Tau aggregation and misfolding are induced by abnormal phosphorylation and proteolytic cleavage. Hyperphosphorylated tau is the main component of NFTs and several kinases and phosphatases have been associated with this. A level of phosphorylation occurs at normal state but in disease state, an abnormal level of phosphorylation is seen and results in a low-binding affinity to tubulin promoting disassembly of microtubules (94, 96).

Although the presence of t-tau and p-tau in CSF has been investigated in several studies, the nature of the protein in CSF is not fully known. A number of studies have suggested the presence of different tau and p-tau fragments in CSF (94, 95) and a recent study has reported that CSF tau and p-tau occur as various N-terminal and mid-domain fragments (67). The level of specific fragments were significantly elevated in AD patients when compared to controls and showed a diagnostic potential but the fragments still remain to be measured in other dementias (67).

Plasma levels of t-tau and tau fragments have only been assessed in few studies. It has been demonstrated that plasma t-tau levels are elevated in AD patients but with an overlap with control subjects (59). Hence, the diagnostic utility of plasma t-tau is not clear. Recently, the presence of protease generated fragments of tau has been shown in serum (75, 100, 101). The fragments have been shown to correlate with symptoms in AD patients and predict the disease progression in early AD (100, 101), indicating the pathological relevance of fragmentations.

It is a possibility that the assays for t-tau may also detect certain fragments of tau and as multiple systems are in use for detecting t-tau, this is most likely different from assay to assay depending on the antibodies used. Unless an assay is constructed as a sandwich ELISA with antibodies detecting the N- and C-terminal sequences, there is this possibility.

Furthermore, it must be noticed that the relative concentration of the protein determined in the clinical studies is a result of the specific calibrators used in the different assays.

In dementia, tau is cleaved by caspases and calpains, but other proteases have also been detected including thrombin, cathepsins, and puromycin-sensitive aminopeptidase (102). It has been found that certain proteolytic fragments of tau are specific for the different tauopathies suggesting that different proteases may be specific to individual tauopathies (102). Several tau fragments have been reported and the most studied are caspase-generated tau fragments cleaved at D13, E391, and D421 as well as a calpain-cleaved fragment of 17 kDa which are associated with AD (66, 103). The majority of the reported fragments have only been analyzed *in vitro*, in AD-affected brains or transgenic animals (94).

Apolipoprotein E

The ε4 allele of ApoE is known to be associated with the risk of developing AD. ApoE is a major transport protein of cholesterols and other lipids in plasma and in the brain. It is most abundant in the brain and the liver (104). In the CNS, ApoE is mainly synthesized in astrocytes but is also present in lower concentration in some neurons, activated microglia, oligodendrocytes, and ependymal layer cells. In neurons, the synthesis of ApoE is induced under neuronal stress and damage and has been detected in cortical and hippocampal neurons (105). In the normal brain, ApoE is associated with the maintenance and repair of neurons and involved in the cholesterol homeostasis (106). ApoE is a polymorphic protein with the main isoforms being ε2, ε3, and ε4. The three isoforms differ by single amino acid substitutions at positions 112 and 158 (104, 107). The ApoE ε4 allele is a risk factor for late-onset familial and sporadic AD (18, 108). Around 10–15% of the general population has the ε4 allele, whereas the prevalence is 40–65% in AD patients. The majority of the general population is homozygous for the ApoE ε3 allele. The third common isoforms ε2 is present in 5–10% of the population. The ApoE ε2 allele has protective effects on the cognition and has been associated with reduced AD-related disease burden (109, 110).

Homozygosity for ApoE ε4 leads to a 50–90% risk of developing AD by the age 85, whereas individuals with one copy have a risk of 45%. For individuals with no ApoE ε4 alleles the risk is about 20% (18, 111). ApoE has been found to be co-localized with amyloid plaques and NFTs (105). Several mechanisms have been proposed for the role of ApoE ε4 in the pathology of AD including regulation of the deposition and clearance of Aβ and amyloid plaques, regulation of phosphorylation and assembly of tau into NFTs, dysfunction of the neuronal signaling pathways, induction of Aβ-regulated lysosomal leakage, increased atherosclerosis and vascular inflammation in AD, and apoptosis in neurons (105, 112). However, its exact role in the AD pathology still remains unclear (105). Besides AD, the ε4 allele has also been associated with CAA, hemorrhages, tauopathies, DLB, PD, and multiple sclerosis (113–116).

The CSF, ApoE levels have been determined by several studies and some have found decreased levels in CSF of AD patients whereas other studies have shown an increase (117). Increased CSF levels of ApoE were also detected in DLB and PD patients (118).

Plasma ApoE levels have also been reported but as seen with the CSF measurements the results have been inconsistent. A study by Taddei et al. (119) reported increased plasma ApoE levels in AD patients compared to controls. In contrast to this, the Australian Imaging, Biomarkers and Lifestyle (AIBL) study showed decreased plasma levels of ApoE and ApoE ε4 in AD patients and showed a correlation with the disease level (120). Two other studies based on the Rotterdam study and apoEurope Study, respectively, also observed decreased ApoE levels in AD patients compared to controls (121, 122). However, this difference was not significant in the Rotterdam study when adjusted for ApoE genotype, age, and gender (121). Finally, a recent study has shown that low plasma ApoE levels are associated with the risk of developing AD independent of the ApoE genotype, indicating the potential of this biomarker as a preclinical marker (123).

Aberrant proteolytic cleavage of ApoE plays an important role in the AD pathology associated with ApoE. ApoE is subjected to intracellular proteolytic cleavage and generates neurotoxic fragments. The fragments have been detected in cultured neurons and AD brains and have been shown to induce tau phosphorylation and formation of NFT-like aggregates in CNS neurons with p-tau and phosphorylated neurofilaments (124, 125). In addition, the fragments impair the function of mitochondria in neurons and promote neurodegeneration. The level of ApoE fragments is elevated in AD brains compared to cognitively normal controls (68). Importantly, ApoE ε4 is more susceptible to fragmentation than ApoE ε3 (124, 126). Among the fragments, a 22 kDa N-terminally peptide has been detected in brain tissue and CSF. Interestingly, the ApoE ε4-derived 22 kDa fragment has been found to be more neurotoxic than the corresponding ApoE ε3-derived fragment (68). Several C-terminally truncated ApoE fragments of different lengths have also been detected in AD brains. One of these is the apoE4 (Δ272–299) fragment which interacts with p-tau and phosphorylated neurofilament to form inclusions (124). A neuro-specific chymotrypsin like protease has been suggested to be involved in the formation of these fragments but further studies are needed (127).

So far, there are no studies on plasma levels of ApoE fragments and their correlation with AD or other dementias.

α-Synuclein

α-synuclein is a small protein located in both the CNS and the peripheral nervous system. It can be found specifically bound to the membrane of pre-synaptic vesicles and very little α-synuclein is distributed throughout the rest of the nerve (128). α-synuclein is also expressed in other tissues including red blood cells (64), kidney, lung, heart, and liver (129). The specific function of α-synuclein is unknown but it is implicated in a number of dementias including AD, DLB, and PD. α-synuclein aggregates to form a component of Lewy bodies that can be found in the cytoplasm of neurons. These aggregates are observed in the dementias mentioned above except for AD and are believed to be the key step in progression of neurdegeneration in synucleionopathies. There is, however, evidence that suggests α-synuclein plays a role in the aggregation of tau, which is observed in AD (130, 131). Furthermore, increased levels of soluble α-synuclein have been found in AD brains in patients in absence of LBD pathology and the levels showed a correlation with cognitive decline (132).

Cerebrospinal fluid levels of α-synuclein and its oligomers have been assessed in several types of dementia. The differential performance of α-synuclein has been inconsistent in different clinical studies. A number of studies have shown that CSF α-synuclein levels are lower in DLB and PD patients than those with AD and other dementias (43, 44, 133), whereas others have concluded that CSF α-synuclein does not discriminate between dementias (46). The levels of CSF α-synuclein oligomers are increased in DLB and PD compared with controls and AD patients (48).

The plasma levels of α-synuclein and its oligomers have been quantified in DLB and PD patients by several studies. Increased plasma levels of α-synuclein and oligomers were seen in patients with PD when compared to controls (134–137). However, contradictory results were observed in other investigations (138, 139). Similarly, the level of plasma α-synuclein oligomers was higher in DLB patients than controls whereas the α-synuclein levels were lower in DLB than AD patients and controls (134, 139).

A lot of focus has been on aggregation of the intact α-synuclein, however more recently studies suggest that fragmentation of α-synuclein is significant in the pathology of synucleinopathies. Fragments of α-synuclein have been identified in brains of PD and DLB patients (69, 141). One protease of interest is calpain, which has been observed to create cleavage products that can induce aggregation of α-synuclein *in vitro.* Calpain cleaves α-synuclein in the N- and C-terminal regions (140). MMPs also play a role in α-synuclein aggregation and therefore Lewy Body formation. Partial cleavage with either MMP-1 or MMP-3 increases aggregation of the protein (141) and both proteases are elevated in PD brains (142, 143). Neurosin is another protease of interest, especially as it is found within amyloid plaques in AD (144). Neurosin has also been identified in CSF and has been found to be lower in patients with synucleinopathies compared to those with AD and healthy patients (145). Finally, cathepsins are known to be involved in the proteolysis of α-synuclein (146). The presence of α-synuclein fragments in CSF and plasma remains to be investigated.

TAR DNA-Binding Protein 43 and Fused in Sarcoma Protein

TAR DNA-binding protein 43 is a nuclear protein that functions in regulation of transcription and exon splicing (24, 147). TDP-43 is known as the key protein in the pathogenesis of FTLD with ubiquitin-positive, tau-negative inclusions. FTLD is the second most common type of dementia after AD with an onset before 65 years of age (148) and differentiation between AD and FTLD can be challenging as they share several clinical features (149).

In FTLD, TDP-43 is post-translationally modified by aberrant ubiquitination, hyperphosphorylation, and proteolytic cleavage at the N-terminus (24, 25). In addition, TDP-43 is translocated from the nucleus and generates cytoplasmic insoluble inclusions containing ubiquitinated and aberrantly phosphorylated TDP-43 (24).

TAR DNA-binding protein 43 neuronal and glial inclusions have been detected in AD and several types of PD (150). TDP-43 inclusions are found in 25–30% of all sporadic AD patients and 14% of familial AD patients. The presence of TDP-43 in AD brains has been shown to give greater brain atrophy and more deficits when compared to AD patients without TDP-43 inclusions (151). In addition, caspase 3-cleaved TDP-43 has been detected in AD brains and it is proposed to be associated with neurodegeneration (70). This suggests that TDP-43 in combination with specific AD biomarkers can be used to identify patients with the risk to develop severe clinical deficits.

TAR DNA-binding protein 43 levels are detectable in CSF and were found to be elevated in FTLD patients when compared to controls (152, 153). TDP-43 has also been detected in plasma and the levels were increased in FTLD and a subset of AD patients (154, 155).

Fragmentation of TDP-43 has been observed. The N-terminal cleavage of TDP-43 generates C-terminal fragments, but the cleavage sites and their function in the pathology of FTLD are not fully known. In an *in vitro* study, two caspase-generated C-terminal fragments of 25 and 35 kDa were identified (156). The 25 kDa fragment of TDP-43 was found to induce the formation of intra-cellular toxic, insoluble and ubiquitin- and phospho-positive aggregations. Hence, protease cleavage initiates the translocation of TDP-43 from the nucleus to cytoplasm and induces formation of toxic insoluble inclusions (25). Caspase 3, 7, 6, and 8 have all been associated with TDP-43 cleavage (156).

The TDP-43 fragments have not been investigated in CSF or plasma.

TAR DNA-binding protein 43 and its fragments are potential biomarkers for tau-negative FTLD and can be used in the differential diagnosis of dementia and aid in the separation between tau-negative FTLD and tauopathies.

Another protein with implication for the differential diagnosis of dementia is the RNA-binding protein fused in sarcoma. The FUS protein is the pathological protein in 10–20% of sporadic FTLD patients (FTLD-FUS), which are negative for TDP-43 (26, 27, 157). The FUS protein binds to DNA and RNA and is associated with several cellular processes such as cell proliferation, DNA repair, transcription regulation, RNA splicing and transport of RNA (158–162). FUS is ubiquitously expressed in the nucleus and cytoplasm in most cell types and in neurons and glial cells it is primarily expressed in the nucleus (163). In FTLD, the FUS protein is mostly present in the cytoplasm whereas the FUS levels in the nucleus are decreased indicating a delocalization of the protein. The delocalization and accumulation of FUS lead to formation of cytoplasmic inclusions that are the characteristics of FTLD-FUS (26, 150). In addition, a mouse model has shown that overexpression of the FUS protein results in neurodegeneration (164).

To the best our knowledge neither the levels of FUS in CSF and plasma nor its fragmentation have been reported.

Glial Fibrillary Acidic Protein

Glial Fibrillary Acidic Protein is a type III intermediate filament (IF) protein constituting a part of the cytoskeleton in specific cell types. Besides the pivotal role of GFAP in the structural properties of these cells, it is involved in several fundamental cellular activities including motility (165), autophagy (166), synapse formation (167), and myelination (168).

Although it was originally considered an astrocyte-specific marker (169), GFAP has subsequently been demonstrated in glial and non-glial cells of the periphery (170–173). GFAP has been observed in virtually all areas of the brain but is mainly expressed in hippocampal regions (174–176) as well as the subventricular zone and olfactory system of both non-demented elders and patients with dementia (174–177). Multiple splice variants exist and in human hippocampal AD tissue many of these isoforms show differential transcript levels (176).

Differential transcript levels of GFAP isoforms may affect cellular function and/or morphology (165) as analysis of *in vitro* transfection suggests that GFAP isoforms differ in their ability to form functioning IFs (174, 176, 178, 179). In general, little is known about the role of GFAP in AD and other dementias. GFAP is known to interact with proteins involved in cleavage of APP (180, 181) as well as proteins modulating chaperone mediated autophagy (CMA) (166). GFAP may both inhibit and promote CMA and the phosphorylation state of GFAP is suggested to influence this balance (166). Incomplete CMA of tau is suggested to promote tau aggregation (182) which is a hallmark of several tauopathies including AD (103).

Studies have shown a correlation between increased expression levels of GFAP within brain regions involved in memory and the neuropathological changes of AD such as Aβ deposits and NFTs (183–187). Also, disease duration and progression of AD has been shown to correlate strongly with up-regulation of GFAP in the temporal lobe of AD patients (176, 184, 188).

In CSF, levels of GFAP have been observed to be increased in AD patients compared to controls (189–192). Furthermore, GFAP levels were found to increase with AD severity (189). In most studies, increased GFAP levels were independent of age, however, Rosengren et al. (190), observed a correlation between these two parameters (190).

Cerebrospinal fluid GFAP levels are also increased in patients with other neurological disorders and brain injuries such as CJD (191, 192), stroke (193, 194), and traumatic brain injury (195, 196). Regardless of this general increase in GFAP levels observed in these disorders and injuries, GFAP may be applied in context with other biomarkers for differential diagnosis, e.g., GFAP, together with the glial-specific S100 calcium binding protein B (S100β) may hold the potential to distinguish between CJD and AD (191).

In a recent study, GFAP was measured in plasma. Patients covering a broad spectrum of neurological diseases, including several forms of dementia, were included. Plasma levels of GFAP were found to be independent of age and evenly distributed between genders. No disease category displayed consistently increased levels of GFAP (197).

In vitro, GFAP is cleaved by caspase 6 at VELD225. The result is a C-terminal fragment of GFAP unable to assemble into filaments and an N-terminal fragment of GFAP perturbing *in vitro* filament assembling and promoting inter-filament aggregation (198). Caspase 3 is suggested to cleave GFAP at DLTD266. Cleaved GFAP has been shown to co-localize with caspase 3 in apoptotic astrocytes around blood vessels as well as plaque-rich regions of specific areas in the human AD brain (199). Furthermore, studies have shown calpain I-mediated cleavage products of GFAP in human brain as well as in CSF following traumatic brain injury (200, 201). Taken together, these data suggest that GFAP is a target of calpain I, caspase 3, and caspase 6 and that astrocyte injury and damage in the AD brain may involve cleavage of GFAP.

Conclusive Remarks

In the last decades several biomarker candidates have been developed and evaluated for AD and related dementias. Given the multiplicity of proteins involved in AD and related dementias as well as the overlap in pathological features between the different dementias it has to be acknowledged that so far no single biomarker permits an accurate and differential diagnosis. The diagnostic performance of the identified biomarkers could be improved by focusing on the pathological fragmentation of these proteins.

Although further studies are needed to evaluate the performance of protein fragmentation biomarkers, we believe that these biomarkers either alone or in combination with other biomarkers have a clinical potential.

References

1. Wimo A, Prince M. *World Alzheimer Report 2010*. Alzheimer's Disease International (2010).
2. Karantzoulis S, Galvin JE. Distinguishing Alzheimer's disease from other major forms of dementia. *Expert Rev Neurother* (2011) **11**:1579–91. doi:10.1586/ern.11.155
3. Holmes C. Dementia. *Medicine* (2012) **40**:628–31. doi:10.1016/j.mpmed.2012.08.012
4. Borroni B, Di Luca M, Padovani A. Predicting Alzheimer dementia in mild cognitive impairment patients. Are biomarkers useful? *Eur J Pharmacol* (2006) **545**:73–80. doi:10.1016/j.ejphar.2006.06.023
5. Assal F, Cummings JL. Neuropsychiatric symptoms in the dementias. *Curr Opin Neurol* (2002) **15**:445–50. doi:10.1097/00019052-200208000-00007
6. Mistur R, Mosconi L, De Santi S, Guzman M, Li Y, Tsui W, et al. Current challenges for the early detection of Alzheimer's disease: brain imaging and CSF studies. *J Clin Neurol* (2009) **5**:153–66. doi:10.3988/jcn.2009.5.4.153
7. McKhann GM, Knopman DS, Chertkow H, Hyman BT, Jack CR, Kawas CH, et al. The diagnosis of dementia due to Alzheimer's disease: recommendations from the National Institute on Aging-Alzheimer's Association workgroups on diagnostic guidelines for Alzheimer's disease. *Alzheimers Dement* (2011) **7**(3):263–9. doi:10.1016/j.jalz.2011.03.005
8. Cairns NJ, Bigio EH, Mackenzie IRA, Neumann M, Lee VMY, Hatanpaa KJ, et al. "Neuropathologic diagnostic and nosologic criteria for frontotemporal lobar degeneration: Consensus of the Consortium for Frontotemporal Lobar Degeneration,". *Acta Neuropathol* (2007) **114**:5–22. doi:10.1007/s00401-007-0237-2
9. Hohl U, Tiraboschi P, Hansen LA, Thal LJ, Corey-Bloom J. Diagnostic accuracy of dementia with Lewy bodies. *Arch Neurol* (2000) **57**:347–51. doi:10.1001/archneur.57.3.347
10. Woodward M, Jacova C, Black SE, Kertesz A, Mackenzie IR, Feldman H, et al. "Differentiating the frontal variant of Alzheimer's disease,". *Int J Geriatr Psychiatry* (2010) **25**:732–8. doi:10.1002/gps.2415
11. Kalaria RN, Ballard C. Overlap between pathology of Alzheimer disease and vascular dementia. *Alzheimer Dis Assoc Disord* (1999) **13**(Suppl 3):S115–23. doi:10.1097/00002093-199912003-00017
12. Cummings JL. Biomarkers in Alzheimer's disease drug development. *Alzheimers Dement* (2011) **7**(3):e13–44. doi:10.1016/j.jalz.2010.06.004
13. Blennow K. Biomarkers in Alzheimer's disease drug development. *Nat Med* (2010) **16**:1218–22. doi:10.1038/nm.2221
14. Schneider P, Hampel H, Buerger K. Biological marker candidates of Alzheimer's disease in blood, plasma, and serum. *CNS Neurosci Ther* (2009) **15**:358–74. doi:10.1111/j.1755-5949.2009.00104.x
15. Henriksen K, O'Bryant SE, Hampel H, Trojanowski JQ, Montine TJ, Jeromin A, et al. The future of blood-based biomarkers for Alzheimer's disease. *Alzheimers Dement* (2014) **10**:115–31. doi:10.1016/j.jalz.2013.01.013
16. Ingelsson M, Hyman BT. Disordered proteins in dementia. *Ann Med* (2002) **34**:259–71. doi:10.1080/078538902320322529
17. Blennow K. Cerebrospinal fluid protein biomarkers for Alzheimer's disease. *NeuroRx* (2004) **1**:213–25. doi:10.1602/neurorx.1.2.213
18. Corder EH, Saunders AM, Strittmatter WJ, Schmechel DE, Gaskell PC, Small GW, et al. Gene dose of apolipoprotein E type 4 allele and the risk of Alzheimer's disease in late onset families. *Science* (1993) **261**:921–3. doi:10.1126/science.8346443
19. Mukaetova-Ladinska EB, Milne J, Andras A, Abdel-All Z, Cerejeira J, Greally E, et al. Alpha- and gamma-synuclein proteins are present in cerebrospinal fluid and are increased in aged subjects with neurodegenerative and vascular changes. *Dement Geriatr Cogn Disord* (2008) **26**:32–42. doi:10.1159/000141039
20. Schoonenboom NSM, Reesink FE, Verwey NA, Kester MI, Teunissen CE, Van De Ven PM, et al. Cerebrospinal fluid markers for differential dementia diagnosis in a large memory clinic cohort. *Neurology* (2012) **78**(1):47–54. doi:10.1212/WNL.0b013e31823ed0f0
21. Kaerst L, Kuhlmann A, Wedekind D, Stoeck K, Lange P, Zerr I. Cerebrospinal fluid biomarkers in Alzheimer's disease, vascular dementia and ischemic stroke patients: a critical analysis. *J Neurol* (2013) **260**:2722–7. doi:10.1007/s00415-013-7047-3
22. Josephs KA, Petersen RC, Knopman DS, Boeve BF, Whitwell JL, Duffy JR, et al. Clinicopathologic analysis of frontotemporal and corticobasal degenerations and PSP. *Neurology* (2006) **66**:41–8. doi:10.1212/01.wnl.0000191307.69661.c3
23. Tokuda T, Qureshi MM, Ardah MT, Varghese S, Shehab SA, Kasai T, et al. Detection of elevated levels of alpha-synuclein oligomers in CSF from patients with Parkinson disease. *Neurology* (2010) **75**:1766–72. doi:10.1212/WNL.0b013e3181fd613b
24. Igaz LM, Kwong LK, Chen-Plotkin A, Winton MJ, Unger TL, Xu Y, et al. Expression of TDP-43 C-terminal fragments in vitro recapitulates pathological features of TDP-43 proteinopathies. *J Biol Chem* (2009) **284**:8516–24. doi:10.1074/jbc.M809462200
25. Zhang Y-J, Xu Y-F, Cook C, Gendron TF, Roettges P, Link CD, et al. Aberrant cleavage of TDP-43 enhances aggregation and cellular toxicity. *Proc Natl Acad Sci U S A* (2009) **106**:7607–12. doi:10.1073/pnas.0900688106
26. Neumann M, Rademakers R, Roeber S, Baker M, Kretzschmar HA, MacKenzie IRA. A new subtype of frontotemporal lobar degeneration with FUS pathology. *Brain* (2009) **132**:2922–31. doi:10.1093/brain/awp214
27. Roeber S, Mackenzie IRA, Kretzschmar HA, Neumann M. TDP-43-negative FTLD-U is a significant new clinico-pathological subtype of FTLD. *Acta Neuropathol* (2008) **116**:147–57. doi:10.1007/s00401-008-0395-x
28. Bateman RJ, Xiong C, Benzinger TLS, Fagan AM, Goate A, Fox NC, et al. Clinical and biomarker changes in dominantly inherited Alzheimer's disease. *N Engl J Med* (2012) **367**:795–804. doi:10.1056/NEJMoa1202753
29. Wang Y, Sørensen MG, Zheng Q, Zhang C, Karsdal MA, Henriksen K. Will posttranslational modifications of brain proteins provide novel serological markers for dementias? *Int J Alzheimers Dis* (2012) **2012**:209409. doi:10.1155/2012/209409
30. Blennow K, Hampel H. CSF markers for incipient Alzheimer's disease. *Lancet Neurol* (2003) **2**:605–13. doi:10.1016/S1474-4422(03)00530-1

31. Mattsson N, Blennow K, Zetterberg H. CSF biomarkers: pinpointing Alzheimer pathogenesis. *Ann N Y Acad Sci* (2009) **1180**:28–35. doi:10.1111/j.1749-6632.2009.04944.x
32. Hansson O, Zetterberg H, Buchhave P, Londos E, Blennow K, Minthon L. Association between CSF biomarkers and incipient Alzheimer's disease in patients with mild cognitive impairment: a follow-up study. *Lancet Neurol* (2006) **5**:228–34. doi:10.1016/S1474-4422(06)70355-6
33. Thinakaran G, Koo EH. Amyloid precursor protein trafficking, processing, and function. *J Biol Chem* (2008) **283**:29615–9. doi:10.1074/jbc.R800019200
34. Hampel H, Teipel SJ. Total and phosphorylated tau proteins: evaluation as core biomarker candidates in frontotemporal dementia. *Dement Geriatr Cogn Disord* (2004) **17**(4):350–4. doi:10.1159/000077170
35. Shaw LM, Vanderstichele H, Knapik-Czajka M, Clark CM, Aisen PS, Petersen RC, et al. Cerebrospinal fluid biomarker signature in Alzheimer's disease neuroimaging initiative subjects. *Ann Neurol* (2009) **65**:403–13. doi:10.1002/ana.21610
36. Duits FH, Teunissen CE, Bouwman FH, Visser PJ, Mattsson N, Zetterberg H, et al. The cerebrospinal fluid 'Alzheimer profile': easily said, but what does it mean? *Alzheimers Dement* (2014) **10**(6):713–23.e2. doi:10.1016/j.jalz.2013.12.023
37. Hampel H, Teipel SJ, Fuchsberger T, Andreasen N, Wiltfang J, Otto M, et al. Value of CSF beta-amyloid1-42 and tau as predictors of Alzheimer's disease in patients with mild cognitive impairment. *Mol Psychiatry* (2004) **9**:705–10. doi:10.1038/sj.mp.4001473
38. Snider BJ, Fagan AM, Roe C, Shah AR, Grant EA, Xiong C, et al. Cerebrospinal fluid biomarkers and rate of cognitive decline in very mild dementia of the Alzheimer type. *Arch Neurol* (2009) **66**:638–45. doi:10.1001/archneurol.2009.55
39. Andreasen N, Vanmechelen E, Vanderstichele H, Davidsson P, Blennow K. Cerebrospinal fluid levels of total-tau, phospho-tau and A-beta 42 predicts development of Alzheimer's disease in patients with mild cognitive impairment. *Acta Neurol Scand Suppl* (2003) **179**:47–51. doi:10.1034/j.1600-0404.107.s179.9.x
40. Hulstaert F, Blennow K, Ivanoiu A, Schoonderwaldt HC, Riemenschneider M, De Deyn PP, et al. Improved discrimination of AD patients using beta-amyloid(1-42) and tau levels in CSF. *Neurology* (1999) **52**:1555–62. doi:10.1212/WNL.52.8.1555
41. Maddalena A, Papassotiropoulos A, üller-Tillmanns BM, Jung HH, Hegi T, Nitsch RM, et al. Biochemical diagnosis of Alzheimer disease by measuring the cerebrospinal fluid ratio of phosphorylated tau protein to beta-amyloid peptide42. *Arch Neurol* (2003) **60**:1202–6. doi:10.1001/archneur.60.9.1202
42. Fagan AM, Roe CM, Xiong C, Mintun MA, Morris JC, Holtzman DM. Cerebrospinal fluid tau/beta-amyloid(42) ratio as a prediction of cognitive decline in nondemented older adults. *Arch Neurol* (2007) **64**:343–9. doi:10.1001/archneur.64.3.noc60123
43. Tokuda T, Salem SA, Allsop D, Mizuno T, Nakagawa M, Qureshi MM, et al. Decreased-alpha-synuclein in cerebrospinal fluid of aged individuals and subjects with Parkinson's disease. *Biochem Biophys Res Commun* (2006) **349**:162–6. doi:10.1016/j.bbrc.2006.08.024
44. Mollenhauer B, Cullen V, Kahn I, Krastins B, Outeiro TF, Pepivani I, et al. Direct quantification of CSF α-synuclein by ELISA and first cross-sectional study in patients with neurodegeneration. *Exp Neurol* (2008) **213**:315–25. doi:10.1016/j.expneurol.2008.06.004
45. Aerts MB, Esselink RAJ, Abdo WF, Bloem BR, Verbeek MM. CSF-alpha-synuclein does not differentiate between parkinsonian disorders. *Neurobiol Aging* (2012) **33**:430.e1–3. doi:10.1016/j.neurobiolaging.2010.12.001
46. Spies PE, Melis RJF, Sjögren MJC, Rikkert MGMO, Verbeek MM. Cerebrospinal fluid α-synuclein does not discriminate between dementia disorders. *J Alzheimers Dis* (2009) **16**:363–9. doi:10.3233/JAD-2009-0955
47. Reesink FE, Lemstra AW, Van Dijk KD, Berendse HW, Van De Berg WDJ, Klein M, et al. CSF-alpha-synuclein does not discriminate dementia with Lewy bodies from Alzheimer's disease. *J Alzheimers Dis* (2010) **22**:87–95. doi:10.3233/JAD-2010-100186
48. Hansson O, Hall S, Öhrfelt A, Zetterberg H, Blennow K, Minthon L, et al. Levels of cerebrospinal fluid α-synuclein oligomers are increased in Parkinson's disease with dementia and dementia with Lewy bodies compared to Alzheimer's disease. *Alzheimers Res Ther* (2014) **6**:25. doi:10.1186/alzrt255
49. Parnetti L, Chiasserini D, Persichetti E, Eusebi P, Varghese S, Qureshi MM, et al. Cerebrospinal fluid lysosomal enzymes and alpha-synuclein in Parkinson's disease. *Mov Disord* (2014) **29**:1019–27. doi:10.1002/mds.25772
50. Slaets S, Vanmechelen E, Le Bastard N, Decraemer H, Vandijck M, Martin JJ, et al. Increased CSF-alpha-synuclein levels in Alzheimer's disease: correlation with tau levels. *Alzheimers Dement* (2014) **10**(5 Suppl):S290–8. doi:10.1016/j.jalz.2013.10.004
51. Rosén C, Hansson O, Blennow K, Zetterberg H. Fluid biomarkers in Alzheimer's disease - current concepts. *Mol Neurodegener* (2013) **8**:20. doi:10.1186/1750-1326-8-20
52. Mattsson N, Andreasson U, Persson S, Arai H, Batish SD, Bernardini S, et al. The Alzheimer's Association external quality control program for cerebrospinal fluid biomarkers. *Alzheimers Dement* (2011) **7**:386–95.e6. doi:10.1016/j.jalz.2011.05.2243
53. Snyder HM, Carrillo MC, Grodstein F, Henriksen K, Jeromin A, Lovestone S, et al. Developing novel blood-based biomarkers for Alzheimer's disease. *Alzheimers Dement* (2014) **10**:109–14. doi:10.1016/j.jalz.2013.10.007
54. Marques F, Sousa JC, Sousa N, Palha JA. Blood – brain-barriers in aging and in Alzheimer's disease. *Mol Neurodegener* (2013) **8**(1):38. doi:10.1186/1750-1326-8-38
55. Sharma HS, Castellani RJ, Smith MA, Sharma A. The blood-brain barrier in Alzheimer's disease. Novel therapeutic targets and nanodrug delivery. *Int Rev Neurobiol* (2012) **102**:47–90. doi:10.1016/B978-0-12-386986-9.00003-X
56. Desai BS, Monahan AJ, Carvey PM, Hendey B. Blood-brain barrier pathology in Alzheimer's and Parkinson's disease: implications for drug therapy. *Cell Transplant* (2007) **16**:285–99. doi:10.3727/000000007783464731
57. Reiber H. Proteins in cerebrospinal fluid and blood: barriers, CSF flow rate and source-related dynamics. *Restor Neurol Neurosci* (2003) **21**:79–96.
58. Duong T, Pommier EC, Scheibel AB. Immunodetection of the amyloid P component in Alzheimer's disease. *Acta Neuropathol* (1989) **78**:429–37. doi:10.1007/BF00688180
59. Zetterberg H, Wilson D, Andreasson U, Minthon L, Blennow K, Randall J, et al. Plasma tau levels in Alzheimer's disease. *Alzheimers Res Ther* (2013) **5**:9. doi:10.1186/alzrt163
60. Chiu MJ, Chen YF, Chen TF, Yang SY, Yang FPG, Tseng TW, et al. Plasma tau as a window to the brain-negative associations with brain ume and memory function in mild cognitive impairment and early Alzheimer's disease. *Hum Brain Mapp* (2014) **35**:3132–42. doi:10.1002/hbm.22390
61. Randall J, Mörtberg E, Provuncher GK, Fournier DR, Duffy DC, Rubertsson S, et al. Tau proteins in serum predict neurological outcome after hypoxic brain injury from cardiac arrest: results of a pilot study. *Resuscitation* (2013) **84**(3):351–6. doi:10.1016/j.resuscitation.2012.07.027
62. Hansson O, Stomrud E, Vanmechelen E, Östling S, Gustafson DR, Zetterberg H, et al. Evaluation of plasma Aβ as predictor of Alzheimer's disease in older individuals without dementia: a population-based study. *J Alzheimers Dis* (2012) **28**:231–8. doi:10.3233/JAD-2011-111418
63. Zetterberg H, Blennow K. Plasma Abeta in Alzheimer's disease-up or down? *Lancet Neurol* (2006) **5**:638–9. doi:10.1016/S1474-4422(06)70503-8
64. Barbour R, Kling K, Anderson JP, Banducci K, Cole T, Diep L, et al. Red blood cells are the major source of alpha-synuclein in blood. *Neurodegener Dis* (2008) **5**:55–9. doi:10.1159/000112832
65. Karsdal MA, Henriksen K, Leeming DJ, Woodworth T, Vassiliadis E, Bay-Jensen AC. Novel combinations of post-translational modification (PTM) neo-epitopes provide tissue-specific biochemical markers-are they the cause or the consequence of the disease? *Clin Biochem* (2010) **43**(10–11):793–804. doi:10.1016/j.clinbiochem.2010.03.015
66. Martin L, Latypova X, Terro F. Post-translational modifications of tau protein: implications for Alzheimer's disease. *Neurochem Int* (2011) **58**:458–71. doi:10.1016/j.neuint.2010.12.023
67. Meredith JE, Sankaranarayanan S, Guss V, Lanzetti AJ, Berisha F, Neely RJ, et al. Characterization of novel CSF tau and ptau biomarkers for Alzheimer's disease. *PLoS One* (2013) **8**:e76523. doi:10.1371/journal.pone.0076523
68. Marques MA, Tolar M, Harmony JA, Crutcher KA. A thrombin cleavage fragment of apolipoprotein E exhibits isoform-specific neurotoxicity. *Neuroreport* (1996) **7**:2529–32. doi:10.1097/00001756-199611040-00025
69. Liu CW, Giasson BI, Lewis KA, Lee VM, Demartino GN, Thomas PJ. A precipitating role for truncated alpha-synuclein and the proteasome in

alpha-synuclein aggregation: implications for pathogenesis of Parkinson disease. *J Biol Chem* (2005) **280**:22670–8. doi:10.1074/jbc.M501508200
70. Rohn TT. Caspase-cleaved TAR DNA-binding protein-43 is a major pathological finding in Alzheimer's disease. *Brain Res* (2008) **1228**:189–98. doi:10.1016/j.brainres.2008.06.094
71. Shayo M, McLay RN, Kastin AJ, Banks WA. The putative blood-brain barrier transporter for the beta-amyloid binding protein apolipoprotein j is saturated at physiological concentrations. *Life Sci* (1997) **60**:L115–8. doi:10.1016/S0024-3205(96)00685-6
72. Mackic JB, Bading J, Ghiso J, Walker L, Wisniewski T, Frangione B, et al. Circulating amyloid-beta peptide crosses the blood-brain barrier in aged monkeys and contributes to Alzheimer's disease lesions. *Vascul Pharmacol* (2002) **38**:303–13. doi:10.1016/S1537-1891(02)00198-2
73. Kastin AJ, Pan W, Maness LM, Banks WA. Peptides crossing the blood-brain barrier: some unusual observations. *Brain Res* (1999) **848**:96–100. doi:10.1016/S0006-8993(99)01961-7
74. Pan W, Kastin AJ. Polypeptide delivery across the blood-brain barrier. *Curr Drug Targets CNS Neurol Disord* (2004) **3**:131–6. doi:10.2174/1568007043482525
75. Shahim P, Linemann T, Inekci D, Karsdal MA, Blennow K, Tegner Y, et al. Serum tau fragments predict return to play in concussed professional ice hockey players. *J Neurotrauma* (2015). doi:10.1089/neu.2014.3741
76. Brunholz S, Sisodia S, Lorenzo A, Deyts C, Kins S, Morfini G. Axonal transport of APP and the spatial regulation of APP cleavage and function in neuronal cells. *Exp Brain Res* (2012) **217**:353–64. doi:10.1007/s00221-011-2870-1
77. De Strooper B. Proteases and proteolysis in Alzheimer disease: a multifactorial view on the disease process. *Physiol Rev* (2010) **90**:465–94. doi:10.1152/physrev.00023.2009
78. Zhang Y, Thompson R, Zhang H, Xu H. APP processing in Alzheimer's disease. *Mol Brain* (2011) **4**:3. doi:10.1186/1756-6606-4-3
79. Buchhave P, Minthon L, Zetterberg H, Wallin AK, Blennow K, Hansson O. Cerebrospinal fluid levels of beta-amyloid 1-42, but not of Tau, are fully changed already 5 to 10 years before the onset of Alzheimer dementia. *Arch Gen Psychiatry* (2012) **69**:98–106. doi:10.1001/archgenpsychiatry.2011.155
80. Jack CR, Knopman DS, Jagust WJ, Petersen RC, Weiner MW, Aisen PS, et al. Tracking pathophysiological processes in Alzheimer's disease: an updated hypothetical model of dynamic biomarkers. *Lancet Neurol* (2013) **12**(2):207–16. doi:10.1016/S1474-4422(12)70291-0
81. Zou K, Kim D, Kakio A, Byun K, Gong J-S, Kim J, et al. Amyloid beta-protein (Abeta)1-40 protects neurons from damage induced by Abeta1-42 in culture and in rat brain. *J Neurochem* (2003) **87**:609–19. doi:10.1046/j.1471-4159.2003.02018.x
82. Verbeek MM, Kremer BPH, Rikkert MO, Van Domburg PHMF, Skehan ME, Greenberg SM. Cerebrospinal fluid amyloid beta(40) is decreased in cerebral amyloid angiopathy. *Ann Neurol* (2009) **66**(2):245–9. doi:10.1002/ana.21694
83. Bogner S, Bernreuther C, Matschke J, Barrera-Ocampo A, Sepulveda-Falla D, Leypoldt F, et al. Immune activation in amyloid-β-related angiitis correlates with decreased parenchymal amyloid-β plaque load. *Neurodegener Dis* (2013) **13**(1):38–44. doi:10.1159/000352020
84. Piazza F, Greenberg SM, Savoiardo M, Gardinetti M, Chiapparini L, Raicher I, et al. Anti-amyloid β autoantibodies in cerebral amyloid angiopathy-related inflammation: implications for amyloid-modifying therapies. *Ann Neurol* (2013) **73**(4):449–58. doi:10.1002/ana.23857
85. Boncoraglioa GB, Piazza F, Savoiardod M, Farinad L, DiFrancescobe JC, Prionif S, et al. Prodromal Alzheimer's disease presenting as cerebral amyloid angiopathy-related inflammation with spontaneous amyloid-related imaging abnormalities and high cerebrospinal fluid anti-beta autoantibodies. *J Alzheimers Dis* (2015) **45**:363–7. doi:10.3233/JAD-142376
86. Bibl M, Gallus M, Welge V, Esselmann H, Wiltfang J. Aminoterminally truncated and oxidized amyloid-β peptides in the cerebrospinal fluid of Alzheimer's disease patients. *J Alzheimers Dis* (2012) **29**(4):809–16. doi:10.3233/JAD-2012-111796
87. Larner AJ. Hypothesis: amyloid beta-peptides truncated at the N-terminus contribute to the pathogenesis of Alzheimer 's disease. *Neurobiol Aging* (1999) **20**:65–9.
88. Portelius E, Tran AJ, Andreasson U, Persson R, Brinkmann G, Zetterberg H, et al. Characterization of amyloid-beta peptides in cerebrospinal fluid by an automated immunoprecipitation procedure followed by mass spectrometry. *J Proteome Res* (2007) **6**:4433–9. doi:10.1021/pr0703627
89. Portelius E, Bogdanovic N, Gustavsson MK, Kmann I, Brinkmalm G, Zetterberg H, et al. Mass spectrometric characterization of brain amyloid beta isoform signatures in familial and sporadic Alzheimer's disease. *Acta Neuropathol* (2010) **120**:185–93. doi:10.1007/s00401-010-0690-1
90. Portelius E, Mattsson N, Andreasson U, Blennow K, Zetterberg H. Novel Aβ isoforms in Alzheimer's disease – their role in diagnosis and treatment. *Curr Pharm Des* (2011) **17**:2594–602. doi:10.2174/138161211797416039
91. Portelius E, Price E, Brinkmalm G, Stiteler M, Olsson M, Persson R, et al. A novel pathway for amyloid precursor protein processing. *Neurobiol Aging* (2011) **32**:1090–8. doi:10.1016/j.neurobiolaging.2009.06.002
92. Thambisetty M, Lovestone S. Blood-based biomarkers of Alzheimer's disease: challenging but feasible. *Biomark Med* (2010) **4**:65–79. doi:10.2217/bmm.09.84
93. Perez-Grijalba SM, Pesini V, Allue P, Sarasa JA, Montanes L, Lacosta M, et al. A-beta (1-17) is a major amyloid-beta fragment isoform in cerebrospinal fluid and blood with possible diagnostic value in Alzheimer's disease. *J Alzheimers Dis* (2015) **43**(1):47–56. doi:10.3233/JAD-140156
94. Iqbal K, Del A, Alonso C, Chen S, Chohan MO, El-Akkad E, et al. Tau pathology in Alzheimer disease and other tauopathies. *Biochim Biophys Acta* (2005) **1739**:198–210. doi:10.1016/j.bbadis.2004.09.008
95. Buée L, Bussière T, Buée-Scherrer V, Delacourte A, Hof PR. Tau protein isoforms, phosphorylation and role in neurodegenerative disorders. *Brain Res Rev* (2000) **33**:95–130. doi:10.1016/S0165-0173(00)00019-9
96. Spillantini MG, Goedert M. Tau pathology and neurodegeneration. *Lancet Neurol* (2013) **12**:609–22. doi:10.1016/S1474-4422(13)70090-5
97. Espinoza M, de Silva R, Dickson DW, Davies P. Differential incorporation of tau isoforms in Alzheimer's disease. *J Alzheimers Dis* (2008) **14**:1–16.
98. Buée L, Delacourte A. Comparative biochemistry of tau in progressive supranuclear palsy, corticobasal degeneration, FTDP-17 and Pick's disease. *Brain Pathol* (1999) **9**:681–93. doi:10.1111/j.1750-3639.1999.tb00550.x
99. Mohamed NV, Herrou T, Plouffe V, Piperno N, Leclerc N. Spreading of tau pathology in Alzheimer's disease by cell-to-cell transmission. *Eur J Neurosci* (2013) **37**:1939–48. doi:10.1111/ejn.12229
100. Henriksen K, Byrjalsen I, Christiansen C, Karsdal MA. Relationship between serum levels of tau fragments and clinical progression of Alzheimer ' s disease,". *J Alzheimers Dis* (2015) **43**(4):1331–41. doi:10.3233/JAD-140984
101. Henriksen K, Wang Y, Sørensen MG, Barascuk N, Suhy J, Pedersen JT, et al. An enzyme-generated fragment of tau measured in serum shows an inverse correlation to cognitive function. *PLoS One* (2013) **8**(5):e64990. doi:10.1371/journal.pone.0064990
102. Hanger DP, Wray S. Tau cleavage and tau aggregation in neurodegenerative disease. *Biochem Soc Trans* (2010) **38**(4):1016–20. doi:10.1042/BST0381016
103. Wang Y, Garg S, Mandelkow E-M, Mandelkow E. Proteolytic processing of tau. *Biochem Soc Trans* (2010) **38**:955–61. doi:10.1042/BST0380955
104. Mahley RW. Apolipoprotein E: cholesterol transport protein with expanding role in cell biology. *Science* (1988) **240**:622–30. doi:10.1126/science.3283935
105. Huang Y, Weisgraber K, Mucke L, Mahley R. Apolipoprotein E. *J Mol Neurosci* (2004) **23**:189–204. doi:10.1385/JMN:23:3:189
106. Leduc V, Jasmin-Bélanger S, Poirier J. APOE and cholesterol homeostasis in Alzheimer's disease. *Trends Mol Med* (2010) **16**:469–77. doi:10.1016/j.molmed.2010.07.008
107. Hatters DM, Peters-Libeu CA, Weisgraber KH. Apolipoprotein E structure: insights into function. *Trends Biochem Sci* (2006) **31**:445–54. doi:10.1016/j.tibs.2006.06.008
108. Bertram L, Tanzi RE. Thirty years of Alzheimer's disease genetics: the implications of systematic meta-analyses. *Nat Rev Neurosci* (2008) **9**:768–78. doi:10.1038/nrn2494
109. Suri S, Heise V, Trachtenberg AJ, Mackay CE. The forgotten APOE allele: a review of the evidence and suggested mechanisms for the protective effect of APOE e2. *Neurosci Biobehav Rev* (2013) **37**(10):2878–86. doi:10.1016/j.neubiorev.2013.10.010
110. Serrano-Pozo A, Qian J, Monsell SE, Betensky RA, Hyman BT. APOEε2 is associated with milder clinical and pathological Alzheimer's disease. *Ann Neurol* (2015). doi:10.1002/ana.24369
111. Harris FM, Tesseur I, Brecht WJ, Xu Q, Mullendorff K, Chang SJ, et al. Astroglial regulation of apolipoprotein E expression in neuronal cells – implications for Alzheimer's disease. *J Biol Chem* (2004) **279**:3862–8. doi:10.1074/jbc.M309475200

112. Tibolla G, Norata GD, Meda C, Arnaboldi L, Uboldi P, Piazza F, et al. Increased atherosclerosis and vascular inflammation in APP transgenic mice with apolipoprotein E deficiency. *Atherosclerosis* (2010) **210**(1):78–87. doi:10.1016/j.atherosclerosis.2009.10.040
113. Greenberg SM, Briggs ME, Hyman BT, Kokoris GJ, Takis C, Kanter DS, et al. Apolipoprotein E epsilon 4 is associated with the presence and earlier onset of hemorrhage in cerebral amyloid angiopathy. *Stroke* (1996) **27**:1333–7. doi:10.1161/01.STR.27.8.1333
114. Pinholt M, Frederiksen JL, Christiansen M. The association between apolipoprotein E and multiple sclerosis. *Eur J Neurol* (2006) **13**:573–80. doi:10.1111/j.1468-1331.2006.01360.x
115. Josephs KA, Tsuboi Y, Cookson N, Watt H, Dickson DW. Apolipoprotein E epsilon 4 is a determinant for Alzheimer-type pathologic features in tauopathies, synucleinopathies, and frontotemporal degeneration. *Arch Neurol* (2004) **61**:1579–84. doi:10.1001/archneur.61.10.1579
116. Martinez M, Brice A, Vaughan JR, Zimprich A, Breteler MMB, Meco G, et al. Apolipoprotein E4 is probably responsible for the chromosome 19 linkage peak for Parkinson's disease. *Am J Med Genet B Neuropsychiatr Genet* (2005) **136B**:72–4. doi:10.1002/ajmg.b.30196
117. Hesse C, Larsson H, Fredman P, Minthon L, Andreasen N, Davidsson P, et al. Measurement of apolipoprotein E (apoE) in cerebrospinal fluid. *Neurochem Res* (2000) **25**:511–7. doi:10.1023/A:1007516210548
118. Vijayaraghavan S, Maetzler W, Reimold M, Lithner CU, Liepelt-Scarfone I, Berg D, et al. High apolipoprotein E in cerebrospinal fluid of patients with Lewy body disorders is associated with dementia. *Alzheimers Dement* (2014) **10**:530–40. doi:10.1016/j.jalz.2013.03.010
119. Taddei K, Clarnette R, Gandy SE, Martins RN. Increased plasma apolipoprotein E (apoE) levels in Alzheimer's disease. *Neurosci Lett* (1997) **223**:29–32. doi:10.1016/S0304-3940(97)13394-8
120. Gupta VB, Laws SM, Villemagne VL, Ames D, Bush AI, Ellis KA, et al. Plasma apolipoprotein e and Alzheimer disease risk: the AIBL study of aging. *Neurology* (2011) **76**:1091–8. doi:10.1212/WNL.0b013e318211c352
121. Slooter AJC, De Knijff P, Hofman A, Cruts M, Breteler MMB, Van Broeckhoven C, et al. Serum apolipoprotein e level is not increased in Alzheimer's disease: the Rotterdam study. *Neurosci Lett* (1998) **248**:21–4. doi:10.1016/S0304-3940(98)00339-5
122. Siest G, Bertrand P, Qin B, Herbeth B, Serot JM, Masana L, et al. Apolipoprotein E polymorphism and serum concentration in Alzheimer's disease in nine European centres: the ApoEurope study. ApoEurope group. *Clin Chem Lab Med* (2000) **38**:721–30. doi:10.1515/CCLM.2000.102
123. Rasmussen KL, Tybjaerg-Hansen A, Nordestgaard BG, Frikke-Schmidt R. Plasma levels of apolipoprotein E and risk of dementia in the general population. *Ann Neurol* (2015) **77**:301–11. doi:10.1002/ana.24326
124. Huang Y, Liu XQ, Wyss-Coray T, Brecht WJ, Sanan DA, Mahley RW. Apolipoprotein E fragments present in Alzheimer's disease brains induce neurofibrillary tangle-like intracellular inclusions in neurons. *Proc Natl Acad Sci U S A* (2001) **98**:8838–43. doi:10.1073/pnas.151254698
125. Wellnitz S, Friedlein A, Bonanni C, Anquez V, Goepfert F, Loetscher H, et al. A 13 kDa carboxy-terminal fragment of ApoE stabilizes Abeta hexamers. *J Neurochem* (2005) **94**:1351–60. doi:10.1111/j.1471-4159.2005.03295.x
126. Brecht WJ, Harris FM, Chang S, Tesseur I, Yu G-Q, Xu Q, et al. "Neuron-specific apolipoprotein e4 proteolysis is associated with increased tau phosphorylation in brains of transgenic mice.,". *J Neurosci* (2004) **24**:2527–34. doi:10.1523/JNEUROSCI.4315-03.2004
127. Tamboli IY, Heo D, Rebeck GW. Extracellular proteolysis of apolipoprotein e (apoE) by secreted serine neuronal protease. *PLoS One* (2014) **9**:e93120. doi:10.1371/journal.pone.0093120
128. Iwai A, Masliah E, Yoshimoto M, Ge N, Flanagan L, de Silva HA, et al. The precursor protein of non-A beta component of Alzheimer's disease amyloid is a presynaptic protein of the central nervous system. *Neuron* (1995) **14**:467–75. doi:10.1016/0896-6273(95)90302-X
129. Ltic S, Perovic M, Mladenovic A, Raicevic N, Ruzdijic S, Rakic L, et al. Alpha-synuclein is expressed in different tissues during human fetal development. *J Mol Neurosci* (2004) **22**:199–204. doi:10.1385/JMN:22:3:199
130. Jensen PH, Hager H, Nielsen MS, Højrup P, Gliemann J, Jakes R. α-synuclein binds to tau and stimulates the protein kinase A-catalyzed tau phosphorylation of serine residues 262 and 356. *J Biol Chem* (1999) **274**:25481–9. doi:10.1074/jbc.274.36.25481
131. Iqbal K, Flory M, Khatoon S, Soininen H, Pirttila T, Lehtovirta M, et al. Subgroups of Alzheimer's disease based on cerebrospinal fluid molecular markers. *Ann Neurol* (2005) **58**:748–57. doi:10.1002/ana.20639
132. Larson ME, Sherman MA, Greimel S, Kuskowski M, Schneider JA, Bennett DA, et al. Soluble alpha-synuclein is a novel modulator of Alzheimer's disease pathophysiology. *J Neurosci* (2012) **32**:10253–66. doi:10.1523/JNEUROSCI.0581-12.2012
133. Kasuga K, Tokutake T, Ishikawa A, Uchiyama T, Tokuda T, Onodera O, et al. Differential levels of alpha-synuclein, beta-amyloid42 and tau in CSF between patients with dementia with Lewy bodies and Alzheimer's disease. *J Neurol Neurosurg Psychiatry* (2010) **81**:608–10. doi:10.1136/jnnp.2009.197483
134. El-Agnaf OMA, Salem SA, Paleologou KE, Curran MD, Gibson MJ, Court JA, et al. Detection of oligomeric forms of alpha-synuclein protein in human plasma as a potential biomarker for Parkinson's disease. *FASEB J* (2006) **20**:419–25. doi:10.1096/fj.03-1449com
135. Lee PH, Lee G, Park HJ, Bang OY, Joo IS, Huh K. The plasma alpha-synuclein levels in patients with Parkinson's disease and multiple system atrophy. *J Neural Transm* (2006) **113**:1435–9. doi:10.1007/s00702-005-0427-9
136. Duran R, Barrero FJ, Morales B, Luna JD, Ramirez M, Vives F. Plasma alpha-synuclein in patients with Parkinson's disease with and without treatment. *Mov Disord* (2010) **25**:489–93. doi:10.1002/mds.22928
137. Foulds PG, Mitchell JD, Parker A, Turner R, Green G, Diggle P, et al. Phosphorylated alpha-synuclein can be detected in blood plasma and is potentially a useful biomarker for Parkinson's disease. *FASEB J* (2011) **25**(12):4127–37. doi:10.1096/fj.10-179192
138. Park MJ, Cheon SM, Bae HR, Kim SH, Kim JW. Elevated levels of α-synuclein oligomer in the cerebrospinal fluid of drug-naïve patients with Parkinson's disease. *J Clin Neurol* (2011) **7**:215–22. doi:10.3988/jcn.2011.7.4.215
139. Laske C, Fallgatter AJ, Stransky E, Hagen K, Berg D, Maetzler W. Decreased alpha-synuclein serum levels in patients with Lewy body dementia compared to Alzheimer's disease patients and control subjects. *Dement Geriatr Cogn Disord* (2011) **31**:413–6. doi:10.1159/000329763
140. Dufty BM, Warner LR, Hou ST, Jiang SX, Gomez-Isla T, Leenhouts KM, et al. Calpain-cleavage of alpha-synuclein: connecting proteolytic processing to disease-linked aggregation. *Am J Pathol* (2007) **170**:1725–38. doi:10.2353/ajpath.2007.061232
141. Levin J, Giese A, Boetzel K, Israel L. T. Högen, G. Nübling, H. Kretzschmar, and S. Lorenzl, "Increased α-synuclein aggregation following limited cleavage by certain matrix metalloproteinases,". *Exp Neurol* (2009) **215**:201–8. doi:10.1016/j.expneurol.2008.10.010
142. Lorenzl S, Albers DS, Narr S, Chirichigno J, Beal MF. Expression of MMP-2, MMP-9, and MMP-1 and their endogenous counterregulators TIMP-1 and TIMP-2 in postmortem brain tissue of Parkinson's disease. *Exp Neurol* (2002) **178**:13–20. doi:10.1006/exnr.2002.8019
143. Kim YS, Choi DH, Block ML, Lorenzl S, Yang L, Kim YJ, et al. A pivotal role of matrix metalloproteinase-3 activity in dopaminergic neuronal degeneration via microglial activation. *FASEB J* (2007) **21**:179–87. doi:10.1096/fj.06-5865com
144. Ogawa K, Yamada T, Tsujioka Y, Taguchi J, Takahashi M, Tsuboi Y, et al. Localization of a novel type trypsin-like serine protease, neurosin, in brain tissues of Alzheimer's disease and Parkinson's disease. *Psychiatry Clin Neurosci* (2000) **54**:419–26. doi:10.1046/j.1440-1819.2000.00731.x
145. Wennström M, Surova Y, Hall S, Nilsson C, Minthon L, Boström F, et al. Low CSF levels of both α-synuclein and the α-synuclein cleaving enzyme neurosin in patients with synucleinopathy. *PLoS One* (2013) **8**:e53250. doi:10.1371/journal.pone.0053250
146. Cookson MR. α-Synuclein and neuronal cell death. *Mol Neurodegener* (2009) **4**:9. doi:10.1186/1750-1326-4-9
147. Hu WT, Grossman M. TDP-43 and frontotemporal dementia. *Curr Neurol Neurosci Rep* (2009) **9**:353–8. doi:10.1007/s11910-009-0052-3
148. Snowden JS. Frontotemporal dementia. *Br J Psychiatry* (2002) **180**:140–3. doi:10.1192/bjp.180.2.140
149. Rascovsky K, Hodges JR, Knopman D, Mendez MF, Kramer JH, Neuhaus J, et al. Sensitivity of revised diagnostic criteria for the behavioural variant of frontotemporal dementia. *Brain* (2011) **134**:2456–77. doi:10.1093/brain/awr179

150. Lagier-Tourenne C, Polymenidou M, Cleveland DW. TDP-43 and FUS/TLS: emerging roles in RNA processing and neurodegeneration. *Hum Mol Genet* (2010) **19**:R46–64. doi:10.1093/hmg/ddq137
151. Wilson AC, Dugger BN, Dickson DW, Wang D-S. TDP-43 in aging and Alzheimer's disease - a review. *Int J Clin Exp Pathol* (2011) **4**:147–55.
152. Steinacker P, Hendrich C, Sperfeld AD, Jesse S, von Arnim CAF, Lehnert S, et al. TDP-43 in cerebrospinal fluid of patients with frontotemporal lobar degeneration and amyotrophic lateral sclerosis. *Arch Neurol* (2008) **65**:1481–7. doi:10.1001/archneur.65.11.1481
153. Kasai T, Tokuda T, Ishigami N, Sasayama H, Foulds P, Mitchell DJ, et al. Increased TDP-43 protein in cerebrospinal fluid of patients with amyotrophic lateral sclerosis. *Acta Neuropathol* (2009) **117**:55–62. doi:10.1007/s00401-008-0456-1
154. Foulds PG, Davidson Y, Mishra M, Hobson DJ, Humphreys KM, Taylor M, et al. Plasma phosphorylated-TDP-43 protein levels correlate with brain pathology in frontotemporal lobar degeneration. *Acta Neuropathol* (2009) **118**:647–58. doi:10.1007/s00401-009-0594-0
155. Foulds P, McAuley E, Gibbons L, Davidson Y, Pickering-Brown SM, Neary D, et al. TDP-43 protein in plasma may index TDP-43 brain pathology in Alzheimer's disease and frontotemporal lobar degeneration. *Acta Neuropathol* (2008) **116**:141–6. doi:10.1007/s00401-008-0389-8
156. De Marco G, Lomartire A, Mandili G, Lupino E, Buccinnà B, Ramondetti C, et al. Reduced cellular Ca2+ availability enhances TDP-43 cleavage by apoptotic caspases. *Biochim Biophys Acta* (2014) **1843**:725–34. doi:10.1016/j.bbamcr.2014.01.010
157. Mackenzie IRA, Foti D, Woulfe J, Hurwitz TA. Atypical frontotemporal lobar degeneration with ubiquitin-positive, TDP-43-negative neuronal inclusions. *Brain* (2008) **131**:1282–93. doi:10.1093/brain/awn061
158. Zinszner H, Sok J, Immanuel D, Yin Y, Ron D. TLS (FUS) binds RNA in vivo and engages in nucleo-cytoplasmic shuttling. *J Cell Sci* (1997) **110**(Pt 1):1741–50.
159. Perrotti D, Bonatti S, Trotta R, Martinez R, Skorski T, Salomoni P, et al. TLS/FUS, a pro-oncogene inved in multiple chromosomal translocations, is a novel regulator of BCR/ABL-mediated leukemogenesis. *EMBO J* (1998) **17**:4442–55. doi:10.1093/emboj/17.15.4442
160. Bertrand P, Akhmedov AT, Delacote F, Durrbach A, Lopez BS. Human POMp75 is identified as the pro-oncoprotein TLS/FUS: both POMp75 and POMp100 DNA homologous pairing activities are associated to cell proliferation. *Oncogene* (1999) **18**:4515–21. doi:10.1038/sj.onc.1203048
161. Baechtold H, Kuroda M, Sok J, Ron D, Lopez BS, Akhmedov AT. Human 75-kDa DNA-pairing protein is identical to the pro-oncoprotein TLS/FUS and is able to promote D-loop formation. *J Biol Chem* (1999) **274**:34337–42. doi:10.1074/jbc.274.48.34337
162. Yang L, Embree LJ, Tsai S, Hickstein DD. Oncoprotein TLS interacts with serine-arginine proteins inved in RNA splicing. *J Biol Chem* (1998) **273**:27761–4. doi:10.1074/jbc.273.43.27761
163. Andersson MK, Ståhlberg A, Arvidsson Y, Olofsson A, Semb H, Stenman G, et al. The multifunctional FUS, EWS and TAF15 proto-oncoproteins show cell type-specific expression patterns and invement in cell spreading and stress response. *BMC Cell Biol* (2008) **9**:37. doi:10.1186/1471-2121-9-37
164. Mitchell JC, McGoldrick P, Vance C, Hortobagyi T, Sreedharan J, Rogelj B, et al. Overexpression of human wild-type FUS causes progressive motor neuron degeneration in an age- and dose-dependent fashion. *Acta Neuropathol* (2013) **125**:273–88. doi:10.1007/s00401-012-1043-z
165. Yoshida T, Tomozawa Y, Arisato T, Okamoto Y, Hirano H, Nakagawa M. The functional alteration of mutant GFAP depends on the location of the domain: morphological and functional studies using astrocytoma-derived cells. *J Hum Genet* (2007) **52**:362–9. doi:10.1007/s10038-007-0124-7
166. Bandyopadhyay U, Sridhar S, Kaushik S, Kiffin R, Cuervol AM. *Identification of regulators of chaperone-mediated autophagy Mol Cell* (2010) **39**:535–47. doi:10.1016/j.molcel.2010.08.004
167. Emirandetti A, Graciele ZR, Sabha M Jr., de Oliveira AL. Astrocyte reactivity influences the number of presynaptic terminals apposed to spinal motoneurons after axotomy. *Brain Res* (2006) **1095**:35–42. doi:10.1016/j.brainres.2006.04.021
168. Giménez YRM, Langa F, Menet V, Privat A. Comparative anatomy of the cerebellar cortex in mice lacking vimentin, GFAP, and both vimentin and GFAP. *Glia* (2000) **31**:69–83. doi:10.1002/(sici)1098-1136(200007)31:1<69::aid-glia70>3.0.co;2-w
169. Eliasson C, Sahlgren C, Berthold CH, Stakeberg J, Celis JE, Betsholtz C, et al. Intermediate filament protein partnership in astrocytes. *J Biol Chem* (1999) **274**:23996–4006. doi:10.1074/jbc.274.34.23996
170. Kato H, Yamamoto T, Yamamoto H, Ohi R, So N, Iwasaki Y. Immunocytochemical characterization of supporting cells in the enteric nervous system in Hirschsprung's disease. *J Pediatr Surg* (1990) **25**:514–9. doi:10.1016/0022-3468(90)90563-O
171. Riol H, Tardy M, Rolland B, Levesque G, Murthy MR. Detection of the peripheral nervous system (PNS)-type glial fibrillary acidic protein (GFAP) and its mRNA in human lymphocytes. *J Neurosci Res* (1997) **48**:53–62. doi:10.1002/(SICI)1097-4547(19970401)48:1%3C53::AID-JNR5%3E3.0.CO;2-D
172. Hainfellner JA, Voigtlander T, Strobel T, Mazal PR, Maddalena AS, Aguzzi A, et al. Fibroblasts can express glial fibrillary acidic protein (GFAP) in vivo. *J Neuropathol Exp Neurol* (2001) **60**:449–61.
173. Carotti S, Morini S, Corradini SG, Burza MA, Molinaro A, Carpino G, et al. Glial fibrillary acidic protein as an early marker of hepatic stellate cell activation in chronic and posttransplant recurrent hepatitis C. *Liver Transpl* (2008) **14**:806–14. doi:10.1002/lt.21436
174. Roelofs RF, Fischer DF, Houtman SH, Sluijs JA, Van Haren W, van Leeuwen FW, et al. Adult human subventricular, subgranular, and subpial zones contain astrocytes with a specialized intermediate filament cytoskeleton. *Glia* (2005) **52**:289e300. doi:10.1002/glia.20243
175. Middeldorp J, van den Berge SA, Aronica E, Speijer D, Hol EM. Specific human astrocyte subtype revealed by affinity purified GFAP+1 antibody. *Unpurified serum cross-reacts with neurofilament-L in Alzheimer PLoS One* (2009) **4**:e7663. doi:10.1371/journal.pone.0007663
176. Kamphuis W, Middeldorp J, Kooijman L, Sluijs JA, Kooi EJ, Moeton M, et al. Glial fibrillary acidic protein isoform expression in plaque related astrogliosis in Alzheimer's disease. *Neurobiol Aging* (2014) **35**:492–510. doi:10.1016/j.neurobiolaging.2013.09.035
177. van den Berge SA, Middeldorp J, Eleana ZC, Curtis MA, Leonard BW, Mastroeni D, et al. Longterm quiescent cells in the aged human subventricular neurogenic system specifically express GFAP-delta. *Aging Cell* (2010) **9**:313–26. doi:10.1111/j.1474-9726.2010.00556.x
178. Perng MD, Wen SF, Gibbon T, Middeldorp J, Sluijs J, Hol EM, et al. Glial fibrillary acidic protein filaments can tolerate the incorporation of assembly-compromised GFAP-delta, but with consequences for filament organization and alphaB-crystallin association. *Mol Biol Cell* (2008) **19**:4521–33. doi:10.1091/mbc.E08-03-0284
179. Blechingberg J, Holm IE, Nielsen KB, Jensen TH, Jorgensen AL, Nielsen AL. Identification and characterization of GFAPkappa, a novel glial fibrillary acidic protein isoform. *Glia* (2007) **55**:497–507. doi:10.1002/glia.20475
180. Nielsen AL, Holm IE, Johansen M, Bonven B, Jorgensen P, Jorgensen ALA. new splice variant of glial fibrillary acidic protein. *GFAP epsilon, interacts with the presenilin proteins J Biol Chem* (2002) **277**:29983–91. doi:10.1074/jbc.M112121200
181. Zhang Z, Nadeau P, Song W, Donoviel D, Yuan M, Bernstein A, et al. Presenilins are required for gamma-secretase cleavage of beta-APP and transmembrane cleavage of Notch-1. *Nature Cell Biol* (2000) **2**:463–5. doi:10.1038/35017108
182. Wang Y, Martinez-Vicente M, Krüger U, Kaushik S, Wong E, Mandelkow EM, et al. Tau fragmentation, aggregation and clearance: the dual role of lysosomal processing. *Hum Mol Genet* (2009) **18**(21):4153–70. doi:10.1093/hmg/ddp367
183. Wharton SB, O'Callaghan JP, Savva GM, Nicoll JA, Matthews F, Simpson JE, et al. Population variation in Glial fibrillary acidic protein levels in brain ageing: relationship to Alzheimer-type pathology and dementia. *Dement Geriatr Cogn Disord* (2009) **27**:465–73. doi:10.1159/000217729
184. Muramori F, Kobayashi K, Nakamura IA. quantitative study of neurofibrillary tangles, senile plaques and astrocytes in the hippocampal subdivisions and entorhinal cortex in Alzheimer's disease, normal controls and non-Alzheimer neuropsychiatric diseases. *Psychiatry Clin Neurosci* (1998) **52**:593–9. doi:10.1111/j.1440-1819.1998.tb02706.x
185. Porchet R, Probst A, Bouras C, Draberova E, Draber P, Riederer BM. Analysis of glial acidic fibrillary protein in the human entorhinal cortex during aging and in Alzheimer's disease. *Proteomics* (2003) **3**:1476–85. doi:10.1002/pmic.200300456
186. Simpson JE, Ince PG, Lace G, Forster G, Shaw PJ, Matthews F, et al. Astrocyte phenotype in relation to Alzheimer-type pathology in the ageing

brain. *Neurobiol Aging* (2010) **31**:578–90. doi:10.1016/j.neurobiolaging.2008.05.015

187. Johnson GV, Seubert P, Cox TM, Motter R, Brown JP, Galasko D. The tau protein in human cerebrospinal fluid in Alzheimer's disease consists of proteolytically derived fragments. *J Neurochem* (1997) **68**:430–3. doi:10.1046/j.1471-4159.1997.68010430.x
188. Ingelsson M, Fukumoto H, Newell KL, Growdon JH, Hedley-Whyte ET, Frosch MP, et al. Early Abeta accumulation and progressive synaptic loss, gliosis, and tangle formation in AD brain. *Neurology* (2004) **62**:925–31. doi:10.1212/01.WNL.0000115115.98960.37
189. Fukuyama R, Izumoto T, Fushiki S. The cerebrospinal fluid level of glial fibrillary acidic protein is increased in cerebrospinal fluid from Alzheimer's disease patients and correlates with severity of dementia. *Eur Neurol* (2001) **46**(1):35–8. doi:10.1159/000050753
190. Rosengren LE, Wikkelsø C, Hagberg L. A sensitive ELISA for glial fibrillary acidic protein: application in CSF of adults.;". *J Neurosci Methods* (1994) **51**(2):197–204. doi:10.1016/0165-0270(94)90011-6
191. Jesse S, Steinacker P, Cepek L, Arnim CV, Tumani H, Lehnert S, et al. Glial fibrillary acidic protein and protein S-100B: different concentration pattern of glial proteins in cerebrospinal fluid of patients with Alzheimer's disease and Creutzfeldt-Jakob disease. *J Alzheimers Dis* (2009) **17**(3):541–51. doi:10.3233/JAD-2009-1075
192. Van Eijk JJ, Van Everbroeck B, Abdo WF, Kremer BPH, Verbeek MM. CSF neurofilament proteins levels are elevated in sporadic Creutzfeldt-Jakob disease. *J Alzheimers Dis* (2010) **21**(2):569–76. doi:10.3233/JAD-2010-090649
193. Brouns R, De Vil B, Cras P, De Surgeloose D, Mariën P, De Deyn PP. Neurobiochemical markers of brain damage in cerebrospinal fluid of acute ischemic stroke patients. *Clin Chem* (2010) **56**(3):451–8. doi:10.1373/clinchem.2009.134122
194. Aurell A, Rosengren LE, Karlsson B, Olsson JE, Zbornikova V, Haglid KG. Determination of S-100 and glial fibrillary acidic protein concentrations in cerebrospinal fluid after brain infarction. *Stroke* (1991) **22**(10):1254–8. doi:10.1161/01.STR.22.10.1254
195. Neselius S, Brisby H, Theodorsson A, Blennow K, Zetterberg H, Marcusson J. Csf-biomarkers in olympic boxing: diagnosis and effects of repetitive head trauma. *PLoS One* (2012) **7**(4):e33606. doi:10.1371/journal.pone.0033606
196. Fraser DD, Close TE, Rose KL, Ward R, Mehl M, Farrell C, et al. Severe traumatic brain injury in children elevates glial fibrillary acidic protein in cerebrospinal fluid and serum. *Pediatr Crit Care Med* (2011) **12**(3):319–24. doi:10.1097/PCC.0b013e3181e8b32d
197. Mayer CA, Brunkhorst R, Niessner M, Pfeilschifter W, Steinmetz H, Foerch C. Blood levels of glial fibrillary acidic protein (GFAP) in patients with neurological diseases. *PLoS One* (2013) **8**(4):e62101. doi:10.1371/journal.pone.0062101
198. Chen MH, Hagemann TL, Quinlan RA, Messing A, Perng MD. Caspase cleavage of GFAP produces an assembly-compromised proteolytic fragment that promotes filament aggregation. *ASN Neuro* (2013) **5**(5):e00125. doi:10.1042/AN20130032
199. Mouser PE, Head E, Ha KH, Rohn TT. Caspase-mediated cleavage of glial fibrillary acidic protein within degenerating astrocytes of the Alzheimer's disease brain. *Am J Pathol* (2006) **168**:936–46. doi:10.2353/ajpath.2006.050798
200. Lee YB, Du S, Rhim H, Lee EB, Markelonis GJ, Oh TH. Rapid increase in immunoreactivity to GFAP in astrocytes in vitro induced by acidic pH is mediated by calcium influx and calpain I. *Brain Res* (2000) **864**(2):220–9. doi:10.1016/S0006-8993(00)02180-6
201. Zoltewicz JS, Scharf D, Yang B, Chawla A, Newsom KJ, Fang L. Characterization of antibodies that detect human GFAP after traumatic brain injury. *Biomark Insights* (2012) **7**:71–9. doi:10.4137/BMI.S9873

2

Cerebrospinal fluid P-tau$_{181P}$: biomarker for improved differential dementia diagnosis

Hanne Struyfs[1], Ellis Niemantsverdriet[1], Joery Goossens[1], Erik Fransen[2], Jean-Jacques Martin[3], Peter P. De Deyn[1,3,4,5] and Sebastiaan Engelborghs[1,4]*

[1] Reference Center for Biological Markers of Dementia (BIODEM), Institute Born-Bunge, University of Antwerp, Antwerp, Belgium, [2] StatUa Center for Statistics, University of Antwerp, Antwerp, Belgium, [3] Biobank, Institute Born-Bunge, University of Antwerp, Antwerp, Belgium, [4] Department of Neurology and Memory Clinic, Hospital Network Antwerp (ZNA) Middelheim and Hoge Beuken, Antwerp, Belgium, [5] Department of Neurology and Alzheimer Research Center, University Medical Center Groningen (UMCG), Groningen, Netherlands

Edited by:
Sylvain Lehmann, Montpellier University Hospital, France

Reviewed by:
Zhihui Yang, University of Florida, USA
Davide Chiasserini, University of Perugia, Italy

***Correspondence:**
Sebastiaan Engelborghs, Reference Center for Biological Markers of Dementia (BIODEM), University of Antwerp, Universiteitsplein 1, Antwerp 2610, Belgium sebastiaan.engelborghs@uantwerpen.be

The goal of this study is to investigate the value of tau phosphorylated at threonine 181 (P-tau$_{181P}$) in the Alzheimer's disease (AD) cerebrospinal fluid (CSF) biomarker panel for differential dementia diagnosis in autopsy confirmed AD and non-AD patients. The study population consisted of 140 autopsy confirmed AD and 77 autopsy confirmed non-AD dementia patients. CSF concentrations of amyloid-β peptide of 42 amino acids (Aβ_{1-42}), total tau protein (T-tau), and P-tau$_{181P}$ were determined with single analyte ELISA-kits (INNOTEST®, Fujirebio, Ghent, Belgium). Diagnostic accuracy was assessed through receiver operating characteristic (ROC) curve analyses to obtain area under the curve (AUC) values and to define optimal cutoff values to discriminate AD from pooled and individual non-AD groups. ROC curve analyses were only performed on biomarkers and ratios that differed significantly between the groups. Pairwise comparison of AUC values was performed by means of DeLong tests. The Aβ_{1-42}/P-tau$_{181P}$ ratio (AUC = 0.770) performed significantly better than Aβ_{1-42} (AUC = 0.677, P = 0.004), T-tau (AUC = 0.592, P < 0.001), and Aβ_{1-42}/T-tau (AUC = 0.678, P = 0.001), while P-tau$_{181P}$ (AUC = 0.720) performed significantly better than T-tau (AUC = 0.592, P < 0.001) to discriminate between AD and the pooled non-AD group. When comparing AD and the individual non-AD diagnoses, Aβ_{1-42}/P-tau$_{181P}$ (AUC = 0.894) discriminated AD from frontotemporal dementia significantly better than Aβ_{1-42} (AUC = 0.776, P = 0.020) and T-tau (AUC = 0.746, P = 0.004), while P-tau$_{181P}$/T-tau (AUC = 0.958) significantly improved the differentiation between AD and Creutzfeldt-Jakob disease as compared to Aβ_{1-42} (AUC = 0.688, P = 0.004), T-tau (AUC = 0.874, P = 0.040), and Aβ_{1-42}/P-tau$_{181P}$ (AUC = 0.760, P = 0.003). In conclusion, this study demonstrates P-tau$_{181P}$ is an essential component of the AD CSF biomarker panel, and combined assessment of Aβ_{1-42}, T-tau, and P-tau$_{181P}$ renders, to present date, the highest diagnostic power to discriminate between AD and non-AD dementias.

Keywords: Alzheimer's disease, dementia, differential diagnosis, biomarkers, cerebrospinal fluid, neuropathology, tau

Introduction

The clinical diagnosis of Alzheimer's disease (AD) is mainly based on the exclusion of other diseases (1). Relative to autopsy confirmation, the clinical diagnostic criteria of AD (1) reach on average 81% sensitivity and 70% specificity (2). However, these figures mostly originate from specialized clinical centers and from diagnoses based on follow-up periods of several years. In the earliest stages of the disease and when the diagnostic work-up is performed in non-specialized centers, far lower diagnostic accuracy can be expected. Diagnosis of definite AD can therefore only be made through postmortem pathological examination of the brain.

Analyzing cerebrospinal fluid (CSF) levels of amyloid-β peptide of 42 amino acids ($A\beta_{1-42}$), total tau protein (T-tau) and tau phosphorylated at threonine 181 (P-tau_{181P}) increases diagnostic certainty for AD (3). Based on autopsy confirmation, it was shown that in the majority of patients with a clinically ambiguous diagnosis (when the clinical diagnostic work-up was not able to discriminate between AD and a non-AD dementia), a correct diagnosis would have been established in 82% by using these CSF biomarkers, indicating that CSF biomarkers may have a particular added diagnostic value in patients with ambiguous clinical diagnoses (4).

Compared to controls, decreased $A\beta_{1-42}$ and increased T-tau and/or P-tau_{181P} concentrations are found in AD. However, when compared to non-AD dementias, the differences are less obvious as the concentrations in patients with non-AD dementias are generally intermediate compared to those found between controls and AD patients, thus pointing to an overlap between AD and non-AD patients, especially in dementia with Lewy bodies (DLB) and to a lesser extent in frontotemporal dementia (FTD), vascular dementia (VaD), and Creutzfeldt-Jakob's disease (CJD) (5). This overlap may partly be explained by the presence of mixed pathologies as well as the low sensitivity and specificity of the clinical diagnosis as most biomarker studies rely on clinically diagnosed patients.

The goal of this study is to investigate the value of P-tau_{181P} in the AD CSF biomarker panel for differential dementia diagnosis in autopsy confirmed AD and non-AD patients.

Materials and Methods

Study Population

In brief, the study population consisted of 140 and 77 CSF samples from dementia patients with pathologically confirmed diagnoses of AD and non-AD, respectively. All CSF samples were selected from the Biobank, Institute Born-Bunge, Antwerp, Belgium. Samples from 173 dementia patients were collected in the Memory Clinic of the Hospital Network Antwerp (ZNA, Antwerp, Belgium) between January 1992 and May 2008, whereas samples from 44 dementia patients were collected in referring centers between April 1992 and May 2005.

The study was approved by the local ethics committee (CME Middelheim) and all subjects gave written informed consent.

Pathological Criteria

All pathological diagnoses were established according to standard neuropathological criteria by the same neuropathologist (Jean-Jacques Martin). Although the neuropathologist was blinded for the CSF biomarker data, he had access to all neuroimaging data and the clinical files of the patients included. For the diagnosis of AD, VaD ($n = 18$), and DLB ($n = 24$), the neuropathological criteria of Montine et al. (6) were applied. FTD ($n = 17$) was neuropathologically diagnosed according to the Cairns criteria (7) and Mackenzie criteria (8, 9). CJD ($n = 13$) was diagnosed according to the criteria of Markesbery (10). Mixed dementia (MXD) was diagnosed when the patient fulfilled the neuropathological criteria of AD in combination with minor pathology suggestive of cerebrovascular disease ($n = 12$), DLB ($n = 1$), or Parkinson's disease ($n = 1$). For statistical analyses, the MXD group ($n = 14$) was pooled with the AD group. The pooled non-AD group furthermore consisted of few patients with progressive nuclear palsy ($n = 3$), spinocerebellar ataxia ($n = 1$), and normal pressure hydrocephalus combined with VaD ($n = 1$). Neuropathology was performed on the right hemisphere of the brain.

CSF Analyses

All subjects underwent a lumbar puncture (LP) in order to collect CSF. LP was performed between the intervertebral space L3/L4 or L4/L5 (11). CSF was sampled according to a standard protocol (12). All samples were stored in polypropylene vials to avoid adsorption of Aβ to the wall of the vial. The samples were frozen in liquid nitrogen and stored at −80°C until analysis.

CSF concentrations of $A\beta_{1-42}$, T-tau, and P-tau_{181P} were determined with commercially available single analyte ELISA-kits (respectively, INNOTEST® β-AMYLOID$_{(1-42)}$, INNOTEST® hTAU-Ag, and INNOTEST® PHOSPHO-TAU$_{(181P)}$; Fujirebio, Ghent, Belgium). A complete description of the CSF analysis has been published previously (13).

Statistical Analyses

Statistical analyses were performed using SPSS 20. As most variables were not normally distributed, non-parametric tests were used. To compare gender distribution between the groups, a Chi-square test was performed. Subsequently, Mann–Whitney *U* tests were performed to compare clinical and biomarker data between the groups. Receiver operating characteristic (ROC) curve analyses were used to obtain area under the curve (AUC) values and to define optimal cutoff values to discriminate AD from the pooled and individual non-AD groups. ROC curve analyses were only performed on biomarkers and ratios that were significantly different ($P < 0.05$), based on the Mann–Whitney *U* tests. The cutoff values were determined by calculating the maximal sum of sensitivity and specificity (i.e., maximizing the Youden index). In order to pairwise compare AUC values, DeLong tests were performed using the pROC package (14) in the statistical software package R (R Core Team).

Systematic Review

To be able to compare the results of this study, a systematic review on the diagnostic accuracy of P-tau_{181P} for differential dementia diagnosis was performed. A PubMed search (until May 2015) was performed using the following terms: (Cerebrospinal fluid OR CSF) AND diagnos* AND (Alzheimer* OR AD OR dementia) AND (tau OR beta amyloid OR abeta) AND (sensitivity OR specificity). Only publications in the English language were

TABLE 1 | Demographic, clinical, and biomarker data of the study population.

	AD	Non-AD	*P*-value
N (M/F)	140 (71/69)	77 (45/32)	0.275
Age at sampling (years)	76 (71–85)	72 (65–76)	**0.001**
MMSE (/30)	14 (9–19) ($n = 98$)	16 (9–21) ($n = 51$)	0.228
Years between sampling and death	0.0 (0.0–2.5)	0.0 (0.0–2.0)	0.452
$A\beta_{1-42}$ (pg/mL)	361 (264–485)	514 (369–695)	**<0.001**
T-tau (pg/mL)	581 (335–872)	379 (242–787)	**0.025**
P-tau_{181P} (pg/mL)	73.2 (51.6–100.0)	45.0 (31.9–65.9)	**<0.001**
$A\beta_{1-42}$/T-tau	0.682 (0.399–1.100)	1.273 (0.719–2.257)	**<0.001**
$A\beta_{1-42}$/P-tau_{181P}	4.982 (3.174–7.802)	10.535 (6.522–16.711)	**<0.001**
P-tau_{181P}/T-tau	0.138 (0.113–0.171)	0.141 (0.090–0.158)	0.094

All data are median values with 25th and 75th quartiles between brackets, except for N. To compare gender distribution between the groups, a Chi-square test was performed, while Mann–Whitney U tests were used to compare clinical and biomarker data between the groups.

AD, Alzheimer's disease; non-AD, dementia not due to Alzheimer's disease; MMSE, mini-mental state examination; $A\beta_{1-42}$, amyloid-β peptide of 42 amino acids; T-tau, total tau-protein; P-tau_{181P}, tau phosphorylated at threonine 181.

Bold values show statistically significant P-values ($P < 0.05$).

evaluated. Subsequently, relevant publications were searched for in reference lists. Publications were included when: (a) their aim was to improve the diagnostic accuracy of diagnosis of dementia by means of CSF biomarkers, (b) AD patients and pooled non-AD patients or patients with DLB, FTD, VaD and/or CJD were included, (c) P-tau_{181P} together with $A\beta_{1-42}$ and/or T-tau was measured in CSF, and (d) diagnostic accuracy values were reported (AUC, sensitivity, and/or specificity). Publications comparing only AD to healthy control subjects were not considered.

Results

Table 1 shows the demographic, clinical, and biomarker data of the studied population. The AD and non-AD groups were not age-matched. However, based on co-variate analyses, confounding effects of age on differences in biomarker concentrations were excluded. Therefore, no corrections for age were included in the subsequent analyses. Boxplots of the individual biomarkers and ratios are presented in **Figure 1**.

The diagnostic powers to discriminate between AD and non-AD of the individual biomarkers and ratios that were significantly different are shown in **Table 2**. Based on the DeLong tests

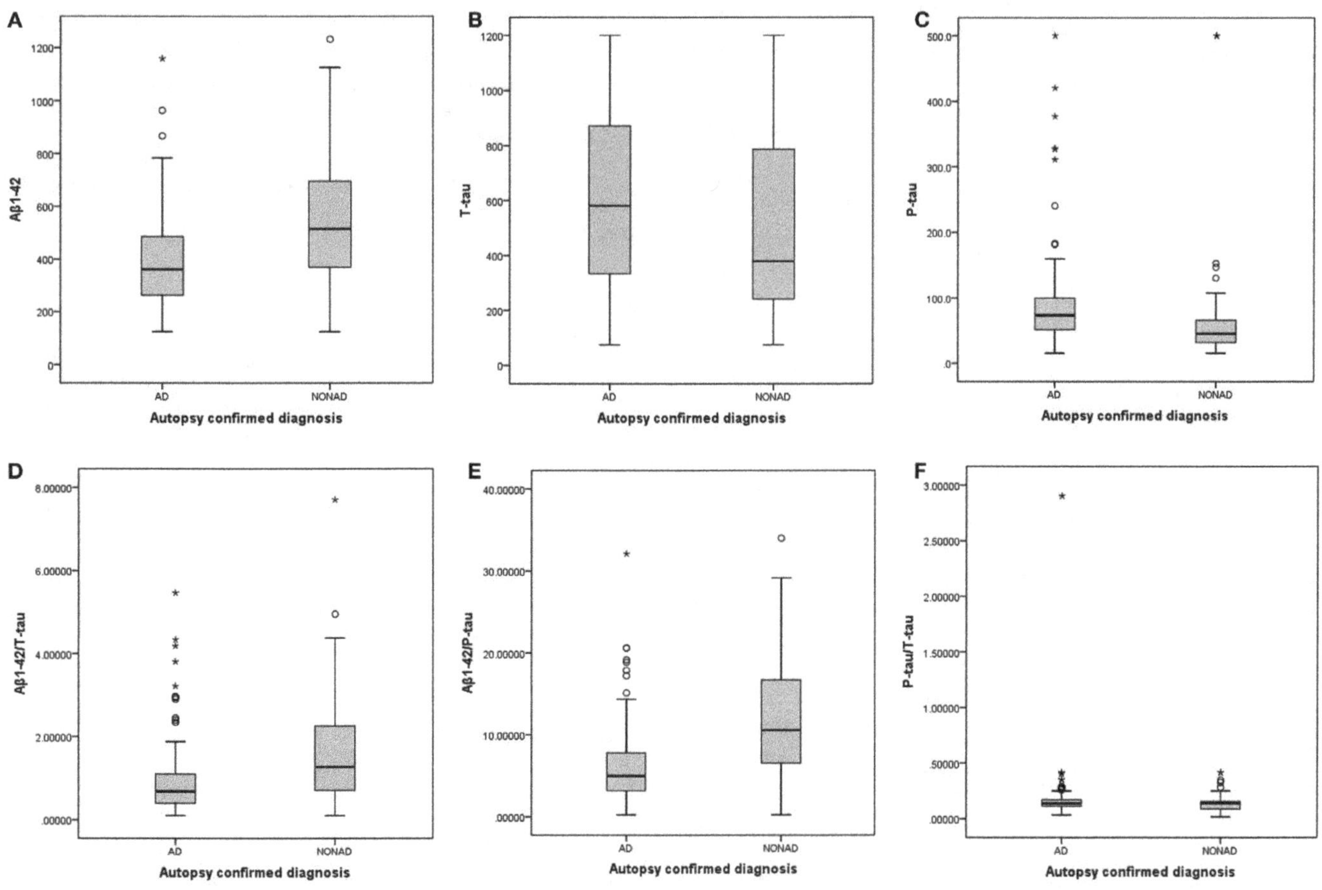

FIGURE 1 | Boxplots of the individual biomarkers and ratios, comparing AD and non-AD. (A) $A\beta_{1-42}$; **(B)** T-tau; **(C)** P-tau_{181P}; **(D)** $A\beta_{1-42}$/T-tau; **(E)** $A\beta_{1-42}$/P-tau_{181P}; **(F)** P-tau_{181P}/T-tau. AD, Alzheimer's disease; non-AD, dementia not due to Alzheimer's disease; $A\beta_{1-42}$, amyloid-β peptide of 42 amino acids; T-tau, total tau-protein; P-tau_{181P}, tau phosphorylated at threonine 181.

TABLE 2 | Diagnostic power of the significantly different individual biomarkers and ratios to discriminate between AD and non-AD, measured by ROC curve analyses.

AD vs. non-AD	AUC	95% CI	Cutoff	Sens (%)	Spec (%)
$A\beta_{1-42}$	0.677	0.597–0.757	500.27	79.3	53.2
T-tau	0.592	0.508–0.675	472.35	62.1	63.6
$P\text{-tau}_{181P}$	0.720	0.648–0.792	50.35	77.9	61.0
$A\beta_{1-42}$/T-tau	0.678	0.601–0.755	1.08	75.0	57.1
$A\beta_{1-42}/P\text{-tau}_{181P}$	0.770	0.703–0.837	9.11	82.9	59.7

AD, Alzheimer's disease; non-AD, dementia not due to Alzheimer's disease; AUC, area under the curve; CI, confidence interval; sens, sensitivity; spec, specificity; $A\beta_{1-42}$, amyloid-β peptide of 42 amino acids; T-tau, total tau-protein; $P\text{-tau}_{181P}$, tau phosphorylated at threonine 181.

TABLE 3 | *P* values of pairwise comparisons of AUC values of the ROC curve analyses to discriminate between AD and non-AD, using DeLong tests.

	$P\text{-tau}_{181P}$	$A\beta_{1-42}/P\text{-tau}_{181P}$
$A\beta_{1-42}$	0.450	**0.004**
T-tau	**<0.001**	**<0.001**
$A\beta_{1-42}$/T-tau	0.290	**0.001**
$A\beta_{1-42}/P\text{-tau}_{181P}$	0.100	NA

$A\beta_{1-42}$, amyloid-β peptide of 42 amino acids; T-tau, total tau-protein; $P\text{-tau}_{181P}$, tau phosphorylated at threonine 181; NA, not applicable.
Bold values show statistically significant P-values ($P < 0.05$).

TABLE 4 | *P* values of pairwise comparisons of the individual biomarkers and ratios, measured by Mann–Whitney *U* tests.

	AD vs. FTD	AD vs. DLB	AD vs. CJD	AD vs. VaD
$A\beta_{1-42}$	**<0.001**	0.068	**0.025**	0.078
T-tau	**0.001**	0.051	**<0.001**	**0.019**
$P\text{-tau}_{181P}$	**<0.001**	**0.011**	0.081	**0.001**
$A\beta_{1-42}$/T-tau	**<0.001**	**0.008**	0.054	**0.010**
$A\beta_{1-42}/P\text{-tau}_{181P}$	**<0.001**	**0.002**	**0.002**	**0.003**
$P\text{-tau}_{181P}$/T-tau	0.096	0.232	**<0.001**	0.932

AD, Alzheimer's disease; FTD, frontotemporal dementia; DLB, dementia with Lewy bodies; CJD, Creutzfeldt-Jakob disease; VaD, vascular dementia; $A\beta_{1-42}$, amyloid-β peptide of 42 amino acids; T-tau, total tau-protein; $P\text{-tau}_{181P}$, tau phosphorylated at threonine 181.
Bold values show statistically significant P-values ($P < 0.05$).

(**Table 3**), the AUC of the $A\beta_{1-42}/P\text{-tau}_{181P}$ ratio was significantly different from those of $A\beta_{1-42}$, T-tau, and $A\beta_{1-42}$/T-tau, while the AUC of $P\text{-tau}_{181P}$ differed significantly from the AUC of T-tau.

When comparing AD and the different non-AD diagnoses, the $A\beta_{1-42}/P\text{-tau}_{181P}$ ratio was significantly different in every differential diagnosis (**Table 4**). This also held true for $P\text{-tau}_{181P}$, except for AD vs. CJD. On the other hand, $P\text{-tau}_{181P}$/T-tau was found to be significantly different when comparing AD to CJD.

The diagnostic powers to discriminate between AD and the different non-AD diagnoses of the individual biomarkers and ratios that differed significantly are shown in **Table 5**. Based on the DeLong tests (**Table 6**), the $A\beta_{1-42}/P\text{-tau}_{181P}$ ratio performed significantly better than $A\beta_{1-42}$ and T-tau to discriminate AD from FTD, while the AUC of $P\text{-tau}_{181P}$/T-tau was significantly better than those of $A\beta_{1-42}$, T-tau, and $A\beta_{1-42}/P\text{-tau}_{181P}$ to differentiate between AD and CJD.

The results of the systematic review are summarized in Table S1 in Supplementary Material. Only results comparing AD to non-AD, FTD, DLB, CJD, and/or VaD were included in this table.

TABLE 5 | Diagnostic power of the significantly different individual biomarkers and ratios to discriminate between AD and individual non-AD diagnoses, measured by ROC curve analyses.

	AUC	95% CI	Cutoff	Sens (%)	Spec (%)
AD vs. FTD					
$A\beta_{1-42}$	0.776	0.652–0.900	385.31	57.1	88.2
T-tau	0.746	0.654–0.838	423.00	67.9	82.4
$P\text{-tau}_{181P}$	0.810	0.710–0.910	47.25	81.4	76.5
$A\beta_{1-42}$/T-tau	0.863	0.794–0.931	0.97	70.1	94.1
$A\beta_{1-42}/P\text{-tau}_{181P}$	0.894	0.823–0.965	9.77	86.4	82.4
AD vs. DLB					
$P\text{-tau}_{181P}$	0.664	0.539–0.788	59.05	65.7	70.8
$A\beta_{1-42}$/T-tau	0.670	0.539–0.802	0.80	60.7	75.0
$A\beta_{1-42}/P\text{-tau}_{181P}$	0.694	0.565–0.824	8.46	80.0	58.3
AD vs. CJD					
$A\beta_{1-42}$	0.688	0.521–0.855	440.12	66.4	69.2
T-tau	0.874	0.775–0.973	>1200	84.3	92.3
$A\beta_{1-42}/P\text{-tau}_{181P}$	0.760	0.634–0.886	6.84	67.9	84.6
$P\text{-tau}_{181P}$/T-tau	0.958	0.925–0.991	0.1030	84.3	100.0
AD vs. VaD					
T-tau	0.670	0.534–0.807	467.93	62.1	72.2
$P\text{-tau}_{181P}$	0.733	0.599–0.867	49.85	78.6	66.7
$A\beta_{1-42}$/T-tau	0.687	0.569–0.804	0.72	56.4	77.8
$A\beta_{1-42}/P\text{-tau}_{181P}$	0.718	0.598–0.838	5.30	55.7	77.8

AD, Alzheimer's disease; FTD, frontotemporal dementia; DLB, dementia with Lewy bodies; CJD, Creutzfeldt-Jakob disease; VaD, vascular dementia; AUC, area under the curve; CI, confidence interval; sens, sensitivity; spec, specificity; $A\beta_{1-42}$, amyloid-β peptide of 42 amino acids; T-tau, total tau-protein; $P\text{-tau}_{181P}$, tau phosphorylated at threonine 181.

TABLE 6 | *P* values of pairwise comparisons of AUC values of the ROC curve analyses to discriminate between AD and individual non-AD diagnoses, using DeLong tests.

	$P\text{-tau}_{181P}$	$A\beta_{1-42}/P\text{-tau}_{181P}$	$P\text{-tau}_{181P}$/T-tau
AD vs. FTD			
$A\beta_{1-42}$	0.700	**0.020**	NA
T-tau	0.120	**0.004**	NA
$A\beta_{1-42}$/T-tau	0.280	0.280	NA
AD vs. DLB			
$A\beta_{1-42}$/T-tau	0.890	0.360	NA
AD vs. CJD			
$A\beta_{1-42}$	NA	0.327	**0.004**
T-tau	NA	0.220	**0.040**
$A\beta_{1-42}/P\text{-tau}_{181P}$	NA	NA	**0.003**
AD vs. VaD			
T-tau	0.370	0.600	NA
$A\beta_{1-42}$/T-tau	0.600	0.610	NA

AD, Alzheimer's disease; FTD, frontotemporal dementia; DLB, dementia with Lewy bodies; CJD, Creutzfeldt-Jakob disease; VaD, vascular dementia; $A\beta_{1-42}$, amyloid-β peptide of 42 amino acids; T-tau, total tau-protein; $P\text{-tau}_{181P}$, tau phosphorylated at threonine 181; NA, not applicable.
Bold values show statistically significant P-values ($P < 0.05$).

Discussion

The goal of this study was to investigate the value of $P\text{-tau}_{181P}$ in the AD biomarker panel for differential dementia diagnosis. First of all, the ratio of $A\beta_{1-42}/P\text{-tau}_{181P}$ was shown to have a significantly higher diagnostic power than $A\beta_{1-42}$, T-tau, and the $A\beta_{1-42}$/T-tau ratio, while $P\text{-tau}_{181P}$ was found to perform significantly better than T-tau to discriminate between AD and non-AD dementia. This clearly signifies the importance of $P\text{-tau}_{181P}$ in the biomarker panel for differential dementia diagnosis. Our results are in line with previously reported findings of (combinations with) P-tau$_{181P}$ having most power to discriminate between AD and non-AD dementias (12, 15–29).

However, in contrast to former studies performed in clinically diagnosed AD and pooled non-AD dementia patients (15, 21, 22, 26–28), the AUC, sensitivity, and specificity of neither P-tau$_{181P}$ nor Aβ_{1-42}/P-tau$_{181P}$ reached the minimal level of 0.80, as established by the Consensus Report of the Working Group on Molecular and Biochemical Markers of AD (30). This is probably not due to the accuracy of the diagnoses used in this study, as autopsy confirmation was used. A possible explanation of the discrepancy in accuracy levels between this study and former studies could be the composition of the non-AD groups. As shown in this study, the accuracy levels of, for example, AD vs. FTD are substantially higher than those of AD vs. DLB. Therefore, if a non-AD group is primarily composed of FTD patients, the AUC levels may be higher than when DLB patients prevail in the non-AD group.

When focusing on the discrimination between AD and FTD, our results showed that the diagnostic power of Aβ_{1-42}/P-tau$_{181P}$ was significantly higher than those of Aβ_{1-42} and T-tau. These results confirm earlier studies performed in clinically diagnosed AD and FTD patients (16, 17, 24, 25, 29).

With regard to the differentiation between AD and CJD, the diagnostic power of P-tau$_{181P}$/T-tau was significantly higher than those of Aβ_{1-42}, T-tau, and Aβ_{1-42}/P-tau$_{181P}$. Our results confirm those of former studies performed in clinically diagnosed AD and CJD patients, and partly performed in autopsy confirmed cases (31–34).

In these latter two comparisons with individual non-AD groups, the AUCs did reach the minimal level of 0.80. This indicates that the pathophysiological variability in the pooled non-AD group lowers the diagnostic accuracy of the CSF biomarkers.

It should be noted that the ratios and other combinations of the AD CSF biomarkers should be used with care. Due to (pre-)analytical issues (35), concentrations differ exceedingly between laboratories. External quality controls and reference material might be able to reduce this variability, which would enable the general use of the same cutoff that was validated in a multicenter setting. At this moment, cutoffs for individual biomarkers as well as ratios and other combinations should be validated in-house before they can be used in clinical practice (36, 37).

In order to further increase diagnostic accuracy, other biomarkers should be included in the biomarker panel in the future. Examples of possible fluid biomarkers for features of Aβ processing in AD are β-site APP cleaving enzyme-1 (BACE1) activity (38–44), soluble amyloid precursor protein (sAPP) α and β (42, 44–51), and Aβ oligomers (52–60). Some fluid biomarkers that are still being investigated seem more specific for non-AD dementias and could also increase diagnostic accuracy when added to the biomarker panel. Examples of possible such non-AD biomarkers are TAR DNA-binding protein 43 (TDP-43) (61–63), TPD-43 phosphorylated at S409 (pTDP-43) (63), and progranulin (64–66) for FTD, α-synuclein (67–71) and neurosin (72) for DLB, metalloproteinases-9 for VaD (73, 74), and total CSF prion protein for CJD (75). For reviews on these biomarkers, see Ref. (76–80). Most of these biomarkers need extensive validation as well as validated ready-to-use analytical methods before they can be used in combination with Aβ_{1-42}, T-tau, and P-tau$_{181P}$ for differential dementia diagnosis in clinical practice.

Another highly promising approach is combining fluid biomarkers and imaging, such as magnetic resonance imaging (MRI) and positron emission tomography (PET) imaging. Several studies have shown that combinations of fluid and imaging biomarkers render higher diagnostic power than these modalities alone (81–85).

In conclusion, this study demonstrates P-tau$_{181P}$ is a fundamental component of the AD biomarker panel and the combined assessment of Aβ_{1-42}, T-tau, and P-tau$_{181P}$ renders, to present date, the highest diagnostic power to discriminate between AD and non-AD dementias. New biomarkers more specifically targeted at non-AD dementia pathology should further increase diagnostic power in the future.

Acknowledgments

This work was supported by the University of Antwerp Research Fund; the Alzheimer Research Foundation (SAO-FRA); the central Biobank facility of the Institute Born-Bunge/University Antwerp; the Research Foundation Flanders (FWO); the Agency for Innovation by Science and Technology (IWT); the Belgian Science Policy Office Interuniversity Attraction Poles (IAP) program; the Flemish Government initiated Methusalem excellence grant; the University of Antwerp Research Fund, Belgium. This work is part of the BIOMARKAPD project within the EU Joint Programme for Neurodegenerative Disease Research (JPND). The research leading to these results has received support from the Innovative Medicines Initiative Joint Undertaking under grant agreement no. 115372, resources of which are composed of financial contribution from the European Union's Seventh Framework Programme (FP7/2007-2013) and EFPIA companies' in kind contribution.

References

1. Mckhann G, Drachman D, Folstein M, Katzman R, Price D, Stadlan EM. Clinical diagnosis of Alzheimer's disease: report of the NINCDS-ADRDA work group under the auspices of department of health and human services task force on Alzheimer's disease. *Neurology* (1984) **34**:939–44. doi:10.1212/WNL.34.7.939
2. Knopman DS, Dekosky ST, Cummings JL, Chui H, Corey-Bloom J, Relkin N, et al. Practice parameter: diagnosis of dementia (an evidence-based review). Report of the quality standards subcommittee of the american academy of neurology. *Neurology* (2001) **56**:1143–53. doi:10.1212/WNL.56.9.1143
3. Blennow K, Hampel H, Weiner M, Zetterberg H. Cerebrospinal fluid and plasma biomarkers in Alzheimer disease. *Nat Rev Neurol* (2010) **6**:131–44. doi:10.1038/nrneurol.2010.4

4. Le Bastard N, Martin JJ, Vanmechelen E, Vanderstichele H, De Deyn PP, Engelborghs S. Added diagnostic value of CSF biomarkers in differential dementia diagnosis. *Neurobiol Aging* (2010) **31**:1867–76. doi:10.1016/j.neurobiolaging.2008.10.017
5. Engelborghs S, Le Bastard N. The impact of cerebrospinal fluid biomarkers on the diagnosis of Alzheimer's disease. *Mol Diagn Ther* (2012) **16**:135–41. doi:10.2165/11634170-000000000-00000
6. Montine TJ, Phelps CH, Beach TG, Bigio EH, Cairns NJ, Dickson DW, et al. National Institute on Aging-Alzheimer's Association guidelines for the neuropathologic assessment of Alzheimer's disease: a practical approach. *Acta Neuropathol* (2012) **123**:1–11. doi:10.1007/s00401-011-0910-3
7. Cairns NJ, Bigio EH, Mackenzie IR, Neumann M, Lee VM, Hatanpaa KJ, et al. Neuropathologic diagnostic and nosologic criteria for frontotemporal lobar degeneration: consensus of the consortium for frontotemporal lobar degeneration. *Acta Neuropathol* (2007) **114**:5–22. doi:10.1007/s00401-007-0237-2
8. Mackenzie IR, Neumann M, Bigio EH, Cairns NJ, Alafuzoff I, Kril J, et al. Nomenclature and nosology for neuropathologic subtypes of frontotemporal lobar degeneration: an update. *Acta Neuropathol* (2010) **119**:1–4. doi:10.1007/s00401-009-0612-2
9. Mackenzie IR, Neumann M, Baborie A, Sampathu DM, Du Plessis D, Jaros E, et al. A harmonized classification system for FTLD-TDP pathology. *Acta Neuropathol* (2011) **122**:111–3. doi:10.1007/s00401-011-0845-8
10. Markesbery WR. *Neuropathology of Dementing Disorders*. London: Arnold (1998).
11. Niemantsverdriet E, Struyfs H, Duits F, Teunissen C, Engelborghs S. Techniques, contraindications and complications of CSF collection procedures. In: Deisenhammer F, Sellebjerg F, Teunissen CE, Tumani H, editors. *Cerebrospinal Fluid in Clinical Neurology*. Cham, Switzerland: Springer International Publishing (2015). p. 35–57.
12. Engelborghs S, De Vreese K, Van De Casteele T, Vanderstichele H, Van Everbroeck B, Cras P, et al. Diagnostic performance of a CSF-biomarker panel in autopsy-confirmed dementia. *Neurobiol Aging* (2008) **29**:1143–59. doi:10.1016/j.neurobiolaging.2007.02.016
13. Le Bastard N, Aerts L, Sleegers K, Martin JJ, Van Broeckhoven C, De Deyn PP, et al. Longitudinal stability of cerebrospinal fluid biomarker levels: fulfilled requirement for pharmacodynamic markers in Alzheimer's disease. *J Alzheimers Dis* (2013) **33**:807–22. doi:10.3233/JAD-2012-110029
14. Robin X, Turck N, Hainard A, Tiberti N, Lisacek F, Sanchez JC, et al. pROC: an open-source package for R and S+ to analyze and compare ROC curves. *BMC Bioinformatics* (2011) **12**:77. doi:10.1186/1471-2105-12-77
15. Maddalena A, Papassotiropoulos A, Muller-Tillmanns B, Jung HH, Hegi T, Nitsch RM, et al. Biochemical diagnosis of Alzheimer disease by measuring the cerebrospinal fluid ratio of phosphorylated tau protein to beta-amyloid peptide42. *Arch Neurol* (2003) **60**:1202–6. doi:10.1001/archneur.60.9.1202
16. Schoonenboom NS, Pijnenburg YA, Mulder C, Rosso SM, Van Elk EJ, Van Kamp GJ, et al. Amyloid beta(1-42) and phosphorylated tau in CSF as markers for early-onset Alzheimer disease. *Neurology* (2004) **62**:1580–4. doi:10.1212/01.WNL.0000123249.58898.E0
17. Blasko I, Lederer W, Oberbauer H, Walch T, Kemmler G, Hinterhuber H, et al. Measurement of thirteen biological markers in CSF of patients with Alzheimer's disease and other dementias. *Dement Geriatr Cogn Disord* (2006) **21**:9–15. doi:10.1159/000089137
18. De Jong D, Jansen RW, Kremer BP, Verbeek MM. Cerebrospinal fluid amyloid beta42/phosphorylated tau ratio discriminates between Alzheimer's disease and vascular dementia. *J Gerontol A Biol Sci Med Sci* (2006) **61**:755–8. doi:10.1093/gerona/61.7.755
19. Vanderstichele H, De Vreese K, Blennow K, Andreasen N, Sindic C, Ivanoiu A, et al. Analytical performance and clinical utility of the INNOTEST PHOSPHO-TAU181P assay for discrimination between Alzheimer's disease and dementia with Lewy bodies. *Clin Chem Lab Med* (2006) **44**:1472–80. doi:10.1515/CCLM.2006.258
20. Reijn TS, Rikkert MO, Van Geel WJ, De Jong D, Verbeek MM. Diagnostic accuracy of ELISA and xMAP technology for analysis of amyloid beta(42) and tau proteins. *Clin Chem* (2007) **53**:859–65. doi:10.1373/clinchem.2006.081679
21. Welge V, Fiege O, Lewczuk P, Mollenhauer B, Esselmann H, Klafki HW, et al. Combined CSF tau, p-tau181 and amyloid-beta 38/40/42 for diagnosing Alzheimer's disease. *J Neural Transm* (2009) **116**:203–12. doi:10.1007/s00702-008-0177-6
22. Yakushev I, Bartenstein P, Siessmeier T, Hiemke C, Scheurich A, Lotz J, et al. Cerebrospinal fluid tau protein levels and 18F-fluorodeoxyglucose positron emission tomography in the differential diagnosis of Alzheimer's disease. *Dement Geriatr Cogn Disord* (2010) **30**:245–53. doi:10.1159/000320206
23. Aerts MB, Esselink RA, Claassen JA, Abdo WF, Bloem BR, Verbeek MM. CSF tau, Abeta42, and MHPG differentiate dementia with Lewy bodies from Alzheimer's disease. *J Alzheimers Dis* (2011) **27**:377–84. doi:10.3233/JAD-2011-110482
24. De Souza LC, Lamari F, Belliard S, Jardel C, Houillier C, De Paz R, et al. Cerebrospinal fluid biomarkers in the differential diagnosis of Alzheimer's disease from other cortical dementias. *J Neurol Neurosurg Psychiatry* (2011) **82**:240–6. doi:10.1136/jnnp.2010.207183
25. Gabelle A, Roche S, Geny C, Bennys K, Labauge P, Tholance Y, et al. Decreased sAbetaPPbeta, Abeta38, and Abeta40 cerebrospinal fluid levels in frontotemporal dementia. *J Alzheimers Dis* (2011) **26**:553–63. doi:10.3233/JAD-2011-110515
26. Gabelle A, Dumurgier J, Vercruysse O, Paquet C, Bombois S, Laplanche JL, et al. Impact of the 2008-2012 French Alzheimer Plan on the use of cerebrospinal fluid biomarkers in research memory center: the PLM Study. *J Alzheimers Dis* (2013) **34**:297–305. doi:10.3233/JAD-121549
27. Shea YF, Chu LW, Zhou L, Li WM, Lin OY, Chan MN, et al. Cerebrospinal fluid biomarkers of Alzheimer's disease in Chinese patients: a pilot study. *Am J Alzheimers Dis Other Demen* (2013) **28**:769–75. doi:10.1177/1533317513504615
28. Duits FH, Teunissen CE, Bouwman FH, Visser PJ, Mattsson N, Zetterberg H, et al. The cerebrospinal fluid "Alzheimer profile": easily said, but what does it mean? *Alzheimers Dement* (2014) **10**(713–723):e712. doi:10.1016/j.jalz.2013.12.023
29. Ewers M, Mattsson N, Minthon L, Molinuevo JL, Antonell A, Popp J, et al. CSF biomarkers for the differential diagnosis of Alzheimer's disease. A large-scale international multicenter study. *Alzheimers Dement* (2015). doi:10.1016/j.jalz.2014.12.006
30. The Ronald and Nancy Reagan Research Institute of the Alzheimer's Association and the National Institute on Aging Working Group. Consensus report of the working group on: "molecular and biochemical markers of Alzheimer's disease". *Neurobiol Aging* (1998) **19**:109–16.
31. Riemenschneider M, Wagenpfeil S, Vanderstichele H, Otto M, Wiltfang J, Kretzschmar H, et al. Phospho-tau/total tau ratio in cerebrospinal fluid discriminates Creutzfeldt-Jakob disease from other dementias. *Mol Psychiatry* (2003) **8**:343–7. doi:10.1038/sj.mp.4001220
32. Satoh K, Shirabe S, Eguchi H, Tsujino A, Eguchi K, Satoh A, et al. 14-3-3 protein, total tau and phosphorylated tau in cerebrospinal fluid of patients with Creutzfeldt-Jakob disease and neurodegenerative disease in Japan. *Cell Mol Neurobiol* (2006) **26**:45–52. doi:10.1007/s10571-006-9370-z
33. Bahl JM, Heegaard NH, Falkenhorst G, Laursen H, Hogenhaven H, Molbak K, et al. The diagnostic efficiency of biomarkers in sporadic Creutzfeldt-Jakob disease compared to Alzheimer's disease. *Neurobiol Aging* (2009) **30**:1834–41. doi:10.1016/j.neurobiolaging.2008.01.013
34. Skillback T, Rosen C, Asztely F, Mattsson N, Blennow K, Zetterberg H. Diagnostic performance of cerebrospinal fluid total tau and phosphorylated tau in Creutzfeldt-Jakob disease: results from the Swedish mortality registry. *JAMA Neurol* (2014) **71**:476–83. doi:10.1001/jamaneurol.2013.6455
35. Le Bastard N, De Deyn PP, Engelborghs S. Importance and impact of preanalytical variables on Alzheimer disease biomarker concentrations in cerebrospinal fluid. *Clin Chem* (2015) **61**:734–43. doi:10.1373/clinchem.2014.236679
36. Lehmann S, Gabelle A, Paquet C. Can we rely only on ratios of cerebrospinal fluid biomarkers for AD biological diagnosis? *Alzheimers Dement* (2014). doi:10.1016/j.jalz.2014.09.003
37. Lehmann S, Delaby C, Paquet C, Gabelle A. Analytical challenges related to the use of biomarker ratios for the biological diagnosis of Alzheimer's disease. *Clin Chem Lab Med* (2015). doi:10.1515/cclm-2014-1232
38. Holsinger RM, Mclean CA, Collins SJ, Masters CL, Evin G. Increased beta-secretase activity in cerebrospinal fluid of Alzheimer's disease subjects. *Ann Neurol* (2004) **55**:898–9. doi:10.1002/ana.20144
39. Holsinger RM, Lee JS, Boyd A, Masters CL, Collins SJ. CSF BACE1 activity is increased in CJD and Alzheimer disease versus [corrected] other dementias. *Neurology* (2006) **67**:710–2. doi:10.1212/01.wnl.0000229925.52203.4c
40. Verheijen JH, Huisman LG, Van Lent N, Neumann U, Paganetti P, Hack CE, et al. Detection of a soluble form of BACE-1 in human cerebrospinal fluid by

a sensitive activity assay. *Clin Chem* (2006) **52**:1168–74. doi:10.1373/clinchem.2006.066720
41. Zhong Z, Ewers M, Teipel S, Burger K, Wallin A, Blennow K, et al. Levels of beta-secretase (BACE1) in cerebrospinal fluid as a predictor of risk in mild cognitive impairment. *Arch Gen Psychiatry* (2007) **64**:718–26. doi:10.1001/archpsyc.64.6.718
42. Zetterberg H, Andreasson U, Hansson O, Wu G, Sankaranarayanan S, Andersson ME, et al. Elevated cerebrospinal fluid BACE1 activity in incipient Alzheimer disease. *Arch Neurol* (2008) **65**:1102–7. doi:10.1001/archneur.65.8.1102
43. Mulder SD, Van Der Flier WM, Verheijen JH, Mulder C, Scheltens P, Blankenstein MA, et al. BACE1 activity in cerebrospinal fluid and its relation to markers of AD pathology. *J Alzheimers Dis* (2010) **20**:253–60. doi:10.3233/JAD-2010-1367
44. Rosen C, Andreasson U, Mattsson N, Marcusson J, Minthon L, Andreasen N, et al. Cerebrospinal fluid profiles of amyloid beta-related biomarkers in Alzheimer's disease. *Neuromolecular Med* (2012) **14**:65–73. doi:10.1007/s12017-012-8171-4
45. Olsson A, Hoglund K, Sjogren M, Andreasen N, Minthon L, Lannfelt L, et al. Measurement of alpha- and beta-secretase cleaved amyloid precursor protein in cerebrospinal fluid from Alzheimer patients. *Exp Neurol* (2003) **183**:74–80. doi:10.1016/S0014-4886(03)00027-X
46. Gabelle A, Roche S, Geny C, Bennys K, Labauge P, Tholance Y, et al. Correlations between soluble alpha/beta forms of amyloid precursor protein and Abeta38, 40, and 42 in human cerebrospinal fluid. *Brain Res* (2010) **1357**:175–83. doi:10.1016/j.brainres.2010.08.022
47. Hertze J, Minthon L, Zetterberg H, Vanmechelen E, Blennow K, Hansson O. Evaluation of CSF biomarkers as predictors of Alzheimer's disease: a clinical follow-up study of 4.7 years. *J Alzheimers Dis* (2010) **21**:1119–28. doi:10.3233/JAD-2010-100207
48. Lewczuk P, Kamrowski-Kruck H, Peters O, Heuser I, Jessen F, Popp J, et al. Soluble amyloid precursor proteins in the cerebrospinal fluid as novel potential biomarkers of Alzheimer's disease: a multicenter study. *Mol Psychiatry* (2010) **15**:138–45. doi:10.1038/mp.2008.84
49. Johansson P, Mattsson N, Hansson O, Wallin A, Johansson JO, Andreasson U, et al. Cerebrospinal fluid biomarkers for Alzheimer's disease: diagnostic performance in a homogeneous mono-center population. *J Alzheimers Dis* (2011) **24**:537–46. doi:10.3233/JAD-2011-101878
50. Perneczky R, Tsolakidou A, Arnold A, Diehl-Schmid J, Grimmer T, Forstl H, et al. CSF soluble amyloid precursor proteins in the diagnosis of incipient Alzheimer disease. *Neurology* (2011) **77**:35–8. doi:10.1212/WNL.0b013e318221ad47
51. Lewczuk P, Popp J, Lelental N, Kolsch H, Maier W, Kornhuber J, et al. Cerebrospinal fluid soluble amyloid-beta protein precursor as a potential novel biomarkers of Alzheimer's disease. *J Alzheimers Dis* (2012) **28**:119–25. doi:10.3233/JAD-2011-110857
52. Pitschke M, Prior R, Haupt M, Riesner D. Detection of single amyloid beta-protein aggregates in the cerebrospinal fluid of Alzheimer's patients by fluorescence correlation spectroscopy. *Nat Med* (1998) **4**:832–4. doi:10.1038/nm0798-832
53. Georganopoulou DG, Chang L, Nam JM, Thaxton CS, Mufson EJ, Klein WL, et al. Nanoparticle-based detection in cerebral spinal fluid of a soluble pathogenic biomarker for Alzheimer's disease. *Proc Natl Acad Sci U S A* (2005) **102**:2273–6. doi:10.1073/pnas.0409336102
54. Shankar GM, Li S, Mehta TH, Garcia-Munoz A, Shepardson NE, Smith I, et al. Amyloid-beta protein dimers isolated directly from Alzheimer's brains impair synaptic plasticity and memory. *Nat Med* (2008) **14**:837–42. doi:10.1038/nm1782
55. Fukumoto H, Tokuda T, Kasai T, Ishigami N, Hidaka H, Kondo M, et al. High-molecular-weight beta-amyloid oligomers are elevated in cerebrospinal fluid of Alzheimer patients. *FASEB J* (2010) **24**:2716–26. doi:10.1096/fj.09-150359
56. Gao CM, Yam AY, Wang X, Magdangal E, Salisbury C, Peretz D, et al. Abeta40 oligomers identified as a potential biomarker for the diagnosis of Alzheimer's disease. *PLoS One.* (2010) **5**:e15725. doi:10.1371/journal.pone.0015725
57. Santos AN, Ewers M, Minthon L, Simm A, Silber RE, Blennow K, et al. Amyloid-beta oligomers in cerebrospinal fluid are associated with cognitive decline in patients with Alzheimer's disease. *J Alzheimers Dis* (2012) **29**:171–6. doi:10.3233/JAD-2012-111361
58. Bruggink KA, Jongbloed W, Biemans EA, Veerhuis R, Claassen JA, Kuiperij HB, et al. Amyloid-beta oligomer detection by ELISA in cerebrospinal fluid and brain tissue. *Anal Biochem* (2013) **433**:112–20. doi:10.1016/j.ab.2012.09.014
59. Handoko M, Grant M, Kuskowski M, Zahs KR, Wallin A, Blennow K, et al. Correlation of specific amyloid-beta oligomers with tau in cerebrospinal fluid from cognitively normal older adults. *JAMA Neurol* (2013) **70**:594–9. doi:10.1001/jamaneurol.2013.48
60. Yang T, Hong S, O'malley T, Sperling RA, Walsh DM, Selkoe DJ. New ELISAs with high specificity for soluble oligomers of amyloid beta-protein detect natural Abeta oligomers in human brain but not CSF. *Alzheimers Dement* (2013) **9**:99–112. doi:10.1016/j.jalz.2012.11.005
61. Steinacker P, Hendrich C, Sperfeld AD, Jesse S, Von Arnim CA, Lehnert S, et al. TDP-43 in cerebrospinal fluid of patients with frontotemporal lobar degeneration and amyotrophic lateral sclerosis. *Arch Neurol* (2008) **65**:1481–7. doi:10.1001/archneur.65.11.1481
62. Feneberg E, Steinacker P, Lehnert S, Schneider A, Walther P, Thal DR, et al. Limited role of free TDP-43 as a diagnostic tool in neurodegenerative diseases. *Amyotroph Lateral Scler Frontotemporal Degener* (2014) **15**:351–6. doi:10.3109/21678421.2014.905606
63. Suarez-Calvet M, Dols-Icardo O, Llado A, Sanchez-Valle R, Hernandez I, Amer G, et al. Plasma phosphorylated TDP-43 levels are elevated in patients with frontotemporal dementia carrying a C9orf72 repeat expansion or a GRN mutation. *J Neurol Neurosurg Psychiatry* (2014) **85**:684–91. doi:10.1136/jnnp-2013-305972
64. Ghidoni R, Benussi L, Glionna M, Franzoni M, Binetti G. Low plasma progranulin levels predict progranulin mutations in frontotemporal lobar degeneration. *Neurology* (2008) **71**:1235–9. doi:10.1212/01.wnl.0000325058.10218.fc
65. Van Damme P, Van Hoecke A, Lambrechts D, Vanacker P, Bogaert E, Van Swieten J, et al. Progranulin functions as a neurotrophic factor to regulate neurite outgrowth and enhance neuronal survival. *J Cell Biol* (2008) **181**:37–41. doi:10.1083/jcb.200712039
66. Philips T, De Muynck L, Thu HN, Weynants B, Vanacker P, Dhondt J, et al. Microglial upregulation of progranulin as a marker of motor neuron degeneration. *J Neuropathol Exp Neurol* (2010) **69**:1191–200. doi:10.1097/NEN.0b013e3181fc9aea
67. Mollenhauer B, El-Agnaf OM, Marcus K, Trenkwalder C, Schlossmacher MG. Quantification of alpha-synuclein in cerebrospinal fluid as a biomarker candidate: review of the literature and considerations for future studies. *Biomark Med* (2010) **4**:683–99. doi:10.2217/bmm.10.90
68. Shi M, Bradner J, Hancock AM, Chung KA, Quinn JF, Peskind ER, et al. Cerebrospinal fluid biomarkers for Parkinson disease diagnosis and progression. *Ann Neurol* (2011) **69**:570–80. doi:10.1002/ana.22311
69. Aerts MB, Esselink RA, Abdo WF, Bloem BR, Verbeek MM. CSF alpha-synuclein does not differentiate between parkinsonian disorders. *Neurobiol Aging* (2012) **33**(430):e431–3. doi:10.1016/j.neurobiolaging.2010.12.001
70. Kapaki E, Paraskevas GP, Emmanouilidou E, Vekrellis K. The diagnostic value of CSF alpha-synuclein in the differential diagnosis of dementia with Lewy bodies vs. normal subjects and patients with Alzheimer's disease. *PLoS One* (2013) **8**:e81654. doi:10.1371/journal.pone.0081654
71. Slaets S, Vanmechelen E, Le Bastard N, Decraemer H, Vandijck M, Martin JJ, et al. Increased CSF alpha-synuclein levels in Alzheimer's disease: correlation with tau levels. *Alzheimers Dement* (2014) **10**(5 Suppl):S290–8. doi:10.1016/j.jalz.2013.10.004
72. Wennstrom M, Surova Y, Hall S, Nilsson C, Minthon L, Bostrom F, et al. Low CSF levels of both alpha-synuclein and the alpha-synuclein cleaving enzyme neurosin in patients with synucleinopathy. *PLoS One* (2013) **8**:e53250. doi:10.1371/journal.pone.0053250
73. Adair JC, Charlie J, Dencoff JE, Kaye JA, Quinn JF, Camicioli RM, et al. Measurement of gelatinase B (MMP-9) in the cerebrospinal fluid of patients with vascular dementia and Alzheimer disease. *Stroke* (2004) **35**:e159–62. doi:10.1161/01.STR.0000127420.10990.76
74. Rosenberg GA. Matrix metalloproteinases and their multiple roles in neurodegenerative diseases. *Lancet Neurol* (2009) **8**:205–16. doi:10.1016/S1474-4422(09)70016-X
75. Dorey A, Tholance Y, Vighetto A, Perret-Liaudet A, Lachman I, Krolak-Salmon P, et al. Association of cerebrospinal fluid prion protein levels and the distinction between Alzheimer disease and Creutzfeldt-Jakob disease. *JAMA Neurol* (2015) **72**:267–75. doi:10.1001/jamaneurol.2014.4068
76. Fagan AM, Perrin RJ. Upcoming candidate cerebrospinal fluid biomarkers of Alzheimer's disease. *Biomark Med* (2012) **6**:455–76. doi:10.2217/bmm.12.42

77. Rosen C, Hansson O, Blennow K, Zetterberg H. Fluid biomarkers in Alzheimer's disease – current concepts. *Mol Neurodegener* (2013) **8**:20. doi:10.1186/1750-1326-8-20
78. Roh JH, Lee JH. Recent updates on subcortical ischemic vascular dementia. *J Stroke* (2014) **16**:18–26. doi:10.5853/jos.2014.16.1.18
79. Schade S, Mollenhauer B. Biomarkers in biological fluids for dementia with Lewy bodies. *Alzheimers Res Ther* (2014) **6**:72. doi:10.1186/s13195-014-0072-3
80. Oeckl P, Steinacker P, Feneberg E, Otto M. Cerebrospinal fluid proteomics and protein biomarkers in frontotemporal lobar degeneration: current status and future perspectives. *Biochim Biophys Acta* (2015) **1854**:757–68. doi:10.1016/j.bbapap.2014.12.010
81. Schoonenboom NS, Van Der Flier WM, Blankenstein MA, Bouwman FH, Van Kamp GJ, Barkhof F, et al. CSF and MRI markers independently contribute to the diagnosis of Alzheimer's disease. *Neurobiol Aging* (2008) **29**:669–75. doi:10.1016/j.neurobiolaging.2006.11.018
82. Brys M, Glodzik L, Mosconi L, Switalski R, De Santi S, Pirraglia E, et al. Magnetic resonance imaging improves cerebrospinal fluid biomarkers in the early detection of Alzheimer's disease. *J Alzheimers Dis* (2009) **16**:351–62. doi:10.3233/JAD-2009-0968
83. Vos S, Van R I, Burns L, Knol D, Scheltens P, Soininen H, et al. Test sequence of CSF and MRI biomarkers for prediction of AD in subjects with MCI. *Neurobiol Aging* (2012) **33**:2272–81. doi:10.1016/j.neurobiolaging.2011.12.017
84. Westman E, Muehlboeck JS, Simmons A. Combining MRI and CSF measures for classification of Alzheimer's disease and prediction of mild cognitive impairment conversion. *Neuroimage* (2012) **62**:229–38. doi:10.1016 j.neuroimage.2012.04.056
85. Shaffer JL, Petrella JR, Sheldon FC, Choudhury KR, Calhoun VD, Coleman RE, et al. Predicting cognitive decline in subjects at risk for Alzheimer disease by using combined cerebrospinal fluid, MR imaging, and PET biomarkers. *Radiology* (2013) **266**:583–91. doi:10.1148/radiol.12120010

3

CSF neurofilament light chain but not FLT3 ligand discriminates parkinsonian disorders

Megan K. Herbert[1,2], *Marjolein B. Aerts*[1,3], *Marijke Beenes*[1,2], *Niklas Norgren*[4], *Rianne A. J. Esselink*[1,3], *Bastiaan R. Bloem*[1,3], *H. Bea Kuiperij*[1,2] and *Marcel M. Verbeek*[1,2,3]*

[1] Department of Neurology and Parkinson Center, Donders Institute for Brain, Cognition and Behaviour, Radboud University Medical Centre, Nijmegen, Netherlands, [2] Department of Laboratory Medicine, Radboud University Medical Centre, Nijmegen, Netherlands, [3] Parkinson Center, Nijmegen, Netherlands, [4] UmanDiagnostics, Umeå, Sweden

Edited by:
Sylvain Lehmann,
Montpellier University Hospital, France

Reviewed by:
Steve M. Gentleman,
Imperial College London, UK
Yadong Huang,
University of California San Francisco, USA

***Correspondence:**
Marcel M. Verbeek,
Neurochemistry Laboratory,
Department of Neurology, Radboud University Medical Centre, 830 TML, P.O. Box 9101, Nijmegen 6500 HB, Netherlands
marcel.verbeek@radboudumc.nl

The differentiation between multiple system atrophy (MSA) and Parkinson's disease (PD) is difficult, particularly in early disease stages. Therefore, we aimed to evaluate the diagnostic value of neurofilament light chain (NFL), fms-like tyrosine kinase ligand (FLT3L), and total tau protein (t-tau) in cerebrospinal fluid (CSF) as biomarkers to discriminate MSA from PD. Using commercially available enzyme-linked immunosorbent assays, we measured CSF levels of NFL, FLT3L, and t-tau in a discovery cohort of 36 PD patients, 27 MSA patients, and 57 non-neurological controls and in a validation cohort of 32 PD patients, 25 MSA patients, 15 PSP patients, 5 CBS patients, and 56 non-neurological controls. Cut-offs obtained from individual assays and binary logistic regression models developed from combinations of biomarkers were assessed. CSF levels of NFL were substantially increased in MSA and discriminated between MSA and PD with a sensitivity of 74% and specificity of 92% (AUC = 0.85) in the discovery cohort and with 80% sensitivity and 97% specificity (AUC = 0.94) in the validation cohort. FLT3L levels in CSF were significantly lower in both PD and MSA compared to controls in the discovery cohort, but not in the validation cohort. t-tau levels were significantly higher in MSA than PD and controls. Addition of either FLT3L or t-tau to NFL did not improve discrimination of PD from MSA above NFL alone. Our findings show that increased levels of NFL in CSF offer clinically relevant, high accuracy discrimination between PD and MSA.

Keywords: Parkinson's disease, multiple system atrophy, neurofilament light chain, FLT3 ligand, cerebrospinal fluid

Introduction

Parkinson's disease (PD) is the most common movement disorder with typical age of onset around 60 years although some patients (~3–5%) develop PD before the age of 40 (1). PD is characterized by four cardinal motor features: involuntary tremor, postural instability, bradykinesia, and rigidity (2). Non-motor features such as cognitive disturbances, depression, mild autonomic dysfunction (including orthostatic hypotension), and disordered sleep commonly accompany these motor symptoms (3).

Multiple system atrophy (MSA) is a relatively rare and sporadic adult-onset disease characterized by a variable combination of parkinsonism, cerebellar ataxia, autonomic dysfunction (particularly orthostatic hypotension), and pyramidal signs (4). MSA is commonly misdiagnosed as PD, particularly in early disease stages, because of overlapping symptoms, occasionally good responsiveness to dopaminergic treatment in MSA, and similar age of onset, typically around 60 years (1, 4). However, MSA progresses more rapidly than PD and is associated with a much poorer quality of life (5). Moreover, the response to levodopa, although variable, is generally poor and may lead to worsening of orthostatic hypotension in some MSA patients (6). A reliable biomarker capable of clearly distinguishing between MSA and PD would have great clinical and diagnostic value.

Two recent studies have investigated the utility of fms-like tyrosine kinase ligand (FLT3L) as a potential cerebrospinal fluid (CSF) biomarker to differentiate MSA from PD but had conflicting results. While one paper reported that CSF levels of FLT3L could differentiate between MSA and PD with high accuracy (7) another showed no significant differences in FLT3L levels between MSA and PD (8). However, there is currently no literature available investigating the biological significance of FLT3L in PD. Therefore, additional studies are required to ascertain the utility of FLT3L as a biomarker and, if its utility in distinguishing PD from MSA can be confirmed, further studies investigating its biological significance would be highly warranted.

Neurofilament proteins are highly phosphorylated neuronal cytoskeleleton proteins composed of three subunits of which the smallest, the 68 kDa neurofilament light chain (NFL), forms the backbone and is essential for neurofilament assembly (9). Elevated levels of CSF NFL in atypical parkinsonisms compared with PD and controls have been observed and may reflect more extensive neuronal damage in AP than in PD. Similarly, tau has an important function in providing structural stability to axonal microtubules. Mutations in the MAPT gene have been associated with PD and thus mark tau as a potential biomarker for PD (10). As might be expected, CSF levels of NFL and total tau protein (t-tau) have been shown to discriminate PD from atypical parkinsonisms (11–14) but these studies require further validation. In the current study, we aimed to determine which CSF biomarker (NFL, t-tau, or FLT3L), or combination of biomarkers, could provide optimal discrimination of MSA from PD.

Materials and Methods

Patients

The present study was performed at the Radboud University Medical Centre (Nijmegen, the Netherlands). We studied patients initially referred to our tertiary movement disorder center between December 2000 and November 2008 (**Figure 1**), with a hypokinetic rigid syndrome of uncertain diagnosis at presentation, and who received a subsequent diagnosis of PD or MSA. The initial clinical diagnosis (at presentation) was established by a neurologist specialized in movement disorders according to current diagnostic criteria for PD (15) and MSA (16). Patients underwent extensive neurological examination and a subset of the patients were included from a previous study in which they were studied prospectively for three years (57% of MSA and 86.8% of PD patients) (17). For these patients, diagnosis was established by

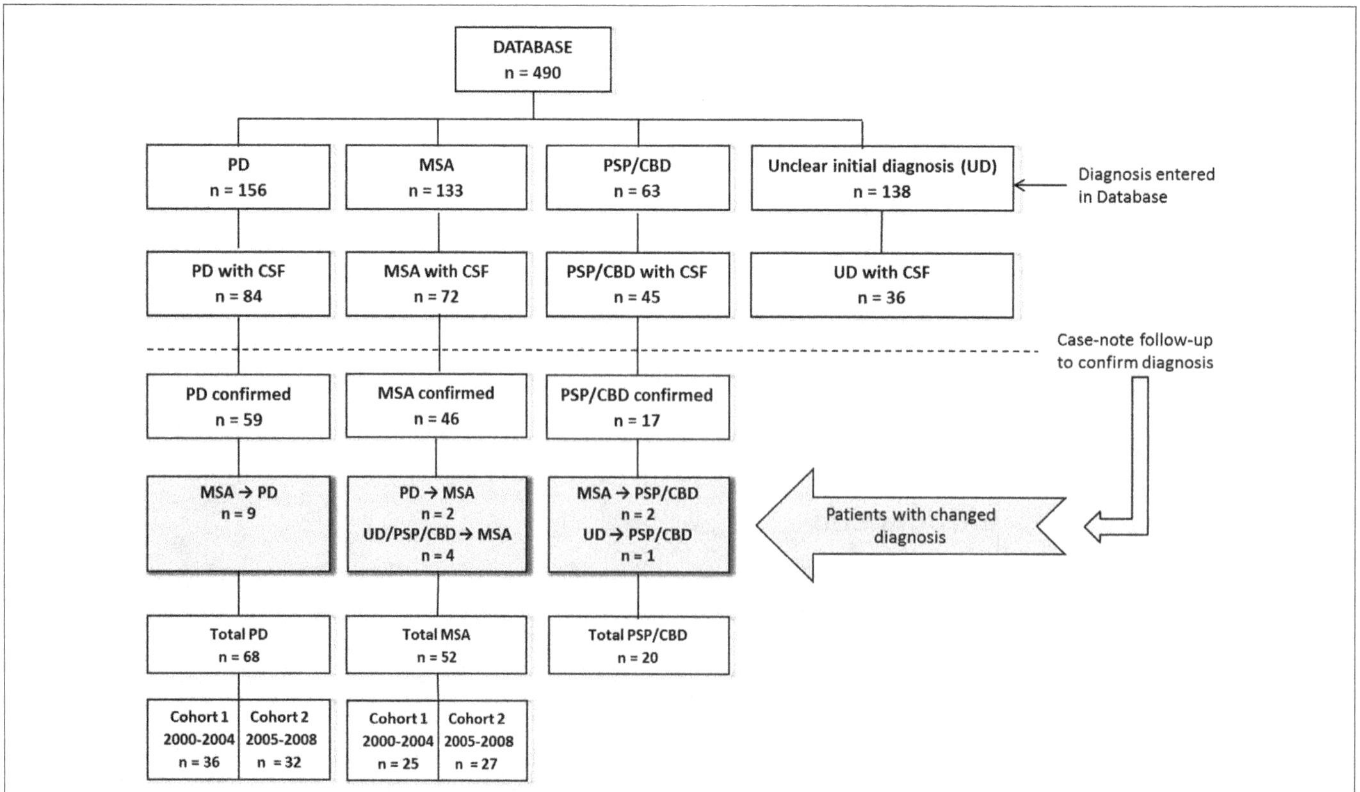

FIGURE 1 | Flowchart of patient inclusion in this study. PD, Parkinson's disease; MSA, multiple system atrophy; PSP, progressive supranuclear palsy; CBD, corticobasal degeneration; CSF, cerebrospinal fluid; *n*, number. CSF was obtained during the initial diagnostic assessment upon presentation.

two neurologists specialized in movement disorders and patients underwent extensive neurological examination and imaging studies at initial visit and again after 3 years (Supplementary Material). Ten MSA patients and five PD patients have been described earlier (14, 18) but the CSF parameters reported in the current study were not previously reported. The remaining eight MSA and four PD patients were incidental cases for whom case review follow-up was performed by a neurologist (author Marjolein B. Aerts).

Disease severity was established using the (modified) Hoehn and Yahr (H&Y) (19) stages and unified Parkinson's disease rating scale (UPDRS) (20); ataxia severity was assessed using the International Cooperative Ataxia Rating Scale (ICARS) (21). Final diagnosis was confirmed by case review up to 9 years after initial visit. Controls consisted of patients referred to our Neurology Department during the period 2001–2009, who underwent lumbar puncture as part of the diagnostic process, and who had been confirmed as having no neurological disease.

For the discovery group, we analyzed CSF samples from PD and MSA patients obtained between 2001 and 2004, and controls consisted of patients with lumbar punctures obtained between 2001 and 2006. To validate our findings, we examined CSF in additional MSA and PD patients with lumbar punctures obtained between 2005 and 2008, and control CSFs obtained between 2007 and 2010. Additional patients diagnosed with progressive supranuclear palsy (PSP, $n = 15$) and corticobasal syndrome (CBS, $n = 5$) with previously unreported, retrospective CSF NFL levels were included to show differences in NFL levels between PD patients and other atypical parkinsonisms (**Figure 1**; Table S5 in Supplementary Material). Initial clinical diagnosis for these patients was established by a movement disorders specialist using current diagnostic criteria for PSP (22) and CBS (23). Lumbar puncture samples from all MSA and PD patients were analyzed for all CSF parameters to determine and validate the utility of these parameters in discriminating PD from MSA. Controls in the discovery group were tested for all CSF parameters for comparison with PD and MSA patients. NFL and FLT3L levels in a second group of controls in the validation cohort provided additional reference values for these parameters.

Ethical Statement

The following applies to 59/68 PD patients and 32/52 MSA patients: written informed consent was obtained from the participants prior to participation of the study. All clinical investigations have been conducted according to the principles expressed in the Declaration of Helsinki. In case patients were unable to consent (defined as MMSE score below 25), written informed consent was obtained from a next of kin of the patient. The local institutional review board ("Commissie Mensgebonden Onderzoek region Arnhem-Nijmegen") approved of this study. For the remaining patients (i.e., 9/68 of PD patients, 20/52 MSA patients, and all controls), CSF samples were obtained as part of the clinical diagnostic work-up of a patient. Patients were informed that their data, including CSF, could be used for further scientific purposes and were given the option to object against this use, in which case their data were not used. This procedure has been approved as well.

CSF Samples and Analysis

Cerebrospinal fluid samples obtained by lumbar puncture were collected in polypropylene tubes, centrifuged (5 min, $860 \times g$ at room temperature), and stored at −80°C. Patient information was decoded to maintain confidentiality. Undiluted CSF samples were measured in duplicate using commercially available enzyme-linked immunosorbent assays (ELISAs) for Human FLT3L (R&D Systems, Abingdon, UK), NFL (NF-light® Neurofilament ELISA RUO; a gift from UmanDiagnostics, Sweden), and t-tau (INNOTEST® hTau, Innogenetics N.V., Ghent, Belgium). ELISAs were performed according to manufacturer's instructions except the capture antibody for the FLT3L ELISA was used at 1 g/mL.

Statistical Analysis

Cerebrospinal fluid parameters with non-Gaussian distribution were log transformed and between-group differences were tested using one-way analysis of variance (ANOVA) followed by Tukey's *post hoc* test. Mann–Whitney *U* tests were used to compare data with a non-Gaussian distribution (NFL levels in the discovery group). Spearman rank correlation was used to determine correlations. We performed analysis of covariance (ANCOVA) to control for possible confounding variables (e.g., age, gender, disease duration, and disease severity). Binary logistic regression was used to identify variables contributing to discrimination of MSA from PD and receiver–operator curves (ROCs) were used to determine the diagnostic accuracy of CSF parameters and models developed from the binary logistic regression. Statistical analyses were performed using GraphPad PRISM 5 software (San Diego, CA, USA) and SPSS software version 20.0 (Chicago, IL, USA). Comparison of the ROC curves was performed using MedCalc® software version 12.5.0.0. Bootstrapping analyses using data from both cohorts were also performed for additional validation of the measures using Medcalc 12.7.0 9 Trial version.

Results

Patient Characteristics

We analyzed 233 CSF samples: 52 MSA patients, 68 PD patients, and 113 non-neurological controls. Of these, 61% (32/52) of the MSA and 87% (59/68) of the PD patients had been studied prospectively for 3 years. The discovery group consisted of 36 PD, 27 MSA, and 57 controls. Patient characteristics and CSF parameters are reported in **Table 1**. CSF samples from controls were used to obtain reference values for NFL, FLT3L, and t-tau. In order to confirm the use of NFL, FLT3L, and t-tau in discriminating between PD and MSA, we included a validation group consisting of 32 PD and 25 MSA patients. Since CSF measures of NFL and FLT3L are rather novel, we included 56 additional controls to obtain additional reference values.

NFL, t-tau, and FLT3L Levels in CSF of the Discovery Cohort

In the discovery group, CSF FLT3L levels were significantly lower in PD (38.4 ± 11.9 ng/L; $p < 0.01$) and MSA (39.3 ± 12.4 ng/L; $p < 0.05$) compared with controls (47.8 ± 14.3 ng/L) but similar in MSA and PD (**Figure 2A**). We found significantly higher levels

TABLE 1 | Patient demographic and baseline characteristics – discovery cohort.

	PD ($n = 36$)	MSA ($n = 27$)	Controls ($n = 57$)
Age in years (SD)[b]	60.1 (10.4)	62.6 (9.0)	57.0 (11.5)
Number of males (%)	22 (61.1)	15 (55.6)	37 (64.9)
Years of follow-up (range)	5.5 (0–9.2)	2.9 (0–7.9)	N/A
NFL (ng/L)	1350 (915)	4548 (3206)	1503 (619)
FLT3L (ng/L)	38.4 (11.9)	39.3 (12.4)	47.8 (14.3)
t-tau (ng/L)	242 (190)	335 (164)	251 (110)
Disease duration, months (range)[c]	PD ($n = 28$) 43.8 (6–158)	MSA ($n = 14$) 43.7 (8–96)	***p*-Value[a]** $p = 0.508$
Disease severity[c]	PD ($n = 32$)	MSA ($n = 14$)	***p*-Value[a]**
H&Y	2.0 (0.60); $n = 32$	2.7 (1.2); $n = 14$	$p = 0.014$
UPDRS; mean (SD)	30.3 (11.5); $n = 27$	32.5 (16.7); $n = 14$	$p = 0.627$
ICARS; mean (SD)	2.9 (4.8); $n = 20$	12.1 (9.5); $n = 9$	$p = 0.020$
Cognitive function	PD ($n = 28$)	MSA ($n = 14$)	***p*-Value[a]**
MMSE; mean (SD)	28.5 (1.6)	27.5 (3.5)	$p > 0.05$

SD, standard deviation; H&Y, Hoehn and Yahr score; ICARS, International Cooperative Ataxia Rating Scale; UPDRS, unified Parkinson's disease rating scale; N/A, not applicable.
[a]Student's t-test p-values for PD versus MSA.
[b]At time of lumbar puncture.
[c]At time of inclusion.

of CSF NFL in MSA (4548 ± 3206 ng/L) compared with both PD (1350 ± 915 ng/L, $p < 0.001$) and controls (1503 ± 619 ng/L, $p < 0.001$) but not between PD and controls (**Figure 2B**). CSF t-tau levels were significantly higher for MSA (335 ± 164 ng/L) than PD (242 ± 190 ng/L; $p < 0.05$; **Figure 2C**) and, compared with our reference values for t-tau in healthy controls, 46% of MSA patients and 11% of PD patients had elevated ($\geq$350 ng/L) t-tau levels.

FLT3L correlated with both NFL and t-tau for PD and controls but not MSA. There was a moderate correlation between NFL and t-tau in PD ($r = 0.39$, $p < 0.05$) but not MSA ($r = 0.34$, $p = 0.11$) or controls ($r = 0.43$, $p = 0.08$). Details of the correlation data are provided in Table S1 in Supplementary Material. Four of the PD patients exhibited levels of t-tau that were markedly different from the remainder of the group (**Figure 2C**) but this was not correlated with MMSE since individual MMSE scores were 30 for 1 patient, 29 for 2 patients, and 26 for 1 patient. Despite long-term clinical follow-up (3–8.8 years), we can neither rule out, nor confirm, subclinical tauopathy in these patients.

Neurofilament light chain alone provided high discrimination (AUC 0.85) between MSA and PD with 74.1% sensitivity and 91.7% specificity. Logistic regression models of combination biomarkers were then analyzed (summarized in **Table 2**). The combination of t-tau and NFL developed in our previous study (12) (Model 1: $y = \text{NFL} + 0.15^*\text{t-tau}$; AUC = 0.89) yielded similar sensitivity (75.0%) and specificity (91.2%; AUC = 0.90) for discriminating MSA from PD whereas the combination of FLT3L and NFL (Model 2: $y = -1.646 + 0.001^*\text{NFL-}0.0308^*\text{FLT3L}$) yielded a sensitivity of 81.8% and specificity of 94.8% (AUC = 0.89). The combination of NFL, FLT3L, and t-tau (Model 3: $y = -3.054\text{–}0.001^*\text{NFL} + 0.003^*\text{t-tau} - 0.028^*\text{FLT3L}$) yielded a higher AUC (0.92) with increased sensitivity (94.7%) but reduced specificity (83.3%). Comparison of the ROC analyses showed that this improvement was not significantly better at discriminating between MSA from PD than NFL alone ($p > 0.05$).

Gender was not correlated with CSF parameters for any group. Age was correlated with, or tended to be correlated with, all CSF parameters in PD and controls but not in MSA (Table S2 in Supplementary Material). Disease duration and severity (ICARS and H&Y) were not correlated with CSF parameters for either PD or MSA in the discovery cohort. UPDRS was not correlated with CSF parameters in the PD group but, intriguingly, showed a significant negative correlation with NFL ($r = -0.57$, $p < 0.05$) in MSA. Details of these correlations are provided in Table S3 in Supplementary Material. When we repeated our analyses controlling for age, gender, UPDRS, and disease duration using ANCOVA, significance levels were maintained for NFL but not FLT3L or t-tau, suggesting that NFL levels are robust but FLT3L and t-tau levels may be influenced by other factors that give rise to heterogeneous values.

Validation of the Diagnostic Markers

In the validation cohort, we confirmed higher levels of CSF NFL in MSA (5938 ± 4267 ng/L) compared with PD (1103 ± 442 ng/L; $p < 0.001$) and controls (1290 ± 664 ng/L; $p < 0.001$; Table S4 in Supplementary Material). CSF NFL levels were also significantly higher in other atypical parkinsonsisms (AP; 15 PSP and 5 CBS) than in PD and controls (Table S5 in Supplementary Material). This significance was maintained after controlling for age, gender, and disease duration with AUC $\geq$ 0.9 (Figure S1 in Supplementary Material). FLT3L levels were non-significantly lower in both PD and MSA compared with the controls although a small significant difference between MSA and controls was found after controlling for age, gender, disease duration, and disease severity ($p < 0.05$). As with the discovery group, we also observed higher levels of t-tau in MSA than PD but this failed to reach significance ($p = 0.06$). We noted that t-tau levels in both PD and MSA in the validation groups were overall lower than in the discovery group and for MSA the difference in t-tau levels in discovery (335 ± 164 ng/L) versus validation (244 ± 93 ng/L) was significant ($p < 0.05$). The methodology used to measure t-tau (Innotest ELISAs) was the same for all patients but CSF samples collected prior to 2004 were analyzed retrospectively, which may have influenced our results.

Disease duration was significantly shorter in PD (25.1 months; range 6–84) than MSA (39.0 months; range 12–106) in the validation group, but controlling for this variable using ANCOVA did not alter the significance level for the CSF parameters.

The models developed using the CSF parameters from the discovery group were applied to the validation group and diagnostic values were calculated using cut-offs obtained from the discovery group. We could correctly identify the majority of MSA patients (sensitivity = 80% and specificity = 97%) using NFL alone (AUC = 0.94). Again, ROC curve comparison showed that none of the models significantly improved the discrimination of MSA from PD.

Bootstrapping analysis of the combined data to further validate our result, produced an ROC curve for NFL (PD versus MSA) that was highly comparable with ROC curves from the individual cohorts (AUC = 0.90; sensitivity = 77%; specificity = 96%, cut-off

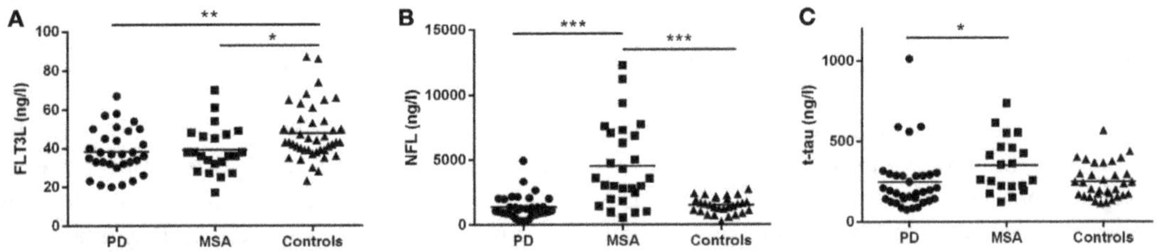

FIGURE 2 | Cerebrospinal fluid concentrations of FLT3L, NFL, and t-tau for the MSA, PD, and control groups: discovery cohort. (A) FLT3L levels are significantly reduced in MSA and PD as compared to controls. NFL **(B)** and t-tau **(C)** concentrations are significantly increased in the MSA group compared with the PD group. MSA, multiple system atrophy; PD, Parkinson's disease; NS, non-significant difference; mean values are indicated by horizontal lines.

TABLE 2 | Comparison of models for discriminating MSA from PD.

CSF variables	Number of patients[a]	Cut-off[b] point	Sensitivity (%)	Specificity (%)	AUC	Youden index[c]	Likelihood ratio[d]
DISCOVERY							
NFL	PD = 36, MSA = 27	>2315	74.1	91.7	0.854	65.7	8.9
Model 1[e]	PD = 34, MSA = 20	>2388	75.0	91.2	0.879	70.6	8.5
Model 2[f]	PD = 31, MSA = 22	>−0. 925	81.8	94.8	0.887	68.9	6.3
Model 3[g]	PD = 29, MSA = 15	>−1.604	94.7	83.3	0.921	78.1	5.7
VALIDATION							
NFL	PD = 32, MSA = 25	>2315	80.0	96.9	0.938	76.9	25.6
Model 1[e]	PD = 32, MSA = 24	>2388	76.1	96.9	0.932	76.1	25.3
Model 2[f]	PD = 32, MSA = 23	>−0. 925	82.6	96.9	0.969	79.5	26.4
Model 3[g]	PD = 32, MSA = 22	>−1.604	81.8	96.9	0.948	75.6	26.2

[a] *Due to missing data points, not all CSF parameters were available in all patients.*
[b] *Cut-off refers to the selected value of the individual biomarker or the combination where the two groups can be separated at the indicated sensitivity and specificity.*
[c] *Youden index: sensitivity + specificity − 100.*
[d] *Likelihood ratio: sensitivity/(1 − specificity).*
[e] *Model 1: y = NFL + 0.15*t-tau.*
[f] *Model 2: y = −1.646 + 0.001*NFL-0.03*FLT3L.*
[g] *Model 3: y = −3.054–0.001*NFL + 0.003*t-tau − 0.028*FLT3L.*

>2174 ng/L). Bootstrapping of the combined FLT3L data revealed significantly lower levels of FLT3L in both the PD and MSA groups compared with controls as was observed in the discovery group but not the validation group. We found no significant differences in CSF FLT3L levels between PD and MSA patients in the individual cohorts nor when using bootstrapping of the combined data.

Discussion

In the current study, we showed that CSF levels of NFL can be used for clinically relevant discrimination of MSA from PD. These results confirm our previous findings using a different method of detection for NFL (14) and the findings of a more recent study using the same ELISA method (12). However, unlike these previous case-control studies, we recruited most of our patients from a prospective study with long clinical follow-up. Higher t-tau levels for MSA patients in this study confirm similar observation in other studies (12, 14, 18) but the contribution of t-tau to the overall discrimination of PD from MSA was not significant. We noted high t-tau values in around 11% of our PD patients and 46% of our MSA patients in the discovery group. However, very few patients in the validation group had high t-tau levels (3% of PD and 8% of MSA). Since the diagnostic value of our previously developed model combining NFL and t-tau (Model 1), did not differ between the discovery and validation groups, this variation probably did not adversely influence our results.

We found significantly decreased CSF FLT3L levels in PD and MSA compared to controls in our discovery cohort but not in the validation cohort. Bootstrapping of the combined data was consistent with the discovery group, revealing significantly lower levels of FLT3L in both PD and MSA compared with controls but we and others (10) found no significant differences in CSF FLT3L levels between PD and MSA. These results contradict an earlier study showing high accuracy discrimination between PD and MSA using FLT3L but we have used a different method of detection for FLT3L than the original paper (7) and our results agree with a more recent study using the same methodology as the original paper (9).

Unlike the first study (7), we did not attempt to exclude patients with possible familial PD, although genetic causes of PD were not identified in our cohorts. Variance could be partly attributable to inclusion of younger PD patients (<50 years in 15/52 PD patients) since we observed a strong correlation between age and FLT3L levels in both PD and controls. After subdivision of PD and MSA for age (i.e., >50 and <50 years), differences between PD and MSA were maintained and we found no differences between young versus old PD or MSA patients (data not shown).

Neurofilament proteins are essential for maintaining the neuronal cytoskeleton and increased levels of NFL in the CSF of

MSA patients likely reflects extensive axonal degeneration. In keeping with earlier findings (12, 14), CSF NFL was increased in MSA and aided discrimination of MSA from PD and, in the current study, NFL alone provided the best tool for discriminating between MSA and PD. The addition of FLT3L and t-tau to NFL analysis improved this discrimination only slightly. However, we observed strong correlations between NFL and FLT3L in PD and controls in both the discovery and validation phases that warrant further investigation to determine the potential function of FLT3L in the central nervous system. The lack of correlation between NFL and FLT3L in the MSA patients suggests that increased levels of NFL were not dependent on changes in FLT3L or vice versa and does not support a role for FLT3L in the pathology of MSA.

FLT3L is a hematopoietic growth factor expressed in various tissues including the brain (24) and has an important role in hematopoietic stem cell survival and proliferation (25). Although FLT3L has a neurotrophic function contributing to increased survival of a subset of post-mitotic neurons (24), its role in neurodegenerative diseases is unknown. In amyotrophic lateral sclerosis (ALS), CSF levels of FLT3L are elevated compared with healthy controls (26). Nerve growth factor (NGF), which normally synergizes with FLT3L to exert its neurotrophic effect, also increases the expression of NFL. Since both NGF and NFL are increased in ALS (27, 28), NGF may contribute to elevated levels of FLT3L and NFL as observed in ALS (27, 29, 30). In PD, levels of NGF are reduced (29) and possibly contribute to observed reductions in CSF FLT3L and NFL levels in some patients. However, contrary to previous observations, CSF FLT3L levels alone do not serve as a biomarker for differentiation of MSA from PD.

A major strength of our study is that diagnosis was made prospectively for the majority of PD and MSA patients using detailed neurological examination in combination with imaging studies, and final diagnosis was confirmed after long follow-up by case review. Our findings emphasize a consistency with other studies (12–14, 31) showing that CSF NFL levels could be a useful adjunct to clinical diagnosis for distinguishing PD from MSA and other atypical parkinsonisms. Since both ours and previous studies have shown significantly increased CSF NFL levels in atypical parkinsonism disorders other than MSA, including PSP and CBS (12, 13, 31), CSF NFL levels do not represent a specific marker for MSA but rather, may be more generally useful for distinguishing PD from atypical parkinsonisms (12, 14). Our results will require confirmation in larger cohorts in future research, with (eventual) pathological confirmation of disease. Further, additional studies will also be required to determine whether NFL levels are influenced by other extraneous influences such as other non-neurological diseases (e.g., cancer) (32, 33) or familial versus sporadic forms of PD, and to determine whether increased NFL levels will be useful for differentiating PD from other APs at early stages of disease.

Following the successful identification of the CSF biomarkers t-tau, p-tau, and Aβ42 that support the clinical diagnosis of Alzheimer's disease, there has been a growing interest in the discovery of similarly specific CSF biomarkers for PD and AP. Many studies have been reported on the quantification of α-synuclein in CSF. Although there is a general consistency that decreased concentrations of this protein are observed in PD and AP with α-synuclein pathology, large overlap between these patient groups and neurological controls has hindered the introduction of its quantification into clinical practice (34, 35). Similarly, a large degree of overlap is seen for levels of oligomeric α-synuclein and lysosomal enzyme levels in PD versus controls (36). Yet another approach, using proteomics discovery in CSF, did not yield a biomarker that could be applied in clinical practice since a panel of a minimum of five proteins was required to differentiate PD from controls at reasonable AUC (0.87) and the AUC of single markers did not exceed 0.79 (37). Therefore, a clinically useful CSF biomarker has not yet been identified for PD. In contrast, however, our study supports the concept that one (NFL) or two (NFL + t-tau) CSF biomarkers may reliably predict AP and PD in a population of patients with parkinsonism at a high AUC (>0.90). This combination of biomarkers also has a better clinical performance than the recently described CSF biomarker UCH-L1 (38), which differentiates PD from AP at an AUC of 0.69. In conclusion, currently the most progress has been made in identifying CSF biomarkers for AP, with NFL, either in combination with t-tau, being the most promising biomarker so far.

Acknowledgments

This study was supported by the following grants: an EU Joint Programme – Neurodegenerative Disease Research (JPND; www.jpnd.eu) project, through funding by the Ministry of Education for Netherlands: ZonMw (The Netherlands Organisation for Health Research and Development); the "Stichting Internationaal Parkinson Fonds"; and the "van Alkemade Keuls fonds." We thank Alexandra Versleijen and other technicians of the Department of Laboratory Medicine for performing the CSF analyses.

Supplementary Material

The Supplementary Material for this article can be found online at http://journal.frontiersin.org/article/10.3389/fneur.2015.00091

References

1. de Lau LM, Breteler MM. Epidemiology of Parkinson's disease. *Lancet Neurol* (2006) **5**(6):525–35. doi:10.1016/S1474-4422(06)70471-9
2. Rodriguez-Oroz MC, Jahanshahi M, Krack P, Litvan I, Macias R, Bezard E, et al. Initial clinical manifestations of Parkinson's disease: features and pathophysiological mechanisms. *Lancet Neurol* (2009) **8**(12):1128–39. doi:10.1016/S1474-4422(09)70293-5
3. Poewe W. Non-motor symptoms in Parkinson's disease. *Eur J Neurol* (2008) **15**:14–20. doi:10.1111/j.1468-1331.2008.02056.x
4. Stefanova N, Bücke P, Duerr S, Wenning GK. Multiple system atrophy: an update. *Lancet Neurol* (2009) **8**(12):1172–8. doi:10.1016/S1474-4422(09)70288-1
5. Schrag A, Geser F, Stampfer-Kountchev M, Seppi K, Sawires M, Köllensperger M, et al. Health-related quality of life in multiple system atrophy. *Mov Disord* (2006) **21**(6):809–15. doi:10.1002/mds.20808

6. Flabeau O, Meissner WG, Tison F. Multiple system atrophy: current and future approaches to management. *Ther Adv Neurol Disord* (2010) **3**(4):249–63. doi:10.1177/1756285610375328
7. Shi M, Movius J, Dator R, Aro P, Zhao Y, Pan C, et al. Cerebrospinal fluid peptides as potential Parkinson disease biomarkers: a staged pipeline for discovery and validation. *Mol Cell Proteomics* (2015) **14**(3):544–55. doi:10.1074/mcp.M114.040576
8. Silajdžić E, Constantinescu R, Holmberg B, Björkqvist M, Hansson O. Flt3 ligand does not differentiate between parkinsonian disorders. *Mov Disord* (2014) **29**(10):1319–22. doi:10.1002/mds.25948
9. Lasec R. Studying the intrinsic determinants of neuronal form and function. In: Lasec RJ, Black MM, editors. *Intrinsic Determinants of Neuronal Form and Function*. New York, NY: Alan R. Liss Inc (1988). p. 1–60.
10. Vandrovcova J, Pittman AM, Malzer E, Abou-Sleiman PM, Lees AJ, Wood NW, et al. Association of MAPT haplotype-tagging SNPs with sporadic Parkinson's disease. *Neurobiol Aging* (2009) **30**(9):1477–82. doi:10.1016/j.neurobiolaging.2007.11.019
11. Bech S, Hjermind LE, Salvesen L, Nielsen JE, Heegaard NH, Jørgensen HL, et al. Amyloid-related biomarkers and axonal damage proteins in parkinsonian syndromes. *Parkinsonism Relat Disord* (2012) **18**(1):69–72. doi:10.1016/j.parkreldis.2011.08.012
12. Hall S, Öhrfelt A, Constantinescu R, Andreasson U, Surova Y, Bostrom F, et al. Accuracy of a panel of 5 cerebrospinal fluid biomarkers in the differential diagnosis of patients with dementia and/or parkinsonian disorders. *Arch Neurol* (2012) **69**(11):1445–52. doi:10.1001/archneurol.2012.1654
13. Constantinescu R, Rosengren L, Johnels B, Zetterberg H, Holmberg B. Consecutive analyses of cerebrospinal fluid axonal and glial markers in Parkinson's disease and atypical parkinsonian disorders. *Parkinsonism Relat Disord* (2010) **16**(2):142–5. doi:10.1016/j.parkreldis.2009.07.007
14. Abdo WF, Bloem BR, Van Geel WJ, Esselink RAJ, Verbeek MM. CSF neurofilament light chain and tau differentiate multiple system atrophy from Parkinson's disease. *Neurobiol Aging* (2007) **28**(5):742–7. doi:10.1016/j.neurobiolaging.2006.03.010
15. Hughes AJ, Daniel SE, Ben-Shlomo Y, Lees AJ. The accuracy of diagnosis of parkinsonian syndromes in a specialist movement disorder service. *Brain* (2002) **125**(4):861–70. doi:10.1093/brain/awf080
16. Gilman S, Wenning GK, Low PA, Brooks DJ, Mathias CJ, Trojanowski JQ, et al. Second consensus statement on the diagnosis of multiple system atrophy. *Neurology* (2008) **71**(9):670–6. doi:10.1212/01.wnl.0000324625.00404.15
17. Aerts MB, Esselink RA, Abdo WF, Meijer FJ, Drost G, Norgren N, et al. Ancillary investigations to diagnose parkinsonism: a prospective clinical study. *J Neurol* (2015) **262**(2):346–56. doi:10.1007/s00415-014-7568-4
18. Abdo WF, van de Warrenburg BP, Kremer HP, Bloem BR, Verbeek MM. CSF biomarker profiles do not differentiate between the cerebellar and parkinsonian phenotypes of multiple system atrophy. *Parkinsonism Relat Disord* (2007) **13**(8):480–2. doi:10.1016/j.parkreldis.2007.02.002
19. Hoehn MM, Yahr MD. Parkinsonism: onset, progression, and mortality. *Neurology* (2001) **57**(10):S11–26.
20. Fahn S, Elton RL. Unified Parkinson's disease rating scale. In: Fahn S, Marsden CD, Calne D, editors. *Recent Developments in Parkinson's Disease*. Florham Park, NJ: MacMillan Healthcare Information (1987). p. 153–63.
21. Trouillas P, Takayanagi T, Hallett M, Currier RD, Subramony SH, Wessel K, et al. International Cooperative Ataxia Rating Scale for pharmacological assessment of the cerebellar syndrome. *J Neurol Sci* (1997) **145**(2):205–11. doi:10.1016/S0022-510X(96)00231-6
22. Litvan I, Agid Y, Calne D, Campbell G, Dubois B, Duvoisin RC, et al. Clinical research criteria for the diagnosis of progressive supranuclear palsy (Steele-Richardson-Olszewski syndrome): report of the NINDS-SPSP International Workshop*. *Neurology* (1996) **47**(1):1–9. doi:10.1212/WNL.47.1.1
23. Boeve BF, Lang AE, Litvan I. Corticobasal degeneration and its relationship to progressive supranuclear palsy and frontotemporal dementia. *Ann Neurol* (2003) **54**(S5):S15–9. doi:10.1002/ana.10570
24. Brazel CY, Ducceschi MH, Pytowski B, Levison SW. The FLT3 tyrosine kinase receptor inhibits neural stem/progenitor cell proliferation and collaborates with NGF to promote neuronal survival. *Mol Cell Neurosci* (2001) **18**(4):381–93. doi:10.1006/mcne.2001.1033
25. Shurin MR, Esche C, Lotze MT. FLT3: receptor and ligand. Biology and potential clinical application. *Cytokine Growth Factor Rev* (1998) **9**(1):37–48. doi:10.1016/S1359-6101(97)00035-X
26. Iłzecka J. Cerebrospinal fluid Flt3 ligand level in patients with amyotrophic lateral sclerosis. *Acta Neurol Scand* (2006) **114**(3):205–9. doi:10.1111/j.1600-0404.2006.00704.x
27. Casaccia-Bonnefil P, Carter BD, Dobrowsky RT, Chao MV. Death of oligodendrocytes mediated by the interaction of nerve growth factor with its receptor p75. *Nature* (1996) **383**(6602):716–9. doi:10.1038/383716a0
28. Mutoh T, Tokuda A, Miyadai T, Hamaguchi M, Fujiki N. Ganglioside GM1 binds to the Trk protein and regulates receptor function. *Proc Natl Acad Sci U S A* (1995) **92**(11):5087–91. doi:10.1073/pnas.92.11.5087
29. Chaturvedi RK, Shukla S, Seth K, Agrawal AK. Nerve growth factor increases survival of dopaminergic graft, rescue nigral dopaminergic neurons and restores functional deficits in rat model of Parkinson's disease. *Neurosci Lett* (2006) **398**(1–2):44–9. doi:10.1016/j.neulet.2005.12.042
30. Reijn T, Abdo W, Schelhaas H, Verbeek M. CSF neurofilament protein analysis in the differential diagnosis of ALS. *J Neurol* (2009) **256**(4):615–9. doi:10.1007/s00415-009-0131-z
31. Holmberg B, Johnels B, Ingvarsson P, Eriksson B, Rosengren L. CSF-neurofilament and levodopa tests combined with discriminant analysis may contribute to the differential diagnosis of parkinsonian syndromes. *Parkinsonism Relat Disord* (2001) **8**(1):23–31. doi:10.1016/S1353-8020(00)00083-3
32. Li X-Q, Li L, Xiao C-H, Feng Y-M. NEFL mRNA expression level is a prognostic factor for early-stage breast cancer patients. *PLoS One* (2012) **7**(2):e31146. doi:10.1371/journal.pone.0031146
33. Emi M, Fujiwara Y, Nakajima T, Tsuchiya E, Tsuda H, Hirohashi S, et al. Frequent loss of heterozygosity for loci on chromosome 8p in hepatocellular carcinoma, colorectal cancer, and lung cancer. *Cancer Res* (1992) **52**(19):5368–72.
34. Parnetti L, Castrioto A, Chiasserini D, Persichetti E, Tambasco N, El-Agnaf O, et al. Cerebrospinal fluid biomarkers in Parkinson disease. *Nat Rev Neurol* (2013) **9**(3):131–40. doi:10.1038/nrneurol.2013.10
35. Kang J, Irwin DJ, Chen-Plotkin AS, Siderowf A, Caspell C, Coffey CS, et al. Association of cerebrospinal fluid β-amyloid 1-42, t-tau, p-tau181, and α-synuclein levels with clinical features of drug-naive patients with early parkinson disease. *JAMA Neurol* (2013) **70**(10):1277–87. doi:10.1001/jamaneurol.2013.3861
36. Parnetti L, Chiasserini D, Persichetti E, Eusebi P, Varghese S, Qureshi MM, et al. Cerebrospinal fluid lysosomal enzymes and alpha-synuclein in Parkinson's disease. *Mov Disord* (2014) **29**(8):1019–27. doi:10.1002/mds.25772
37. Shi M, Bradner J, Hancock AM, Chung KA, Quinn JF, Peskind ER, et al. Cerebrospinal fluid biomarkers for Parkinson disease diagnosis and progression. *Ann Neurol* (2011) **69**(3):570–80. doi:10.1002/ana.22311
38. Mondello S, Constantinescu R, Zetterberg H, Andreasson U, Holmberg B, Jeromin A. CSF α-synuclein and UCH-L1 levels in Parkinson's disease and atypical parkinsonian disorders. *Parkinsonism Relat Disord* (2014) **20**(4):382–7. doi:10.1016/j.parkreldis.2014.01.011

4

Differential roles of environmental enrichment in Alzheimer's type of neurodegeneration and physiological aging

*Vladimir V. Salmin[1], Yulia K. Komleva[2,3], Natalia V. Kuvacheva[2,3], Andrey V. Morgun[4], Elena D. Khilazheva[2,3], Olga L. Lopatina[2,3], Elena A. Pozhilenkova[2,3], Konstantin A. Shapovalov[1], Yulia A. Uspenskaya[3] and Alla B. Salmina[2,3]**

[1] Department of Medical and Biological Physics, Krasnoyarsk State Medical University named after Prof. V.F. Voino-Yasenetsky, Krasnoyarsk, Russia, [2] Department of Biochemistry, Medical, Pharmaceutical and Toxicological Chemistry, Krasnoyarsk State Medical University named after Prof. V.F. Voino-Yasenetsky, Krasnoyarsk, Russia, [3] Research Institute of Molecular Medicine and Pathobiochemistry, Krasnoyarsk State Medical University named after Prof. V.F. Voino-Yasenetsky, Krasnoyarsk, Russia, [4] Department of Pediatrics, Krasnoyarsk State Medical University named after Prof. V.F. Voino-Yasenetsky, Krasnoyarsk, Russia

Edited by:
Athanasios Alexiou,
Novel Global Community Educational Foundation (NGCEF), Hebersham, Australia

Reviewed by:
Daniel Ortuño-Sahagún,
Centro Universitario de Ciencias de la Salud, Mexico
Maik Gollasch,
Charité Universitätsmedizin Berlin, Germany

****Correspondence:***
Alla B. Salmina
allasalmina@mail.ru

Impairment of hippocampal adult neurogenesis in aging or degenerating brain is a well-known phenomenon caused by the shortage of brain stem cell pool, alterations in the local microenvironment within the neurogenic niches, or deregulation of stem cell development. Environmental enrichment (EE) has been proposed as a potent tool to restore brain functions, to prevent aging-associated neurodegeneration, and to cure neuronal deficits seen in neurodevelopmental and neurodegenerative disorders. Here, we report our data on the effects of environmental enrichment on hippocampal neurogenesis *in vivo* and neurosphere-forming capacity of hippocampal stem/progenitor cells *in vitro.* Two models – Alzheimer's type of neurodegeneration and physiological brain aging – were chosen for the comparative analysis of EE effects. We found that environmental enrichment greatly affects the expression of markers specific for stem cells, progenitor cells and differentiated neurons (Pax6, Ngn2, NeuroD1, NeuN) in the hippocampus of young adult rats or rats with Alzheimer's disease (AD) model but less efficiently in aged animals. Application of time-lag mathematical model for the analysis of impedance traces obtained in real-time monitoring of cell proliferation *in vitro* revealed that EE could restore neurosphere-forming capacity of hippocampal stem/progenitor cells more efficiently in young adult animals (fourfold greater in the control group comparing to the AD model group) but not in the aged rats (no positive effect of environmental enrichment at all). In accordance with the results obtained *in vivo*, EE was almost ineffective in the recovery of hippocampal neurogenic reserve *in vitro* in aged, but not in amyloid-treated or young adult, rats. Therefore, EE-based neuroprotective strategies effective in Aβ-affected brain could not be directly extrapolated to aged brain.

Keywords: environmental enrichment, neurogenesis, neurosphere, Alzheimer's disease, aging, time-lag model

INTRODUCTION

Environmental enrichment (EE) is considered as an environment with numerous sensorimotor, cognitive, and social stimulations able to affect brain plasticity, to restore brain functional reserves, and to facilitate establishment of novel connections actual for preventive or rehabilitation strategies. Modeling EE is currently widely used in experiments aimed to study synaptogenesis, neurogenesis, and brain connectivity (Komleva Iu et al., 2013). EE stimulates neurogenesis and synapse turnover, integration of newly-formed cells into neuronal ensembles, modifies epigenetic mechanisms controlling resistance to oxidative stress, modulates production of neurotransmitters and molecules with neurotrophic activity, prevents apoptosis, suppresses neuroinflammation, affects neuron-glia interactions, thereby enhancing cognition, learning, and social communications in animals or humans with or without brain pathology (Herring et al., 2011; Cotel et al., 2012; Komleva Iu et al., 2013; Leger et al., 2015; Grinan-Ferre et al., 2016; Stuart et al., 2017). These effects well-correspond to those observed in people practicing so-called cognitive training because of their professional duties or personal habits and demonstrating good preservation of cognitive functions even at the eldest period of life (Mora, 2013). However, action of EE depends on experimental conditions, duration of exposure, severity of brain injury, age, gender etc., thereby, the observed effects of EE on neuroplasticity might be different and even unexpected (Ming and Song, 2011; Valero-Aracama et al., 2015).

Growing number of experimental and clinical findings suggest that EE might serve as an effective strategy to restore the functional capacity of damaged brain, i.e., in Alzheimer's disease (AD), in neurodevelopmental disorders, after stroke, etc. (Janssen et al., 2014; Polito et al., 2014; Cioni et al., 2016; Rosbergen et al., 2016). Particularly, prevention or treatment of Alzheimer-type neurodegeneration is one of the most challenging questions in the modern neuroscience which is directly linked to the controlled modulation of hippocampal plasticity (Balietti et al., 2012) In such context, EE provides a lot of premises for its effective application: prevention of hippocampal astroglial dysfunction in the AD transgenic mice (Rodriguez et al., 2013), up-regulation of brain-derived growth factor expression in the hippocampus of senescence-accelerated prone mice (Yuan et al., 2012), prevention of amyloid β (Aβ) deposition and memory impairment in AD model mice (Maesako et al., 2012), modulation of hippocampal synaptic proteins expression (Barak et al., 2013).

In contrast, EE action in aging brain is not deciphered in detail, even aging itself is the certain risk for AD development (Avila et al., 2010). Moreover, precise molecular mechanisms of EE effects on neuroplasticity in aged or AD brain remain to be unclear or even contradictory (Herring et al., 2011; Cotel et al., 2012; Bezzina et al., 2015; Huttenrauch et al., 2016). Impairment of hippocampal adult neurogenesis in aging is a well-known phenomenon caused by the shortage of brain stem cell pool, alterations in the local microenvironment within the neurogenic niches, or deregulation of stem cell development (Ali et al., 2015; Moraga et al., 2015). It is well-known that there is an obvious contrast between Alzheimer-type neurodegeneration and physiological aging, however, both of them are associated with progressive cognitive deficits and impairment of brain plasticity. Healthy aging brain is characterized by moderate decline in neurogenesis affecting the structure and function of the entorhinal-hippocampal circuit which is in the focus of neurodegeneration seen in AD due to the toxic action of Aβ, oxidative stress, excitotoxicity, and neuroinflammation (Hollands et al., 2016). In physiologically aging brain, no significant changes in the number of neural stem cells (NSCs) residing within the hippocampal neurogenic niche have been detected (Hattiangady and Shetty, 2008). In contrast, gradual decrease of NSCs and neural progenitor cells (NPCs) number has been reported in the experimental APP/PS1/nestin-GFP triple transgenic mouse model of AD (Zeng et al., 2016). Thus, the earliest stages of adult neurogenesis (stem cell maintenance, self-renewal, and proliferation) are significantly affected in AD neurodegeneration but not in healthy aging. Since enhancing neurogenesis was proposed as a therapeutic approach in neurodegeneration (Hollands et al., 2016), one may assume that EE could produce different effects on aging-associated and AD-compromised hippocampal neurogenesis. Despite several experimental and clinical observations on EE action in elderly subjects with or without AD, little information is available on the comparative efficacy of EE in AD and healthy aging.

So, whether EE-induced changes are equally beneficial in aging brain and in AD? The subject has received increased attention with the deciphering the biological mechanisms of late-life brain alterations: reduced neurogenesis and synapse turnover (Mostany et al., 2013), suppressed release of neuropeptides and neurotrophic factors (Forlenza et al., 2015), appearance of white matter lesions and pathological blood–brain barrier permeability (Marin-Padilla and Knopman, 2011; Firbank et al., 2012). Several studies suggest that EE affects epigenetic mechanisms controlling neuroplasticity, promotes remyelination, or reduces glia-supported neuroinflammation in the neurogenic niches in the aged brain (Williamson et al., 2012; Yang et al., 2012; Neidl et al., 2016). However, alterations in neurogenesis and the capacity of so-called "neurogenic reserve" may have different patterns and degree of progression in normal aging and in AD (Esiri and Chance, 2012).

Assessment of neurogenesis represents an appropriate system to analyze the activity of factors with presumptive neuroprotective properties. *In vivo*, neurogenesis can be studied with the approach based on the detection of markers expression in cells at different stages of development within the neurogenic niches or along their migratory paths in the brain (Roybon et al., 2009). Apart from this, some neurogenesis-associated events are easily reproduced *in vitro* due to ability of neurogenic non-differentiated cells to produce non-adherent spherical clusters of cells known as neurospheres (NS). NS-forming capacity is a parameter which is widely used for the assessment of neurogenic potential of neural stem/progenitor cells as well as the action of regulatory molecules, neurotoxic substances, or drug candidates (Pacey et al., 2006). Positive effects of EE on neurogenesis *in vivo* have been shown (Monteiro et al., 2014; Clemenson et al., 2015), however, there are very limited data on NS development *in vitro* in AD or aging (Heo et al., 2007; Diaz-Moreno et al., 2013).

Recently, we have demonstrated EE-mediated enhancement of neurosphere-forming capacity of NSCs obtained from the brains of AD rat model (Kuvacheva et al., 2015). It should be mentioned that analysis of data obtained with NS culture systems is hampered by the relative shortage of tools for adequate interpretation within the context of cell cycle- and proliferation-related events. Modeling the cell growth kinetics has been in the focus of researchers for a long time (Baker et al., 1998), but mathematic analysis of kinetic features of stem cells behavior in several subsequent NS generations *in vitro* was undertaken in few studies only (Ma et al., 2007). Development of correct mathematical models of NS establishment in the short-term experimental conditions (when reduction of cell population due to cell death might be contingently neglected) would provide new opportunities for rapid and effective analysis of endogenous and exogenous stimuli targeting neurogenesis. Moreover, current achievements in the application of NS cultures for AD modeling *in vitro* (Choi et al., 2013; Ghate et al., 2014) or novel attempts to restore brain functions with NSCs transplantation therapy (Waldau and Shetty, 2008) determine the needs in the appropriate mathematical modeling of NS-generation *in vitro* to clarify mechanisms underlying neurogenesis modulation in a given microenvironment.

Thus, we may entertain the hypothesis that: (i) effects of EE on neurogenesis are different in healthy brain aging and in brain affected by Alzheimer's type of neurodegeneration; (ii) combination of *in vivo* and *in vitro* approaches to the assessment of neurogenesis with the mathematical modeling of neurogenic reserve could help us to identify the neurogenesis stage which is a main "target" for the action of EE in normal and damaged brain. Therefore, the goal of this study was to compare the effects of *in vivo* EE in the Alzheimer's type of neurodegeneration and physiological brain aging with the special focus on hippocampal neurogenesis *in vivo* and NS-forming capacity of hippocampal stem/progenitor cells *in vitro*.

Experimental Procedures

Modeling Environmental Enrichment *In Vivo*

Wistar male rats ($n = 64$) were maintained in standard cages with water and standard diet with free access to food and water. The following groups of animals were included in the experiment: (i) young adult rats, 7–9 months old ($n = 40$) kept under standard conditions (SC, $n = 20$) or in the environmental enrichment (EE, $n = 20$); (ii) elderly rats, 23–25 months old ($n = 24$) kept under SC or in the EE. In SC, rats were housing in the cages sized 50 cm × 30 cm × 18 cm (five animals in one cage). In EE, rats were housing for 60 days in cages sized 78 cm × 48 cm × 39 cm (10 animals in one cage) equipped with various devices to provide extensive physical and explanatory activity (tunnels, houses, hammocks, stairs, boxes, wheels) (Jankowsky et al., 2003).

Modeling Alzheimer-Type Neurodegeneration

In the group of young adult rats, 10 animals kept under SC and 10 animals kept in EE have been used for modeling AD with intracerebral bilateral stereotaxic-guided (Narishige Scientific Instrument Lab) injections of 5 μl (2 μg/μl) aggregated Aβ1-42 (Sigma-Aldrich) into CA1 zones of hippocampus at the day 60 of SC or EE housing according to the protocol described (Li et al., 2011). For this procedure, anesthesia with chloral hydrate (0.35 g/kg) has been applied, and the following stereotaxic coordinates have been chosen: A/P = 3.0 mm, M/L = ± 2.2 mm, D/V = 2.8 mm. Establishment of AD model (Aβ deposition and cognitive impairment) has been confirmed with Thioflavin S staining of brain tissue and neurobehavioral phenotyping of animals (data not shown).

Assessment of Hippocampal Neurogenesis

Expression of markers in NSCs, progenitor cells and differentiated neurons (Pax6, Neurogenin 2, NeuroD1, NeuN) was assessed in the hippocampus of animals in all experimental groups according to the standard protocol of immunohistochemistry with antigen unmasking (proteinase K) procedure. Briefly, 2 μm hippocampal slices were obtained after transcardial perfusion of anesthesized rats with 0.1 M PBS (pH 7.4) and 4% PFA followed by hippocampus fixation in 10% buffered PFA for 24 h. The following primary antibodies have been used: Pax-6 (Abcam, ab78545, mouse monoclonal), 1:100, Neurogenin2 (Abcam, ab26190, rabbit polyclonal), 1:50, NeuroD1 (Abcam, ab60704, mouse monoclonal), 1:100, NeuN (Millipore, ABN78, rabbit polyclonal), 1:500. Alexa-conjugated secondary antibodies were used in 1:500 dilution: Alexa Fluor 488 chicken anti-mouse (for Pax6 detection), Alexa Fluor 488 donkey anti-rabbit (for Neurogenin2 detection), NeuN (rabbit polyclonal) – Alexa Fluor 488 donkey anti-rabbit (for NeuroD1 detection), and Alexa Fluor 488 chicken anti-rabbit (for NeuN detection) on slices. Images were visualized with Olympus CX41 microscope and analyzed with Image J software. Corrected total cell fluorescence (CTCF) was calculated for all the images.

Isolation of Adult Hippocampal Cells with the NS-Forming Capacity

At the day 70 of housing (10 days after AD modeling in the corresponding group of animals), isolation of hippocampus was performed in anesthesized rats according to the standard protocol described (Kuvacheva et al., 2015). After brain tissue dissociation and isolation of hippocampal cells, counting of the cells for further adjusting the viable cell concentrations was done with the Scepter CellCounter (Millipore). Assessment of proliferation of obtained hippocampal cells *in vitro* has been performed by culturing them in NeuroCult®NS-A Proliferation Medium with bFGF and EGF (Stemcell). On the next day after cell plating, development of neurospheres as transparent free-floating cell aggregates with surface microspikes was assessed with phase-contrast microscopy. At the day 3 of NS culture, cells were carefully harvested from the flasks, centrifuged, and suspended in the fresh NeuroCult®NS-A Proliferation Medium.

Real-Time Analysis of Cell Proliferation *In Vitro*

Further real-time analysis of cell proliferation kinetics was done using xCElligence system (Roche) with the gold microelectrode-covered microtiter plates. This method allows electrical impedance monitoring in the real-time manner. For this,

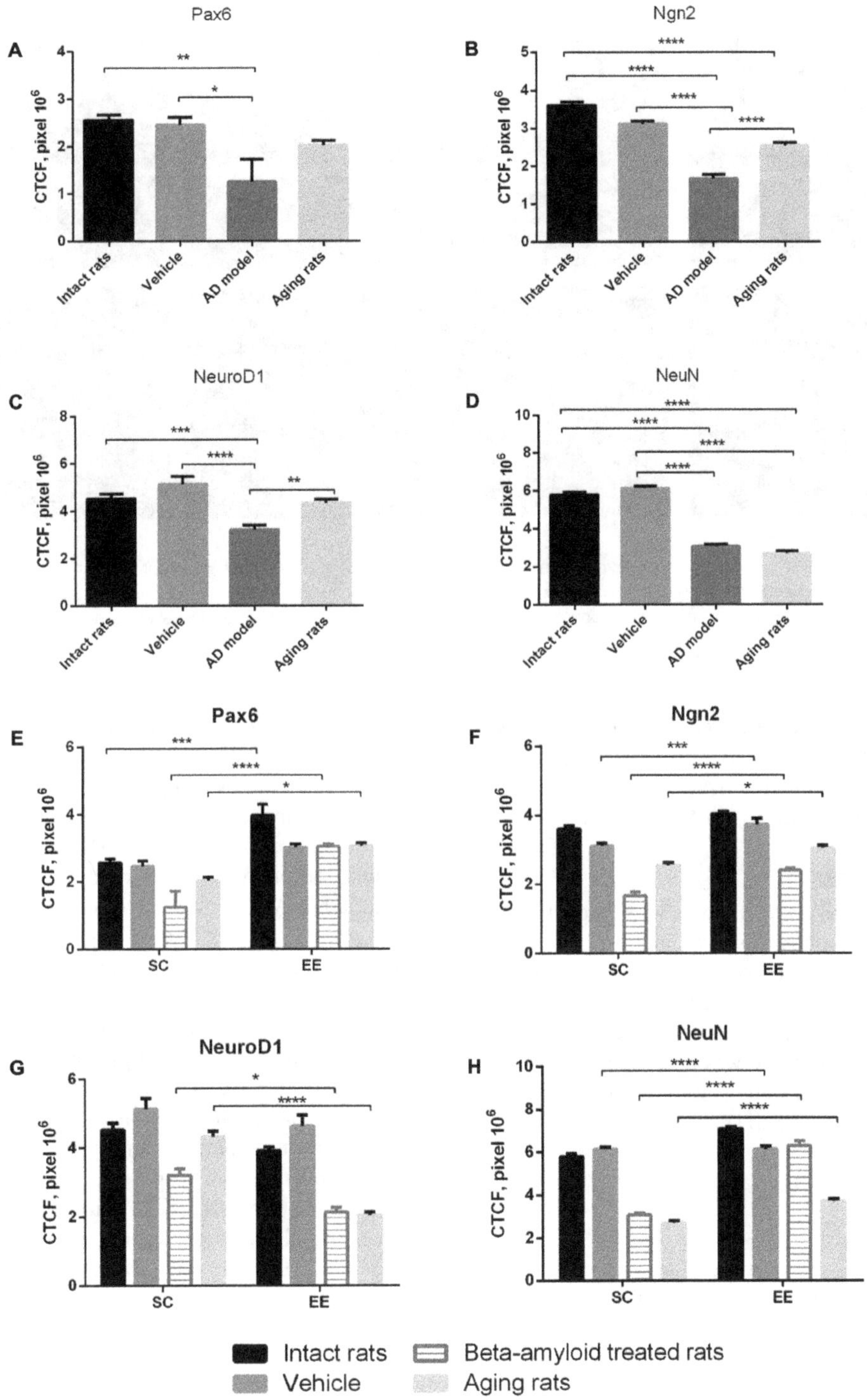

FIGURE 1 | Neurogenesis in the subgranular and granular layers of the dentate gyrus in experimental groups (intact rats, vehicle – sham-operated rats, AD model – Aβ-treated rats, aging rats, SC – standard conditions, EE – environmental enrichment). **(A–D)** Measurement of the CTCF index of different neurogenesis markers between groups under standards conditions (*N* = 10/per group, one-way ANOVA; Turkey's multiple comparisons test was run between groups). **(A)** Pax6 CTCF index ($p < 0.01$; one-way ANOVA). **(B)** Ngn2 CTCF index ($p < 0.0001$; one-way ANOVA). **(C)** NeuroD1 CTCF index ($p < 0.0001$; one-way ANOVA). **(D)** NeuN CTCF index ($p < 0.0001$; one-way ANOVA). Asterisks indicate statistical differences between groups. *$p < 0.05$; **$p < 0.01$; ***$p < 0.001$; ****$p < 0.0001$. **(E–H)** Measurement of the CTCF index of different neurogenesis markers between groups under standards conditions compared to environmental enrichment (*N* = 10/per group, statistical significance was determined by two-way ANOVA with a Sidak's test multiple comparisons test). **(E)** Pax6 CTCF index [Interaction $p < 0.05$, $F(3,72) = 2.573$, two-way ANOVA]. **(F)** Ngn2 CTCF index [Interaction ns; environmental factor $p < 0.0001$, $F(1,72) = 68.85$, group factor $p < 0.0001$, $F(3,72) = 130.7$, two-way ANOVA]. **(G)** NeuroD1 CTCF index [Interaction $p = 0.0001$, $F(3,72) = 7.91$, two-way ANOVA]. **(H)** NeuN CTCF index [Interaction $p < 0.0001$, $F(3,72) = 47.92$, two-way ANOVA]. Asterisks indicate statistical differences between groups. *$p < 0.05$; ***$p < 0.001$; ****$p < 0.0001$.

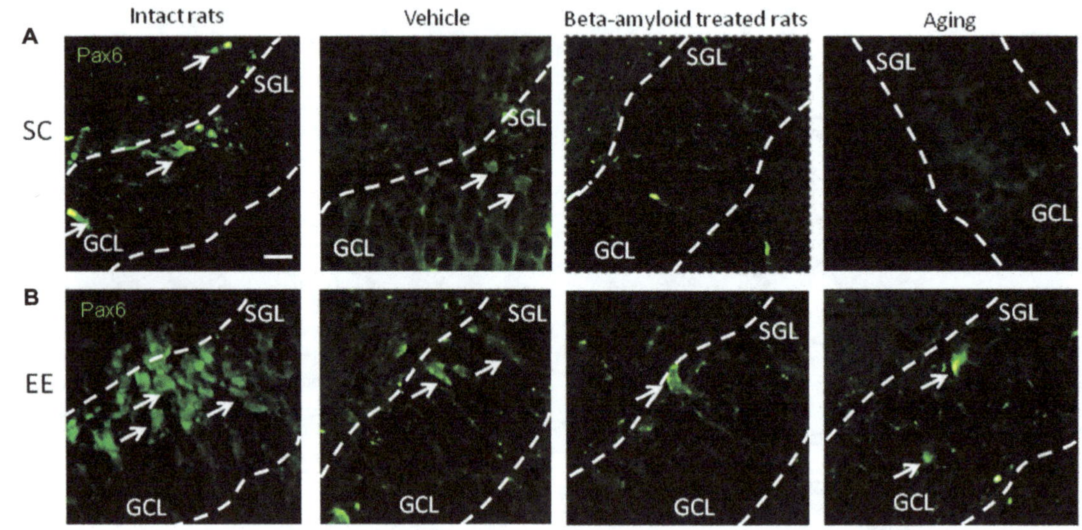

FIGURE 2 | Immunohistochemical (IHC) detection of Pax6 expression in intact, vehicle-, Aβ-treated, and aged rats kept under standard conditions (SC) **(A)** and environmental enrichment (EE) **(B)**. Representative photomicrographs show Pax6 immunostaining in the granular cell layer (GCL) and subgranular layer (SGL) of dentate gyrus. Pax6 was visualized using primary anti-Pax6 monoclonal antibody and secondary chicken anti-mouse IgG conjugated with green fluorescent dye Alexa Fluor 488.

1.2–2.5 × 10^4 cells/ml were cultured in NeuroCult®NS-A Proliferation Medium (100 μl per well, four wells for each series) at +37°C, 5% CO_2 with the measurements intervals of 5 min (from time 0 to 4.5 h) and 15 min (from 4.5 to 24 h).

Statistical Analysis

Non-linear regression analysis was done with the Origin 8.5 software (OriginLab). We applied user-defined function models. All regression models indicate the confidence coefficient χ^2 not worsen than 10^{-4}, and determination coefficient R^2 not less than 0.99. Statistical analysis was performed with the GraphPad Prism 6.0 software. Statistical significance was determined by one-way or two-way ANOVA with a Sidak's test multiple comparisons test. The data are presented as mean and standard deviation.

RESULTS

Immunohistochemical analysis of molecular markers expression in cells at different stages of neurogenesis (Pax6, Neurogenin 2, NeuroD1, NeuN) in the hippocampus revealed that their levels were dramatically affected in Aβ-treated rats and in the group of aging animals (**Figures 1A–D**). Noteworthy, EE did not affect the expression of the markers in the hippocampus of intact or sham-operated rats. EE demonstrated pronounced restorative effect on the impaired neurogenesis in the animals with AD model comparing with the elderly rats (**Figures 1E–H**). Among all the markers, most prominent changes were observed in the expression of NeuroD1 (reduction in all the tested animals subjected to EE).

Expression of Pax6 was efficiently restored by EE in all the groups tested (**Figure 2**). It is well-known that Pax6 is a transcription factor controlling proliferation of multipotent stem/progenitor cells in hippocampus and cortex being predominantly expressed by radial glia. High expression of Pax6 is usually followed by the elevated expression of Neurogenin 2 in amplifying unipotent progenitors, which is later replaced with the expression of NeuroD1 in neuronally committed cells of hippocampus where it is required for their survival (Roybon et al., 2009). At the final stage of neurogenesis, mature neurons in the granule zone of hippocampus are highly enriched in NeuN with the evident elevation in animals kept in EE, particularly in those having AD-type of neurodegeneration (**Figure 3**).

To analyze plausible mechanisms of the observed effect of EE at the initial stage of hippocampal adult neurogenesis, we further used the experimental model suitable for the assessing the kinetic parameters of cell proliferation *in vitro*. Evaluation of NS-forming capacity of hippocampal stem/progenitor cells is rather reliable tool to get the integral pattern of neurogenic cells proliferation and differentiation in the controlled conditions where cell cluster formation and development resemble the events occurring *in vivo* (Malik et al., 2015), particularly at the earliest steps of neurogenesis that were more sensitive to the action of EE *in vivo* (as shown above). We found that being cultured *in vitro*, adult hippocampal stem/progenitor cells produce NS whose appearance could be detected and analyzed with real-time impedance measurements. Recently, we have presented actual impedance traces for NS obtained from the animals with AD model kept under SC or EE (Kuvacheva et al., 2015). For analyzing the kinetic parameters of cell proliferation we applied several assumptions shown below.

Cell index (C) which is the impedance value corresponds to the number of adherent cells, therefore, cell sedimentation leads to the elevation of cell index. If the medium viscosity is not changed, then cell sedimentation to the microplate bottom

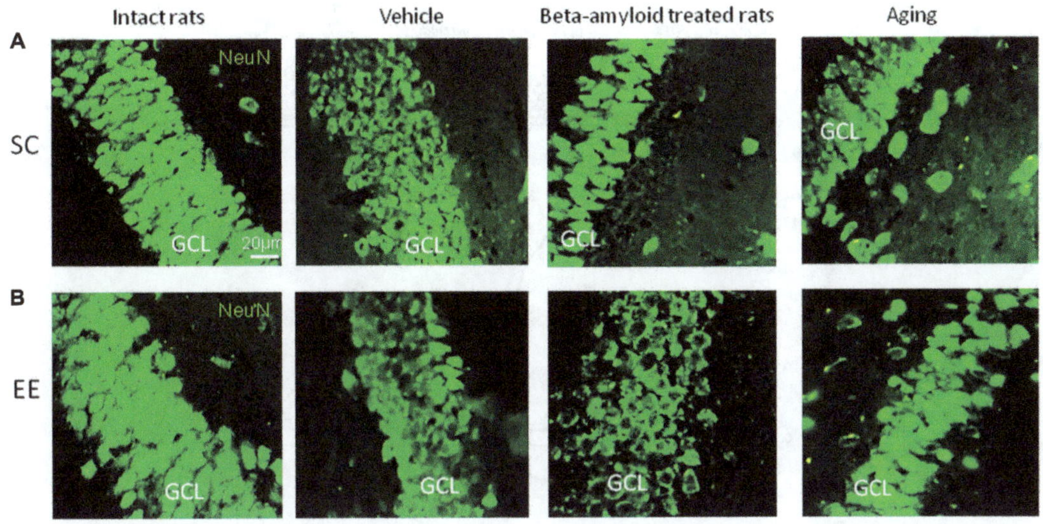

FIGURE 3 | Immunohistochemical (IHC) detection of NeuN expression in intact, vehicle-, Aβ-treated, and aged rats kept under standard conditions (SC) **(A)** and environmental enrichment (EE) **(B)**. Representative photomicrographs show NeuN immunostaining in the granular cell layer (GCL) of dentate gyrus. NeuN was visualized using primary anti-NeuN antibody and secondary donkey anti-rabbit IgG conjugated with green fluorescent dye Alexa Fluor 488.

demonstrates constant velocity, and C is progressively rising at the initial phase of cell culture with the linear dependence on the time:

$$C = \eta t + C_0.$$

Constant parameter η characterizes velocity of cell sedimentation, C_0 is the cell index obtained for the adherent cells at the initial point of measurements. The described process corresponds to the phase A (attachment of cells to the plate). Let assume that cells might be at any phase of cell cycle at this period. Phase I_1 of the impedance trace corresponds to the period after the complete cell adhesion (interphase of the cell cycle) when maximal value of cell index (C_{max}) is not changed. It is well-known that just before mitosis cell adhesion is weakened, and flattened cells acquire round shape (VanHook, 2014), therefore formation of NS leads to decrease of C value. This process corresponds to the mitotic phase M_1. Phase I_2 (interphase) demonstrates stable C value established just before entering mitosis in the 2nd generation of cells. This period is followed by reducing cell adhesion in the 2nd cell generation which corresponds to the mitotic phase M_2 (**Figure 4A**).

Thus, we postulate that in the given experimental conditions: (i) cell proliferation is synchronized; (ii) mitosis-associated loss of cell adhesion leads to C decline; (iii) two generations of cells are present in the system during 24 h of cell culture on microelectrode-covered microplates.

To exclude the impact of cell sedimentation velocity on C kinetics, lets adopt the cell index value as $C{=}C_{max}$ at the initial phase A. We may use the parameter shown below to take into account all the changes in C caused by the decreasing number of adherent cells:

$$C_N = C_{max} - C$$

Normalization of cell index changes (c_N) allows considering some deviations in cell concentrations in the microplate wells:

$$c_N = \frac{C_N}{C_{N\,max}}$$

Typical curve for c_N kinetics is shown in **Figure 4B**.

In order to analyze the observed changes in c_N, we may apply a lag model developed for explaining the proliferative kinetics of cell population with the synchronized growth (Baker et al., 1998). For this purpose we must use bell-shaped distribution of cells along the different phases of cell cycle. Let's propose that the probability of cell detachment out of microelectrode caused by alterations in adhesion mechanisms would have Boltzmann's distribution of time, whereas normalized changes in c_N value could be covered by the following equation:

$$c_N = c_0 + \frac{A_1}{1 + \exp\left(\frac{t_C - t}{t_M}\right)},$$

where c_0 – value of normalized changes of cell index at the initial point of measurements $t = 0$, A_1 – amplitude of normalized changes of cell index at the point of completing the 1st cycle of proliferation, t_c – duration of cell cycle, t_M – duration of phase M_1 (**Figure 2B**), presumably, corresponding to the duration of mitotic phase in the synchronously proliferating cell population.

The equation given above does not account for any time delay between the cell cycle initiation and beginning of cell index changes. To do this we will introduce another parameter – time-lag t_L, and we will consider a shift from the half-time of mitotic phase duration in the previous cell division (before the

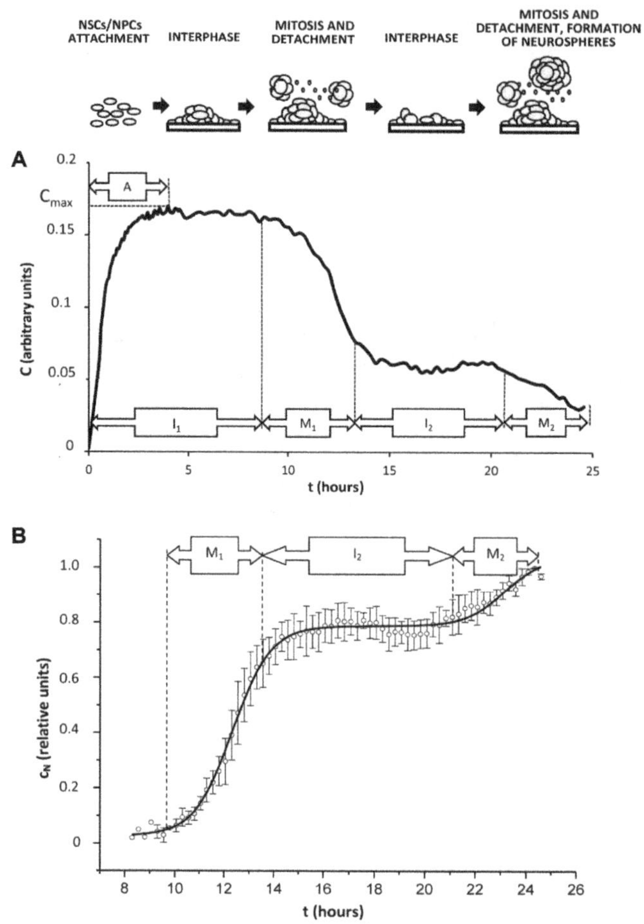

FIGURE 4 | Typical kinetics of cell index in the conditions promoting generation of neurospheres *in vitro*. Cells (NSCs, NPCs) isolated from rat hippocampus were plated in the microelectrode-covered plates of xCELLigence system for impedance measurements as described in Section "Experimental Procedures." Time of incubation is shown as t, hours. **(A)** A representative curve of cell index kinetics (indicated as C, arbitrary units) reflects real impedance trace obtained from the xCELLigence system during 24 h of cell culture. Cell index kinetics corresponds to changes in the number of attached cells during cell cycle progression. A – attachment phase, $I_{1,2}$ – interphase of 1st or 2nd cell cycle (interphasic cells attach to the microelectrode-covered plate), $M_{1,2}$ – mitosis in the 1st or 2nd cell cycle (mitotic cells detach from the microelectrode-covered plate). Corresponding changes in the cell culture are shown schematically at the top of the figure.
(B) Normalized and approximated cell index (indicated as c_n, relative units) was calculated from the real cell index C as shown in Section "Results," and relates to the number of detached cells. Solid curve corresponds to the best regression model.

measurements). Then, the equation covering cell index changes due to 1st mitosis would be as follows:

$$c_N = c_0 + \frac{A_1}{1 + \exp\left(\frac{t_C - t_L - 0.5t_M - t}{t_M}\right)}$$

Second mitosis will be accounted by introducing the second summand:

$$c_N = c_0 + \frac{A_1}{1 + \exp\left(\frac{t_C - t_L - 0.5t_M - t}{t_M}\right)} + \frac{A_2}{1 + \exp\left(\frac{2 * t_C - t_L - 0.5t_M - t}{t_M}\right)}$$

We have used this equation for non-linear regression analysis of experimental data. **Figure 4B** shows regression solid curve corresponding to the applied model for the cells isolated from young adult rats exposed to EE.

At the first round of regression analysis, we determined the mean value of cell cycle duration t_C with kinetic curves for the normalized changes of cell index for the groups of cells with the well-identified phase of 2nd division. This group included data obtained from EE-treated rats as well as from aged rats housed in SC. Then, the obtained value of cell cycle duration for all the cell types was as follows:

$$t_C = 10.8 \pm 2.5 \text{ hr}.$$

At the second round of regression analysis, we fixed the cell cycle duration t_C, and values of t_M have been estimated for all the cell types. The data obtained for the duration of "mitotic phase" t_M are presented in **Table 1**.

Supposing t_M duration as a time of cell cycle "mismatch" in the synchronously proliferating population, we may assume that when the number of cell generations is $N_g = \frac{t_C}{t_M}$ full

TABLE 1 | Parameters of NS-forming capacity of hippocampal progenitors in rats with the Alzheimer-type neurodegeneration (AD) or physiological aging housed in the standard conditions (SC) or in the environmental enrichment (EE).

Experimental group	t_M *(hours)*	*Ng*	*Nc*	*K*
Young adult rats (SC)	1.23 ± 0.07	9	512	
Young adult rats (EE)	0.77 ± 0.03	14	16,384	32
AD model rats (SC)	2.23 ± 0.07	5	32	
AD model rats (EE)	1.42 ± 0.05	8	256	8
Elderly rats (SC)	1.66 ± 0.06	7	128	
Elderly rats (EE)	1.57 ± 0.08	7	128	1

t_M – duration of mitotic phase M.
N_g – number of cell generations produced before full desynchronization of cell growth.
N_c – maximal cluster size obtained before full desynchronization of cell growth.
K – coefficient of cluster size enlargement due to effect of EE.

desynchronization would happen, thereby affecting cells microenvironment and their proliferative capacity. Under the given experimental conditions, desynchronization is most obvious in the cell culture obtained from the group of elderly rats.

Supposing doubling of cell number in every next cell generation, we may adopt that maximal cluster size (number of cells in an aggregate) which might be formed before full desynchronization of cell cycle in the culture is:

$$N_C = 2^{N_g}$$

Therefore, maximal cluster size Nc should be interpreted as neurosphere-forming capacity. It is clearly shown (**Table 1**) that it is dramatically reduced in the elderly rats and – even more visibly – in the rats with AD-type of neurodegeneration. Since NS-forming ability marks the general neurogenic potential (or neurogenic reserve) of cells involved into adult hippocampal neurogenesis, we may conclude that Aβ treatment of young adult rats produces more prominent suppression of neurogenesis than healthy aging. However, the restorative potential of EE might be easily calculated using coefficient K describing changes in Nc:

$$K = \frac{N_C(EE)}{N_C(SC)}$$

As might be expected from our *in vivo* experiments, EE restored Nc more efficiently in young adult animals (fourfold greater in the control group comparing to the AD model group) but not in the elderly rats (no positive effect of EE at all). Thus, 60 days in the conditions of EE produced no any preventive effect on the aging-associated suppression of hippocampal neurogenesis *in vitro*, being, however, relatively effective in the Alzheimer's type of neurodegeneration. This finding well-corresponds to the number of NeuN+ mature neurons in the dentate gyrus in rats kept in SC or EE (**Figure 1H**) where prominent restoration of mature neurons number was evident in the group of amyloid-treated rats but not in the group of aged animals.

DISCUSSION

Our findings clearly indicate that EE restores neurogenesis affected by the toxic action of Aβ or by aging at the earliest stage of niche cell development (before neuronal fate specification) as was evident both *in vivo* and *in vitro*. In contrast to aging brain, amyloid-affected brain was much more susceptible to the action of EE on the neurogenic capacity of cells. These findings confirm our hypothesis that EE may have different efficacy in AD-type of neurodegeneration and healthy aging brain in the context of neurogenesis improvement.

In accordance to previously published data (Hattiangady and Shetty, 2008) we found that expression of Pax6 within the neurogenic niche was not dramatically decreased in aging animals, but demonstrated prominent decline in AD model. However, the number of NeuN-immunopositive mature neurons was reduced both in healthy aging brain and in AD-affected brain in a similar manner. Therefore, it was not surprising that the earliest stages of neurogenesis both *in vivo* and *in vitro* were more sensitive to the action of EE. Particularly, Pax6 expression was greatly improved by EE exposure *in vivo* in Aβ-treated or aging rats, and the expression pattern of the same marker confirmed the highest neurogenic reserve in young adult rats exposed to long-lasting EE.

Unexpectedly, EE promoted obvious reduction in NeuroD1 expression in the hippocampus in AD group or aged group, whereas in the group of young adult animals no significant changes in NeuroD1 expression have been observed upon action of EE. It is known that NeuroD1 controls survival and maturation of neurons born in the adult brain (Gao et al., 2009) being under the control of Wnt-regulated activity of Sox2 and HDAC1 in NSCs (Chen and Do, 2012). This transcription factor may also direct reprogramming of glial cells into functional neurons *in vivo*, particularly, in AD brain (Guo et al., 2014). NeuroD1 overexpression could reduce functional deficits in newly-formed hippocampal neurons in the experimental model of AD (Richetin et al., 2015). In the aging brain, NeuroD expression declines in the hippocampal neurogenic niche (Uittenbogaard and Chiaramello, 2000). Thus, taking into the consideration the role of NeuroD1 in controlling cell fate and differentiation in hippocampal neurogenesis, one may assume that EE-induced reduction of NeuroD1 expression in Aβ-treated or aged rats could relate to some kind of preservation of neurogenic cells in the non-differentiated state, particularly, in the group of aging rats where elevation of NeuN+ neurons number was less evident than in the group with AD model. Since such effect on NeuroD1 expression was not found in young adult animals, changes in NeuroD1-controled cell differentiation might be considered as a "marker" of EE action in Alzheimer-type neurodegeneration or in healthy brain aging.

It should be noted that EE-mediated decline in NeuroD1 expression is in the contrast to the majority of reports on EE-induced expression of main neurogenesis markers, including NeuroD (Terada et al., 2008). However, similar effect was reported in Manuel et al. (2015) where it was attributed to the inhibition of avoidance behavior in fish subjected to EE. Thus, we may conclude that EE-induced reduction in NeuroD1 hippocampal expression in Aβ-treated or aging rats could reflect some adaptive behavioral reactions needed in further investigation.

We also should point out that housing in standard conditions revealed that NeuroD1 expression in healthy aging brain was well-preserved comparing with Aβ-affected brain. In EE-exposed rats, NeuroD1 expression underwent dramatic decline, particularly in the group of aging animals. Different sensitivity of NeuroD1-expressing cells to the action of EE in aging and AD is consistent with the observed effect of EE on the number of NeuN-immunopositive hippocampal mature neurons: stimulatory action of EE was considerably stronger in Aβ-treated rats.

In sum, EE efficiently improves neurogenesis impaired in the Alzheimer-type neurodegeneration (at least in the AD model used in our study) but produces relatively weak effect on neurogenesis in physiologically aging brain. In both cases, earliest stages of neurogenesis (stimuli-induced proliferation of stem cells and progenitors) *in vivo* represent the periods with higher sensitivity to the action of EE.

The essential question now is whether this effect might be reproduced and quantitatively explained *in vitro*? Analysis of neurogenesis *in vivo* is commonly complemented with *in vitro* studies. Along this way, establishment of NS culture *in vitro* is very useful for assessing proliferative and differentiating properties of stem cells and their progeny, however, quantitative insight into the process of NS development and evolution is highly required (Pacey et al., 2006). Characteristic behavior of NSCs/NPCs in NS culture could not be easy interpreted with simple observations and routine statistics. This problem is further complicated when a number of kinetic data appears in the conditions enabling action of various factors *in vivo* (before cell isolation) or *in vitro* (during cell clusters expansion and development). Therefore, we applied original algorithm to produce comparative analysis of EE effects on the neurogenic reserve of NSCs/NPCs obtained from all the tested groups.

We found that mathematical modeling allowed analyzing the kinetics of cell proliferation *in vitro* with high accuracy and in a good correspondence to the data obtained *in vivo*. Moreover, we were able to get the integral parameter (Nc) reflecting neurogenic reserve of stem/progenitor hippocampal cells affected by different factors (aging, amyloid treatment, EE) *in vivo*. We demonstrated that NS-forming capacity of brain stem and progenitor cells was positively affected by EE in young adult animals, aging animals, but not in elderly rats. The observed difference in the effects of EE on aging- or AD-associated impairment of neurospheres generation *in vitro* might be linked to the very recently reported age-related alterations in the duration of cell cycle (particularly, abnormal extension of G1 phase of the cell cycle not associated with a differentiation commitment) in the hippocampal stem cells resulting in neurogenesis decline (Daynac et al., 2016). A rough analogy might be found with G1-lengthening and alterations in G1/S transition in embryonic stem cells leading to imbalance between self-renewal and differentiation (Coronado et al., 2013). Therefore, the observed prevalence of desynchronization-related changes in the neurosphere-forming capacity in the group of elderly rats is very likely caused by the analogous mechanism of cell cycle impairment. Moreover, such alterations in the cell cycle progression that are evident in neurogenic cells derived from the aged brain might contribute to the relative inefficacy of EE in the context of neurogenesis recovery in aging.

In contrast to physiological aging, Aβ is able to increase NSC activity at the earliest steps of AD pathogenesis followed by later decline (Heo et al., 2007; Diaz-Moreno et al., 2013). Furthermore, EE was reported to increase Aβ accumulation in the transgenic AD model mice due to extensive synaptic activity (Jankowsky et al., 2003). Here, we will note that neurospheres-generating capacity of hippocampal stem/progenitor cells might be enhanced by neuronal excitation due to recruitment of latent stem cells into adult neurogenesis (Walker et al., 2008). That is why Aβ-induced alterations in the adult neurogenesis seem to be more profound but at the same time more sensitive to the restorative capacity of EE-provided neuronal excitation than in the healthy aging brain. Thus, it is reasonable to suggest that long-lasting exposure to EE preceding Aβ neurotoxic action results in excitation-mediated mobilization of latent stem cells and partial restoration of neurosphere-forming capacity *in vitro*. However, this effect is less prominent in Aβ-treated rats than in intact young adult animals. In the group of elderly rats, alterations in the duration of cell cycle diminish EE-induced changes in the stem/progenitor cells pool.

Previously, several attempts have been done to get a mathematical model of neurogenesis (Ashbourn et al., 2012; Ziebell et al., 2014). In this study we propose a mathematical model describing early processes in NSCs/NPCs development *in vitro*. Our time-lag model is based on several assumptions and simplifications but proves our data obtained *in vivo* and provides quantitative parameter (Nc) which is suitable for comparative analysis of effects produced by different factors (i.e., age, housing conditions, neurotoxic stimuli). Thus, combination of *in vivo* and *in vitro* approaches with mathematical modeling reveals some important characteristics of EE action on hippocampal neurogenesis in healthy aging brain or in Alzheimer-type neurodegeneration. It is tempting to speculate that the same approach might be further applied for assessing neurogenesis-targeting activity of drug-candidates in preclinical studies.

There is a growing interest to the restoration of impaired neurogenesis and prevention of neurological deficits in physiological aging (Marr et al., 2010; Mattson, 2015), but differential sensitivity of aging brain and Alzheimer's brain to the conditions of EE should be carefully taken into the consideration. Coming back to our initial hypothesis, we may conclude that: (i) early stages of adult hippocampal neurogenesis are more sensitive to the action of EE in the experimental model of Alzheimer-type neurodegeneration or in aging; (ii) EE differently affects neurogenesis in physiological aging and in experimental AD, particularly, Aβ-affected brain is more susceptible to the action of EE comparing with healthy aging brain; (iii) different outcomes of EE action on NSCs/NPCs in AD or in healthy aging brain can be reliably detected with NS-forming assay *in vitro* and time-lag model of synchronized growth.

Thus, it is clear that EE-based neuroprotective strategies effective in the amyloid-affected brain could not be directly extrapolated to neurodegenerative processes associated with physiological brain aging. Therefore, application of EE strategy aimed to enhance adult neurogenesis should be considered as a personalized and pathogenetically based preventive or therapeutic intervention.

ETHICS STATEMENT

All animal experiments were performed in accordance with the principles of humanity set out in the Directive of the European Community (2010/63/EU). Protocols were reviewed and approved by the Local ethics committee of the Krasnoyarsk State Medical University named after Prof. V.F. Voino-Yasenetsky (35/2011).

AUTHOR CONTRIBUTIONS

VS, YK, and AS conceived and designed the research. All authors performed experiments. VS, YK, NK, AM, EK, and KS analyzed data. VS, YK, OL, and EP prepared figures. VS, YK, YU, EP, and AS prepared the initial draft; VS, YK, OL, and AS revised the manuscript. All authors reviewed the final manuscript and approved its publication.

ACKNOWLEDGMENT

The study is supported by the grant given by the President of Russian Federation for the Leading Scientific Teams (N 10241.2016.7).

REFERENCES

Ali, A. A. H., Schwarz-Herzke, B., Stahr, A., Prozorovski, T., Aktas, O., and von Gall, C. (2015). Premature aging of the hippocampal neurogenic niche in adult Bmal1-deficient mice. *Aging* 7, 435–449. doi: 10.18632/aging.100764

Ashbourn, J. M. A., Miller, J. J., Reumers, V., Baekelandt, V., and Geris, L. (2012). A mathematical model of adult subventricular neurogenesis. *J. R. Soc. Interface* 9, 2414–2423. doi: 10.1098/rsif.2012.0193

Avila, J., Insausti, R., and Del Rio, J. (2010). Memory and neurogenesis in aging and Alzheimer's Disease. *Aging Dis.* 1, 30–36.

Baker, C. T., Bocharov, G. A., Paul, C. A., and Rihan, F. A. (1998). Modelling and analysis of time-lags in some basic patterns of cell proliferation. *J. Math. Biol.* 37, 341–371. doi: 10.1007/s002850050133

Balietti, M., Tamagnini, F., Fattoretti, P., Burattini, C., Casoli, T., Platano, D., et al. (2012). Impairments of synaptic plasticity in aged animals and in animal models of Alzheimer's disease. *Rejuvenation Res.* 15, 235–238. doi: 10.1089/rej.2012.1318

Barak, B., Shvarts-Serebro, I., Modai, S., Gilam, A., Okun, E., Michaelson, D. M., et al. (2013). Opposing actions of environmental enrichment and Alzheimer's disease on the expression of hippocampal microRNAs in mouse models. *Transl. Psychiatry* 3:e304. doi: 10.1038/tp.2013.77

Bezzina, C., Verret, L., Halley, H., Dahan, L., and Rampon, C. (2015). Environmental enrichment does not influence hypersynchronous network activity in the Tg2576 mouse model of Alzheimer's disease. *Front. Aging Neurosci.* 7:178. doi: 10.3389/fnagi.2015.00178

Chen, M., and Do, H. (2012). Wnt Signaling in neurogenesis during aging and physical activity. *Brain Sci.* 2, 745–768. doi: 10.3390/brainsci2040745

Choi, Y. J., Park, J., and Lee, S.-H. (2013). Size-controllable networked neurospheres as a 3D neuronal tissue model for Alzheimer's disease studies. *Biomaterials* 34, 2938–2946. doi: 10.1016/j.biomaterials.2013.01.038

Cioni, G., Inguaggiato, E., and Sgandurra, G. (2016). Early intervention in neurodevelopmental disorders: underlying neural mechanisms. *Dev. Med. Child Neurol.* 58(Suppl. 4), 61–66. doi: 10.1111/dmcn.13050

Clemenson, G. D., Deng, W., and Gage, F. H. (2015). Environmental enrichment and neurogenesis: from mice to humans. *Curr. Opin. Behav. Sci.* 4, 56–62. doi: 10.1016/j.cobeha.2015.02.005

Coronado, D., Godet, M., Bourillot, P.-Y., Tapponnier, Y., Bernat, A., Petit, M., et al. (2013). A short G1 phase is an intrinsic determinant of naïve embryonic stem cell pluripotency. *Stem Cell Res.* 10, 118–131. doi: 10.1016/j.scr.2012.10.004

Cotel, M. C., Jawhar, S., Christensen, D. Z., Bayer, T. A., and Wirths, O. (2012). Environmental enrichment fails to rescue working memory deficits, neuron loss, and neurogenesis in APP/PS1KI mice. *Neurobiol. Aging* 33, 96–107. doi: 10.1016/j.neurobiolaging.2010.02.012

Daynac, M., Morizur, L., Chicheportiche, A., Mouthon, M.-A., and Boussin, F. D. (2016). Age-related neurogenesis decline in the subventricular zone is associated with specific cell cycle regulation changes in activated neural stem cells. *Sci. Rep.* 6:21505. doi: 10.1038/srep21505

Diaz-Moreno, M., Hortiguela, R., Goncalves, A., Garcia-Carpio, I., Manich, G., Garcia-Bermudez, E., et al. (2013). Abeta increases neural stem cell activity in senescence-accelerated SAMP8 mice. *Neurobiol. Aging* 34, 2623–2638. doi: 10.1016/j.neurobiolaging.2013.05.011

Esiri, M. M., and Chance, S. A. (2012). Cognitive reserve, cortical plasticity and resistance to Alzheimer's disease. *Alzheimers Res. Ther.* 4:7. doi: 10.1186/alzrt105

Firbank, M. J., Teodorczuk, A., van der Flier, W. M., Gouw, A. A., Wallin, A., Erkinjuntti, T., et al. (2012). Relationship between progression of brain white matter changes and late-life depression: 3-year results from the LADIS study. *Br. J. Psychiatry* 201, 40–45. doi: 10.1192/bjp.bp.111.098897

Forlenza, O. V., Miranda, A. S., Guimar, I., Talib, L. L., Diniz, B. S., Gattaz, W. F., et al. (2015). Decreased neurotrophic support is associated with cognitive decline in non-demented subjects. *J. Alzheimers. Dis.* 46, 423–429. doi: 10.3233/jad-150172

Gao, Z., Ure, K., Ables, J. L., Lagace, D. C., Nave, K.-A., Goebbels, S., et al. (2009). Neurod1 is essential for the survival and maturation of adult-born neurons. *Nat. Neurosci.* 12, 1090–1092. doi: 10.1038/nn.2385

Ghate, P. S., Sidhar, H., Carlson, G. A., and Giri, R. K. (2014). Development of a novel cellular model of Alzheimer's disease utilizing neurosphere cultures derived from B6C3-Tg(APPswe,PSEN1dE9)85Dbo/J embryonic mouse brain. *Springerplus* 3, 161. doi: 10.1186/2193-1801-3-161

Grinan-Ferre, C., Puigoriol-Illamola, D., Palomera-Avalos, V., Perez-Caceres, D., Companys-Alemany, J., Camins, A., et al. (2016). Environmental enrichment modified epigenetic mechanisms in SAMP8 mouse hippocampus by reducing oxidative stress and inflammaging and achieving neuroprotection. *Front. Aging Neurosci.* 8:241. doi: 10.3389/fnagi.2016.00241

Guo, Z., Zhang, L., Wu, Z., Chen, Y., Wang, F., and Chen, G. (2014). In vivo direct reprogramming of reactive glial cells into functional neurons after brain injury and in an Alzheimer's disease model. *Cell Stem Cell* 14, 188–202. doi: 10.1016/j.stem.2013.12.001

Hattiangady, B., and Shetty, A. K. (2008). Aging does not alter the number or phenotype of putative stem/progenitor cells in the neurogenic region of the hippocampus. *Neurobiol. Aging* 29, 129–147. doi: 10.1016/j.neurobiolaging.2006.09.015

Heo, C., Chang, K. A., Choi, H. S., Kim, H. S., Kim, S., Liew, H., et al. (2007). Effects of the monomeric, oligomeric, and fibrillar Abeta42 peptides on the proliferation and differentiation of adult neural stem cells from subventricular zone. *J. Neurochem.* 102, 493–500. doi: 10.1111/j.1471-4159.2007.04499.x

Herring, A., Lewejohann, L., Panzer, A. L., Donath, A., Kroll, O., Sachser, N., et al. (2011). Preventive and therapeutic types of environmental enrichment counteract beta amyloid pathology by different molecular mechanisms. *Neurobiol. Dis.* 42, 530–538. doi: 10.1016/j.nbd.2011.03.007

Hollands, C., Bartolotti, N., and Lazarov, O. (2016). Alzheimer's Disease and Hippocampal adult neurogenesis; exploring shared mechanisms. *Front. Neurosci.* 10:178. doi: 10.3389/fnins.2016.00178

Huttenrauch, M., Walter, S., Kaufmann, M., Weggen, S., and Wirths, O. (2016). Limited effects of prolonged environmental enrichment on the pathology of 5XFAD Mice. *Mol. Neurobiol.* doi: 10.1007/s12035-016-0167-x [Epub ahead of print].

Jankowsky, J. L., Xu, G., Fromholt, D., Gonzales, V., and Borchelt, D. R. (2003). Environmental enrichment exacerbates amyloid plaque formation in a transgenic mouse model of Alzheimer disease. *J. Neuropathol. Exp. Neurol.* 62, 1220–1227. doi: 10.1093/jnen/62.12.1220

Janssen, H., Ada, L., Bernhardt, J., McElduff, P., Pollack, M., Nilsson, M., et al. (2014). An enriched environment increases activity in stroke patients undergoing rehabilitation in a mixed rehabilitation unit: a pilot non-randomized controlled trial. *Disabil. Rehabil.* 36, 255–262. doi: 10.3109/09638288.2013.788218

Komleva Iu, K., Salmina, A. B., Prokopenko, S. V., Shestakova, L. A., Petrova, M. M., Malinovskaia, N. A., et al. (2013). Changes in structural and functional plasticity of the brain induced by environmental enrichment. *Vestn. Ross. Akad. Med. Nauk.* 39–48.

Kuvacheva, N. V., Morgun, A. V., Komleva, Y. K., Khilazheva, E. D., Gorina, Y. V., Lopatina, O. L., et al. (2015). In Vitro modeling of brain progenitor cell development under the effect of environmental factors. *Bull. Exp. Biol. Med.* 159, 546–549. doi: 10.1007/s10517-015-3012-8

Leger, M., Paizanis, E., Dzahini, K., Quiedeville, A., Bouet, V., Cassel, J. C., et al. (2015). Environmental enrichment duration differentially affects behavior and neuroplasticity in adult mice. *Cereb. Cortex* 25, 4048–4061. doi: 10.1093/cercor/bhu119

Li, X., Yuan, H. F., Quan, Q. K., Wang, J. J., Wang, N. N., and Li, M. (2011). Scavenging effect of Naoerkang on amyloid beta-peptide deposition in the hippocampus in a rat model of Alzheimer's disease. *Chin. J. Integr. Med.* 17, 847–853. doi: 10.1007/s11655-011-0896-7

Ma, B. F., Liu, X. M., Zhang, A. X., Wang, P., Zhang, X. M., Li, S. N., et al. (2007). Mathematical models for the proliferation of neural stem/progenitor cells in clonogenic culture. *Rejuvenation Res.* 10, 205–214. doi: 10.1089/rej.2006.0532

Maesako, M., Uemura, K., Kubota, M., Kuzuya, A., Sasaki, K., Asada, M., et al. (2012). Environmental enrichment ameliorated high-fat diet-induced Abeta deposition and memory deficit in APP transgenic mice. *Neurobiol. Aging* 33, 1011.e11–e23. doi: 10.1016/j.neurobiolaging.2011.10.028

Malik, A., Jamasbi, R. J., Kondratov, R. V., and Geusz, M. E. (2015). Development of circadian oscillators in neurosphere cultures during adult neurogenesis. *PLoS ONE* 10:e0122937. doi: 10.1371/journal.pone.0122937

Manuel, R., Gorissen, M., Stokkermans, M., Zethof, J., Ebbesson, L. O., van de Vis, H., et al. (2015). The effects of environmental enrichment and age-related differences on inhibitory avoidance in zebrafish (Danio rerio Hamilton). *Zebrafish* 12, 152–165. doi: 10.1089/zeb.2014.1045

Marin-Padilla, M., and Knopman, D. S. (2011). Developmental aspects of the intracerebral microvasculature and perivascular spaces: insights into brain response to late-life diseases. *J. Neuropathol. Exp. Neurol.* 70, 1060–1069. doi: 10.1097/NEN.0b013e31823ac627

Marr, R. A., Thomas, R. M., and Peterson, D. A. (2010). Insights into neurogenesis and aging: potential therapy for degenerative disease? *Future Neurol.* 5, 527–541. doi: 10.2217/fnl.10.33

Mattson, M. P. (2015). Lifelong brain health is a lifelong challenge: from evolutionary principles to empirical evidence. *Ageing Res. Rev.* 20, 37–45. doi: 10.1016/j.arr.2014.12.011

Ming, G.-L., and Song, H. (2011). Adult neurogenesis in the mammalian brain: significant answers and significant questions. *Neuron* 70, 687–702. doi: 10.1016/j.neuron.2011.05.001

Monteiro, B. M., Moreira, F. A., Massensini, A. R., Moraes, M. F., and Pereira, G. S. (2014). Enriched environment increases neurogenesis and improves social memory persistence in socially isolated adult mice. *Hippocampus* 24, 239–248. doi: 10.1002/hipo.22218

Mora, F. (2013). Successful brain aging: plasticity, environmental enrichment, and lifestyle. *Dialogues Clin. Neurosci.* 15, 45–52.

Moraga, A., Pradillo, J. M., García-Culebras, A., Palma-Tortosa, S., Ballesteros, I., Hernández-Jiménez, M., et al. (2015). Aging increases microglial proliferation, delays cell migration, and decreases cortical neurogenesis after focal cerebral ischemia. *J. Neuroinflamm.* 12, 87. doi: 10.1186/s12974-015-0314-8

Mostany, R., Anstey, J. E., Crump, K. L., Maco, B., Knott, G., and Portera-Cailliau, C. (2013). Altered synaptic dynamics during normal brain aging. *J. Neurosci.* 33, 4094–4104. doi: 10.1523/jneurosci.4825-12.2013

Neidl, R., Schneider, A., Bousiges, O., Majchrzak, M., Barbelivien, A., de Vasconcelos, A. P., et al. (2016). Late-life environmental enrichment induces acetylation events and nuclear factor kappaB-dependent regulations in the hippocampus of aged rats showing improved plasticity and learning. *J. Neurosci.* 36, 4351–4361. doi: 10.1523/jneurosci.3239-15.2016

Pacey, L., Stead, S., Gleave, J., Tomczyk, K., and Doering, L. (2006). Neural stem cell culture: neurosphere generation, microscopical analysis and cryopreservation. *Protoc. Exch.* doi: 10.1038/nprot.2006.215

Polito, L., Chierchia, A., Tunesi, M., Bouybayoune, I., Kehoe, P. G., Albani, D., et al. (2014). Environmental enrichment lessens cognitive decline in APP23 mice without affecting brain sirtuin expression. *J. Alzheimers. Dis.* 42, 851–864. doi: 10.3233/jad-131430

Richetin, K., Leclerc, C., Toni, N., Gallopin, T., Pech, S., Roybon, L., et al. (2015). Genetic manipulation of adult-born hippocampal neurons rescues memory in a mouse model of Alzheimer's disease. *Brain* 138(Pt 2), 440–455. doi: 10.1093/brain/awu354

Rodriguez, J. J., Terzieva, S., Olabarria, M., Lanza, R. G., and Verkhratsky, A. (2013). Enriched environment and physical activity reverse astrogliodegeneration in the hippocampus of AD transgenic mice. *Cell Death Dis.* 4:e678. doi: 10.1038/cddis.2013.194

Rosbergen, I. C. M., Grimley, R. S., Hayward, K. S., Walker, K. C., Rowley, D., Campbell, A. M., et al. (2016). The effect of an enriched environment on activity levels in people with stroke in an acute stroke unit: protocol for a before-after pilot study. *Pilot Feasibility Stud.* 2:36. doi: 10.1186/s40814-016-0081-z

Roybon, L., Hjalt, T., Stott, S., Guillemot, F., Li, J.-Y., and Brundin, P. (2009). Neurogenin2 directs granule neuroblast production and amplification while NeuroD1 specifies neuronal fate during hippocampal neurogenesis. *PLoS ONE* 4:e4779. doi: 10.1371/journal.pone.0004779

Stuart, K. E., King, A. E., Fernandez-Martos, C. M., Dittmann, J., Summers, M. J., and Vickers, J. C. (2017). Mid-life environmental enrichment increases synaptic density in CA1 in a mouse model of Abeta-associated pathology and positively influences synaptic and cognitive health in healthy ageing. *J. Comp. Neurol.* 525, 1797–1810. doi: 10.1002/cne.24156

Terada, M., Kuzumaki, N., Hareyama, N., Imai, S., Niikura, K., Narita, M., et al. (2008). Suppression of enriched environment-induced neurogenesis in a rodent model of neuropathic pain. *Neurosci. Lett.* 440, 314–318. doi: 10.1016/j.neulet.2008.05.078

Uittenbogaard, M., and Chiaramello, A. (2000). Differential expression patterns of the basic helix-loop-helix transcription factors during aging of the murine brain. *Neurosci. Lett.* 280, 95–98. doi: 10.1016/S0304-3940(00)00761-8

Valero-Aracama, M. J., Sauvage, M. M., and Yoshida, M. (2015). Environmental enrichment modulates intrinsic cellular excitability of hippocampal CA1 pyramidal cells in a housing duration and anatomical location-dependent manner. *Behav. Brain Res.* 292, 209–218. doi: 10.1016/j.bbr.2015.05.032

VanHook, A. M. (2014). De-adhesion for mitotic progression. *Sci. Signal.* 7, ec337. doi: 10.1126/scisignal.aaa3737

Waldau, B., and Shetty, A. K. (2008). Behavior of neural stem cells in the Alzheimer brain. *Cell. Mol. Life Sci.* 65, 2372–2384. doi: 10.1007/s00018-008-8053-y

Walker, T. L., White, A., Black, D. M., Wallace, R. H., Sah, P., and Bartlett, P. F. (2008). Latent stem and progenitor cells in the hippocampus are activated by neural excitation. *J. Neurosci.* 28, 5240–5247. doi: 10.1523/jneurosci.0344-08.2008

Williamson, L. L., Chao, A., and Bilbo, S. D. (2012). Environmental enrichment alters glial antigen expression and neuroimmune function in the adult rat hippocampus. *Brain Behav. Immun.* 26, 500–510. doi: 10.1016/j.bbi.2012.01.003

Yang, S., Lu, W., Zhou, D. S., and Tang, Y. (2012). Enriched environment and white matter in aging brain. *Anat. Rec. (Hoboken)* 295, 1406–1414. doi: 10.1002/ar.22526

Yuan, Z., Wang, M., Yan, B., Gu, P., Jiang, X., Yang, X., et al. (2012). An enriched environment improves cognitive performance in mice from the senescence-accelerated prone mouse 8 strain: role of upregulated neurotrophic factor expression in the hippocampus. *Neural Regen. Res.* 7, 1797–1804. doi: 10.3969/j.issn.1673-5374.2012.23.006

Zeng, Q., Zheng, M., Zhang, T., and He, G. (2016). Hippocampal neurogenesis in the APP/PS1/nestin-GFP triple transgenic mouse model of Alzheimer's disease. *Neuroscience* 314, 64–74. doi: 10.1016/j.neuroscience.2015.11.054

Ziebell, F., Martin-Villalba, A., and Marciniak-Czochra, A. (2014). Mathematical modelling of adult hippocampal neurogenesis: effects of altered stem cell dynamics on cell counts and bromodeoxyuridine-labelled cells. *J. R. Soc. Interface* 11, 20140144. doi: 10.1098/rsif.2014.0144

5

Application of an amyloid beta oligomer standard in the sFIDA assay

Katja Kühbach[1], Maren Hülsemann[1], Yvonne Herrmann[1], Kateryna Kravchenko[1], Andreas Kulawik[1], Christina Linnartz[1], Luriano Peters[1], Kun Wang[1], Johannes Willbold[1], Dieter Willbold[1,2] and Oliver Bannach[1,2]*

[1] ICS-6 Structural Biochemistry, Forschungszentrum Jülich GmbH, Jülich, Germany, [2] Institut für Physikalische Biologie, Heinrich-Heine-Universität Düsseldorf, Düsseldorf, Germany

Edited by:
Charlotte Elisabeth Teunissen,
VU University Medical Center
Amsterdam, Netherlands

Reviewed by:
Xifei Yang,
Shenzhen Center for Disease Control and Prevention, China
Mary Josephine Savage,
Merck and Company, USA

***Correspondence:**
Oliver Bannach
o.bannach@fz-juelich.de

Still, there is need for significant improvements in reliable and accurate diagnosis for Alzheimer's disease (AD) at early stages. It is widely accepted that changes in the concentration and conformation of amyloid-β (Aβ) appear several years before the onset of first symptoms of cognitive impairment in AD patients. Because Aβ oligomers are possibly the major toxic species in AD, they are a promising biomarker candidate for the early diagnosis of the disease. To date, a variety of oligomer-specific assays have been developed, many of them ELISAs. Here, we demonstrate the sFIDA assay, a technology highly specific for Aβ oligomers developed toward single particle sensitivity. By spiking stabilized Aβ oligomers to buffer and to body fluids from control donors, we show that the sFIDA readout correlates with the applied concentration of stabilized oligomers diluted in buffer, cerebrospinal fluid (CSF), and blood plasma over several orders of magnitude. The lower limit of detection was calculated to be 22 fM of stabilized oligomers diluted in PBS, 18 fM in CSF, and 14 fM in blood plasma.

Keywords: Alzheimer's disease, amyloid-β peptide, diagnostic biomarker, early diagnosis, sFIDA, surface-based fluorescence intensity distribution analysis, stabilized oligomers, standard molecule

INTRODUCTION

Worldwide 5–7% of people older than 60 years are affected by dementia, with Alzheimer's disease (AD) being the most common type. Due to the aging population, the total number of demented people is predicted to increase even further (Prince et al., 2013). There is neither a cure nor a sufficiently reliable laboratory diagnostic test available for this fatal neurodegenerative disease (Lansdall, 2014). Early diagnosis of AD, however, is of great importance for the development of therapeutics and their future application at an early stage of the disease. It is believed that AD can be treated most effectively in preclinical stages, before cognitive functions become impaired and neurons and synapses are damaged irreversibly (Golde et al., 2011). Hitherto, the definitive diagnosis can only be made after the patients' death based on neuropathological hallmarks, like amyloid plaques, neurodegeneration and neurofibrillary tangles (Ballard et al., 2011).

The main component of amyloid plaques is amyloid β peptide (Aβ), which is formed from the amyloid precursor protein (APP) by β- and γ-secretases (Haass et al., 2012). Once released from the precursor, the Aβ peptide is prone to aggregation and can assemble into oligomeric structures and amyloid fibrils. It is widely accepted that soluble Aβ oligomers but not monomers are highly neurotoxic and that the pathological process in AD starts already years before the onset of clinical manifestation (Braak and Braak, 1991; McLean et al., 1999; Cleary et al., 2004; Lesné et al., 2006).

Currently, the total concentration of Aβ_{42} in cerebrospinal fluid (CSF), which is lower in AD patients compared to healthy persons (Sunderland et al., 2003; Shaw et al., 2009), is used as a biomarker in clinical trials or academic settings to increase the accuracy of AD diagnosis. At the current stage of biomarker development, however, the total concentration of Aβ_{42} in CSF, even in combination with other biomarkers such as tau protein, does not allow a clear distinction of AD patients from healthy controls or patients with other dementias (Humpel, 2011). Therefore, the development of more accurate biomarkers is of utmost importance.

Since Aβ oligomeric species are known to be directly involved in AD pathology or even to trigger the disease (Haass and Selkoe, 2007), Aβ oligomers are considered as promising biomarker for AD (Blennow et al., 2010). The main challenges for Aβ oligomer-based diagnostics in body fluids are the presumably very low concentrations of Aβ oligomers and the high background of monomeric Aβ (Rosén et al., 2013). To meet those requirements, we have previously developed an assay called sFIDA (surface-based fluorescence intensity distribution analysis; Birkmann et al., 2007; Funke et al., 2007, 2010; Bannach et al., 2012). The principle of sFIDA is illustrated in **Figure 1**. The biochemical setup of sFIDA resembles a conventional sandwich ELISA. All Aβ species are immobilized on a functionalized glass surface via Aβ-specific capture antibodies. After immobilization, Aβ aggregates are multiply loaded by at least two detection antibodies, each of them labeled with a different fluorochrome. Because capture and detection antibodies recognize the same or an overlapping epitope on Aβ, Aβ monomers cannot bind any detection antibodies while bound to the capture antibody. In contrast to a classical ELISA, the result of the measurement is not a single readout for the whole sample. Instead, the surface is imaged by high-resolution fluorescence microscopy, such as dual-color total internal reflection fluorescence microscopy (TIRFM). Only those pixels that show signal intensities above the background noise in both channels are counted. Thus, the number of colocalized pixels above the background noise is expected to correlate with the concentration of Aβ oligomers in the sample.

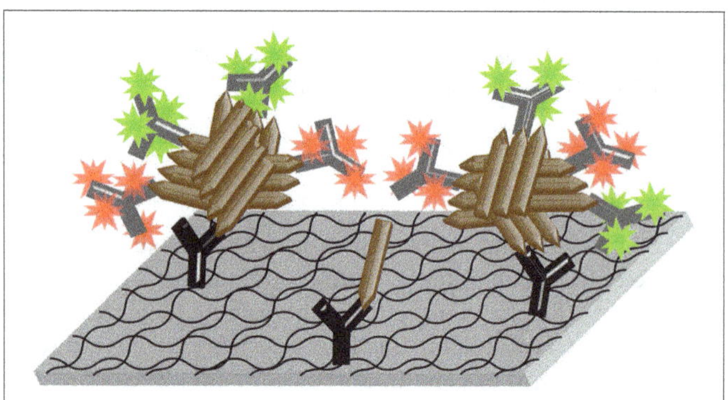

FIGURE 1 | Scheme of the sFIDA assay. Aβ-specific capture antibodies (dark gray Y symbols) are immobilized on a functionalized glass surface. Aβ oligomers (brown rods) present in the sample bind to the capture antibodies and are detected by fluorescence labeled (colored stars) anti-Aβ-antibodies (light gray Y symbols). The surface is then imaged by dual-color microscopy. In this version of the assay, all three of the applied antibodies (one capture and two different detection antibodies labeled with two different fluorochromes) bind to overlapping epitopes at the N-terminus of Aβ, which corresponds to the spiky ends of the brown rods in the scheme above. Thereby, only oligomers with multiple epitopes, but not monomers, are able to bind detection antibodies while bound to the capture and thus yield detectable signals.

Results showing increased sFIDA readouts for AD patients compared to non-demented controls have been reported previously (Wang-Dietrich et al., 2013). However, in this study no reliable Aβ oligomer standard was available to determine absolute concentrations from the assay readout. Due to both the dynamic aggregation and dissociation of Aβ, non-stabilized oligomers are not suited as standard in oligomer-based diagnostic assays.

Here, we demonstrate application of stabilized Aβ oligomers as standard molecules in the sFIDA assay. The sFIDA readout correlates with the applied oligomer concentration over five magnitudes down to a femtomolar range, which will allow the quantification of natural Aβ oligomer concentrations in body fluids.

MATERIALS AND METHODS

Biological Samples and PBS Spiked with Stabilized Oligomers

Four individual human EDTA-anticoagulated plasma samples (Zen-Bio, Research Triangle Park, USA) and one pooled human EDTA-anticoagulated plasma sample from three healthy donors were centrifuged for 15 min at 15,000 × *g*. The supernatant was collected and equal volumes from each sample were combined to obtain one large pool from several donors (from here on referred to as "plasma fraction"). Human cerebrospinal fluid sample (CSF; pooled from healthy donors/mixed gender) was purchased from Biochemed (Winchester, USA). Stabilized Aβ oligomers (Crossbeta Biosciences B.V., Utrecht, the Netherlands), from here on called "oligomers", were serially diluted from the stock solution (10 nM) to concentrations of 1 nM, 100 pM, 10 pM, 1 pM, 100 fM, 10 fM, and 1 fM in PBS (GE Healthcare, Chalfont St. Giles, UK), CSF or the plasma fraction as described above. All concentrations of Aβ oligomers in this publication refer to oligomer particle concentrations, if not stated otherwise. The oligomers consist of approximately 220 Aβ_{1-42} monomers (manufacturer's data); further characterization of the stabilized oligomers, including data on the size homogeneity and stability, are available on the manufacturer's homepage (Crossbeta Biosciences, 2015).

sFIDA

Plate Preparation

384-well plates (SensoPlate Plus with 175 μm glass bottom; Greiner Bio-One, Kremsmünster, Austria) were used for sFIDA. Functionalization of the glass surface was performed as previously described in Janissen et al. (2009). The surface was treated with 5 M NaOH (AppliChem, Darmstadt, Germany) for 15 min, washed three times with water, neutralized with 1 M HCl (AppliChem, Darmstadt, Germany; 15 min), washed again three times with water and then twice with 70% ethanol (VWR International, Langenfeld, Germany). After drying the plate at room temperature, the wells were incubated in

10 M ethanolamine in DMSO (Sigma-Aldrich, St. Louis, USA) overnight. Afterwards, the wells were washed three times with DMSO, twice with 70% ethanol and the plate was dried again at room temperature. A solution of 50 mM SC-PEG-CM (MW 5000 Da, Laysan Bio, Arab, USA) in DMSO was heated shortly to 70°C until the PEG dissolved. After the solution cooled down, 2% (v/v) triethylamin (Fluka, Buchs, Switzerland) were added, the solution was quickly vortexed and 15 μl were applied per well. After an incubation time of 1 h the wells were washed five times with water.

The carboxymethyl groups of SC-PEG-CM on the glass surface were then activated by addition of 30 μl of 100 mM EDC (Fluka, Buchs, Switzerland)/100 mM NHS (Aldrich, Milwaukee, USA) in 0.1 M MES buffer, pH 3.5 (AppliChem) per well for 30 min. After flushing the wells three times quickly with MES buffer, 15 μl of 10 ng/μl capture antibody Nab228 in PBS (the supernatant after centrifuging 10 min at 18,000 g) was added to the surface. After incubating for 90 min, unbound antibody was removed and wells were washed three times with PBST (PBS + 0.05% Tween20, AppliChem Panreac, Darmstadt, Germany) and three times with PBS. Then 50 μl of blocking solution (SmartBlock, CANDOR Biosciences, Wangen, Germany) per well were incubated for 1 h. After washing the wells three times with PBST and three times with PBS, 15 μl sample was applied to each well and incubated overnight. The wells were washed once with PBST and twice with PBS. The detection antibodies 6E10 labeled with Alexa Fluor 488 (Covance, Princeton, USA) and Nab228 labeled with Alexa Fluor 647 (Santa Cruz, Dallas, USA) were combined to each 1.25 μg/ml in PBS and centrifuged for 1 h (100,000 g, 4°C). The supernatant was mixed and added to the wells (15 μl/well, 1 h). Finally, the wells were washed once with PBST and twice with PBS. The buffer was removed and 100 μl of water were applied to each well for image acquisition on TIRFM (AM TIRF MC, Leica microsystems, Wetzlar, Germany).

Image Data Acquisition

Using TIRF microscopy, 25 positions per well were imaged in two different channels (14 bit gray scale; channel 0: excitation at 635 nm, emission filter 705/72 nm; channel 1: excitation at 488 nm, emission filter 525/36 nm). Each image contains 1000 × 1000 pixels and represents an area of 116 × 116 μm. In total, 3.15% of the well surface was imaged.

Image Data Analysis

Prior to data analysis, images showing inhomogeneous surfaces, e.g., due to mechanical damage of the surface or impurities, were excluded from the analysis by automated artifact detection, which is briefly described in the following: Each original image was converted to a binary image by replacing all pixels having intensities above or equal the mean pixel intensity of the regarding image plus one standard deviation with the number one, all others with the number zero. In the next step, erosion was applied to these binary images by using a rectangular structuring element with a size of 31 × 31 pixels. After erosion, the binary image was dilated using the same structuring element as for erosion. Each cluster that consisted of connected pixels with the intensity one in the binary image after dilatation was then analyzed in the original image. Clusters showing either a mean pixel intensity of above 4000, a standard deviation of pixel intensities above 2800, or a skewness of <0 in the original images were defined as artificial and the whole image was excluded from the analysis. Images that had a mean pixel intensity of 16,383 over the whole image in at least one channel were included for image analysis although they were excluded by the artifact detection, because those images are estimated as being saturated, but not artificial.

To account for inhomogeneous illumination, only the central "region of interest" containing 500 × 500 pixels of each image were used for further analysis.

The remaining images were analyzed for colocalization: For both channels, intensity cutoffs for exclusion of background signal were determined. As the background signal might differ from one matrix (i.e., PBS, CSF, and plasma fraction) to another, the cutoff values were determined for each matrix individually, but—in order to compare sFIDA readouts achieved by diluting oligomers in the different matrices—in a reliable and unbiased way. The cutoff for each channel and each matrix was determined from the unspiked control sample to be the value, which is exceeded by only 0.01% of total image pixels. This value represents a reasonable compromise between efficient background removal and retention of assay sensitivity. For cutoffs used in this study, see **Table 1**.

Colocalized pixels with intensity values above the cutoffs in both channels were counted for each image. The number of colocalized pixels was determined for each picture and the average pixel count from all pictures from the same sample was referred to as "sFIDA readout". Please note that the sFIDA readout cannot exceed 250,000, which corresponds to the total number of pixels per analyzed image section.

Calculation of Calibration Curves

For the calibration of assay readout (number of colocalized pixels) to molecule concentration a weighted linear regression analysis was performed with Matlab (The MathWorks, Natick, USA) from experimental data points within the linear detection range (CSF: 100 pM to 10 fM; PBS: 10 pM to 10 fM; plasma fraction: 10 pM to 10 fM) with respective weights calculated as 1/readout. In cases of readout = 0 the weight was determined as 1.

Statistics

In order to statistically assess differences between sFIDA readouts of different concentrations of oligomers diluted in the same matrix, two-way omnibus Kruskal-Wallis test was used for comparison of more than two groups. *Post-hoc*

TABLE 1 | Cutoffs for the different body fluids.

Matrix	Cutoff channel 635 nm	Cutoff channel 488 nm
CSF	3268	2339
PBS	4082	2773
Plasma fraction	4259	2028

Cutoffs were obtained for each channel and matrix by allowing only 0.01% of all pixels to be above background signal for negative controls.

analysis was performed by using two-tailed Mann-Whitney-U test and *p*-value adjustment according to Benjamini and Hochberg (1995) in order to account for multiple testing. By Mann-Whitney-U test, sFIDA readouts from each concentration were compared to the next lower one. Additionally, sFIDA readouts from blank samples were compared to readouts from 10 to 100 fM. The false discovery rate controlling procedure after Benjamini and Hochberg was calculated for 0.05 (for significant results, indicated with *) and 0.01 (for very significant results, indicated with **). Kruskal-Wallis and Mann-Whitney-U test were calculated using the statistical software Origin (OriginLab Corporation, Northampton, USA), false discovery rate controlling procedure after Benjamini and Hochberg was calculated in Microsoft Excel (Microsoft Corporation, Redmond, USA).

RESULTS

Detection of Stabilized Oligomers by sFIDA

In a first set of experiments we sought to find out if the stabilized oligomers can be sensitively detected by the sFIDA assay. Therefore, a log10 dilution series of oligomers in PBS with concentrations ranging from 1 nM to 1 fM was subjected to sFIDA analysis in quadruplicate determination. As can be seen in **Figure 2**, the sFIDA readout correlated well with the applied concentration of stabilized oligomers in the range of 100 pM down to 1 fM. The readouts from 1 nM to 100 pM oligomers in PBS reached saturation, which means that all pixels were above cutoff in both channels. At the lower end of the dilution series, the sFIDA readout of the lowest oligomer concentration (1 fM) did not differ significantly from the readouts from 10 fM oligomers and the blank control. However, there was a significant difference in the sFIDA readouts from 10 fM oligomers and the blank control.

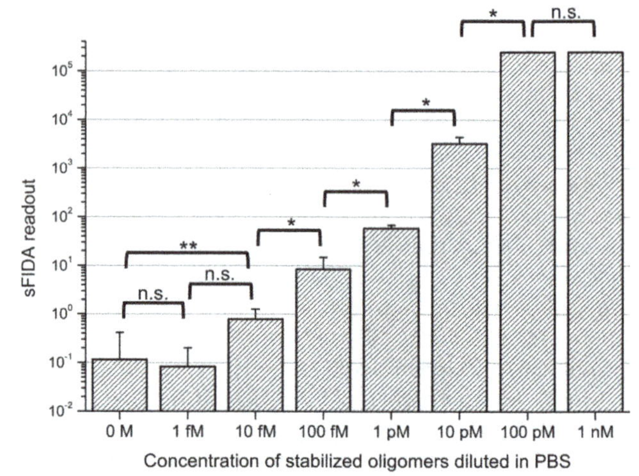

FIGURE 2 | sFIDA readout of stabilized oligomers diluted in PBS. Columns and error bars represent the mean values and standard deviations calculated from a fourfold determination of samples containing oligomers. The blank was determined 21-fold. Cutoffs for each channel were set to discard virtually all background from control samples except for 25 pixels, which are 0.01% of all pixels. This led to the following cutoff values (channel 635 nm/channel 488 nm): 4082/2773. Please note that the number of colocalized pixels (sFIDA readout) is lower than the number of pixels above background in the single channels. n.s., not significant; $^{*}p \leq 0.05$; $^{**}p \leq 0.01$.

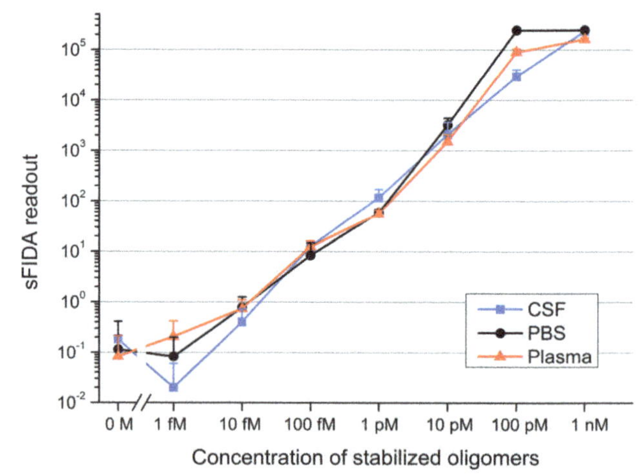

FIGURE 3 | sFIDA readout of stabilized oligomers diluted in CSF, PBS, and a plasma fraction. Shown are mean values and standard deviations from fourfold (samples containing stabilized oligomers) or 21-fold (all blanks) determinations. Cutoffs for channel 635 nm/channel 488 nm: CSF, 3268/2339; PBS, 4082/2773; plasma fraction, 4259/2028.

Spiking of CSF, PBS, and EDTA Plasma Fraction with Stabilized Oligomers

After demonstrating the ability to detect even femtomolar concentrations of stabilized oligomers diluted in buffer, we investigated if different body fluid environments affect the sensitivity of oligomer detection by sFIDA. To check for matrix effects that possibly attenuate the specific signal of Aβ oligomers, the oligomers were spiked into CSF and blood plasma from healthy, non-demented control subjects. All samples containing oligomers were determined fourfold by sFIDA analysis, while each blank sample was measured 21-fold. **Figure 3** shows the mean sFIDA readouts for all samples.

The sFIDA readout correlated well with the oligomer concentration down to 1 fM. However, there was no significant difference in the readouts of 10 fM as compared to 1 fM, as well as in the readouts from the blank sample compared to 1 and 10 fM oligomers spiked into CSF. sFIDA readouts from 100 fM and the blank sample differed significantly.

For plasma samples, there was even a very significant difference between the sFIDA readouts of 10 fM and blank sample.

Lower Limits of Detection and Lower Limits of Quantification for Stabilized Oligomers Diluted in PBS, CSF, and the Plasma Fraction

As the concentration of Aβ oligomers in body fluids like CSF and blood is presumably very low (Bruggink et al., 2013; Höltta et al., 2013; Savage et al., 2014), the lower limit of detection (LLOD) is an important characteristic of every assay for the determination of Aβ oligomer concentration. To identify the LLOD for each matrix used in this report, each blank sample was determined 21-fold. The LLOD was calculated as the mean sFIDA readout from all blank samples plus three times the standard deviation. By establishing a calibration curve from the dilution series, the Aβ oligomer concentration corresponding to the calculated sFIDA readout was then determined. The resulting LLODs were 22 fM for stabilized oligomers diluted in PBS, 18 fM in CSF, and 14 fM in the plasma fraction.

The lower limits of quantification (LLOQ) were calculated as the mean sFIDA readout from all blank samples plus ten times the standard deviation. The same calibration curves as used for determination of LLOD were applied, leading to the following concentrations: 32 fM for stabilized oligomers diluted in PBS, 24 fM for dilution in CSF, and 22 fM for dilution in the plasma fraction.

DISCUSSION

In the present work we applied stabilized Aβ oligomers as standard in the sFIDA assay. For dilutions in PBS, CSF from control donors, and blood plasma from control donors, the sFIDA readout correlated with the oligomer concentration over five to six orders of magnitude. Although oligomer concentrations in the upper picomolar range are presumably not physiologically relevant, the observed linearity over several orders of magnitude is useful to check assay functionality and to facilitate assay calibration. The calculated LLODs for oligomers diluted in PBS, CSF, and a plasma fraction were in the range of 14–22 fM particle concentration. We can exclude that endogenous Aβ oligomers, which are possibly present also in healthy subjects, contribute significantly to the assay readout, since the intensity cutoff was determined based on the non-spiked control samples.

For the lower concentrations from 1 pM down to 1 fM, a linear relation between the sFIDA readout and concentrations of Aβ oligomers was observed. We expect that to be the relevant concentration range for analysis of biological samples, as published concentrations of oligomers in CSF are in the femtomolar to low picomolar range (stated as monomeric concentrations of Aβ; oligomeric concentrations are even lower; Bruggink et al., 2013; Hölttä et al., 2013; Savage et al., 2014).

LLODs often refer to the concentration or mass of the total applied peptide, although the actual portion of oligomerized Aβ and the size of Aβ oligomers in the preparations is mostly unknown (Santos et al., 2007; Sancesario et al., 2012). The concentration of 14 fM of the stabilized oligomers used in this study corresponds to 3.1 pM (13.9 ng/L) monomeric $A\beta_{1-42}$. The LLOD given in mass per volume is roughly in the same range or above the limits of detection published for some Aβ oligomer specific ELISA (Fukumoto et al., 2010; Bruggink et al., 2013; Hölttä et al., 2013; Savage et al., 2014). In principle, sFIDA allows detection and quantification of single particles of oligomers consisting of approximately 220 Aβ monomers.

Although the stabilized oligomers used in this study might not accurately reflect the properties of native Aβ oligomers in terms of composition, mass, and structural heterogeneity, they are nevertheless a valuable tool for assay development, assay calibration, and determination of inter- and intra-assay variation due to their stability and homogenous size. While heterogeneous Aβ oligomer standards would resemble endogenous conditions more closely, it is hardly possible to reliably produce such standards with minimal batch-to-batch-variations thus limiting their use in assay validation.

The stabilized oligomers are advantageous with regard to long term stability and they can easily be distributed to compare inter-laboratory results. This enables to thoroughly validate and calibrate an assay, which is a very important feature in assay development. However, the applicability of this standard for biological samples will have to be addressed in future studies. Quantification of very small oligomers in body fluids might emphasize the need for even smaller standard oligomers than the ones used in this study.

We have previously shown that monomers of synthetic Aβ give not rise to significant signals in the sFIDA assay by using overlapping epitopes in the capture and detection system (Wang-Dietrich et al., 2013). When analyzing native CSF samples in diagnostic setups, however, experimental conditions (i.e., pH, incubation times, freeze/thaw cycles) have to be carefully adjusted to avoid false-positive signals due to artificial aggregation of endogenous Aβ monomers.

In the present version of the assay, two N-terminal antibodies were used for capturing and detection of Aβ, i.e., Nab228 (epitope Aβ1-11) and 6E10 (epitope Aβ3-8). By using alternative capture and probe antibodies, it is not only possible to detect oligomers composed of different Aβ isoforms, but also to detect hybrid aggregates composed of different peptides or proteins. Therefore, sFIDA assay can in future be applied for scientific purpose in order to investigate the presence and pathological relevance of different oligomeric species in body fluids or brain homogenates of patients with different neurodegenerative diseases, such as AD. Additionally, after thorough investigation and validation of the assay and the measured targets, sFIDA might either give extra information useful for diagnostics or even measure oligomeric biomarkers that allow a reliable diagnosis, and might be useful for disease monitoring in clinical trials during treatment.

AUTHOR CONTRIBUTIONS

KKU, MH, YH, KKR, AK, CL, LP, KW, JW conducted experiments. KKU, DW, and OB designed experiments and wrote the manuscript.

ACKNOWLEDGMENTS

This work was supported by the Federal Ministry of Education and Research within the projects VIP (03V0641), KNDD (01GI1010A), and JPND/BIOMARKAPD (01ED1203H).

REFERENCES

Ballard, C., Gauthier, S., Corbett, A., Brayne, C., Aarsland, D., and Jones, E. (2011). Alzheimer's disease. *Lancet* 377, 1019–1031. doi: 10.1016/S0140-6736(10)61349-9

Bannach, O., Birkmann, E., Reinartz, E., Jaeger, K. E., Langeveld, J. P., Rohwer, R. G., et al. (2012). Detection of prion protein particles in blood plasma of scrapie infected sheep. *PLoS ONE* 7:e36620. doi: 10.1371/journal.pone.0036620

Benjamini, Y., and Hochberg, Y. (1995). Controlling the false discovery rate: a practical and powerful approach to multiple testing. *J. R. Stat. Soc. B* 57, 289–300.

Birkmann, E., Henke, F., Weinmann, N., Dumpitak, C., Groschup, M., Funke, A., et al. (2007). Counting of single prion particles bound to a capture-antibody surface (surface-FIDA). *Vet. Microbiol.* 123, 294–304. doi: 10.1016/j.vetmic.2007.04.001

Blennow, K., Hampel, H., Weiner, M., and Zetterberg, H. (2010). Cerebrospinal fluid and plasma biomarkers in Alzheimer disease. *Nat. Rev. Neurol.* 6, 131–144. doi: 10.1038/nrneurol.2010.4

Braak, H., and Braak, E. (1991). Neuropathological stageing of Alzheimer-related changes. *Acta Neuropathol.* 82, 239–259. doi: 10.1007/BF00308809

Bruggink, K. A., Jongbloed, W., Biemans, E. A. L. M., Veerhuis, R., Claassen, J. A. H. R., Verbeek, M. M., et al. (2013). Amyloid-β oligomer detection by ELISA in cerebrospinal fluid and brain tissue. *Anal. Biochem.* 433, 112–120. doi: 10.1016/j.ab.2012.09.014

Cleary, J. P., Walsh, D. M., Hofmeister, J. J., Shankar, G. M., Kuskowski, M. A., Selkoe, D. J., et al. (2004). Natural oligomers of the amyloid-β protein specifically disrupt cognitive function. *Nat. Neurosci.* 8, 79–84. doi: 10.1038/nn1372

Crossbeta Biosciences (2015). *Crossbeta Oligomer Publications* [Online]. Available online at: http://www.crossbeta.com/technology/publications/ (Accessed December 07, 2015).

Fukumoto, H., Tokuda, T., Kasai, T., Ishigami, N., Hidaka, H., Kondo, M., et al. (2010). High-molecular-weight β-amyloid oligomers are elevated in cerebrospinal fluid of Alzheimer patients. *FASEB J.* 24, 2716–2726. doi: 10.1096/fj.09-150359

Funke, S. A., Birkmann, E., Henke, F., Görtz, P., Lange-Asschenfeldt, C., Riesner, D., et al. (2007). Single particle detection of Abeta aggregates associated with Alzheimer's disease. *Biochem. Biophys. Res. Commun.* 364, 902–907. doi: 10.1016/j.bbrc.2007.10.085

Funke, S. A., Wang, L., Birkmann, E., and Willbold, D. (2010). Single-particle detection system for Aβ aggregates: adaptation of surface-fluorescence intensity distribution analysis to laser scanning microscopy. *Rejuvenation Res.* 13, 206–209. doi: 10.1089/rej.2009.0925

Golde, T. E., Schneider, L. S., and Koo, E. H. (2011). Anti-aβ therapeutics in Alzheimer's disease: the need for a paradigm shift. *Neuron* 69, 203–213. doi: 10.1016/j.neuron.2011.01.002

Haass, C., Kaether, C., Thinakaran, G., and Sisodia, S. (2012). Trafficking and proteolytic processing of APP. *Cold Spring Harb. Perspect. Med.* 2:a006270. doi: 10.1101/cshperspect.a006270

Haass, C., and Selkoe, D. J. (2007). Soluble protein oligomers in neurodegeneration: lessons from the Alzheimer's amyloid β-peptide. *Nat. Rev. Mol. Cell Biol.* 8, 101–112. doi: 10.1038/nrm2101

Hölttä, M., Hansson, O., Andreasson, U., Hertze, J., Minthon, L., Nägga, K., et al. (2013). Evaluating amyloid-β oligomers in cerebrospinal fluid as a biomarker for Alzheimer's disease. *PLoS ONE* 8:e66381. doi: 10.1371/journal.pone.0066381

Humpel, C. (2011). Identifying and validating biomarkers for Alzheimer's disease. *Trends Biotechnol.* 29, 26–32. doi: 10.1016/j.tibtech.2010.09.007

Janissen, R., Oberbarnscheidt, L., and Oesterhelt, F. (2009). Optimized straight forward procedure for covalent surface immobilization of different biomolecules for single molecule applications. *Colloids Surf. B Biointerfaces* 71, 200–207. doi: 10.1016/j.colsurfb.2009.02.011

Lansdall, C. J. (2014). An effective treatment for Alzheimer's disease must consider both amyloid and tau. *Biosci. Horizons* 7:hzu002. doi: 10.1093/biohorizons/hzu002

Lesné, S., Koh, M. T., Kotilinek, L., Kayed, R., Glabe, C. G., Yang, A., et al. (2006). A specific amyloid-β protein assembly in the brain impairs memory. *Nature* 440, 352–357. doi: 10.1038/nature04533

McLean, C. A., Cherny, R. A., Fraser, F. W., Fuller, S. J., Smith, M. J., Vbeyreuther, K., et al. (1999). Soluble pool of Aβ amyloid as a determinant of severity of neurodegeneration in Alzheimer's disease. *Ann. Neurol.* 46, 860–866.

Prince, M., Bryce, R., Albanese, E., Wimo, A., Ribeiro, W., and Ferri, C. P. (2013). The global prevalence of dementia: a systematic review and metaanalysis. *Alzheimer's Dement.* 9, 63–75. doi: 10.1016/j.jalz.2012.11.007

Rosén, C., Hansson, O., Blennow, K., and Zetterberg, H. (2013). Fluid biomarkers in Alzheimer's disease - current concepts. *Mol. Neurodegener.* 8:20. doi: 10.1186/1750-1326-8-20

Sancesario, G. M., Cencioni, M. T., Esposito, Z., Borsellino, G., Nuccetelli, M., Martorana, A., et al. (2012). The load of amyloid-β oligomers is decreased in the cerebrospinal fluid of Alzheimer's disease patients. *J. Alzheimers Dis.* 31, 865–878. doi: 10.3233/JAD-2012-120211

Santos, A. N., Torkler, S., Nowak, D., Schlittig, C., Goerdes, M., Lauber, T., et al. (2007). Detection of amyloid-β oligomers in human cerebrospinal fluid by flow cytometry and fluorescence resonance energy transfer. *J. Alzheimers Dis.* 11, 117–125.

Savage, M. J., Kalinina, J., Wolfe, A., Tugusheva, K., Korn, R., Cash-Mason, T., et al. (2014). A sensitive Aβ oligomer assay discriminates alzheimer's and aged control cerebrospinal fluid. *J. Neurosci.* 34, 2884–2897. doi: 10.1523/JNEUROSCI.1675-13.2014

Shaw, L. M., Vanderstichele, H., Knapik-Czajka, M., Clark, C. M., Aisen, P. S., Petersen, R. C., et al. (2009). Cerebrospinal fluid biomarker signature in Alzheimer's disease neuroimaging initiative subjects. *Ann. Neurol.* 65, 403–413. doi: 10.1002/ana.21610

Sunderland, T., Linker, G., Mirza, N., Putnam, K. T., Friedman, D. L., Kimmel, L. H., et al. (2003). Decreased β-amyloid1-42 and increased tau levels in cerebrospinal fluid of patients with Alzheimer disease. *JAMA* 289, 2094–2103. doi: 10.1001/jama.289.16.2094

Wang-Dietrich, L., Funke, S. A., Kühbach, K., Wang, K., Besmehn, A., Willbold, S., et al. (2013). The amyloid-β oligomer count in cerebrospinal fluid is a biomarker for Alzheimer's disease. *J. Alzheimers Dis.* 34, 985–994. doi: 10.3233/JAD-122047

6

Fluid biomarkers in clinical trials of Alzheimer's disease therapeutics

Aaron Ritter and Jeffrey Cummings*

Cleveland Clinic Lou Ruvo Center for Brain Health, Las Vegas, NV, USA

Edited by:
Charlotte Elisabeth Teunissen, VU University Medical Center Amsterdam, Netherlands

Reviewed by:
Ricardo Insausti, University of Castilla-La Mancha, Spain
Douglas Galasko, University of California San Diego, USA

****Correspondence:***
Aaron Ritter, Cleveland Clinic Lou Ruvo Center for Brain Health, 888 West Bonneville Avenue, Las Vegas, NV 89016, USA
rittera@ccf.org

With the demographic shift of the global population toward longer life expectancy, the number of people living with Alzheimer's disease (AD) has rapidly expanded and is projected to triple by the year 2050. Current treatments provide symptomatic relief but do not affect the underlying pathology of the disease. Therapies that prevent or slow the progression of the disease are urgently needed to avoid this growing public health emergency. Insights gained from decades of research have begun to unlock the pathophysiology of this complex disease and have provided targets for disease-modifying therapies. In the last decade, few therapeutic agents designed to modify the underlying disease process have progressed to clinical trials and none have been brought to market. With the focus on disease modification, biomarkers promise to play an increasingly important role in clinical trials. Six biomarkers have now been included in diagnostic criteria for AD and are regularly incorporated into clinical trials. Three biomarkers are neuroimaging measures – hippocampal atrophy measured by magnetic resonance imaging (MRI), amyloid uptake as measured by Pittsburg compound B positron emission tomography (PiB-PET), and decreased fluorodeoxyglucose (18F) uptake as measured by PET (FDG-PET) – and three are sampled from fluid sources – cerebrospinal fluid levels of amyloid β42 (Aβ42), total tau, and phosphorylated tau. Fluid biomarkers are important because they can provide information regarding the underlying biochemical processes that are occurring in the brain. The purpose of this paper is to review the literature regarding the existing and emerging fluid biomarkers and to examine how fluid biomarkers have been incorporated into clinical trials.

Keywords: Alzheimer's disease, amyloid cascade hypothesis, amyloid beta, tau, clinical trials, drugs

Introduction

Alzheimer's disease (AD), the most common cause of dementia, is a progressive neurodegenerative disorder that becomes more prevalent with increasing age. Currently, there are more than 44 million people worldwide living with dementia (1). As the demographics of the global population shift toward longer life, it is projected that this number will be more than triple by the year 2050. With the estimated cost of dementia already exceeding 1% of the world's gross domestic product (1), this rapid increase constitutes a looming public health emergency. Available therapies for AD were approved based on their ability to improve the symptoms of the disease but do not alter underlying pathophysiologic processes (2). In order to ease the public health burden posed by AD, drugs with disease-modifying properties are urgently needed.

Insights gained from decades of AD research have begun to elucidate the pathophysiology underlying this complex disease. It is now widely accepted that the chain of biochemical events thought to be responsible for AD are triggered many years prior to symptom onset (3). While an enhanced understanding of the two characteristic pathological changes seen in AD – plaques composed of amyloid β (Aβ) and neurofibrillary tangles (NFTs) composed of hyperphosphorylated tau – have yielded targets that may be amenable to pharmacological intervention, no therapeutics with potentially disease-modifying properties have advanced past Phase III trials. A number of theories have been proposed to explain this failure: (1) selection of patients based on clinical diagnosis can be inaccurate, leading to the inclusion of large number of patients without AD in clinical trials (4): (2) the timing of interventions designed to clear amyloid – at stages when subjects have already begun to manifest the symptoms of mild to moderate dementia – is too late in the disease course to affect cognitive change (5, 6): (3) the progression of the disease is too gradual to demonstrate drug–placebo differences in "typical length" drug trials (7): (4) candidate agents have been permitted to advance to Phase III trials without strong evidence of target engagement or disease modification from preclinical models or early clinical trials (8).

New strategies are needed to address the high failure rate in AD drug development. New trial designs, centralized rating and review, more predictive models in preclinical testing, improved clinical outcome measures, and more stringent testing of drugs in Phase II are all strategies that may improve success rates. While proof of efficacy of AD treatments will ultimately depend on demonstration of benefit on clinical measures, biological markers (biomarkers) of underlying disease processes will take on enhanced significance, especially as trials move toward enrolling subjects earlier in the disease process.

Aided by the development of biomarkers, AD is now considered one clinical disease with a continuum through several clinical stages (5). Reflecting this change in disease conception, several biomarkers have now been accepted widely enough that they have been incorporated into the two most recent research criteria (9–12). Three of these biomarkers are imaging biomarkers: hippocampal atrophy as detected by structural magnetic resonance imaging (MRI); decreased uptake of (18F) in characteristic regions on positron emission tomography (FDG-PET); and increased amyloid tracer retention on PET (PiB-PET). Three biomarkers are cerebrospinal fluid (CSF) protein levels: low CSF levels of amyloid β42 (Aβ42) and elevated CSF levels of total (t-tau) and phosphorylated tau (p-tau). Imaging biomarkers are important because they can provide crucial information about topographical changes in the brain. There are a number of excellent reviews describing their use in both clinical practice and drug trials (13). They will not be described here. The focus of this contribution is fluid biomarkers. The purpose of this paper is to review the literature regarding the existing and emerging fluid biomarkers and to examine how fluid biomarkers have been incorporated into clinical trials.

Fluid Biomarkers Regularly Incorporated into Clinical Trials

CSF Aβ42

A picture of the complex chain of events leading to AD has emerged over the last three decades. The leading theory to explain the pathophysiological changes in AD is the amyloid cascade hypothesis (14). Based largely on models derived from familial cases of AD – in which, one of three autosomal dominantly inherited mutations results in pathological aggregation and accumulation of Aβ – the amyloid cascade hypothesis posits that the pathological accumulation of amyloid triggers a complex sequence of biochemical events ultimately leading to widespread synaptic dysfunction, neuronal dysfunction, and cell death. An overview of the initial steps involved in Aβ production is provided in **Figure 1**.

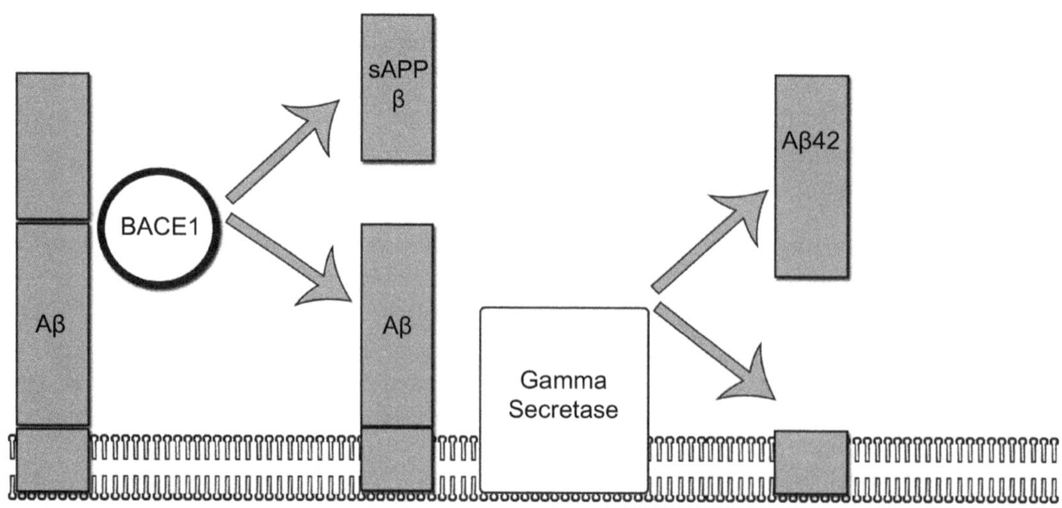

FIGURE 1 | The amyloidogenic pathway. In the amyloidogenic pathway, The amyloid precursor protein (APP) is processed in two sequential steps: (1) in the first step, APP is cleaved by BACE1 yielding a membrane-bound fragment and releasing sAPP into the interstitial space. (2) In the second step, gamma secretase cleaves the remaining membrane-bound fragment releasing an abeta 42 fragment.

The amount of Aβ in the brain is determined by a balance between Aβ production and degradation/clearance mechanisms (15). Several enzymes, such as neprilysin, insulin-degrading enzyme, plasminogen inhibitor, break down Aβ in the interstitial space (16). Fragments that are not degraded in the brain are actively transported across the blood–brain barrier (BBB) or diffuse into the CSF space (17). The two transport proteins responsible for Aβ efflux from the brain are the low density lipoprotein receptor related protein-1 (LRP-1) and Apo J (15). Once in blood, Aβ is rapidly taken up by plasma proteins and transported to the liver for further degradation. A dynamic equilibrium exists between the amount of Aβ in the CSF and the amount of Aβ in the plasma space, and a small amount of non-neuronal Aβ is found in the CSF. A transport protein known as the receptor for advanced end products (RAGE) is responsible for the influx of Aβ from the serum into the CNS. The amount of amyloid in the brain is a highly regulated process and it is estimated that the entire load of soluble Aβ is turned over twice per day (17).

In AD, there is a significant decrease in Aβ clearance (18) resulting in dramatic increases (100–1,000 fold) in the amount of Aβ in the brain (17). Aβ fragments consisting of 42 amino acids (Aβ42) are particularly prone to aggregation (19). As amyloid concentrations rise, Aβ42 fragments rapidly aggregate into oligomers of various sizes and conformations (20). Aβ oligomers are neurotoxic and have been shown to inhibit memory, disrupt long-term potentiation, and impair synaptic function in animal models (21, 22). Emerging data is beginning to clarify the role that Aβ oligomers play in triggering AD pathophysiology (23). In addition to oligomerizing, Aβ fragments also fibrillize into cross-β-sheets, forming the insoluble plaques that constitute the main neuropathological finding in AD. The primary role of amyloid plaques seems to be to serve as large reservoirs of soluble amyloid (the amount of insoluble fibrillar Aβ is 100-fold greater than the amount of soluble Aβ in the brain) (24). Plaques may serve to buffer any changes in the amount of circulating amyloid. Plaques, however, are not entirely benign species as array tomography has revealed that they are surrounded by a ring of dystrophic and disfigured neurons (25), implying that they exert local neurotoxic effects (26). Plaque burden, however, correlates poorly with disease severity (27, 28) and it is now widely thought that Aβ's primary role in the pathogenesis of AD is by triggering another pathological process (29).

Several commercially available, CSF enzyme-linked immunosorbent assays (ELISAs) have been developed that detect CSF Aβ. CSF assays for Aβ detect soluble monomeric species. In AD, levels of CSF Aβ 40 remain stable while Aβ42 levels have consistently been shown drop to <50% of normal (30). The reduction in CSF Aβ42 levels is generally thought to reflect both the sequestration of Aβ42 in insoluble plaques (27) and aggregation into oligomeric species (31). Post-mortem studies have also reported correlations between low CSF Aβ42 and increased amyloid plaque load (32, 33). With the development of amyloid PET imaging (which allows for the direct visualization of fibrillar amyloid), the relationship between low CSF Aβ42 levels and amyloid plaque has been established *in vivo* (34) and has been confirmed in many different studies (35, 36). Although low CSF Aβ42 levels and increased fibrillar uptake on PET scan generally correspond with one another and are often used interchangeably to diagnose AD, it is important to note that they are not detecting the same form of amyloid (CSF assays detect monomeric, soluble amyloid while PET imaging detects fibrillar plaque). The discrepancy between the two measures has been illustrated in several studies (37, 38). A recent study using cross-sectional data found that 20% of cognitively normal subjects had low CSF Aβ42 levels but negative PET scans. This discrepancy was seen in only 6% of subjects with dementia (38). PET scan positivity was also found to correlate closely with increased CSF tau levels. The authors interpreted these findings to suggest that CSF Aβ42 "positivity" comes earlier in the disease progression than amyloid uptake on PET scan. If this finding is verified in longitudinal studies, it would suggest that low levels of CSF Aβ42 may be a marker of early disease processes while amyloid scanning would have utility as a marker of disease progression.

CSF Tau

Neurofibrillary tangles composed of hyperphosphorylated tau are the second major neuropathologic finding in AD. Tau is a ubiquitous intracellular protein that promotes cellular stability through interactions with microtubule proteins (39). Consequently, tau plays a key role in maintaining neuronal integrity, cellular signaling, and axonal transport. The dynamic relationship that exists between tau and microtubule proteins is driven by the phosphorylation state of tau, which is under the control of a variety of kinases and phosphatases (40, 41). In AD, for reasons that remain to be elucidated, the phosphorylation state of tau increases (42). Various theories have been proposed to explain this phenomenon. A leading theory is that it is a direct response to the toxic effects of Aβ accumulation (43); however, other potential causes include neuroinflammation (44), oxidative stress (45), genetic factors (46), or even infection (47). Tau hyperphosphorylation is a key step in the pathogenesis of AD because hyperphorsphorylated tau no longer binds to microtubule proteins (48). This leads to higher cytosolic concentrations of unbound tau. Unbound, hyperphosphorylated tau is susceptible to aggregation, protein trapping, and misfolding (49, 50). Aggregated fibrils consisting of hyperphosphorylaed tau comprise the helical filaments in NFTs. The accumulation of NFTs within neuronal axons is toxic to cells. Both the loss of normal physiological function (i.e., loss of cellular integrity) and the gain of toxicity induced by NFT accretion are thought to contribute to neuronal dysfunction in AD (50).

In AD, NFT accumulation proceeds through the brain in a stereotypical pattern, appearing first in the locus coeruleus and the entorhinal cortex, proceeding next to the hippocampus, and then spreading to the temporal cortex and neocortical association areas (51). Neuropathological studies have reported correlations between NFT formation and neuronal loss, both of which increase in parallel with AD disease progression (52). Understanding the intercellular spread of NFT as it progresses through the brain has been the focus of recent investigation (53, 54). In mouse models, injection of filamentous tau induces NFT formation at the injection site that over time progresses to neighboring and synaptically connected brain regions (55). This finding suggests that tau exhibits prion-like behavior as it spreads from highly focal brain regions to involvement of limbic, paralimbic, and neocortical regions (56).

In AD, CSF levels of t-tau increase to 3× normal (57). Increases in CSF t-tau have been associated with both NFT burden and Braak staging (33). Elevations in CSF t-tau, however, are not specific to AD as transient elevations are found following stroke (58) and traumatic brain injury (TBI) (59). This finding suggests that elevated CSF t-tau levels are reflective of non-specific neuronal injury and cell death. The highest levels of CSF t-tau are found in Creutzfeldt–Jakob disease (CJD), a disease characterized by accelerated neurodegeneration (60). It is also important to note that tau secretion is an active physiological process, occurring independently of neuronal injury (56). In AD, an additional source of CSF tau is the residence of this molecule in extracellular space during its passage from neuron to neuron. More research is needed to fully understand the composition of CSF t-tau levels in AD.

In addition to detecting total tau (t-tau), several ELISAs have been developed that reflect the phosphorylation state of tau. In AD, CSF levels of p-tau increase to approximately twice normal levels. Commonly used assays measure tau phosphorylation at residue either 181 or 231, both of which increase to similar levels in AD (61). Autopsy studies reveal that CSF p-tau correlates with NFT burden in AD (62). Because levels of p-tau are thought to reflect both NFT load and phosphorylation state, elevations in p-tau are generally thought to be a more specific finding in AD than elevations in CSF t-tau (61, 63). Dissociations between high t-tau and normal p-tau levels have been reported in several dementing diseases including CJD (64), frontotemporal dementia, and vascular dementia (61).

Utility of CSF Aβ42, t-Tau, and p-Tau

Used individually, CSF markers (CSF Aβ42 or tau) demonstrate good sensitivity in distinguishing subjects with AD from non-controls (41); however, several studies have reported poor specificity in distinguishing subjects with AD from non-AD dementias (65–67). Diagnostic precision has also been shown to decrease with increasing age (68). Diagnostic accuracy increases considerably when these measures are combined into a so-called "AD signature" consisting of low Aβ42 and elevated total and p-tau. This signature demonstrates 80–95% sensitivity and specificity in identifying subjects with AD in the dementia phase of disease (5) and has been shown to be highly predictive of AD pathology at autopsy (28). The ability of CSF biomarkers to identify subjects harboring AD pathology is considerably better than the accuracy of a diagnosis made on clinical grounds alone. In a study looking at 919 autopsy-confirmed cases of AD that comprise the National Alzheimer's Coordinating Center (NACC) database, clinical diagnosis was 71–88% sensitive but only 44–71% specific in predicting AD pathology at autopsy (69). The challenge of accurately identifying subjects with AD pathology based on clinical diagnosis alone has also been demonstrated in clinical trials that have incorporated amyloid PET scans (4, 70, 71). Data from several clinical trials suggest that a substantial percentage of subjects enrolled in clinical trials do not actually have evidence of AD pathology on PET scan. For example, in the Phase III trial of bapineuzumab >35% of APOE ε4 non-carriers had negative amyloid scans (70). As it is unlikely that compounds with putative anti-AD properties will produce clinical benefits in subjects without AD pathology, inaccurate inclusion rates increase the likelihood of trial failure. Incorporating CSF biomarkers into inclusion criteria is a strategy that can be used to enrich patient samples, increase a trial's statistical power, and ensure that candidate compounds are being accurately tested against the AD substrates they are designed to ameliorate.

The temporal relationship among Aβ42, t-tau, and p-tau levels has been the subject of much exploration and several models have been proposed to explain the complex dynamics that exist between CSF biomarkers and disease progression (43, 72). There is now convincing evidence that CSF Aβ42 and tau levels convert from normal to "pathologic" years before the onset of clinical symptoms, providing a powerful tool to assess which individuals are at risk for developing AD dementia (73). Decreases in CSF Aβ42 are typically appreciated before changes in CSF tau, and in accordance with the amyloid cascade hypothesis, suggest that amyloid accumulation drives tau pathology. Examining a cohort of subjects with autosomal dominant AD, Bateman et al. demonstrated that changes in Aβ42 can be fully appreciated 25 years before expected symptom onset and changes in tau 15 years before expected symptoms onset (3). In cohorts without AD mutations, several studies have reported that decreases in CSF Aβ42 (with or without changes in CSF tau) can be detected in cognitively normal subjects and predict the development of cognitive decline (74) and dementia (75, 76). CSF biomarkers have also showed good sensitivity (83–95%) and specificity (71–90%) in predicting which subjects with mild cognitive impairment (MCI) will progress to develop AD dementia (77–80). The accurate identification of patients in this early stage of the disease is important because MCI is a non-specific syndrome and only around 50% of subjects with MCI are thought to have AD (81). Using CSF biomarkers to accurately identify subjects harboring AD pathology as early as possible in the disease course will allow for testing of candidate compounds earlier in the disease course and at time points that may prove more amenable to pharmacological intervention.

While the CSF biomarkers discussed above provide a powerful window into the pathological processes occurring in AD, several limitations deserve mention. An innate limitation of all fluid biomarkers is that they lack anatomical precision (82). Unlike imaging biomarkers, CSF biomarkers do not provide insight into the topographic distribution of pathological changes in the brain. Another limitation of current CSF biomarkers is that aside from small increases in t-tau (83), they remain fairly stable during the dementia phase of disease (84). Therefore, current CSF biomarkers have limited utility in disease staging or prognosis (73). Furthermore, because only weak associations between CSF biomarkers and clinical measures have been reported (85), it is unknown if drug-induced changes in these measures will result in clinically meaningful effects (16). Unknown variables include when interventions need to be timed and to what degree a biomarker change may be correlated with a clinical outcome (86). An additional limitation of CSF biomarkers is the high degree of variability and lack of assay standardization that exists among laboratories. A 2013 study analyzing data from Alzheimer's

Association quality control program reported a 20–30% discrepancy among laboratories in measuring CSF biomarkers (68). This is too high for globally accepted reference ranges to be assigned (87). Quality control and standardization projects have been initiated with the intent of improving precision and reproducibility across laboratories (5).

Emerging CSF Biomarkers

Given the limitations of the currently used CSF biomarkers, substantial research has been devoted to finding and validating additional CSF biomarkers. Guided by an enhanced understanding of the neurobiological changes in AD, several promising candidate markers have been identified. **Table 1** summarizes the development of CSF candidates.

Amyloid-Related CSF Biomarker Candidates

BACE1

BACE1 is an aspartic protease that catalyzes the rate-limiting step in the generation of Aβ42 (**Figure 1**). BACE1 also plays a role in the processing of other membrane proteins, such as neuregulin (88), and is thought to influence myelination (89) and synaptic plasticity (90). Because of its diverse and important role in normal brain functioning, BACE1 activity is synchronized by a variety of complicated regulatory mechanisms at both the transcriptional and translational levels (91). Increased levels of BACE1 and indicators of BACE1 activity have been found in the brains of patients with AD (92, 93). Elevations in CSF BACE1 have also been detected in the CSF of patients with AD (94, 95) and subjects with MCI who later went on to develop AD (96). Several explanations have been proposed to account for the increases in CSF BACE1 in AD. Increased CSF BACE1 levels have been found to correlate with increases in CSF t-tau (96) and one possibility is that BACE1 release into the CSF is a product of a non-specific release of proteins from injured or dying neurons. New research, however, suggests a more complicated picture, in which, normal regulatory controls on BACE1 activity are lost. Faghihi et al., for example, has reported that a non-coding antisense RNA that stabilizes BACE1 mRNA and results in increased BACE1 activity is increased in the brains of subjects with AD. Furthermore, *in vitro* exposure of cells to Aβ42 induces this antisense RNA, laying the groundwork for a deleterious feed-forward cycle of AD disease progression, in which, increased levels of Aβ induce the expression of increased BACE1 activity and further Aβ production (97). CSF BACE1 will be important in establishing target engagement in compounds with putative BACE1 inhibiting properties.

sAPP-β

The first step in APP processing is the proteolytic cleavage by BACE1. This cleavage yields two products, one of which is the membrane bound fragment (which then undergoes further processing by gamma secretase to eventually form Aβ) and the other, a larger amino acid fragment, sAPP-β, which is secreted into the interstitial space. Levels of CSF sAPP-β may serve as an indirect marker of BACE activity and Aβ production. Studies looking at the clinical correlation between CSF sAPP-β have generally been positive and elevated levels of sAPP-β have been reported in MCI (98), AD (99), and patients with incipient AD (100). However, not all studies have demonstrated meaningful clinical correlations (79). Changes in CSF levels of sAPP-β may eventually be used in clinical trials to provide evidence of target engagement and to monitor for drug effects.

Aβ Oligomers

In vitro exposure of Aβ oligomers to hippocampal neurons quickly impairs synaptic function and is more toxic than

TABLE 1 | Candidate CSF biomarkers.

Biomarker	Role in the pathogenesis of AD	Evidence for clinical utility
CSF BACE1	Transmembrane secretase responsible for the rate-limiting step in the generation of amyloid	Increased CSF BACE in AD in some (94) but not all studies (209) Increased CSF BACE levels predicted which subjects with MCI progressed to dementia (96)
CSF sAPP	Byproduct of BACE activity	Increased CSF levels in MCI (98), AD (99), and incipient AD (100) Elevated CSF levels were not predictive of subjects converting from MCI to dementia (79)
CSF Aβ oligomers	Neurotoxic species that inhibit memory, long-term potentiation, and synaptic function	Low levels make detection difficult (103, 104) (105) Inverse correlation between CSF Aβ oligomers and MMSE score (104, 105)
CSF Aβ38	Aβ fragment consisting of 38 amino acids	Increased CSF levels do not correlate with amyloid uptake on PET scan (110) CSF levels did not discriminate between healthy controls and subjects with AD (111)
CSF visinin-like protein-1 (VILIP-1)	Neuronal calcium sensor protein that functions in membrane trafficking	CSF VILIP-1 levels correlated with elevated CSF t-tau and p-tau and decreased brain volumes (115) Elevated CSF levels predicted cognitive decline in subjects with MCI (117)
CSF F2-isoprostanes	Markers of lipid peroxidation caused by free radicals	Increased CSF levels in AD (121) Increased CSF levels predicted cognitive decline in MCI (122) Increased CSF levels improved diagnostic accuracy when combined with MRI and memory testing (123)
YLK-40	Marker of plaque-associated neuroinflammation secreted by activated microglia	Elevated CSF levels in early AD (126) Elevated CSF levels predicted cognitive decline in MCI (127)
Neurogranin	Synaptic protein involved in plasticity and long-term potentiation	Elevated CSF levels in AD but not MCI (130) Elevated CSF levels predict conversion from MCI to AD and predicted a more rapid rate of decline in subjects with MCI and a positive amyloid PET scan (131)

exposure to monomeric or fibrillar forms of amyloid (101). This finding, in conjunction with reports from several animal models that demonstrate neuroanatomical and behavioral abnormalities before the appearance of plaques (25), has led the field to consider the role of Aβ oligomers in AD pathogenesis. The steady state of Aβ oligomers in the CSF is very low – <0.02% of total CSF Aβ levels (102) – and attempts to detect them standard assays have failed (101) while other attempts have produced variable results (103–105). Recently, Hong et al. were able to demonstrate that Aβ oligomers in the interstitial fluid were quickly sequestered onto cellular membranes, displaying a particular affinity for GM1 gangliosides (102). In this study, Aβ oligomers demonstrated a higher binding affinity for cell membranes than monomeric Aβ species, potentially explaining the low contribution of oligomers to the overall composition of CSF Aβ levels. The authors were also able to detect low levels of GM1-bound Aβ in human CSF. These levels correlated with CSF Aβ42. Further investigation is needed to determine if CSF GM1-bound Aβ will prove useful as a biomarker in AD. It is also important to note that soluble Aβ oligomers may have utility as a progression biomarker, as two studies – one using flow cytometry (105) and the other using ELISA (104) – have reported an inverse correlation between levels of CSF Aβ oligomers and score on MMSE. The challenges of reliably quantifying Aβ oligomers in CSF will need to be overcome before the potential of this biomarker can be fully realized.

Aβ Isoforms

While most Aβ species exist as peptide fragments consisting of either 40 or 42 amino acids, isoforms of varying length have also been detected in the CSF of patients with AD (106–108). One small study reported that a particular CSF amyloid "signature" consisting of Aβ16, Aβ33, Aβ39, and Aβ42 could distinguish subjects with AD from controls with an accuracy of 86% (106). The performance of Aβ38 has been investigated in a number of studies and as an exploratory measure in a phase II trial of avagacestat (109). The utility of CSF Aβ38 appears to be limited given that levels do not correlate with amyloid uptake on PET (110) and did not discriminate controls from subjects with AD in another study (111).

Non-Amyloid CSF Biomarker Candidates

Cerebrospinal fluid markers that reflect processes that occur after amyloid deposition, including neurodegeneration, synapse loss, neuroinflammation, oxidative stress, etc. may also provide diagnostic and prognostic utility. A select group of candidates will be discussed here. For a comprehensive review, the reader is directed to the review by Fagan and Perrin (112).

Visinin-Like Protein-1

Visinin-like protein-1 (VILIP-1) is a neuronal calcium sensor protein that can be detected in most regions of the brain (sparing the caudate and putamen) (113). It belongs to a family of proteins thought to play a role in membrane trafficking (Braunewell Cell Tissue Res) and is thought to play a role in calcium-mediated neuronal death (114). CSF levels of VILIP-1 have shown to correlate with CSF t-tau, p-tau, and brain volumes (115, 116). High levels of CSF VILIP-1 have also been reported to predict the cognitive decline in a cohort of patients with mild AD followed over a period of 2.6 years (117). Several studies have shown that higher levels of CSF VILIP-1 are seen in AD than other dementing diseases, such as dementia with Lewy bodies (114), frontotemporal dementia, and progressive supranuclear palsy (117).

F2-Isoprostanes

There is a growing body of evidence suggesting that oxidative damage plays a key role in the pathogenesis of AD (118). F2-isoprostanes are markers of lipid peroxidation caused by free radicals (119). Increased levels of F2-isoprostanes are found in AD brains (120) and in the CSF of patients with AD (121). Elevated levels of CSF F2-isoprostanes have also been shown to correlate with eventual cognitive decline in MCI (122) and improve diagnostic accuracy of AD when combined with memory testing and MRI (123).

YKL-40

Neuropathological, biochemical, and genetic studies indicate that alterations in neuroinflammatory pathways play a role in the pathogenesis of AD (124). YKL-40 is a marker of plaque-associated neuroinflammation that is secreted by activated microglia (125). Several studies suggest that YKL-40 may be an early marker of AD as levels have been shown to be increased in the preclinical phase (116, 126) and to predict cognitive decline in early stage dementia (127).

Neurogranin

Neurogranin is a synaptic protein that is enriched in forebrain areas (128). It is thought to be involved in synaptic plasticity and long-term potentiation (129). Elevated levels of neurogranin have been reported in the CSF of subjects with AD (but not MCI) (130). Elevated levels of CSF neurogranin have been shown to predict conversion from MCI to AD and to predict a more rapid rate of decline in subjects with MCI and a positive amyloid PET scan (131).

Serum Biomarkers

The process of obtaining CSF fluid by lumbar puncture (LP) is invasive and associated with a small but significant risk of post-LP headache (132). Given the negative public perception of the LP procedure, it is unlikely that all patients in a clinical trial would agree to have CSF sampling. Serum samples are easily obtained and readily accepted by patients. The development of a reliable serum biomarker could potentially be integrated into a multi-stage screening and diagnostic process, to provide valuable information about which patients should proceed to more expensive/invasive testing, and to monitor disease progression (133). Currently, there has been little success in finding reliable serum biomarkers in AD or MCI (41). **Table 2** summarizes the findings regarding candidate serum biomarkers in AD.

Serum Aβ

Despite being the focus of intense investigation, the utility of serum Aβ as AD biomarkers has not been fully defined. Serum

TABLE 2 | Candidate non-CSF biomarkers.

Biomarker	Role in the pathogenesis of AD	Evidence for clinical utility
Serum Aβ40	Major byproduct of APP processing	Associated with increased risk of AD dementia in some but not all studies (134, 135)
Serum Aβ42	Primary component amyloid plaques	Associated with increased risk of AD dementia in some but not all studies (136)
Serum tau	NFTs composed of hyperphosphorylated tau comprise major neuropathological finding in AD	Undetectable by traditional assays (148) Ultra-sensitive assays have detected and report increased levels in AD compared to normal but with considerable overlap; do not discriminate between subjects with MCI who remained stable and those who progressed to AD (150)

Aβ (40,42) levels in AD show considerable overlap with non-AD controls, which limits its use as a diagnostic marker (92). The use of serum Aβ as a marker of risk is also unclear as some studies have reported an increased risk with increased Aβ40 (134, 135) or Aβ42 (136) while others have reported that increased risk is associated with low levels of Aβ42 (137). In addition, several studies have failed to find an association between serum Aβ levels and AD risk (138, 139). One meta-analysis reported that a low Aβ42:Aβ40 ratio was associated with an increased risk of AD (140); however, the generalizability of this analysis is limited by the heterogeneity of included studies. Little is known about the prognostic value of serum levels of Aβ. One study has reported that higher baseline levels of serum Aβ42 were associated with faster rates of cognitive decline over a 1-year period in subjects with AD (141). The small sample size and the lack of follow-up analysis of plasma levels means that additional research is needed to determine if serum levels can be used for patient stratification. Changes in serum Aβ levels have also been detected in several clinical trials and have been used as evidence to support claims of target engagement (71, 142). Further investigation is needed to clarify the association between serum Aβ levels and AD pathophysiology.

One potential explanation for the discrepancy between the performance of CSF Aβ and serum Aβ is that serum levels do not accurately reflect CSF Aβ levels (143). The majority of CSF Aβ is of neuronal origin and is thought to directly reflect Aβ production in the brain. Serum Aβ, on the other hand, is derived from a variety of non-neuronal sources including the liver, bone, muscle, kidney, pancreas, and platelets (66). The physiologic milieu in the CSF is also drastically different from the serum compartment. In the serum, there are 300× more Aβ binding proteins than in the CSF (15) and the majority of Aβ in the serum is protein bound (144).

Serum Tau

Transient elevations in serum tau are detected in response to neuronal injury from ischemic stroke (145), hypoxic brain injury during cardiac arrest (146), and TBI (147). There is considerable evidence that the biochemical regulation of tau is dependent on which biological compartment it resides. For example, following neuronal injury, CSF tau may stay elevated for weeks while in the serum, tau is cleared rapidly, returning to normal levels within hours (58). As a result, serum tau levels are not thought to accurately reflect CSF tau levels. In a small study using a sandwich ELISA, serum tau levels were essentially undetectable in patients with AD despite having elevated CSF t-tau levels (148). More recently, ultra-sensitive assays have been developed that have captured changes in serum tau levels following TBI (146) and cardiac arrest (149). This assay has been tested in one cohort with AD (150). In this study, higher serum tau levels were seen in patients with AD as compared to subjects with MCI and controls; however, a considerable degree of overlap was noted across the three groups, limiting its diagnostic utility (150). Additionally, serum tau levels did not discriminate between subjects with MCI who remained stable and those with MCI who went on to develop AD.

Other Serum Markers

Other novel serum targets for development include F2-isoprostanes (151) and plasma complement factor H (152); however, the results of studies looking at these candidates have been disappointing and do not support their application as diagnostic or prognostic factors at this time.

Proteomic Approaches

An alternative approach to developing serum biomarkers in AD is to identify a characteristic profile of protein markers, which, taken together, would constitute a pathological "fingerprint" (133). Significant interest in proteomic strategies was generated following a study, which identified a characteristic pattern of 18 abnormal plasma signaling and inflammatory proteins in a sample of patients with AD (153). Applied to a pre-existing data set, this profile correctly identified subjects with AD from healthy controls with 90% accuracy. In addition, this profile predicted conversion from MCI to dementia in 20 of 22 patients (followed up to 6 years). With advances in bioinformatics, the numbers of trials employing proteomic approaches have increased. Using pre-existing data sets, a number of proteomic profiles have been identified, which have shown high diagnostic accuracy (154–157). Challenges to the proteomic approach include successful replication of findings across studies (154) and whether profiles can reach appropriate standardization levels to be replicated across laboratories (133). Guidelines designed to approach these challenges have recently been published (158). No consensus has been reached on a specific proteomic profile that provides reliable information in AD.

Urine and Saliva

Urine and saliva are appealing targets for biomarker development due to their ease of collection. Molecules sampled from these sources, however, are subjected to filtration and metabolic processing and may not reflect biochemical changes occurring in the brain. For this reason, AD research has largely ignored these biological compartments (159). One small study detected reduced acetylcholinesterase activity in the saliva of patients with AD compared to normal controls (160) while another found no difference (161). Increased levels of salivary Aβ42 have been demonstrated in patients with mild AD compared to normal controls and patients with Parkinson's disease (162). In another study using mass spectroscopy, an increased salivary p-tau to t-tau ratio was found in AD patients compared to normal controls (163). More research is needed on these readily accessible fluids to determine if they contain meaningful information on brain states.

Use of Fluid Biomarkers in Clinical Trials

The scope of use of fluid biomarkers in clinical trials is described below. Here, we describe the results of several clinical trials in which fluid biomarkers were included among outcome measures. **Table 3** summarizes the results of these studies as well as others that are not described.

Active Amyloid Immunization Strategies

The impetus for the development of amyloid immunotherapy strategies came from a landmark study involving the PDAPP transgenic mouse, which overexpresses mutant human APP. In this study, it was shown that amyloid plaque deposition could be prevented by immunizing mice against Aβ42 (164). Subsequent studies reported that active immunization attenuated memory changes and reduced behavioral impairment (165, 166). Testing in several different models revealed that the greatest benefit was seen when immunization was achieved before the expected age of amyloid deposition (164, 167), signifying that immunization strategies work best in a clearance paradigm (167).

Composed of a full-length synthetic Aβ42 molecule, AN1792 was the first anti-amyloid vaccine evaluated in clinical trials. Despite appearing safe and demonstrating efficacy on an exploratory measure of functional decline in Phase I (168), further development of AN1792 was halted after 6% of subjects developed meningoencephalitis during Phase II testing (169). While the exact cause of this response remains unknown, the type of T-cell response (Th2-biased in the Phase I study and Th1-biased in the Phase II study) differed between the two studies (170). Treatment was terminated early (only 20% developed the predetermined antibody response), but double-blind assessments were continued during the entire 12-month period. Antibody response

TABLE 3 | Fluid biomarkers in clinical trials.

Compound	Mechanism of action	Relevant clinical outcome	Fluid biomarker outcome
AN1792	Active immunization against full-length Aβ42	PII: halted because of the development of meningoencephalitis (169)	PII: reduction in CSF tau; no change in CSF Aβ42 (169)
CAD106	Active immunization against Aβ fragment	PI: well tolerated in subject with AD (176)	PI: no changes in CSF Aβ40, Aβ42, p-tau, or t-tau; increase in total serum plasma Aβ and decrease in free Aβ (176)
Bapineuzumab	Monoclonal antibody directed against N-terminus of Aβ	PII: *post hoc* analysis showed effect on cognition in APOE ε4 non-carriers (185) PIII: two separate studies (one with APOE ε4 carriers and one with non-carriers) failed to reach clinical endpoints (70) Development of MRI changes in ~20% of treated patients (210)	PII: reduction in CSF p-tau and t-tau; no effect on CSF Aβ40 or 42 (186) PIII: decrease in CSF p-tau (carriers); no effect on any CSF measures (Aβ42, p-tau, t-tau) in non-carriers; no effect on Aβ42 in carriers (70)
Solanezumab	Monoclonal antibody against middle portion of Aβ	PIII: two large trials failed to reach clinical endpoints. A pooled analysis of the two trials demonstrated an effect on cognition in subjects with mild dementia (142)	PII: increase in serum and CSF Aβ40 and 42 (190) PIII: increase in both CSF Aβ40 and 42; no effect on CSF p-tau or t-tau; increases in serum Aβ40 and 42 (142)
Crenezumab	Monoclonal antibody against middle portion of Aβ; built on IgG1 backbone	PI: well tolerated in subjects with mild to moderate AD (211)	PI: increase in serum Aβ levels (211)
Gantenerumab	Entirely humanized monoclonal antibody binds the N-terminus of Aβ fibrils	PIII: results not yet published, trial discontinued	No fluid biomarker data have been reported
Ponezumab	Humanized monoclonal antibody binds the C-terminus of Aβ	PI: well tolerated in subjects with AD (212–214)	PI: increase in serum and CSF Aβ levels w/single dose (212)
Tramiprosate	Molecule that binds Aβ and prevents aggregation	PIII: no benefit on clinical endpoints (215)	PII: reduction in CSF Aβ42 (216)
Avagacestat	Gamma secretase inhibitor	PII: well tolerated at low doses; at doses found to have CSF effects, a trend worsening cognition was detected (109)	PII: at higher, poorly tolerated doses, reductions in CSF Aβ 38, 40, and 42 were reported. Non-significant trend toward reduction in CSF p-tau and t-tau at all doses No changes in CSF Aβ at lower doses (109)
Semagacestat	Gamma secretase inhibitor	PIII: preplanned analysis showed an association with worsening cognitive and functional outcomes resulting in early termination (71)	PII: no effect on CSF Aβ40 or 42; reduction in plasma Aβ40 (201) PI: dose-dependent reduction in Aβ production as measured by SILK (18) PIII: no changes in CSF Aβ or t-tau; p-tau remained the same (increased in placebo) dose-dependent reduction in serum Aβ40 and 42 (71)

was associated with two positive clinical effects: improvement on composite scores of memory function and, in an extended follow-up study, significantly less functional decline (171). CSF monitoring in a subset of 11 subjects deemed "antibody responders" showed significant reductions in CSF t-tau (−204 ± pg/mL) at 1 year. Changes in CSF Aβ42 levels were not appreciated (169).

Several post-mortem neuropathological studies have been completed on subjects receiving the AN1792 vaccine (172–175). Because of the small number of participants and lack of information about baseline (or pretreatment) plaque burden, it is difficult to make definitive conclusions about these studies (8). Nonetheless, several interesting findings have been reported including reductions in plaque load (174) and decreased microglial activation (173). Evidence of pathological change was not, however, associated with improvement in survival time or time to severe dementia (174). Only one study (examining five brains) reported evidence of a reduction in tau pathology (175).

It is difficult to make accurate assessments regarding the CSF and neuropathological data from the AN1792 trials given the small sample sizes and the heterogeneity of the reported findings. According to the amyloid hypothesis, an active immune response would likely only be beneficial if achieved prior to the event that triggers the cascade (29). From a fluid biomarker perspective, it is unknown if the dramatic changes in CSF t-tau had any association with the positive signal seen on several clinical metrics. This is one of many unanswered questions that remain after this trial. Clearly, additional study is required to fully inform decisions about whether active immunization strategies can be efficacious in the treatment or prevention of AD. Several vaccines designed to illicit a safer B-cell response, including ACC-001, CAD106, V950, and Affitope AD02, are in various stages of clinical testing (86). The results of both Phase I and IIa testing have been published for CAD106 (176, 177). Although the vaccine appears much safer than AN1792, neither study demonstrated a significant biomarker or clinical effect.

Passive Amyloid Immunization Strategies

Passive immunization strategies involve the infusion of humanized monoclonal antibodies designed to bind amyloid species. Preclinical studies have shown that passively administered antibodies can enter the CNS and bind to various forms of amyloid (178). Compounds in this class differ depending on what domain within the Aβ fragment they bind (179).

Bapineuzumab

Bapineuzumab is a humanized monoclonal antibody directed against the N-terminus of Aβ. Recognition of the N-terminus ensures that bapineuzumab can attach to both soluble and insoluble amyloid species. Several theories have been proposed to explain bapineuzumab's mechanism of action including direct inhibition of plaque formation (180) and antibody-mediated triggering of microglial cells to clear plaques (181). In preclinical models, bapineuzumab-treated PDAPP mice show reduced cortical amyloid plaque burdens (178). As with other amyloid therapies, treatment with bapineuzumab appears most effective for preventing rather than clearing pre-existing plaques (6). One potential explanation for the inability of bapineuzumab to clear existing plaques is proposed by Demattos et al. who hypothesize that in advanced disease, bapineuzumab is unable to bind plaques because it is saturated by soluble amyloid species that surround mature plaques (182). Infusion of bapineuzumab has also been associated with an increased incidence of microhemorrhage, which is thought to be due to its binding to vascular amyloid (183).

A Phase II study was undertaken to assess the safety of bapineuzumab in subjects with mild to moderate AD dementia (184). Higher rates of edema known as amyloid-related imaging abnormalities (ARIA) were seen at higher infusion doses and in subjects possessing the APOE ϵ4 genotype. Although clinical benefits were not initially detected, a *post hoc* analysis using multiple comparisons suggested possible benefits on both cognition and function (185). The biomarker data from Phase II testing also detected a possible disease-modifying signal as CSF data ($n = 27$) showed significant reductions in p-tau (−9.9 pg/mL) and a trend toward reduction in t-tau (−72.3 pg/mL) (186). In a smaller trial using an identical protocol, change in amyloid uptake as measured by PET scan was assessed as a primary outcome. In this trial, treatment with bapineuzumab ($N = 20$) was associated with reduced cortical binding compared with baseline (4).

Based on the positive signals seen in the Phase II trials, bapineuzumab advanced to Phase III testing (9). To reduce the risk of ARIA-E, dose selection was based on APOE ϵ4 status. Included in the secondary analysis was amyloid PET, volumetric MRI, and CSF biomarkers. Results of this study were disappointing as primary endpoints were not met. Although there were some signs of a positive biomarker effect, the signal was much weaker in Phase III testing than had been seen in the Phase II trial. APOE ϵ4 carriers ($N = 127$) experienced significant but small reductions in CSF p-tau (−5.8 pg/mL) compared to the placebo comparison group. In non-carriers, significant reductions in CSF p-tau were reported but only at the highest dose (−8.17 pg/mL). No significant changes were noted in CSF Aβ42 levels or t-tau levels. In both APOE ϵ4 carriers and non-carriers, amyloid uptake (as measured by PET scan) remained unchanged during the course of the trial.

The interpretation of outcome data from the bapineuzumab trials is complicated by the finding that a significant percentage of participants (6% of APOE ϵ4 carriers and 36% of APOE ϵ4 non-carriers) did not have evidence of amyloid pathology on PET scan. Nonetheless, the reduction of CSF p-tau is notable and suggests that passive immunization strategies targeting amyloid may be able to effect key pathological processes. Additional studies are needed to replicate this finding. The preclinical data suggest that bapineuzumab may be more effective when timed earlier in the disease course or at higher doses (182). The candidacy of bapineuzumab, however, is limited by ARIA-E.

Solanezumab

Solanezumab is a humanized monoclonal antibody directed against the middle amino acid section of Aβ. Because this epitope is not accessible on amyloid plaques, solanezumab only binds soluble Aβ species and does not bind Aβ plaques (187) or oligomers (188). In mouse models, infused solanezumab rapidly binds and completely sequesters plasma Aβ (187). By capturing the entire pool of soluble Aβ, solanezumab prevents this pool of amyloid from re-entering the brain, potentially shifting the amyloid gradient toward plaque dissolution and efflux out of the brain (29). According to this hypothesis, solanezumab acts as a "peripheral sink" as it draws amyloid out of the brain. In mouse models, peripheral administration of solanezumab results in rapid, 1,000-fold increases in plasma Aβ and significant reductions in plaque deposition (187). Not all preclinical data on solanezumab has been positive as one study found that treatment neither prevented nor reduced amyloid deposition (189). Unlike bapinezumab, solanezumab has not been associated with ARIA-E in either preclinical or human testing.

In a Phase II testing, treatment with solanezumab was associated with dose-related increases in both plasma and CSF levels of Aβ40 and 42 (190). Notably, both antibody-bound and antibody-free levels of CSF Aβ42 increased. Increases in unbound CSF Aβ42 could be interpreted as evidence of Aβ42 leaving plaques and diffusing down the gradient to replace sequestered plasma Aβ species consistent with the peripheral sink hypothesis. Amyloid PET scanning would have been informative in determining if the source of the increased unbound Aβ42 was in fact from plaque.

Solanezumab advanced to two large Phase III trials known as EXPEDITION 1 and 2 (142). Although both trials failed to meet primary endpoints, identical study designs allowed for pooling of data across the two studies. In the pooled analysis, the subgroup identified as having mild AD showed statistically significant slower rates of cognitive decline and positive trends on functional measures (185). Consistent with the Phase II trial, serum levels of both Aβ40 and 42 increased following infusion and remained significantly elevated during the entire trial. In a smaller subset of patients with CSF data ($N = 44$), significant increases were seen in both total CSF Aβ40 and 42, but unlike the Phase II trial, there were no significant changes in unbound Aβ42. Treatment was also not associated with changes in CSF tau, volumetric MRI, or amyloid PET.

Any interpretation of outcome data from the Phase III study of solanezumab must be tempered by the finding that a significant percentage (>20%) of enrollees who underwent amyloid PET scanning during the trial had negative scans (29). The dramatic increases in both serum and CSF levels of Aβ species in those treated with solanezumab could be interpreted as evidence of amyloid mobilization in the CNS. Whether antibody-mediated sequestration of soluble amyloid is enough to drive deposited amyloid out of plaque is still unknown and was not demonstrated in this trial with PET scanning (187). Clearly, the preclinical evidence regarding solanezumab has suggested a more profound effect on amyloid plaque prevention than clearance, and, as with other anti-amyloid therapies, treatment may prove more effective earlier in the disease course. Two ongoing trials of solanezumab – one enrolling patients with mild AD and the other enrolling cognitively subjects – will hope to shed light on these lingering issues.

Gamma Secretase Inhibitors

Gamma secretase is a multi-unit enzyme complex that facilitates the second enzymatic step in the processing of APP to Aβ. It consists of four subunits: nicastrin, presenilin-1 (PSEN1), anterior pharynx-defective-1, and presenilin-2 (PSEN2). Mutations in the genes that code for PSEN1 or PSEN2 cause early-onset AD by increasing the fractional production of Aβ42 (27). In animal models, compounds that decrease gamma secretase activity have been shown to reduce Aβ42 synthesis and improve behavioral and cognitive symptoms (191, 192). Development of safe gamma secretase inhibitors is complicated by the enzyme's crucial role in the regulation of Notch protein signaling pathways. Notch signaling is involved in cell fate pathways in rapidly dividing cells and disruption of normal Notch protein function can result in adverse gastrointestinal, hematologic, and dermatologic effects (193). Safe gamma secretase inhibitors must show a selective preference for Aβ inhibition over disruption of Notch signaling pathways.

Semagacestat

Semagacestat is a gamma secretase inhibitor that demonstrates selective inhibition of APP processing over Notch inhibition in several *in vitro* studies (194, 195). Not all studies have reported this preference, and in the most recent study (published after the Phase III trials were completed) semagacestat showed greater affinitiy for inhibiting Notch signaling pathways than BACE (196). In animal models, semagacestat reduces soluble Aβ in brain, CSF, and serum. Because studies using microdialysis show significant reductions in interstitial amyloid, there was also hope that gamma secretase inhibition would drive the amyloid gradient and promote the dissolution of amyloid out of plaques and into the interstitial space (197). Data from several mouse models suggested that although gamma secretase reduced soluble Aβ levels and prevented the formation of new plaques, there was little evidence that treatment promoted the clearance of preexisting plaques (198, 199).

Early human testing of semagacestat was enriched by the use of stable isotope labeling kinetics (SILK) (18). By continuously labeling and monitoring soluble Aβ in the CSF, SILK provides an estimation of the production and clearance of Aβ over a specified period of time (200). Using SILK, it was shown that single doses of semagacestat caused dramatic reductions in Aβ production in healthy human subjects. This finding provided convincing evidence of target engagement and semagacestat advanced to additional testing. In a 14 week Phase II study powered to detect safety, treatment was associated with significant reductions in serum Aβ40, but somewhat surprisingly, not with significant changes in either CSF Aβ40 or Aβ42 (*post hoc* analyses suggested a trend toward CSF Aβ40 reduction) (201).

Two large multicenter trials enrolling more than 2,000 patients have been conducted (71). Known as the IDENTITY 1 and IDENTITY 2, both trials were terminated early after a preplanned interim analysis revealed that treatment was associated with an increased incidence of adverse side effects. Patients receiving active treatment experienced skin cancers, GI symptoms, and dermatological side effects at twice the rate of those receiving placebo. In the modified intention-to-treat population, treatment was associated with worsening cognition and functional status. Biomarker from IDENTIY included both serum and CSF biomarkers as well as neuroimaging. Significant dose-dependent reductions in both serum Aβ40 and 42 were seen with treatment. Notably, the reduction in serum Aβ40 was more than twice that seen for Aβ42. CSF monitoring of Aβ (40,42) and tau was done in a smaller subset of patients ($N = 47$). Although no significant changes were seen in either Aβ or t-tau, there was a significant reduction in p-tau levels, which was greater in the lower dose group (8% vs. 4%). Changes in amyloid uptake were not appreciated in 59 patients with multiple amyloid PET scans. Worsening cognition and an increased rate of side effects were also seen in Phase II testing of avagacestat, another gamma secretase inhibitor (109).

Unless gamma secretase inhibitors without Notch signaling inhibition can be developed (and definitively proven *in vitro*), it is unwise to devote further resources to gamma secretase inhibition as a viable treatment for AD. Inhibition of Aβ production, however, remains a promising option for AD therapies. Biomarker data from the semagacestat trial, which showed significant (albeit, modest) reductions in CSF p-tau levels, may indicate that reducing Aβ production may alter the neuropathological process of AD. An alternative pathway to reduce Aβ production is with BACE1 inhibition. Several lines of research support the role of BACE1 activity in the pathogenesis of AD including two studies that have reported allelic variations, that reduce BACE1 activity, are protective against AD (202, 203). A significant barrier to BACE1 inhibitor development is that its large active site requires the development of bulky compounds that do not pass through the BBB into the brain (204). Nonetheless, several BACE1 inhibitors have been developed and are entering clinical testing. Preliminary data suggest that BACE1 inhibitors significantly reduce CSF Aβ42 levels (205).

Conclusion

Aided by the development of several validated biomarkers, the concept of AD has drastically changed over the past 30 years. Reflected in new research criteria, AD is now seen as a disease that progress through several stages (ranging from a prodromal/asymptomatic stage to mildly symptomatic to frank dementia) (5). We now know that the biological processes that lead to the disease are triggered years to decades before the onset of symptoms (9). Fluid biomarkers, which provide a window into the complex biochemical process in the brain, will take on an enhanced role in overcoming the challenges of developing therapeutic agents with disease-modifying properties. Three CSF fluid biomarkers (consisting of low Aβ42 and elevated t-tau and p-tau) are now widely accepted and commonly used in both clinical practice and research. When combined, these three biomarkers constitute an "AD signature" that better predicts the presence of AD pathology on autopsy than a diagnosis made on clinical grounds (73). Because changes in these biomarkers can be detected years before the dementia phase of disease, they have also been shown to demonstrate good accuracy in identifying individuals at risk for disease progression (77). As a result, they should be used to enhance clinical trial enrichment strategies, especially as trials move toward enrolling patients earlier in the disease course. Less is known about their utility in tracking disease progression or monitoring therapeutic responses. There are some data to suggest that CSF tau tracks more closely with disease progression (52) and may be better suited in this role than Aβ. It is still unknown if drug-induced changes in these markers will result in clinically meaningful benefits.

Due to several shortcomings in the current fluid biomarkers, it is imperative that new biomarkers be developed. Several promising new candidates have emerged with good preliminary data to support their further development. These include CSF BACE1 (96), VILIP-1, and YLK-40 (116). The matching of a biomarker with a particular drug designed to modulate that aspect of AD pathophysiology (CSF BACE1 with a BACE1 inhibitor) has the potential to provide information about target engagement, inform dosing decisions, and to monitor for drug effects. Perhaps, the most promising of all emerging approaches is the development of proteomics. With further development of biotechnology that promises to increase the capacity to analyze larger datasets, it seems likely that an "AD fingerprint" composed of several fluid biomarkers will emerge that will enhance our ability to identify, stage, and maybe even chose appropriate treatments for AD.

Several candidate agents with potential disease-modifying properties have advanced to Phase III testing, each has failed to meet clinical endpoints. A few trials have included biomarker data as secondary outcomes. Owing to the heterogeneity of the findings and lack of correlation with clinical metrics, these results are difficult to interpret. The slow progression of the disease, complicated pathophysiology, and difficulty in accurately modeling the pathology of sporadic AD in animal models present formidable challenges to clinical trial design and implementation. Biomarkers, however, have the ability to answer questions more quickly and effectively about target engagement, patient selection, and disease monitoring. In preclinical studies, biomarkers can be used to verify that a candidate agent is having its proposed effect on the biological systems it is designed to target. Because animal models are limited in their ability to replicate all of the behavioral and pathological features of AD (206), testing in multiple animals may improve the predictive value of clinical testing. Preclinical testing should also include biomarker data that are translatable to humans (including both CSF and serum). CSF testing in larger animals like guinea pigs and canines can provide valuable information about a candidate drug's effects in the CSF

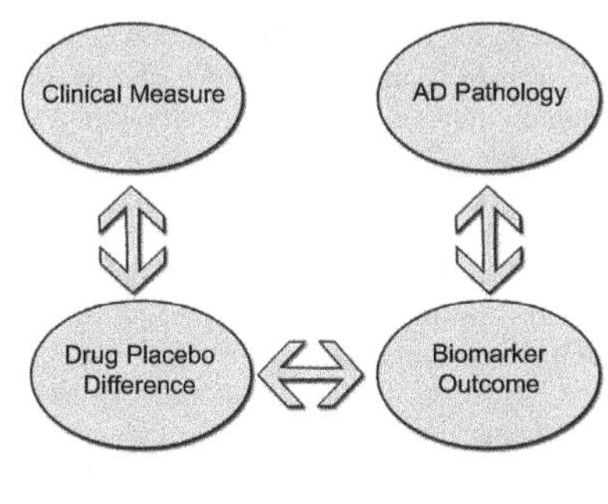

FIGURE 2 | Standard parallel group design to demonstrate disease modification groups receiving active treatment and placebo would be compared on clinical measures while an effect on disease pathology would be demonstrated by showing differences on a biomarker measure of disease progression. A correlation between drug–placebo difference and a biomarker outcome could potentially support a claim of disease modification.

and may improve upon information derived from mouse models (207). As a candidate compound advances to early clinical testing in humans, an early priority should be to confirm that biomarker changes demonstrated in preclinical testing are seen in humans (8). This can be tested with smaller, proof of concept trials that are powered to pre-specified endpoints. It is at this stage that go, no-go decisions can be made about advancing to longer, more expensive trials. If an agent is to be labeled with a claim of disease modification, support may come from biomarker data in Phase III trials. **Figure 2** illustrates a potential model for a standard parallel group design. Groups receiving active treatment and placebo would be compared based on clinical measures and a biomarker known to exert an effect on the underlying pathophysiology. A drug–placebo difference would be supported by differences on clinical measures (cognition, function, or global outcomes); while an effect on disease pathology would be demonstrated by showing a significant difference on biomarker measures of disease progression (for example, CSF t-tau). A statistically significant correlation between these two measures could potentially be used to support a claim for disease modification (208).

References

1. 2013 Alzheimer's disease facts and figures. *Alzheimers Dement* (2013) **9**(2):208–45. doi:10.1016/j.jalz.2013.02.003
2. Cummings JL. Alzheimer's disease. *N Engl J Med* (2004) **351**(1):56–67. doi:10.1056/NEJMra040223
3. Bateman RJ, Xiong C, Benzinger TL, Fagan AM, Goate A, Fox NC, et al. Clinical and biomarker changes in dominantly inherited Alzheimer's disease. *N Engl J Med* (2012) **367**(9):795–804. doi:10.1056/NEJMoa1202753
4. Rinne JO, Brooks DJ, Rossor MN, Fox NC, Bullock R, Klunk WE, et al. 11C-PiB PET assessment of change in fibrillar amyloid-beta load in patients with Alzheimer's disease treated with bapineuzumab: a phase 2, double-blind, placebo-controlled, ascending-dose study. *Lancet Neurol* (2010) **9**(4):363–72. doi:10.1016/S1474-4422(10)70043-0
5. Hampel H, Lista S, Teipel SJ, Garaci F, Nistico R, Blennow K, et al. Perspective on future role of biological markers in clinical therapy trials of Alzheimer's disease: a long-range point of view beyond 2020. *Biochem Pharmacol* (2014) **88**(4):426–49. doi:10.1016/j.bcp.2013.11.009
6. Karran E, Hardy J. Antiamyloid therapy for Alzheimer's disease – are we on the right road? *N Engl J Med* (2014) **370**(4):377–8. doi:10.1056/NEJMe1313943
7. Siemers ER. How can we recognize "disease modification" effects? *J Nutr Health Aging* (2009) **13**(4):341–3. doi:10.1007/s12603-009-0036-7
8. Karran E, Hardy J. A critique of the drug discovery and phase 3 clinical programs targeting the amyloid hypothesis for Alzheimer disease. *Ann Neurol* (2014) **76**(2):185–205. doi:10.1002/ana.24188
9. Dubois B, Feldman HH, Jacova C, Hampel H, Molinuevo JL, Blennow K, et al. Advancing research diagnostic criteria for Alzheimer's disease: the IWG-2 criteria. *Lancet Neurol* (2014) **13**(6):614–29. doi:10.1016/S1474-4422(14)70090-0
10. Sperling RA, Aisen PS, Beckett LA, Bennett DA, Craft S, Fagan AM, et al. Toward defining the preclinical stages of Alzheimer's disease: recommendations from the National Institute on Aging-Alzheimer's Association workgroups on diagnostic guidelines for Alzheimer's disease. *Alzheimers Dement* (2011) **7**(3):280–92. doi:10.1016/j.jalz.2011.03.003
11. Albert MS, DeKosky ST, Dickson D, Dubois B, Feldman HH, Fox NC, et al. The diagnosis of mild cognitive impairment due to Alzheimer's disease: recommendations from the National Institute on Aging-Alzheimer's Association workgroups on diagnostic guidelines for Alzheimer's disease. *Alzheimers Dement* (2011) **7**(3):270–9. doi:10.1016/j.jalz.2011.03.008
12. McKhann GM, Knopman DS, Chertkow H, Hyman BT, Jack CR Jr, Kawas CH, et al. The diagnosis of dementia due to Alzheimer's disease: recommendations from the National Institute on Aging-Alzheimer's Association workgroups on diagnostic guidelines for Alzheimer's disease. *Alzheimers Dement* (2011) **7**(3):263–9. doi:10.1016/j.jalz.2011.03.005
13. Petrella JR. Neuroimaging and the search for a cure for Alzheimer disease. *Radiology* (2013) **269**(3):671–91. doi:10.1148/radiol.13122503
14. Hardy JA, Higgins GA. Alzheimer's disease: the amyloid cascade hypothesis. *Science* (1992) **256**(5054):184–5. doi:10.1126/science.1566067
15. Bates KA, Verdile G, Li QX, Ames D, Hudson P, Masters CL, et al. Clearance mechanisms of Alzheimer's amyloid-beta peptide: implications for therapeutic design and diagnostic tests. *Mol Psychiatry* (2009) **14**(5):469–86. doi:10.1038/mp.2008.96
16. Cummings JL. Biomarkers in Alzheimer's disease drug development. *Alzheimers Dement* (2011) **7**(3):e13–44. doi:10.1016/j.jalz.2010.06.004
17. Bateman RJ, Klunk WE. Measuring target effect of proposed disease-modifying therapies in Alzheimer's disease. *Neurotherapeutics* (2008) **5**(3):381–90. doi:10.1016/j.nurt.2008.05.009
18. Bateman RJ, Siemers ER, Mawuenyega KG, Wen G, Browning KR, Sigurdson WC, et al. A gamma-secretase inhibitor decreases amyloid-beta production in the central nervous system. *Ann Neurol* (2009) **66**(1):48–54. doi:10.1002/ana.21623
19. Burdick D, Soreghan B, Kwon M, Kosmoski J, Knauer M, Henschen A, Assembly and aggregation properties of synthetic Alzheimer's A4/beta amyloid peptide analogs. *J Biol Chem* (1992) **267**(1):546–54.
20. Lee J, Culyba EK, Powers ET, Kelly JW. Amyloid-beta forms fibrils by nucleated conformational conversion of oligomers. *Nat Chem Biol* (2011) **7**(9), 602–9. doi:10.1038/nchembio.624
21. Lesne S, Koh MT, Kotilinek L, Kayed R, Glabe CG, Yang A, et al. A specific amyloid-beta protein assembly in the brain impairs memory. *Nature* (2006) **440**(7082):352–7. doi:10.1038/nature04533
22. Snyder EM, Nong Y, Almeida CG, Paul S, Moran T, Choi EY, et al. Regulation of NMDA receptor trafficking by amyloid-beta. *Nat Neurosci* (2005) **8**(8):1051–8. doi:10.1038/nn1503
23. Lesne SE, Sherman MA, Grant M, Kuskowski M, Schneider JA, Bennett DA, et al. Brain amyloid-beta oligomers in ageing and Alzheimer's disease. *Brain* (2013) **136**(Pt 5):1383–98. doi:10.1093/brain/awt062
24. Mathis CA, Lopresti BJ, Klunk WE. Impact of amyloid imaging on drug development in Alzheimer's disease. *Nucl Med Biol* (2007) **34**(7):809–22. doi:10.1016/j.nucmedbio.2007.06.015
25. Mucke L, Selkoe DJ. Neurotoxicity of amyloid beta-protein: synaptic and network dysfunction. *Cold Spring Harb Perspect Med* (2012) **2**(7):a006338. doi:10.1101/cshperspect.a006338
26. Bezprozvanny I. Amyloid goes global. *Sci Signal* (2009) **2**(63):pe16. doi:10.1126/scisignal.263pe16
27. Haass C, Selkoe DJ. Soluble protein oligomers in neurodegeneration: lessons from the Alzheimer's amyloid beta-peptide. *Nat Rev Mol Cell Biol* (2007) **8**(2):101–12. doi:10.1038/nrm2101
28. Savva GM, Wharton SB, Ince PG, Forster G, Matthews FE, Brayne C. Age, neuropathology, and dementia. *N Engl J Med* (2009) **360**(22):2302–9. doi:10.1056/NEJMoa0806142
29. Karran E, Mercken M, De Strooper B. The amyloid cascade hypothesis for Alzheimer's disease: an appraisal for the development of therapeutics. *Nat Rev Drug Discov* (2011) **10**(9):698–712. doi:10.1038/nrd3505
30. Zetterberg H, Blennow K, Hanse E. Amyloid beta and APP as biomarkers for Alzheimer's disease. *Exp Gerontol* (2010) **45**(1):23–9. doi:10.1016/j.exger.2009.08.002
31. Englund H, Degerman Gunnarsson M, Brundin RM, Hedlund M, Kilander L, Lannfelt L, et al. Oligomerization partially explains the lowering of Abeta42 in Alzheimer's disease cerebrospinal fluid. *Neurodegener Dis* (2009) **6**(4):139–47. doi:10.1159/000225376
32. Strozyk D, Blennow K, White LR, Launer LJ. CSF Abeta 42 levels correlate with amyloid-neuropathology in a population-based autopsy study. *Neurology* (2003) **60**(4):652–6. doi:10.1212/01.WNL.0000046581.81650.D0
33. Tapiola T, Alafuzoff I, Herukka SK, Parkkinen L, Hartikainen P, Soininen H, et al. Cerebrospinal fluid {beta}-amyloid 42 and tau proteins as biomarkers of Alzheimer-type pathologic changes in the brain. *Arch Neurol* (2009) **66**(3):382–9. doi:10.1001/archneurol.2008.596
34. Fagan AM, Mintun MA, Mach RH, Lee SY, Dence CS, Shah AR, et al. Inverse relation between in vivo amyloid imaging load and cerebrospinal

fluid Abeta42 in humans. *Ann Neurol* (2006) **59**(3):512–9. doi:10.1002/ana.20730
35. Weigand SD, Vemuri P, Wiste HJ, Senjem ML, Pankratz VS, Aisen PS, et al. Transforming cerebrospinal fluid Abeta42 measures into calculated Pittsburgh compound B units of brain Abeta amyloid. *Alzheimers Dement* (2011) **7**(2):133–41. doi:10.1016/j.jalz.2010.08.230
36. Tolboom N, van der Flier WM, Yaqub M, Boellaard R, Verwey NA, Blankenstein MA, et al. Relationship of cerebrospinal fluid markers to 11C-PiB and 18F-FDDNP binding. *J Nucl Med* (2009) **50**(9):1464–70. doi:10.2967/jnumed.109.064360
37. Fagan AM. What does it mean to be 'amyloid-positive'? *Brain* (2015) **138**(Pt 3):514–6. doi:10.1093/brain/awu387
38. Mattsson N, Insel PS, Donohue M, Landau S, Jagust WJ, Shaw LM, et al. Independent information from cerebrospinal fluid amyloid-beta and florbetapir imaging in Alzheimer's disease. *Brain* (2015) **138**(Pt 3):772–83. doi:10.1093/brain/awu367
39. Weingarten MD, Lockwood AH, Hwo SY, Kirschner MW. A protein factor essential for microtubule assembly. *Proc Natl Acad Sci U S A* (1975) **72**(5):1858–62. doi:10.1073/pnas.72.5.1858
40. Imahori K, Uchida T. Physiology and pathology of tau protein kinases in relation to Alzheimer's disease. *J Biochem* (1997) **121**(2):179–88.
41. Blennow K, Hampel H, Weiner M, Zetterberg H. Cerebrospinal fluid and plasma biomarkers in Alzheimer disease. *Nat Rev Neurol* (2010) **6**(3):131–44. doi:10.1038/nrneurol.2010.4
42. Tepper K, Biernat J, Kumar S, Wegmann S, Timm T, Hubschmann S, et al. Oligomer formation of tau protein hyperphosphorylated in cells. *J Biol Chem* (2014) **289**(49):34389–407. doi:10.1074/jbc.M114.611368
43. Jack CR Jr, Holtzman DM. Biomarker modeling of Alzheimer's disease. *Neuron* (2013) **80**(6):1347–58. doi:10.1016/j.neuron.2013.12.003
44. Heneka MT, Carson MJ, El Khoury J, Landreth GE, Brosseron F, Feinstein DL, et al. Neuroinflammation in Alzheimer's disease. *Lancet Neurol* (2015) **14**(4):388–405. doi:10.1016/S1474-4422(15)70016-5
45. Bonda DJ, Wang X, Lee HG, Smith MA, Perry G, Zhu X. Neuronal failure in Alzheimer's disease: a view through the oxidative stress looking-glass. *Neurosci Bull* (2014) **30**(2):243–52. doi:10.1007/s12264-013-1424-x
46. Hardy J, Duff K, Hardy KG, Perez-Tur J, Hutton M. Genetic dissection of Alzheimer's disease and related dementias: amyloid and its relationship to tau. *Nat Neurosci* (1998) **1**(5):355–8. doi:10.1038/1565
47. Honjo K, van Reekum R, Verhoeff NP. Alzheimer's disease and infection: do infectious agents contribute to progression of Alzheimer's disease? *Alzheimers Dement* (2009) **5**(4):348–60. doi:10.1016/j.jalz.2008.12.001
48. Iqbal K, Gong CX, Liu F. Hyperphosphorylation-induced tau oligomers. *Front Neurol* (2013) **4**:112. doi:10.3389/fneur.2013.00112
49. Brandt R, Hundelt M, Shahani N. Tau alteration and neuronal degeneration in tauopathies: mechanisms and models. *Biochim Biophys Acta* (2005) **1739**(2–3):331–54. doi:10.1016/j.bbadis.2004.06.018
50. Ballatore C, Lee VM, Trojanowski JQ. Tau-mediated neurodegeneration in Alzheimer's disease and related disorders. *Nat Rev Neurosci* (2007) **8**(9):663–72. doi:10.1038/nrn2194
51. Braak H, Braak E. Neuropathological stageing of Alzheimer-related changes. *Acta Neuropathol* (1991) **82**(4):239–59. doi:10.1007/BF00308809
52. Gomez-Isla T, Hollister R, West H, Mui S, Growdon JH, Petersen RC, et al. Neuronal loss correlates with but exceeds neurofibrillary tangles in Alzheimer's disease. *Ann Neurol* (1997) **41**(1):17–24. doi:10.1002/ana.410410106
53. Dujardin S, Begard S, Caillierez R, Lachaud C, Delattre L, Carrier S, et al. Ectosomes: a new mechanism for non-exosomal secretion of tau protein. *PLoS One* (2014) **9**(6):e100760. doi:10.1371/journal.pone.0100760
54. Stohr J, Condello C, Watts JC, Bloch L, Oehler A, Nick M, et al. Distinct synthetic Abeta prion strains producing different amyloid deposits in bigenic mice. *Proc Natl Acad Sci U S A* (2014) **111**(28):10329–34. doi:10.1073/pnas.1408968111
55. Clavaguera F, Bolmont T, Crowther RA, Abramowski D, Frank S, Probst A, et al. Transmission and spreading of tauopathy in transgenic mouse brain. *Nat Cell Biol* (2009) **11**(7):909–13. doi:10.1038/ncb1901
56. Clavaguera F, Hench J, Goedert M, Tolnay M. Invited review: prion-like transmission and spreading of tau pathology. *Neuropathol Appl Neurobiol* (2015) **41**(1):47–58. doi:10.1111/nan.12197
57. Blennow K. Cerebrospinal fluid protein biomarkers for Alzheimer's disease. *NeuroRx* (2004) **1**(2):213–25. doi:10.1602/neurorx.1.2.213
58. Hesse C, Rosengren L, Andreasen N, Davidsson P, Vanderstichele H, Vanmechelen E, et al. Transient increase in total tau but not phospho-tau in human cerebrospinal fluid after acute stroke. *Neurosci Lett* (2001) **297**(3):187–90. doi:10.1016/S0304-3940(00)01697-9
59. Franz G, Beer R, Kampfl A, Engelhardt K, Schmutzhard E, Ulmer H, et al. Amyloid beta 1-42 and tau in cerebrospinal fluid after severe traumatic brain injury. *Neurology* (2003) **60**(9):1457–61. doi:10.1212/01.WNL.0000063313.57292.00
60. Otto M, Wiltfang J, Cepek L, Neumann M, Mollenhauer B, Steinacker P, et al. Tau protein and 14-3-3 protein in the differential diagnosis of Creutzfeldt-Jakob disease. *Neurology* (2002) **58**(2):192–7. doi:10.1212/WNL.58.2.192
61. Hampel H, Buerger K, Zinkowski R, Teipel SJ, Goernitz A, Andreasen N, et al. Measurement of phosphorylated tau epitopes in the differential diagnosis of Alzheimer disease: a comparative cerebrospinal fluid study. *Arch Gen Psychiatry* (2004) **61**(1):95–102. doi:10.1001/archpsyc.61.1.95
62. Buerger K, Ewers M, Pirttila T, Zinkowski R, Alafuzoff I, Teipel SJ, et al. CSF phosphorylated tau protein correlates with neocortical neurofibrillary pathology in Alzheimer's disease. *Brain* (2006) **129**(Pt 11):3035–41. doi:10.1093/brain/awl269
63. van Harten AC, Kester MI, Visser PJ, Blankenstein MA, Pijnenburg YA, van der Flier WM, et al. Tau and p-tau as CSF biomarkers in dementia: a meta-analysis. *Clin Chem Lab Med* (2011) **49**(3):353–66. doi:10.1515/CCLM.2011.086
64. Buerger K, Otto M, Teipel SJ, Zinkowski R, Blennow K, DeBernardis J, et al. Dissociation between CSF total tau and tau protein phosphorylated at threonine 231 in Creutzfeldt-Jakob disease. *Neurobiol Aging* (2006) **27**(1):10–5. doi:10.1016/j.neurobiolaging.2004.12.003
65. Grossman M, Farmer J, Leight S, Work M, Moore P, Van Deerlin V, et al. Cerebrospinal fluid profile in frontotemporal dementia and Alzheimer's disease. *Ann Neurol* (2005) **57**(5):721–9. doi:10.1002/ana.20477
66. Roher AE, Esh CL, Kokjohn TA, Castano EM, Van Vickle GD, Kalback WM, et al. Amyloid beta peptides in human plasma and tissues and their significance for Alzheimer's disease. *Alzheimers Dement* (2009) **5**(1):18–29. doi:10.1016/j.jalz.2008.10.004
67. Engelborghs S, De Vreese K, Van de Casteele T, Vanderstichele H, Van Everbroeck B, Cras P, et al. Diagnostic performance of a CSF-biomarker panel in autopsy-confirmed dementia. *Neurobiol Aging* (2008) **29**(8):1143–59. doi:10.1016/j.neurobiolaging.2007.02.016
68. Mattsson N, Andreasson U, Persson S, Carrillo MC, Collins S, Chalbot S, et al. CSF biomarker variability in the Alzheimer's Association quality control program. *Alzheimers Dement* (2013) **9**(3):251–61. doi:10.1016/j.jalz.2013.01.010
69. Beach TG, Monsell SE, Phillips LE, Kukull W. Accuracy of the clinical diagnosis of Alzheimer disease at National Institute on Aging Alzheimer Disease Centers, 2005–2010. *J Neuropathol Exp Neurol* (2012) **71**(4):266–73. doi:10.1097/NEN.0b013e31824b211b
70. Salloway S, Sperling R, Fox NC, Blennow K, Klunk W, Raskind M, et al. Two phase 3 trials of bapineuzumab in mild-to-moderate Alzheimer's disease. *N Engl J Med* (2014) **370**(4):322–33. doi:10.1056/NEJMoa1304839
71. Doody RS, Raman R, Farlow M, Iwatsubo T, Vellas B, Joffe S, et al. A phase 3 trial of semagacestat for treatment of Alzheimer's disease. *N Engl J Med* (2013) **369**(4):341–50. doi:10.1056/NEJMoa1210951
72. Young AL, Oxtoby NP, Daga P, Cash DM, Fox NC, Ourselin S, et al. A data-driven model of biomarker changes in sporadic Alzheimer's disease. *Brain* (2014) **137**(Pt 9):2564–77. doi:10.1093/brain/awu176
73. Blennow K, Dubois B, Fagan AM, Lewczuk P, de Leon MJ, Hampel H. Clinical utility of cerebrospinal fluid biomarkers in the diagnosis of early Alzheimer's disease. *Alzheimers Dement* (2015) **11**(1):58–69. doi:10.1016/j.jalz.2014.02.004
74. Stomrud E, Hansson O, Blennow K, Minthon L, Londos E. Cerebrospinal fluid biomarkers predict decline in subjective cognitive function over 3 years in healthy elderly. *Dement Geriatr Cogn Disord* (2007) **24**(2):118–24. doi:10.1159/000105017
75. Skoog I, Davidsson P, Aevarsson O, Vanderstichele H, Vanmechelen E, Blennow K. Cerebrospinal fluid beta-amyloid 42 is reduced before the onset of sporadic dementia: a population-based study in 85-year-olds. *Dement Geriatr Cogn Disord* (2003) **15**(3):169–76. doi:10.1159/000068478
76. van Harten AC, Visser PJ, Pijnenburg YA, Teunissen CE, Blankenstein MA, Scheltens P, et al. Cerebrospinal fluid Abeta42 is the best predictor of clinical progression in patients with subjective complaints. *Alzheimers Dement* (2013) **9**(5):481–7. doi:10.1016/j.jalz.2012.08.004

77. Buchhave P, Minthon L, Zetterberg H, Wallin AK, Blennow K, Hansson O. Cerebrospinal fluid levels of beta-amyloid 1-42, but not of tau, are fully changed already 5 to 10 years before the onset of Alzheimer dementia. *Arch Gen Psychiatry* (2012) **69**(1):98–106. doi:10.1001/archgenpsychiatry.2011.155
78. Mattsson N, Zetterberg H, Hansson O, Andreasen N, Parnetti L, Jonsson M, et al. CSF biomarkers and incipient Alzheimer disease in patients with mild cognitive impairment. *JAMA* (2009) **302**(4):385–93. doi:10.1001/jama.2009.1064
79. Hertze J, Minthon L, Zetterberg H, Vanmechelen E, Blennow K, Hansson O. Evaluation of CSF biomarkers as predictors of Alzheimer's disease: a clinical follow-up study of 4.7 years. *J Alzheimers Dis* (2010) **21**(4):1119–28. doi:10.3233/JAD2010100207
80. Hampel H, Teipel SJ, Fuchsberger T, Andreasen N, Wiltfang J, Otto M, et al. Value of CSF beta-amyloid1-42 and tau as predictors of Alzheimer's disease in patients with mild cognitive impairment. *Mol Psychiatry* (2004) **9**(7):705–10. doi: 10.1038/sj.mp.4001473
81. DeCarli C. Mild cognitive impairment: prevalence, prognosis, aetiology, and treatment. *Lancet Neurol* (2003) **2**(1):15–21. doi:10.1016/S1474-4422(03)00262-X
82. Rosen C, Hansson O, Blennow K, Zetterberg H. Fluid biomarkers in Alzheimer's disease – current concepts. *Mol Neurodegener* (2013) **8**:20. doi:10.1186/1750-1326-8-20
83. Andreasen N, Minthon L, Clarberg A, Davidsson P, Gottfries J, Vanmechelen E, et al. Sensitivity, specificity, and stability of CSF-tau in AD in a community-based patient sample. *Neurology* (1999) **53**(7):1488–94. doi:10.1212/WNL.53.7.1488
84. Buchhave P, Blennow K, Zetterberg H, Stomrud E, Londos E, Andreasen N, et al. Longitudinal study of CSF biomarkers in patients with Alzheimer's disease. *PLoS One* (2009) **4**(7):e6294. doi:10.1371/journal.pone.0006294
85. Vemuri P, Wiste HJ, Weigand SD, Shaw LM, Trojanowski JQ, Weiner MW, et al. MRI and CSF biomarkers in normal, MCI, and AD subjects: diagnostic discrimination and cognitive correlations. *Neurology* (2009) **73**(4):287–93. doi:10.1212/WNL.0b013e3181af79e5
86. Kang JH, Ryoo NY, Shin DW, Trojanowski JQ, Shaw LM. Role of cerebrospinal fluid biomarkers in clinical trials for Alzheimer's disease modifying therapies. *Korean J Physiol Pharmacol* (2014) **18**(6):447–56. doi:10.4196/kjpp.2014.18.6.447
87. Bjerke M, Portelius E, Minthon L, Wallin A, Anckarsater H, Anckarsater R, et al. Confounding factors influencing amyloid beta concentration in cerebrospinal fluid. *Int J Alzheimers Dis* (2010) **2010**:1–11. doi:10.4061/2010/986310
88. Willem M, Garratt AN, Novak B, Citron M, Kaufmann S, Rittger A, et al. Control of peripheral nerve myelination by the beta-secretase BACE1. *Science* (2006) **314**(5799):664–6. doi:10.1126/science.1132341
89. Hu X, Hicks CW, He W, Wong P, Macklin WB, Trapp BD, et al. Bace1 modulates myelination in the central and peripheral nervous system. *Nat Neurosci* (2006) **9**(12):1520–5. doi:10.1038/nn1797
90. Laird FM, Cai H, Savonenko AV, Farah MH, He K, Melnikova T, et al. BACE1, a major determinant of selective vulnerability of the brain to amyloid-beta amyloidogenesis, is essential for cognitive, emotional, and synaptic functions. *J Neurosci* (2005) **25**(50):11693–709. doi:10.1523/JNEUROSCI.2766-05.2005
91. Rossner S, Sastre M, Bourne K, Lichtenthaler SF. Transcriptional and translational regulation of BACE1 expression – implications for Alzheimer's disease. *Prog Neurobiol* (2006) **79**(2):95–111. doi:10.1016/j.pneurobio.2006.06.001
92. Fukumoto H, Tennis M, Locascio JJ, Hyman BT, Growdon JH, Irizarry MC. Age but not diagnosis is the main predictor of plasma amyloid beta-protein levels. *Arch Neurol* (2003) **60**(7):958–64. doi:10.1001/archneur.60.7.958
93. Holsinger RM, McLean CA, Beyreuther K, Masters, CL, Evin G. Increased expression of the amyloid precursor beta-secretase in Alzheimer's disease. *Ann Neurol* (2002) **51**(6):783–6. doi:10.1002/ana.10208
94. Verheijen JH, Huisman LG, van Lent N, Neumann U, Paganetti P, Hack CE, et al. Detection of a soluble form of BACE-1 in human cerebrospinal fluid by a sensitive activity assay. *Clin Chem* (2006) **52**(6):1168–74. doi:10.1373/clinchem.2006.066720
95. Holsinger RM, Lee JS, Boyd A, Masters CL, Collins SJ. CSF BACE1 activity is increased in CJD and Alzheimer disease versus [corrected] other dementias. *Neurology* (2006) **67**(4):710–2. doi:10.1212/01.wnl.0000229925.52203.4c
96. Zetterberg H, Andreasson U, Hansson O, Wu G, Sankaranarayanan S, Andersson ME, et al. Elevated cerebrospinal fluid BACE1 activity in incipient Alzheimer disease. *Arch Neurol* (2008) **65**(8):1102–7. doi:10.1001/archneur.65.8.1102
97. Faghihi MA, Modarresi F, Khalil AM, Wood DE, Sahagan BG, Morgan TE, et al. Expression of a noncoding RNA is elevated in Alzheimer's disease and drives rapid feed-forward regulation of beta-secretase. *Nat Med* (2008) **14**(7):723–30. doi:10.1038/nm1784
98. Olsson A, Hoglund K, Sjogren M, Andreasen N, Minthon L, Lannfelt L, et al. Measurement of alpha- and beta-secretase cleaved amyloid precursor protein in cerebrospinal fluid from Alzheimer patients. *Exp Neurol* (2003) **183**(1):74–80. doi:10.1016/S0014-4886(03)00027-X
99. Lewczuk P, Kamrowski-Kruck H, Peters O, Heuser I, Jessen F, Popp J, et al. Soluble amyloid precursor proteins in the cerebrospinal fluid as novel potential biomarkers of Alzheimer's disease: a multicenter study. *Mol Psychiatry* (2010) **15**(2):138–45. doi:10.1038/mp.2008.84
100. Perneczky R, Tsolakidou A, Arnold A, Diehl-Schmid J, Grimmer T, Forstl H, et al. CSF soluble amyloid precursor proteins in the diagnosis of incipient Alzheimer disease. *Neurology* (2011) **77**(1):35–8. doi:10.1212/WNL.0b013e318221ad47
101. Esparza TJ, Zhao H, Cirrito JR, Cairns NJ, Bateman RJ, Holtzman DM, et al. Amyloid-beta oligomerization in Alzheimer dementia versus high-pathology controls. *Ann Neurol* (2013) **73**(1):104–19. doi:10.1002/ana.23748
102. Hong S, Ostaszewski BL, Yang T, O'Malley TT, Jin M, Yanagisawa K, et al. Soluble Abeta oligomers are rapidly sequestered from brain ISF in vivo and bind GM1 ganglioside on cellular membranes. *Neuron* (2014) **82**(2):308–19. doi:10.1016/j.neuron.2014.02.027
103. Georganopoulou DG, Chang L, Nam JM, Thaxton CS, Mufson EJ, Klein WL, et al. Nanoparticle-based detection in cerebral spinal fluid of a soluble pathogenic biomarker for Alzheimer's disease. *Proc Natl Acad Sci U S A* (2005) **102**(7):2273–6. doi:10.1073/pnas.0409336102
104. Fukumoto H, Tokuda T, Kasai T, Ishigami N, Hidaka H, Kondo M, et al. High-molecular-weight beta-amyloid oligomers are elevated in cerebrospinal fluid of Alzheimer patients. *FASEB J* (2010) **24**(8):2716–26. doi:10.1096/fj.09-150359
105. Santos AN, Ewers M, Minthon L, Simm A, Silber RE, Blennow K, et al. Amyloid-beta oligomers in cerebrospinal fluid are associated with cognitive decline in patients with Alzheimer's disease. *J Alzheimers Dis* (2012) **29**(1):171–6. doi:10.3233/JAD-2012-111361
106. Portelius E, Zetterberg H, Andreasson U, Brinkmalm G, Andreasen N, Wallin A, et al. An Alzheimer's disease-specific beta-amyloid fragment signature in cerebrospinal fluid. *Neurosci Lett* (2006) **409**(3):215–9. doi:10.1016/j.neulet.2006.09.044
107. Lewczuk P, Esselmann H, Meyer M, Wollscheid V, Neumann M, Otto M, et al. The amyloid-beta (Abeta) peptide pattern in cerebrospinal fluid in Alzheimer's disease: evidence of a novel carboxyterminally elongated Abeta peptide. *Rapid Commun Mass Spectrom* (2003) **17**(12):1291–6. doi:10.1002/rcm.1048
108. Schoonenboom NS, Mulder C, Van Kamp GJ, Mehta SP, Scheltens P, Blankenstein MA, et al. Amyloid beta 38, 40, and 42 species in cerebrospinal fluid: more of the same? *Ann Neurol* (2005) **58**(1):139–42. doi:10.1002/ana.20508
109. Coric V, van Dyck CH, Salloway S, Andreasen N, Brody M, Richter RW, et al. Safety and tolerability of the gamma-secretase inhibitor avagacestat in a phase 2 study of mild to moderate Alzheimer disease. *Arch Neurol* (2012) **69**(11):1430–40. doi:10.1001/archneurol.2012.2194
110. Fagan AM, Mintun MA, Shah AR, Aldea P, Roe CM, Mach RH, et al. Cerebrospinal fluid tau and ptau(181) increase with cortical amyloid deposition in cognitively normal individuals: implications for future clinical trials of Alzheimer's disease. *EMBO Mol Med* (2009) **1**(8–9):371–80. doi:10.1002/emmm.200900048
111. Mehta PD, Pirttila T. Increased cerebrospinal fluid A beta38/A beta42 ratio in Alzheimer disease. *Neurodegener Dis* (2005) **2**(5):242–5. doi:10.1159/000090363
112. Fagan AM, Perrin RJ. Upcoming candidate cerebrospinal fluid biomarkers of Alzheimer's disease. *Biomark Med* (2012) **6**(4):455–76. doi:10.2217/bmm.12.42
113. Paterlini M, Revilla V, Grant AL, Wisden W. Expression of the neuronal calcium sensor protein family in the rat brain. *Neuroscience* (2000) **99**(2):205–16. doi:10.1016/S0306-4522(00)00201-3
114. Stejskal D, Sporova L, Svestak M, Karpisek M. Determination of serum visinin like protein-1 and its potential for the diagnosis of brain injury due to

the stroke: a pilot study. *Biomed Pap Med Fac Univ Palacky Olomouc Czech Repub* (2011) **155**(3):263–8. doi:10.5507/bp.2011.049

115. Tarawneh R, D'Angelo G, Macy E, Xiong C, Carter D, Cairns NJ, et al. Visinin-like protein-1: diagnostic and prognostic biomarker in Alzheimer disease. *Ann Neurol* (2011) **70**(2):274–85. doi:10.1002/ana.22448
116. Sutphen CL, Jasielec MS, Shah AR, Macy EM, Xiong C, Vlassenko AG, et al. Longitudinal cerebrospinal fluid biomarker changes in preclinical Alzheimer disease during middle age. *JAMA Neurol* (2015). doi:10.1001/jamaneurol.2015.1285
117. Tarawneh R, Lee JM, Ladenson JH, Morris JC, Holtzman DM. CSF VILIP-1 predicts rates of cognitive decline in early Alzheimer disease. *Neurology* (2012) **78**(10):709–19. doi:10.1212/WNL.0b013e318248e568
118. Sultana R, Baglioni M, Cecchetti R, Cai J, Klein JB, Bastiani P, et al. Lymphocyte mitochondria: toward identification of peripheral biomarkers in the progression of Alzheimer disease. *Free Radic Biol Med* (2013) **65**:595–606. doi:10.1016/j.freeradbiomed.2013.08.001
119. Miller E, Morel A, Saso L, Saluk J. Isoprostanes and neuroprostanes as biomarkers of oxidative stress in neurodegenerative diseases. *Oxid Med Cell Longev* (2014) **2014**:572491. doi:10.1155/2014/572491
120. Pratico D, Lee V MY, Trojanowski JQ, Rokach J, Fitzgerald GA. Increased F2-isoprostanes in Alzheimer's disease: evidence for enhanced lipid peroxidation in vivo. *FASEB J* (1998) **12**(15):1777–83.
121. Montine TJ, Kaye JA, Montine KS, McFarland L, Morrow JD, Quinn JF. Cerebrospinal fluid abeta42, tau, and f2-isoprostane concentrations in patients with Alzheimer disease, other dementias, and in age-matched controls. *Arch Pathol Lab Med* (2001) **125**(4):510–2. doi:10.1043/0003-9985(2001)125<0510:cfataf>2.0.co;2
122. Brys M, Pirraglia E, Rich K, Rolstad S, Mosconi L, Switalski R, et al. Prediction and longitudinal study of CSF biomarkers in mild cognitive impairment. *Neurobiol Aging* (2009) **30**(5):682–90. doi:10.1016/j.neurobiolaging.2007.08.010
123. de Leon MJ, Mosconi L, Li J, De Santi S, Yao Y, Tsui WH, et al. Longitudinal CSF isoprostane and MRI atrophy in the progression to AD. *J Neurol* (2007) **254**(12):1666–75. doi:10.1007/s00415-007-0610-z
124. Eikelenboom P, van Exel E, Hoozemans JJ, Veerhuis R, Rozemuller AJ, van Gool WA. Neuroinflammation – an early event in both the history and pathogenesis of Alzheimer's disease. *Neurodegener Dis* (2010) **7**(1–3):38–41. doi:10.1159/000283480
125. Bonneh-Barkay D, Bissel SJ, Wang G, Fish KN, Nicholl GC, Darko SW, et al. YKL-40, a marker of simian immunodeficiency virus encephalitis, modulates the biological activity of basic fibroblast growth factor. *Am J Pathol* (2008) **173**(1):130–43. doi:10.2353/ajpath.2008.080045
126. Perrin RJ, Craig-Schapiro R, Malone JP, Shah AR, Gilmore P, Davis AE, et al. Identification and validation of novel cerebrospinal fluid biomarkers for staging early Alzheimer's disease. *PLoS One* (2011) **6**(1):e16032. doi:10.1371/journal.pone.0016032
127. Craig-Schapiro R, Perrin RJ, Roe CM, Xiong C, Carter D, Cairns NJ, et al. YKL-40: a novel prognostic fluid biomarker for preclinical Alzheimer's disease. *Biol Psychiatry* (2010) **68**(10):903–12. doi:10.1016/j.biopsych.2010.08.025
128. Gerendasy DD, Herron SR, Watson JB, Sutcliffe JG. Mutational and biophysical studies suggest RC3/neurogranin regulates calmodulin availability. *J Biol Chem* (1994) **269**(35):22420–6.
129. Huang KP, Huang FL, Jager T, Li J, Reymann KG, Balschun D. Neurogranin/RC3 enhances long-term potentiation and learning by promoting calcium-mediated signaling. *J Neurosci* (2004) **24**(47):10660–9. doi:10.1523/JNEUROSCI.2213-04.2004
130. Thorsell A, Bjerke M, Gobom J, Brunhage E, Vanmechelen E, Andreasen N, et al. Neurogranin in cerebrospinal fluid as a marker of synaptic degeneration in Alzheimer's disease. *Brain Res* (2010) **1362**:13–22. doi:10.1016/j.brainres.2010.09.073
131. Kvartsberg H, Duits FH, Ingelsson M, Andreasen N, Ohrfelt A, Andersson K, et al. Cerebrospinal fluid levels of the synaptic protein neurogranin correlates with cognitive decline in prodromal Alzheimer's disease. *Alzheimers Dement* (2014). doi:10.1016/j.jalz.2014.10.009
132. de Almeida SM, Shumaker SD, LeBlanc SK, Delaney P, Marquie-Beck J, Ueland S, et al. Incidence of post-dural puncture headache in research volunteers. *Headache* (2011) **51**(10):1503–10. doi:10.1111/j.1526-4610.2011.01959.x
133. Henriksen K, O'Bryant SE, Hampel H, Trojanowski JQ, Montine TJ, Jeromin A, et al. The future of blood-based biomarkers for Alzheimer's disease. *Alzheimers Dement* (2014) **10**(1):115–31. doi:10.1016/j.jalz.2013.01.013
134. van Oijen M, Hofman A, Soares HD, Koudstaal PJ, Breteler MM. Plasma Abeta(1-40) and Abeta(1-42) and the risk of dementia: a prospective case-cohort study. *Lancet Neurol* (2006) **5**(8):655–60. doi:10.1016/S1474-4422(06)70501-4
135. Mayeux R, Honig LS, Tang MX, Manly J, Stern Y, Schupf N, et al. Plasma A[beta]40 and A[beta]42 and Alzheimer's disease: relation to age, mortality, and risk. *Neurology* (2003) **61**(9):1185–90. doi:10.1212/01.WNL.0000091890.32140.8F
136. Schupf N, Tang MX, Fukuyama H, Manly J, Andrews H, Mehta P, et al. Peripheral Abeta subspecies as risk biomarkers of Alzheimer's disease. *Proc Natl Acad Sci U S A* (2008) **105**(37):14052–7. doi:10.1073/pnas.0805902105
137. Sundelof J, Giedraitis V, Irizarry MC, Sundstrom J, Ingelsson E, Ronnemaa E, et al. Plasma beta amyloid and the risk of Alzheimer disease and dementia in elderly men: a prospective, population-based cohort study. *Arch Neurol* (2008) **65**(2):256–63. doi:10.1001/archneurol.2007.57
138. Lopez OL, Kuller LH, Mehta PD, Becker JT, Gach HM, Sweet RA, et al. Plasma amyloid levels and the risk of AD in normal subjects in the Cardiovascular Health Study. *Neurology* (2008) **70**(19):1664–71. doi:10.1212/01.wnl.0000306696.82017.66
139. Hansson O, Zetterberg H, Vanmechelen E, Vanderstichele H, Andreasson U, Londos E, et al. Evaluation of plasma Abeta(40) and Abeta(42) as predictors of conversion to Alzheimer's disease in patients with mild cognitive impairment. *Neurobiol Aging* (2010) **31**(3):357–67. doi:10.1016/j.neurobiolaging.2008.03.027
140. Koyama A, Okereke OI, Yang T, Blacker D, Selkoe DJ, Grodstein F. Plasma amyloid-beta as a predictor of dementia and cognitive decline: a systematic review and meta-analysis. *Arch Neurol* (2012) **69**(7):824–31. doi:10.1001/archneurol.2011.1841
141. Laske C, Sopova K, Gkotsis C, Eschweiler GW, Straten G, Gawaz M, et al. Amyloid-beta peptides in plasma and cognitive decline after 1 year follow-up in Alzheimer's disease patients. *J Alzheimers Dis* (2010) **21**(4):1263–9. doi:10.3233/JAD2010100510
142. Doody RS, Thomas RG, Farlow M, Iwatsubo T, Vellas B, Joffe S, et al. Phase 3 trials of solanezumab for mild-to-moderate Alzheimer's disease. *N Engl J Med* (2014) **370**(4):311–21. doi:10.1056/NEJMoa1312889
143. Toledo JB, Shaw LM, Trojanowski JQ. Plasma amyloid beta measurements – a desired but elusive Alzheimer's disease biomarker. *Alzheimers Res Ther* (2013) **5**(2):8. doi:10.1186/alzrt162
144. Kuo YM, Emmerling MR, Lampert HC, Hempelman SR, Kokjohn TA, Woods AS, et al. High levels of circulating Abeta42 are sequestered by plasma proteins in Alzheimer's disease. *Biochem Biophys Res Commun* (1999) **257**(3):787–91. doi:10.1006/bbrc.1999.0552
145. Wunderlich MT, Lins H, Skalej M, Wallesch CW, Goertler M. Neuron-specific enolase and tau protein as neurobiochemical markers of neuronal damage are related to early clinical course and long-term outcome in acute ischemic stroke. *Clin Neurol Neurosurg* (2006) **108**(6):558–63. doi:10.1016/j.clineuro.2005.12.006
146. Randall J, Mortberg E, Provuncher GK, Fournier DR, Duffy DC, Rubertsson S, et al. Tau proteins in serum predict neurological outcome after hypoxic brain injury from cardiac arrest: results of a pilot study. *Resuscitation* (2013) **84**(3):351–6. doi:10.1016/j.resuscitation.2012.07.027
147. Liliang PC, Liang CL, Weng HC, Lu K, Wang KW, Chen HJ, et al. Tau proteins in serum predict outcome after severe traumatic brain injury. *J Surg Res* (2010) **160**(2):302–7. doi:10.1016/j.jss.2008.12.022
148. Noguchi-Shinohara M, Hamaguchi T, Nozaki I, Sakai K, Yamada M. Serum tau protein as a marker for the diagnosis of Creutzfeldt-Jakob disease. *J Neurol* (2011) **258**(8):1464–8. doi:10.1007/s00415-011-5960-x
149. Shahim P, Linemann T, Inekci D, Karsdal MA, Blennow K, Tegner Y, et al. Serum tau fragments predict return to play in concussed professional ice hockey players. *J Neurotrauma* (2015). doi:10.1089/neu.2014.3741
150. Zetterberg H, Wilson D, Andreasson U, Minthon L, Blennow K, Randall J, et al. Plasma tau levels in Alzheimer's disease. *Alzheimers Res Ther* (2013) **5**(2):9. doi:10.1186/alzrt163
151. Montine TJ, Quinn J, Kaye J, Morrow JD. F(2)-isoprostanes as biomarkers of late-onset Alzheimer's disease. *J Mol Neurosci* (2007) **33**(1):114–9. doi:10.1007/s12031-007-0044-1

152. Williams MA, Haughton D, Stevenson M, Craig D, Passmore AP, Silvestri G. Plasma complement factor H in Alzheimer's Disease. *J Alzheimers Dis* (2015). doi: 10.3233/JAD-142742
153. Ray S, Britschgi M, Herbert C, Takeda-Uchimura Y, Boxer A, Blennow K, et al. Classification and prediction of clinical Alzheimer's diagnosis based on plasma signaling proteins. *Nat Med* (2007) **13**(11):1359–62. doi:10.1038/nm1653
154. Hu WT, Holtzman DM, Fagan AM, Shaw LM, Perrin R, Arnold SE, et al. Plasma multianalyte profiling in mild cognitive impairment and Alzheimer disease. *Neurology* (2012) **79**(9):897–905. doi:10.1212/WNL.0b013e318266fa70
155. Doecke JD, Laws SM, Faux NG, Wilson W, Burnham SC, Lam CP, et al. Blood-based protein biomarkers for diagnosis of Alzheimer disease. *Arch Neurol* (2012) **69**(10):1318–25. doi:10.1001/archneurol.2012.1282
156. O'Bryant SE, Xiao G, Barber R, Huebinger R, Wilhelmsen K, Edwards M, et al. A blood-based screening tool for Alzheimer's disease that spans serum and plasma: findings from TARC and ADNI. *PLoS One* (2011) **6**(12):e28092. doi:10.1371/journal.pone.0028092
157. Llano DA, Devanarayan V, Simon AJ. Evaluation of plasma proteomic data for Alzheimer disease state classification and for the prediction of progression from mild cognitive impairment to Alzheimer disease. *Alzheimer Dis Assoc Disord* (2013) **27**(3):233–43. doi:10.1097/WAD.0b013e31826d597a
158. O'Bryant SE, Gupta V, Henriksen K, Edwards M, Jeromin A, Lista S, et al. Guidelines for the standardization of preanalytic variables for blood-based biomarker studies in Alzheimer's disease research. *Alzheimers Dement* (2014). doi:10.1016/j.jalz.2014.08.099
159. Zurbig P, Jahn H. Use of proteomic methods in the analysis of human body fluids in Alzheimer research. *Electrophoresis* (2012) **33**(24):3617–30. doi:10.1002/elps.201200360
160. Sayer R, Law E, Connelly PJ, Breen KC. Association of a salivary acetylcholinesterase with Alzheimer's disease and response to cholinesterase inhibitors. *Clin Biochem* (2004) **37**(2):98–104. doi:10.1016/j.clinbiochem.2003.10.007
161. Boston PF, Gopalkaje K, Manning L, Middleton L, Loxley M. Developing a simple laboratory test for Alzheimer's disease: measuring acetylcholinesterase in saliva – a pilot study. *Int J Geriatr Psychiatry* (2008) **23**(4):439–40. doi:10.1002/gps.1882
162. Bermejo-Pareja F, Antequera D, Vargas T, Molina JA, Carro E. Saliva levels of Abeta1-42 as potential biomarker of Alzheimer's disease: a pilot study. *BMC Neurol* (2010) **10**:108. doi:10.1186/1471-2377-10-108
163. Shi M, Sui YT, Peskind ER, Li G, Hwang H, Devic I, et al. Salivary tau species are potential biomarkers of Alzheimer's disease. *J Alzheimers Dis* (2011) **27**(2):299–305. doi:10.3233/JAD-2011-110731
164. Schenk D, Barbour R, Dunn W, Gordon G, Grajeda H, Guido T, Immunization with amyloid-beta attenuates Alzheimer-disease-like pathology in the PDAPP mouse. *Nature* (1999) **400**(6740):173–7. doi:10.1038/22124
165. Morgan D, Diamond DM, Gottschall PE, Ugen KE, Dickey C, Hardy J, A beta peptide vaccination prevents memory loss in an animal model of Alzheimer's disease. *Nature* (2000) **408**(6815):982–5. doi:10.1038/35050116
166. Janus C, Pearson J, McLaurin J, Mathews PM, Jiang Y, Schmidt SD, A beta peptide immunization reduces behavioural impairment and plaques in a model of Alzheimer's disease. *Nature* (2000) **408**(6815):979–82. doi:10.1038/35050110
167. Das P, Murphy MP, Younkin LH, Younkin SG, Golde TE. Reduced effectiveness of Abeta1-42 immunization in APP transgenic mice with significant amyloid deposition. *Neurobiol Aging* (2001) **22**(5):721–7. doi:10.1016/S0197-4580(01)00245-7
168. Bayer AJ, Bullock R, Jones RW, Wilkinson D, Paterson KR, Jenkins L, et al. Evaluation of the safety and immunogenicity of synthetic Abeta42 (AN1792) in patients with AD. *Neurology* (2005) **64**(1):94–101. doi:10.1212/01.WNL.0000148604.77591.67
169. Gilman S, Koller M, Black RS, Jenkins L, Griffith SG, Fox NC, et al. Clinical effects of Abeta immunization (AN1792) in patients with AD in an interrupted trial. *Neurology* (2005) **64**(9):1553–62. doi:10.1212/01.WNL.0000159740.16984.3C
170. Pride M, Seubert P, Grundman M, Hagen M, Eldridge J, Black RS. Progress in the active immunotherapeutic approach to Alzheimer's disease: clinical investigations into AN1792-associated meningoencephalitis. *Neurodegener Dis* (2008) **5**(3-4):194–6. doi:10.1159/000113700
171. Vellas B, Black R, Thal LJ, Fox NC, Daniels M, McLennan G, et al. Long-term follow-up of patients immunized with AN1792: reduced functional decline in antibody responders. *Curr Alzheimer Res* (2009) **6**(2):144–51. doi:10.2174/156720509787602852
172. Masliah E, Hansen L, Adame A, Crews L, Bard F, Lee C, et al. Abeta vaccination effects on plaque pathology in the absence of encephalitis in Alzheimer disease. *Neurology* (2005) **64**(1):129–31. doi:10.1212/01.WNL.0000148590.39911.DF
173. Zotova E, Bharambe V, Cheaveau M, Morgan W, Holmes C, Harris S, et al. Inflammatory components in human Alzheimer's disease and after active amyloid-beta42 immunization. *Brain* (2013) **136**(Pt 9):2677–96. doi:10.1093/brain/awt210
174. Holmes C, Boche D, Wilkinson D, Yadegarfar G, Hopkins V, Bayer A, et al. Long-term effects of Abeta42 immunisation in Alzheimer's disease: follow-up of a randomised, placebo-controlled phase I trial. *Lancet* (2008) **372**(9634):216–23. doi:10.1016/S0140-6736(08)61075-2
175. Serrano-Pozo A, William CM, Ferrer I, Uro-Coste E, Delisle MB, Maurage CA, et al. Beneficial effect of human anti-amyloid-beta active immunization on neurite morphology and tau pathology. *Brain* (2010) **133**(Pt 5):1312–27. doi:10.1093/brain/awq056
176. Winblad B, Andreasen N, Minthon L, Floesser A, Imbert G, Dumortier T, et al. Safety, tolerability, and antibody response of active Abeta immunotherapy with CAD106 in patients with Alzheimer's disease: randomised, double-blind, placebo-controlled, first-in-human study. *Lancet Neurol* (2012) **11**(7):597–604. doi:10.1016/S1474-4422(12)70140-0
177. Farlow MR, Andreasen N, Riviere ME, Vostiar I, Vitaliti A, Sovago J, et al. Long-term treatment with active Abeta immunotherapy with CAD106 in mild Alzheimer's disease. *Alzheimers Res Ther* (2015) **7**(1):23. doi:10.1186/s13195-015-0108-3
178. Bard F, Cannon C, Barbour R, Burke RL, Games D, Grajeda H, et al. Peripherally administered antibodies against amyloid beta-peptide enter the central nervous system and reduce pathology in a mouse model of Alzheimer disease. *Nat Med* (2000) **6**(8):916–9. doi:10.1038/78682
179. Blennow K, Hampel H, Zetterberg H. Biomarkers in amyloid-beta immunotherapy trials in Alzheimer's disease. *Neuropsychopharmacology* (2014) **39**(1):189–201. doi:10.1038/npp.2013.154
180. Legleiter J, Czilli DL, Gitter B, DeMattos RB, Holtzman DM, Kowalewski T. Effect of different anti-Abeta antibodies on Abeta fibrillogenesis as assessed by atomic force microscopy. *J Mol Biol* (2004) **335**(4):997–1006. doi:10.1016/j.jmb.2003.11.019
181. Lemere CA. Developing novel immunogens for a safe and effective Alzheimer's disease vaccine. *Prog Brain Res* (2009) **175**:83–93. doi:10.1016/S0079-6123(09)17506-4
182. Demattos RB, Lu J, Tang Y, Racke MM, Delong CA, Tzaferis JA, et al. A plaque-specific antibody clears existing beta-amyloid plaques in Alzheimer's disease mice. *Neuron* (2012) **76**(5):908–20. doi:10.1016/j.neuron.2012.10.029
183. Schroeter S, Khan K, Barbour R, Doan M, Chen M, Guido T, et al. Immunotherapy reduces vascular amyloid-beta in PDAPP mice. *J Neurosci* (2008) **28**(27):6787–93. doi:10.1523/JNEUROSCI.2377-07.2008
184. Salloway S, Sperling R, Gilman S, Fox NC, Blennow K, Raskind M, et al. A phase 2 multiple ascending dose trial of bapineuzumab in mild to moderate Alzheimer disease. *Neurology* (2009) **73**(24):2061–70. doi:10.1212/WNL.0b013e3181c67808
185. Vellas B, Carrillo MC, Sampaio C, Brashear HR, Siemers E, Hampel H, et al. Designing drug trials for Alzheimer's disease: what we have learned from the release of the phase III antibody trials: a report from the EU/US/CTAD task force. *Alzheimers Dement* (2013) **9**(4):438–44. doi:10.1016/j.jalz.2013.03.007
186. Blennow K, Zetterberg H, Rinne JO, Salloway S, Wei J, Black R, et al. Effect of immunotherapy with bapineuzumab on cerebrospinal fluid biomarker levels in patients with mild to moderate Alzheimer disease. *Arch Neurol* (2012) **69**(8):1002–10. doi:10.1001/archneurol.2012.90
187. DeMattos RB, Bales KR, Cummins DJ, Dodart JC, Paul SM, Holtzman DM. Peripheral anti-A beta antibody alters CNS and plasma A beta clearance and decreases brain A beta burden in a mouse model of Alzheimer's disease. *Proc Natl Acad Sci U S A* (2001) **98**(15):8850–5. doi:10.1073/pnas.151261398
188. Racke MM, Boone LI, Hepburn DL, Parsadainian M, Bryan MT, Ness DK, et al. Exacerbation of cerebral amyloid angiopathy-associated microhemorrhage in amyloid precursor protein transgenic mice by immunotherapy is dependent on antibody recognition of deposited forms of amyloid beta. *J Neurosci* (2005) **25**(3):629–36. doi:10.1523/JNEUROSCI.4337-04.2005

189. Seubert P, Barbour R, Khan K, Motter R, Tang P, Kholodenko D, et al. Antibody capture of soluble Abeta does not reduce cortical Abeta amyloidosis in the PDAPP mouse. *Neurodegener Dis* (2008) **5**(2):65–71. doi:10.1159/000112834

190. Farlow M, Arnold SE, van Dyck CH, Aisen PS, Snider BJ, Porsteinsson AP, et al. Safety and biomarker effects of solanezumab in patients with Alzheimer's disease. *Alzheimers Dement* (2012) **8**(4):261–71. doi:10.1016/j.jalz.2011.09.224

191. Comery TA, Martone RL, Aschmies S, Atchison KP, Diamantidis G, Gong X, et al. Acute gamma-secretase inhibition improves contextual fear conditioning in the Tg2576 mouse model of Alzheimer's disease. *J Neurosci* (2005) **25**(39):8898–902. doi:10.1523/JNEUROSCI.2693-05.2005

192. Martone RL, Zhou H, Atchison K, Comery T, Xu JZ, Huang X, et al. Begacestat (GSI-953): a novel, selective thiophene sulfonamide inhibitor of amyloid precursor protein gamma-secretase for the treatment of Alzheimer's disease. *J Pharmacol Exp Ther* (2009) **331**(2):598–608. doi:10.1124/jpet.109.152975

193. Tong G, Castaneda L, Wang JS, Sverdlov O, Huang SP, Slemmon R, et al. Effects of single doses of avagacestat (BMS-708163) on cerebrospinal fluid Abeta levels in healthy young men. *Clin Drug Investig* (2012) **32**(11):761–9. doi:10.1007/s40261-012-0006-4

194. Li T, Huang Y, Jin S, Ye L, Rong N, Yang X, et al. Gamma-secretase modulators do not induce Abeta-rebound and accumulation of beta-C-terminal fragment. *J Neurochem* (2012) **121**(2):277–86. doi:10.1111/j.1471-4159.2011.07560.x

195. Mitani Y, Yarimizu J, Saita K, Uchino H, Akashiba H, Shitaka Y, et al. Differential effects between gamma-secretase inhibitors and modulators on cognitive function in amyloid precursor protein-transgenic and nontransgenic mice. *J Neurosci* (2012) **32**(6):2037–50. doi:10.1523/JNEUROSCI.4264-11.2012

196. Chavez-Gutierrez L, Bammens L, Benilova I, Vandersteen A, Benurwar M, Borgers M, et al. The mechanism of gamma-secretase dysfunction in familial Alzheimer disease. *EMBO J* (2012) **31**(10):2261–74. doi:10.1038/emboj.2012.79

197. Cirrito JR, May PC, O'Dell MA, Taylor JW, Parsadanian M, Cramer JW, et al. In vivo assessment of brain interstitial fluid with microdialysis reveals plaque-associated changes in amyloid-beta metabolism and half-life. *J Neurosci* (2003) **23**(26):8844–53. doi: 0270-6474/03/238844-10

198. Abramowski D, Wiederhold KH, Furrer U, Jaton AL, Neuenschwander A, Runser MJ, et al. Dynamics of Abeta turnover and deposition in different beta-amyloid precursor protein transgenic mouse models following gamma-secretase inhibition. *J Pharmacol Exp Ther* (2008) **327**(2):411–24. doi:10.1124/jpet.108.140327

199. Garcia-Alloza M, Subramanian M, Thyssen D, Borrelli LA, Fauq A, Das P, et al. Existing plaques and neuritic abnormalities in APP:PS1 mice are not affected by administration of the gamma-secretase inhibitor *LY-411575. Mol Neurodegener* (2009) **4**:19. doi:10.1186/1750-1326-4-19

200. Bateman RJ, Munsell LY, Morris JC, Swarm R, Yarasheski KE, Holtzman DM. Human amyloid-beta synthesis and clearance rates as measured in cerebrospinal fluid in vivo. *Nat Med* (2006) **12**(7):856–61. doi:10.1038/nm1438

201. Fleisher AS, Raman R, Siemers ER, Becerra L, Clark CM, Dean RA, et al. Phase 2 safety trial targeting amyloid beta production with a gamma-secretase inhibitor in Alzheimer disease. *Arch Neurol* (2008) **65**(8):1031–8. doi:10.1001/archneur.65.8.1031

202. Callaway E. Gene mutation defends against Alzheimer's disease. *Nature* (2012) **487**(7406):153. doi:10.1038/487153a

203. Jonsson T, Atwal JK, Steinberg S, Snaedal J, Jonsson PV, Bjornsson S, et al. A mutation in APP protects against Alzheimer's disease and age-related cognitive decline. *Nature* (2012) **488**(7409):96–9. doi:10.1038/nature11283

204. Mikulca JA, Nguyen V, Gajdosik DA, Teklu SG, Giunta EA, Lessa EA, et al. Potential novel targets for Alzheimer pharmacotherapy: II. Update on secretase inhibitors and related approaches. *J Clin Pharm Ther* (2014) **39**(1):25–37. doi:10.1111/jcpt.12112

205. Menting KW, Claassen JA. beta-secretase inhibitor; a promising novel therapeutic drug in Alzheimer's disease. *Front Aging Neurosci* (2014) **6**:165. doi:10.3389/fnagi.2014.00165

206. Kokjohn TA, Roher AE. Amyloid precursor protein transgenic mouse models and Alzheimer's disease: understanding the paradigms, limitations, and contributions. *Alzheimers Dement* (2009) **5**(4):340–7. doi:10.1016/j.jalz.2009.03.002

207. DeMattos RB, Bales KR, Parsadanian M, O'Dell MA, Foss EM, Paul SM, et al. Plaque-associated disruption of CSF and plasma amyloid-beta (Abeta) equilibrium in a mouse model of Alzheimer's disease. *J Neurochem* (2002) **81**(2):229–36. doi:10.1046/j.1471-4159.2002.00889.x

208. Cummings J, Gould H, Zhong K. Advances in designs for Alzheimer's disease clinical trials. *Am J Neurodegener Dis* (2012) **1**(3):205–16. doi: AJND1210001

209. Mulder SD, van der Flier WM, Verheijen JH, Mulder C, Scheltens P, Blankenstein MA, et al. BACE1 activity in cerebrospinal fluid and its relation to markers of AD pathology. *J Alzheimers Dis* (2010) **20**(1):253–60. doi:10.3233/JAD-2010-1367

210. Sperling R, Salloway S, Brooks DJ, Tampieri D, Barakos J, Fox NC, et al. Amyloid-related imaging abnormalities in patients with Alzheimer's disease treated with bapineuzumab: a retrospective analysis. *Lancet Neurol* (2012) **11**(3):241–9. doi:10.1016/S1474-4422(12)70015-7

211. Adolfsson O, Pihlgren M, Toni N, Varisco Y, Buccarello AL, Antoniello K, et al. An effector-reduced anti-beta-amyloid (Abeta) antibody with unique abeta binding properties promotes neuroprotection and glial engulfment of Abeta. *J Neurosci* (2012) **32**(28):9677–89. doi:10.1523/JNEUROSCI.4742-11.2012

212. Burstein AH, Zhao Q, Ross J, Styren S, Landen JW, Ma WW, et al. Safety and pharmacology of ponezumab (PF-04360365) after a single 10-minute intravenous infusion in subjects with mild to moderate Alzheimer disease. *Clin Neuropharmacol* (2013) **36**(1):8–13. doi:10.1097/WNF.0b013e318279bcfa

213. Landen JW, Zhao Q, Cohen S, Borrie M, Woodward M, Billing CB Jr, et al. Safety and pharmacology of a single intravenous dose of ponezumab in subjects with mild-to-moderate Alzheimer disease: a phase I, randomized, placebo-controlled, double-blind, dose-escalation study. *Clin Neuropharmacol* (2013) **36**(1):14–23. doi:10.1097/WNF.0b013e31827db49b

214. Miyoshi I, Fujimoto Y, Yamada M, Abe S, Zhao Q, Cronenberger C, et al. Safety and pharmacokinetics of PF-04360365 following a single-dose intravenous infusion in Japanese subjects with mild-to-moderate Alzheimer's disease: a multicenter, randomized, double-blind, placebo-controlled, dose-escalation study. *Int J Clin Pharmacol Ther* (2013) **51**(12):911–23. doi:10.5414/CP201816

215. Aisen PS, Gauthier S, Ferris SH, Saumier D, Haine D, Garceau D, et al. Tramiprosate in mild-to-moderate Alzheimer's disease – a randomized, double-blind, placebo-controlled, multi-centre study (the Alphase Study). *Arch Med Sci* (2011) **7**(1):102–11. doi:10.5114/aoms.2011.20612

216. Aisen PS, Saumier D, Briand R, Laurin J, Gervais F, Tremblay P, et al. A Phase II study targeting amyloid-beta with 3APS in mild-to-moderate Alzheimer disease. *Neurology* (2006) **67**(10):1757–63. doi:10.1212/01.wnl.0000244346.08950.64

7

The past and the future of Alzheimer's disease CSF biomarkers—a journey toward validated biochemical tests covering the whole spectrum of molecular events

Kaj Blennow and Henrik Zetterberg*

Clinical Neurochemistry Laboratory, Department of Psychiatry and Neurochemistry, Institute of Neuroscience and Physiology, The Sahlgrenska Academy at University of Gothenburg, Mölndal, Sweden

Edited by:
Sylvain Lehmann,
Montpellier University Hospital, France

Reviewed by:
Claudia Cicognola,
University of Perugia, Italy
Julien Dumurgier
Université Paris Diderot - Paris 7, France

****Correspondence:***
Kaj Blennow,
Clinical Neurochemistry Laboratory, Department of Psychiatry and Neurochemistry, Institute of Neuroscience and Physiology, Sahlgrenska University Hospital, The Sahlgrenska Academy at University of Gothenburg, Mölndal Campus, SE-431 80 Mölndal, Sweden
kaj.blennow@neuro.gu.se

This paper gives a short review on cerebrospinal fluid (CSF) biomarkers for Alzheimer's disease (AD), from early developments to high-precision validated assays on fully automated lab analyzers. We also discuss developments on novel biomarkers, such as synaptic proteins and Aβ oligomers. Our vision for the future is that assaying a set of biomarkers in a single CSF tube can monitor the whole spectrum of AD molecular pathogenic events. CSF biomarkers will have a central position not only for clinical diagnosis, but also for the understanding of the sequence of molecular events in the pathogenic process underlying AD and as tools to monitor the effects of novel drug candidates targeting these different mechanisms.

Keywords: Alzheimer disease, biomarker, cerebrospinal fluid, neurogranin, oligomers, synaptic proteins, tau proteins

Laboratory medicine tests influence up to 70% of clinical decisions and thus have a central position in clinical medicine (Beastall and Watson, 2013). Biochemical markers for chronic neurodegenerative disorders are especially important, since the slow progression and diffuse symptomatology results in diagnostic difficulties, and tissue sampling with direct visualization of central nervous system (CNS) pathology is not clinically applicable. For this reason, the Alzheimer's disease (AD) arena is in the good situation that a set of highly validated and specific biomarkers are at hand; in addition to amyloid positron emission tomography (PET) and magnetic resonance imaging (MRI) measurements, a set of cerebrospinal fluid (CSF) tests reflecting key aspects of disease pathology are available. This paper comments on some caveats on the road to develop and validate these CSF biomarkers and some recent developments on novel biochemical tests.

Early Assay Developments

The story on modern AD biomarker development started in 1995 with a series of publications on enzyme-linked immunosorbent assays (ELISA) based on monoclonal antibodies to measure CSF levels of total tau (T-tau) and phosphorylated tau (P-tau) and the 42 amino acid isoform (Aβ42) of β-amyloid (Blennow et al., 1995; Motter et al., 1995). These papers reported a marked increase in CSF T-tau and P-tau accompanied by a marked decrease in Aβ42 in AD (Blennow et al., 1995; Motter et al., 1995). The following years, many research reports consistently showed that the "AD profile" of increased CSF levels of T-tau and P-tau together with decreased Aβ42 had high sensitivity and specificity, both in the range of 85–90%, to identify AD dementia, for review see (Blennow and Hampel, 2003). Since these three CSF biomarkers reflect key elements of AD pathophysiology, i.e., neuronal degeneration (T-tau), tau pathology (P-tau), and amyloid plaques (Aβ42), they are often termed the "core" AD biomarkers (Hampel et al., 2004).

The Problem with Studies Based on Clinical Diagnosis

The vast majority of studies were cross-sectional and the diagnoses were based on the exclusion criteria published in 1984 by the National Institute of Neurological and Communicative Disorders and Stroke and the Alzheimer's Disease and Related Disorders Association (NINCDS-ADRDA). In the studies evaluating the diagnostic performance of CSF biomarkers, the diagnostic entity "probable AD" based on the NINCDS-ADRDA criteria, i.e., an exclusion diagnosis made on pure clinical grounds, was used as gold standard in the evaluation of the CSF biomarkers (McKhann et al., 1984). For logical reasons, the poor diagnostic accuracy of these criteria (Knopman et al., 2001), and the overlap in pathology between AD and other dementias, such as Lewy body dementia and vascular dementia (Blennow et al., 2006), made it impossible to achieve full diagnostic separation between AD and aging or other dementias using biomarkers.

The Issue of Biomarker-positive Elderly

The introduction of amyloid PET in the arsenal of AD biomarkers marked a major change in AD biomarker research, since it became clear that 20–30% of apparently healthy elderly showed positive on scans (Klunk, 2011). In 2006, the first study showed that high amyloid ligand retention on amyloid PET almost completely corresponds to low CSF Aβ42 (Fagan et al., 2006), and vice versa, a finding that has been verified in numerous subsequent studies, for review see Blennow et al. (2015). This knowledge rather quickly changed the view on how to interpret low CSF Aβ42 levels in cognitively intact elderly, from poor assay quality or biomarker performance to an indicator of preclinical AD.

In support of this, reliable biomarkers for cerebral β-amyloidosis also made it possible to follow cognitively normal Aβ-positive individuals over time. Such longitudinal studies are relevant given the fact that many individuals with AD neuropathology could be dementia-free when they died. Longitudinal Aβ biomarker studies suggest that the majority of Aβ-positive individuals followed over many years develop cognitive impairment and eventually dementia. In other words, if the dementia-free individuals with AD neuropathology would have lived 5–10 years longer they would most likely have developed AD (Buchhave et al., 2012).

Turning Direction Toward Early Diagnosis

The failures of Phase 2 and 3 trials testing anti-Aβ disease-modifying drug candidates on AD patients in the dementia stage initiated a discussion on the whether this type of treatment need to be initiated before the dementia phase of the disease, i.e., before the neurodegenerative process is too severe and widespread (Blennow, 2010). An attractive option was therefore to perform further trails on AD patients in the mild cognitive impairment (MCI) stage of the disease. However, this would also introduce diagnostic challenges since MCI is a heterogeneous syndrome that may have many different underlying causes. Around 50–60% of MCI cases have prodromal AD (Dubois et al., 2007), meaning that they have underlying AD pathology and will progress to AD with dementia. MCI symptoms may also be caused by other neurodegenerative disorders such as Lewy body dementia and vascular dementia or be due to age-related benign cognitive disturbances, stress and depression. Further, symptoms in MCI cases are by definition vague and diffuse, which makes it impossible to diagnose AD clinically in unselected MCI cohorts (Petersen et al., 1999). This created a need to test if the CSF biomarkers have value also for early diagnosis.

In 1999, a first paper showed that MCI patients progressing to AD with dementia, which is sometimes called "converting," during the clinical follow-up period had the typical AD CSF profile of high T-tau and P-tau together with low Aβ42, and levels were equally abnormal in the MCI and the dementia stage in cases with longitudinal sampling (Andreasen et al., 1999). In the first studies, no MCI group with long clinical follow-up, which is needed to ascertain that stable MCI cases will not progress, was presented. The first study with an extended clinical follow-up period, showed that the AD CSF profile had a 95% sensitivity for prodromal AD at a specificity of 83–92% against controls and stable MCI cases and MCI cases that proved to have other dementias (Hansson et al., 2006). A series of large multi-center studies could verify such a high diagnostic accuracy of the AD CSF biomarker profile to identify prodromal AD (Mattsson et al., 2009; Shaw et al., 2009; Visser et al., 2009).

Entering Diagnostic Criteria

In 2007, the International Work Group (IWG) published the first research criteria for the diagnosis of prodromal AD for New Research Criteria for the Diagnosis of AD (Dubois et al., 2007). These criteria provided a new conceptual framework stating that AD could be diagnosed based on the combination of a clinical phenotype of episodic memory disturbances and one or more abnormal AD biomarker including CSF biomarkers (Aβ and tau proteins), volumetric MRI and amyloid PET) (Dubois et al., 2007). In 2011, similar, but not identical, criteria for MCI due to AD (Albert et al., 2011) and dementia due to AD (McKhann et al., 2011) were published by the National Institute on Aging—Alzheimer's Association (NIA-AA) workgroups on diagnostic guidelines for AD. The IWG criteria for prodromal AD and NIA–AA criteria for MCI due to AD are similar, and most cases fulfilling one set of criteria will also fulfill the other, but the NIA–AA criteria allow for assessment of the likelihood of being correctly diagnosed, with both amyloid and (neuronal) injury biomarker positive cases having the highest likelihood (Visser et al., 2012). In the updated IWG-2 criteria (Dubois et al., 2014), CSF biomarkers got a more central role, together with amyloid PET, due to their high diagnostic performance (Hansson et al., 2006; Li et al., 2007; Brys et al., 2009; Snider et al., 2009; van Rossum et al., 2012), while downstream topographical AD biomarkers, such as volumetric MRI and FDG- PET, were judged to function better in monitoring disease course in AD.

Cut-offs and Clinical Interpretation

The issue of identifying unified cut-offs for the CSF biomarkers was brought up in the updated IWG-2 criteria (Dubois et al., 2014). For CSF biomarkers, this problem stems from differences in pre-analytical procedures between clinics and in analytical procedures between laboratories, and not the least from variability in manufacturing procedures for the assays, with batch-to-batch variations (Mattsson et al., 2013). To overcome these problems, several standardization initiatives have been launched with the aim to minimize this type of variability, including the Global Biomarker Standardization Consortium (GBSC) and the International Federation of Clinical Chemistry and Laboratory Medicine (IFCC) Work Group for CSF proteins, that aims to develop certified reference materials and methods to serve as "gold standards" for CSF biomarker measurements (Carrillo et al., 2013). These initiatives will, together with novel validated assays produced under rigorous quality control measures and CSF biomarker methods run on fully automated lab analyzers, allow to uniform cut-off levels for diagnosis, and a more widespread use of CSF biomarkers in the routine clinical diagnostic setting.

However, for common age-related disorders such as diabetes type II and hypertension, there is no distinct line between health and disease, and recommended cut-offs must therefore be based on estimations of risk and values in the individual patient must always undergo clinical interpretation. The situation is the same for AD, with an increasing overlap in neuropathological changes (Mountjoy et al., 1983; Mann et al., 1984; Hansen et al., 1988) and in CSF biomarker levels (Andreasen et al., 1999a; Mattsson et al., 2012) between aging and AD with increasing age. Indeed, studies comparing the diagnostic performance of CSF biomarker levels (Aβ42) and amyloid PET show that the overlap around the proposed cut-off for both biomarker modalities (Mattsson et al., 2014) makes it questionable to dichotomize results into biomarker (CSF Aβ42 or amyloid PET) "positive" or "negative." The tradition in Laboratory medicine is to report the actual concentration of a biomarker back to the clinician who based on clinical experience interprets biomarker values near the cut-off with caution.

Ratios such as T-tau/Aβ42, combining one injury and one amyloid biomarker, are commonly evaluated in clinical biomarker studies, and often found to perform better than either biomarker alone. Even if this type of ratios show excellent diagnostic separation in selected AD and control populations, they may be difficult to implement in unselected populations in the clinic. This is since an increase in CSF T-tau in patients with minor stroke, encephalitis or CJD will have a very high ratio despite having normal CSF Aβ42, and thus no indication of amyloid pathology (Blennow et al., 2006).

The Putative *APOE* Dependence of CSF Aβ42

The apolipoprotein E (*APOE*) ε4 allele is the main genetic risk factor for AD (Bertram and Tanzi, 2008). In the late 1990ies, several studies reported that AD patients possessing the *APOE* ε4 allele had lower CSF Aβ42 than those without this gene variant (Galasko et al., 1998; Hulstaert et al., 1999). This association is present also in cognitively normal elderly (Prince et al., 2004). In contrast, CSF tau levels do not depend on the ε4 allele (Andreasen et al., 1999b).

These results raised the question whether the ApoE4 isoform modulates brain and CSF Aβ levels through a physiological mechanism. Some studies on mice found that the ApoE isoforms differentially regulates Aβ clearance, and suggested that the *APOE* genotype contribute to AD risk by differentially regulating clearance of Aβ the brain throughout life (Castellano et al., 2011; Verghese et al., 2013). In a clinical study challenging this hypothesis, MCI patients stratified by for cortical amyloid deposition as evaluated by amyloid PET, amyloid positive cases had low CSF Aβ42 levels, and amyloid negative cases normal Aβ42 levels, independently of ε4 status (Lautner et al., 2014). These findings indicate that the gene-dose dependent association between the *APOE* ε4 allele and Aβ42 is caused by more severe amyloid deposition in patients that are ε4 carriers. In support of this conclusion, there is no association between CSF Aβ42 and the *APOE* ε4 allele in young individuals, that are likely to be free of brain amyloid deposition (Lautner et al., 2014), and thus no evidence of a physiological effect on Aβ clearance in man. In addition, these findings show that there is no need for *APOE* allele-dependent cut-off levels for CSF Aβ42.

Compensating for Differences in Basic Aβ Production—the Aβ42/Aβ42 Ratio

Except for Aβ42, the CSF contains several other Aβ isoforms, the most abundant variant being Aβ40 (Portelius et al., 2006). Even if CSF Aβ40 is relatively unchanged in AD, the CSF Aβ42/Aβ40 has been suggested to have stronger diagnostic accuracy for AD compared to CSF Aβ42 alone (Hansson et al., 2007). The explanation may be that the ratio normalizes individuals according to their Aβ production level, so that low CSF Aβ42 can be more easily detected in "high Aβ producers" and vice versa (Lewczuk et al., 2015). Recent studies show that the CSF Aβ42/Aβ40 ratio is valuable also in the clinical setting (Dumurgier et al., 2015).

The Everlasting Promise of Blood Biomarkers for AD

The CSF is continuous with the brain extracellular space, with a free exchange of molecules that makes it possible to monitor brain biochemistry by CSF analyses. Nevertheless, since blood is more accessible than CSF, for which a lumbar puncture is needed, blood biomarkers are desirable both for clinical diagnosis or screening and for multiple sampling in clinical trials. However, there are several circumstances that make blood a more challenging matrix than CSF for brain biomarkers. First, peripheral blood (plasma and serum) and the brain are separated by the blood-brain barrier, making only a small fraction of brain proteins enter the bloodstream. Second, the minute amounts of brain proteins entering the blood will be diluted in a compartment containing very high levels of other proteins such as albumin and IgG, introducing a high risk of interference in analytical methods (Blennow and Zetterberg, 2015). Third, brain proteins in the bloodstream will be subjected to degradation by proteases, degradation in the liver or clearance in the kidneys, which will introduce a risk of confounding data. As an example, the Australian Imaging Biomarkers and Lifestyle (AIBL) research team have reported that plasma Aβ levels are influenced by inflammatory and renal function covariates and that absolute levels of either Aβ40 or Aβ42 do not associate with AD or neocortical Aβ burden (Rembach et al., 2014). These factors make development of blood biomarkers for chronic neurodegenerative disorders challenging and limits the potential of blood samples as biomarker sources for AD.

One possible approach is to apply hypothesis-free proteomics, lipidomics, and similar methods in the search for AD blood biomarkers. Such studies report combinations of proteins, lipids, metabolites, or other molecules that discriminate AD from controls, and propose such panels as novel AD blood biomarkers, for review see (Henriksen et al., 2014). These studies often screen a high number of unselected molecules, each showing a marked overlap between AD and controls. However, when combining a number of molecules using multivariate statistics, a diagnostic separation is found. This type of studies have several challenges. First, analytical standardization is difficult for a panel of analyses consisting of high number of proteins or molecules with different characteristics (O'Bryant et al., 2015). Second, pre-analytical factors, such as influence of age, gender, other diseases, medications, food-intake, or physical activity may vary considerably between these molecules, or are not known or not examined. Third, patient and control cohort differences may influence outcome, but the panel is often evaluated in a "training" and "validation" set of patients and controls from the same cohort. Last, but not least, the issue of potential statistical over-fitting of data to identify a "biomarker panel" from a very large number of molecules in samples from a specific cohort with limited number of cases may introduce bias. For these reasons, such panels of molecules unrelated to AD pathogenesis often fail to replicate in independent clinical cohorts (Zhao et al., 2015), or alternative protein biomarker panels are proposed in the different studies (Henriksen et al., 2014).

Biochemical Tests Covering the Whole Spectrum of Molecular Events

Despite that the core CSF AD biomarkers reflect central pathogenic mechanisms of the disease, novel biomarkers to monitor additional important molecular mechanisms in AD are constantly sought. Two important aspects of AD pathophysiology are soluble oligomeric Aβ species and synaptic dysfunction and degeneration.

Oligomeric Aβ May Give Clues to Disease Pathogenesis

Amyloid plaques are composed of aggregated Aβ, but research during the last decade has put focus on soluble oligomers of Aβ that may inhibit long-term potentiation (LTP) and cause tau hyperphosphorylation and neuritic dystrophy (Walsh et al., 2002; Jin et al., 2011), possibly by specifically affecting synapses and disturbing synaptic signaling pathways (Pozueta et al., 2013). LTP is thought to be the key mechanism behind memory encoding, the possible causation between Aβ oligomers and synaptic dysfunction and damage has evolved into an active area of research. However, LTP cannot be measured *in vivo* in man, and a key question is whether there is a primary Aβ oligomer-induced deficit in LTP in the early stages of AD, or whether the synaptic degeneration in AD causes memory impairment through other mechanisms, with LTP deficits being downstream consequences of the synaptic dysfunction and loss. Tools to study these molecular mechanisms in man would thus be valuable.

Aβ oligomers, ranging from dimers, trimers, dodecamers, and larger molecular weight species have been found to be present in CSF (Klyubin et al., 2008; Handoko et al., 2013). However, in addition to the molecular heterogeneity, CSF Aβ oligomer levels are very low, making reliable quantification challenging. Indeed, different studies have applied a wide variety of methodologies to allow quantification of these soluble aggregates, such as fluorescence correlation spectroscopy (Pitschke et al., 1998), bio-barcode assay (Georganopoulou et al., 2005), misfolded protein assay (Gao et al., 2010), ELISA with the same monoclonal antibody both for capture and detection (Fukumoto et al., 2010), flow cytometry based assays (Santos et al., 2012), immunoprecipitation and Western blot (Handoko et al., 2013), and ultrasensitive bead-based immunoassays (Savage et al., 2014). Several studies have found increased Aβ oligomer levels in CSF of AD patients (Pitschke et al., 1998; Georganopoulou et al., 2005; Fukumoto et al., 2010; Gao et al., 2010; Handoko et al., 2013; Holtta et al., 2013; Savage et al., 2014), but with large overlap with control groups, while other studies have reported no change (Santos et al., 2012; Bruggink et al., 2013; Jongbloed et al., 2015) or lower levels (Sancesario et al., 2012).

The reason for these contradictory results is unclear, but may include analytical shortcomings, variability in how and in which type of oligomer assemblies are secreted from the brain to the CSF, instability of Aβ oligomers in CSF or during the analytical procedures, or other factors. Nevertheless, if these analytical shortcomings and variability between studies can be overcome, CSF Aβ oligomers measurements may provide important clues to disease pathogenesis when applied in longitudinal studies in the different stages of AD and related to both neuropsychological evaluations and other AD biomarkers such as amyloid PET and MRI measurements. However, the finding in several studies that CSF Aβ oligomer levels correlate with disease severity, with higher CSF levels in more advanced disease (Fukumoto et al., 2010; Santos et al., 2012; Savage et al., 2014), does not support that they are associated with early disease pathogenesis.

Synaptic Biomarkers Enter the Arena

Synapses are the building blocks of neuronal networks. Synapses consist of a pre-synaptic unit with synaptic vesicles containing the neurotransmitters that upon release, regulated by a delicate machinery of pre-synaptic proteins, bind to post-synaptic receptors at the dendritic spines and activate a cascade of molecular events to advance the signal (Jahn and Fasshauer, 2012). Synaptic dysfunction and degeneration is likely the direct cause of the cognitive deterioration in AD. Synaptic degeneration is an early pathogenic event in AD (Masliah et al., 2001; Scheff et al., 2007), with synaptic loss being more tightly correlated with cognitive impairment than either plaque or tangle pathology (DeKosky and Scheff, 1990; Blennow et al., 1996; Sze et al., 1997). Thus, synaptic biomarkers may serve as a tool to study the link between the molecular pathology and cognitive symptoms.

As mentioned above, there is no method to measure LTP in man, but some synaptic proteins such as neurogranin has been shown to play a critical role in LTP (Wu et al., 2002; Huang et al., 2004). Neurogranin is highly concentrated in dendritic spines, and neurogranin levels are markedly reduced in the hippocampus and the frontal cortex in AD, indicating loss of post-synaptic elements (Davidsson and Blennow, 1998; Reddy et al., 2005). A pilot study using immunoprecipitation and Western blot showed increased CSF levels of neurogranin in AD (Thorsell et al., 2010). The first study using a quantitative immunoassay showed a marked increase in CSF neurogranin in AD dementia and high levels predicted progression to AD dementia among MCI patients (Kvartsberg et al., 2014). Further, in amyloid positive MCI cases, high neurogranin correlated with a more rapid cognitive deterioration during clinical follow-up (Kvartsberg et al., 2014). Among proteins specific for the pre-synaptic part of the synapse, SNAP-25 CSF levels are clearly elevated in AD, also in the prodromal phase of the disease (Brinkmalm et al., 2014a), probably reflecting the ongoing destruction of presynaptic terminals (Davidsson and Blennow, 1998; Brinkmalm et al., 2014b).

Concluding Remarks

Three CSF biomarkers reflecting the core pathological features of AD are available: T-tau (neurodegeneration), P-tau (tau hyperphosphorylation and, potentially, tangle formation), and Aβ42 (plaque pathology). According to revised clinical criteria, these markers may help diagnose AD more accurately and open up the possibility of detecting pre-dementia stages of the disease. At present, their most obvious utility is in clinical trials of novel disease-modifying treatments against AD. In the future, they may help selecting the right treatment for individual patients by making it possible to assess which molecular pathology is most likely to cause the patient's symptom at different stages of the disease. Standardization efforts are now moving the CSF tau and Aβ biomarker tests toward automated clinical-grade assays, which hopefully will become as established and standardized as clinical chemistry tests for other common human diseases. In addition, there is considerable promise that CSF biomarkers will provide *in vivo* measurement of a range of additional pathophysiological processes in AD. New biomarkers including synaptic proteins and Aβ oligomers, will broaden the arsenal toward a panel that covers the whole spectrum of molecular events in AD. The application of such panels in longitudinal clinical studies will give essential additional information of the evolution of pathogenic processes in AD.

Acknowledgments

The Torsten Söderberg Foundation at the Royal Swedish Academy of Sciences.

References

Albert, M. S., DeKosky, S. T., Dickson, D., Dubois, B., Feldman, H. H., Fox, N. C., et al. (2011). The diagnosis of mild cognitive impairment due to Alzheimer's disease: recommendations from the National Institute on Aging-Alzheimer's Association workgroups on diagnostic guidelines for Alzheimer's disease. *Alzheimer's Demen.* 7, 270–279. doi: 10.1016/j.jalz.2011.03.008

Andreasen, N., Hesse, C., Davidsson, P., Minthon, L., Wallin, A., Winblad, B., et al. (1999a). Cerebrospinal fluid beta-amyloid(1-42) in Alzheimer disease: differences between early- and late-onset Alzheimer disease and stability during the course of disease. *Archiv. Neurol.* 56, 673–680. doi: 10.1001/archneur.56.6.673

Andreasen, N., Minthon, L., Clarberg, A., Davidsson, P., Gottfries, J., Vanmechelen, E., et al. (1999b). Sensitivity, specificity, and stability of CSF-tau in AD in a community-based patient sample. *Neurology* 53, 1488–1494. doi: 10.1212/WNL.53.7.1488

Andreasen, N., Minthon, L., Vanmechelen, E., Vanderstichele, H., Davidsson, P., Winblad, B., et al. (1999). Cerebrospinal fluid tau and Abeta42 as predictors of development of Alzheimer's disease in patients with mild cognitive impairment. *Neurosci. Lett.* 273, 5–8. doi: 10.1016/S0304-3940(99)00617-5

Beastall, G. H., and Watson, I. D. (2013). Clinical chemistry and laboratory medicine: an appreciation. *Clin. Chem. Lab. Med.* 51, 3–4. doi: 10.1515/cclm-2012-0546

Bertram, L., and Tanzi, R. E. (2008). Thirty years of Alzheimer's disease genetics: the implications of systematic meta-analyses. *Nat. Rev. Neurosci.* 9, 768–778. doi: 10.1038/nrn2494

Blennow, K. (2010). Biomarkers in Alzheimer's disease drug development. *Nat. Med.* 16, 1218–1222. doi: 10.1038/nm.2221

Blennow, K., Bogdanovic, N., Alafuzoff, I., Ekman, R., and Davidsson, P. (1996). Synaptic pathology in Alzheimer's disease: relation to severity of dementia, but not to senile plaques, neurofibrillary tangles, or the ApoE4 allele. *J. Neural Transm.* 103, 603–618. doi: 10.1007/BF01273157

Blennow, K., de Leon, M. J., and Zetterberg, H. (2006). Alzheimer's disease. *Lancet* 368, 387–403. doi: 10.1016/S0140-6736(06)69113-7

Blennow, K., and Hampel, H. (2003). CSF markers for incipient Alzheimer's disease. *Lancet Neurol.* 2, 605–613. doi: 10.1016/S1474-4422(03)00530-1

Blennow, K., Mattsson, N., Scholl, M., Hansson, O., and Zetterberg, H. (2015). Amyloid biomarkers in Alzheimer's disease. *Trends Pharmacol. Sci.* 36, 297–309. doi: 10.1016/j.tips.2015.03.002

Blennow, K., Wallin, A., Agren, H., Spenger, C., Siegfried, J., and Vanmechelen, E. (1995). Tau protein in cerebrospinal fluid: a biochemical marker for axonal degeneration in Alzheimer disease? *Mol. Chem. Neuropathol.* 26, 231–245.

Blennow, K., and Zetterberg, H. (2015). Understanding biomarkers of neurodegeneration: ultrasensitive detection techniques pave the way for mechanistic understanding. *Nat. Med.* 21, 217–219. doi: 10.1038/nm.3810

Brinkmalm, A., Brinkmalm, G., Honer, W. G., Frolich, L., Hausner, L., Minthon, L., et al. (2014a). SNAP-25 is a promising novel cerebrospinal fluid biomarker for synapse degeneration in Alzheimer's disease. *Mol. Neurodegener.* 9:53. doi: 10.1186/1750-1326-9-53

Brinkmalm, A., Brinkmalm, G., Honer, W. G., Moreno, J. A., Jakobsson, J., Mallucci, G. R., et al. (2014b). Targeting synaptic pathology with a novel affinity mass spectrometry approach. *Mol. Cell. Proteom.* 13, 2584–2592. doi: 10.1016/j.neurobiolaging.2011.09.006

Bruggink, K. A., Jongbloed, W., Biemans, E. A., Veerhuis, R., Claassen, J. A., Kuiperij, H. B., et al. (2013). Amyloid-beta oligomer detection by ELISA in cerebrospinal fluid and brain tissue. *Anal. Biochem.* 433, 112–120. doi: 10.1016/j.ab.2012.09.014

Brys, M., Pirraglia, E., Rich, K., Rolstad, S., Mosconi, L., Switalski, R., et al. (2009). Prediction and longitudinal study of CSF biomarkers in mild cognitive impairment. *Neurobiol. Aging.* 30, 682–690. doi: 10.1016/j.neurobiolaging.2007.08.010

Buchhave, P., Minthon, L., Zetterberg, H., Wallin, A. K., Blennow, K., and Hansson, O. (2012). Cerebrospinal fluid levels of beta-amyloid 1-42, but not of tau, are fully changed already 5 to 10 years before the onset of Alzheimer dementia. *Arch. Gen. Psychiatry.* 69, 98–106. doi: 10.1001/archgenpsychiatry.2011.155

Carrillo, M. C., Blennow, K., Soares, H., Lewczuk, P., Mattsson, N., Oberoi, P., et al. (2013). Global standardization measurement of cerebral spinal fluid for Alzheimer's disease: an update from the Alzheimer's Association Global Biomarkers Consortium. *Alzheimer's Demen.* 9, 137–140. doi: 10.1016/j.jalz.2012.11.003

Castellano, J. M., Kim, J., Stewart, F. R., Jiang, H., DeMattos, R. B., Patterson, B. W., et al. (2011). Human apoE isoforms differentially regulate brain amyloid-beta peptide clearance. *Sci. Transl. Med.* 3, 89ra57. doi: 10.1126/scitranslmed.3002156

Davidsson, P., and Blennow, K. (1998). Neurochemical dissection of synaptic pathology in Alzheimer's disease. *Int. Psychogeriatr* 10, 11–23.

DeKosky, S. T., and Scheff, S. W. (1990). Synapse loss in frontal cortex biopsies in Alzheimer's disease: correlation with cognitive severity. *Ann. Neurol.* 27, 457–464. doi: 10.1002/ana.410270502

Dubois, B., Feldman, H. H., Jacova, C., Dekosky, S. T., Barberger-Gateau, P., Cummings, J., et al. (2007). Research criteria for the diagnosis of Alzheimer's disease: revising the NINCDS-ADRDA criteria. *Lancet Neurol.* 6, 734–746. doi: 10.1016/S1474-4422(07)70178-3

Dubois, B., Feldman, H. H., Jacova, C., Hampel, H., Molinuevo, J. L., Blennow, K., et al. (2014). Advancing research diagnostic criteria for Alzheimer's disease: the IWG-2 criteria. *Lancet Neurol.* 13, 614–629. doi: 10.1016/S1474-4422(14)70090-0

Dumurgier, J., Schraen, S., Gabelle, A., Vercruysse, O., Bombois, S., Laplanche, J. L., et al. (2015). Cerebrospinal fluid amyloid-beta 42/40 ratio in clinical setting of memory centers: a multicentric study. *Alzheimer's Res. Ther.* 7, 30. doi: 10.1186/s13195-015-0114-5

Fagan, A. M., Mintun, M. A., Mach, R. H., Lee, S. Y., Dence, C. S., Shah, A. R., et al. (2006). Inverse relation between *in vivo* amyloid imaging load and cerebrospinal fluid Abeta42 in humans. *Ann. Neurol.* 59, 512–519. doi: 10.1002/ana.20730

Fukumoto, H., Tokuda, T., Kasai, T., Ishigami, N., Hidaka, H., Kondo, M., et al. (2010). High-molecular-weight beta-amyloid oligomers are elevated in cerebrospinal fluid of Alzheimer patients. *FASEB J.* 24, 2716–2726. doi: 10.1096/fj.09-150359

Galasko, D., Chang, L., Motter, R., Clark, C. M., Kaye, J., Knopman, D., et al. (1998). High cerebrospinal fluid tau and low amyloid beta42 levels in the clinical diagnosis of Alzheimer disease and relation to apolipoprotein E genotype. *Arch. Neurol.* 55, 937–945. doi: 10.1001/archneur.55.7.937

Gao, C. M., Yam, A. Y., Wang, X., Magdangal, E., Salisbury, C., Peretz, D., et al. (2010). Abeta40 oligomers identified as a potential biomarker for the diagnosis of Alzheimer's disease. *PLoS ONE* 5:e15725. doi: 10.1371/journal.pone.0015725

Georganopoulou, D. G., Chang, L., Nam, J. M., Thaxton, C. S., Mufson, E. J., Klein, W. L., et al. (2005). Nanoparticle-based detection in cerebral spinal fluid of a soluble pathogenic biomarker for Alzheimer's disease. *Proc. Natl. Acad. Sci. U.S.A.* 102, 2273–2276. doi: 10.1073/pnas.0409336102

Hampel, H., Mitchell, A., Blennow, K., Frank, R. A., Brettschneider, S., Weller, L., et al. (2004). Core biological marker candidates of Alzheimer's disease—perspectives for diagnosis, prediction of outcome and reflection of biological activity. *J. Neural Transm.* 111, 247–272. doi: 10.1007/s00702-003-0065-z

Handoko, M., Grant, M., Kuskowski, M., Zahs, K. R., Wallin, A., Blennow, K., et al. (2013). Correlation of specific amyloid-beta oligomers with tau in cerebrospinal fluid from cognitively normal older adults. *JAMA Neurol.* 70, 594–599. doi: 10.1001/jamaneurol.2013.48

Hansen, L. A., DeTeresa, R., Davies, P., and Terry, R. D. (1988). Neocortical morphometry, lesion counts, and choline acetyltransferase levels in the age spectrum of Alzheimer's disease. *Neurology* 38, 48–54. doi: 10.1212/WNL.38.1.48

Hansson, O., Zetterberg, H., Buchhave, P., Andreasson, U., Londos, E., Minthon, L., et al. (2007). Prediction of Alzheimer's disease using the CSF Abeta42/Abeta40 ratio in patients with mild cognitive impairment. *Dement. Geriatr. Cogn. Disord.* 23, 316–320. doi: 10.1159/000100926

Hansson, O., Zetterberg, H., Buchhave, P., Londos, E., Blennow, K., and Minthon, L. (2006). Association between CSF biomarkers and incipient Alzheimer's disease in patients with mild cognitive impairment: a follow-up study. *Lancet Neurol.* 5, 228–234. doi: 10.1016/S1474-4422(06)70355-6

Henriksen, K., O'Bryant, S. E., Hampel, H., Trojanowski, J. Q., Montine, T. J., Jeromin, A., et al. (2014). The future of blood-based biomarkers for Alzheimer's disease. *Alzheimer's Demen.* 10, 115–131. doi: 10.1016/j.jalz.2013.01.013

Holtta, M., Hansson, O., Andreasson, U., Hertze, J., Minthon, L., Nagga, K., et al. (2013). Evaluating amyloid-beta oligomers in cerebrospinal fluid as a biomarker for Alzheimer's disease. *PLoS ONE* 8:e66381. doi: 10.1371/journal.pone.0066381

Huang, K. P., Huang, F. L., Jager, T., Li, J., Reymann, K. G., and Balschun, D. (2004). Neurogranin/RC3 enhances long-term potentiation and learning by promoting calcium-mediated signaling. *J. Neurosci.* 24, 10660–10669. doi: 10.1523/JNEUROSCI.2213-04.2004

Hulstaert, F., Blennow, K., Ivanoiu, A., Schoonderwaldt, H. C., Riemenschneider, M., De Deyn, P. P., et al. (1999). Improved discrimination of AD patients using beta-amyloid(1-42) and tau levels in CSF. *Neurology* 52, 1555–1562. doi: 10.1212/WNL.52.8.1555

Jahn, R., and Fasshauer, D. (2012). Molecular machines governing exocytosis of synaptic vesicles. *Nature* 490, 201–207. doi: 10.1038/nature11320

Jin, M., Shepardson, N., Yang, T., Chen, G., Walsh, D., and Selkoe, D. J. (2011). Soluble amyloid beta-protein dimers isolated from Alzheimer cortex directly induce Tau hyperphosphorylation and neuritic degeneration. *Proc. Natl. Acad. Sci. U.S.A.* 108, 5819–5824. doi: 10.1073/pnas.1017033108

Jongbloed, W., Bruggink, K. A., Kester, M. I., Visser, P. J., Scheltens, P., Blankenstein, M. A., et al. (2015). Amyloid-beta oligomers relate to cognitive decline in Alzheimer's disease. *J. Alzheimer's Dis.* 45, 35–43. doi: 10.3233/JAD-142136

Klunk, W. E. (2011). Amyloid imaging as a biomarker for cerebral beta-amyloidosis and risk prediction for Alzheimer dementia. *Neurobiol. Aging.* 32(Suppl. 1), S20–S36. doi: 10.1016/j.neurobiolaging.2011.09.006

Klyubin, I., Betts, V., Welzel, A. T., Blennow, K., Zetterberg, H., Wallin, A., et al. (2008). Amyloid beta protein dimer-containing human CSF disrupts synaptic plasticity: prevention by systemic passive immunization. *J. Neurosci.* 28, 4231–4237. doi: 10.1523/JNEUROSCI.5161-07.2008

Knopman, D. S., DeKosky, S. T., Cummings, J. L., Chui, H., Corey-Bloom, J., Relkin, N., et al. (2001). Practice parameter: diagnosis of dementia (an evidence-based review). Report of the Quality Standards Subcommittee of the American Academy of Neurology. *Neurology* 56, 1143–1153. doi: 10.1212/WNL.56.9.1143

Kvartsberg, H., Duits, F. H., Ingelsson, M., Andreasen, N., Öhrfelt, A., Andersson, K., et al. (2014). Cerebrospinal fluid levels of the synaptic protein neurogranin correlates with cognitive decline in prodromal Alzheimer's disease. *Alzheimer's Dem.* doi: 10.1016/j.jalz.2014.10.009. [Epub ahead of print].

Lautner, R., Palmqvist, S., Mattsson, N., Andreasson, U., Wallin, A., Palsson, E., et al. (2014). Apolipoprotein E genotype and the diagnostic accuracy of cerebrospinal fluid biomarkers for Alzheimer disease. *JAMA Psychiatry* 71, 1183–1191. doi: 10.1001/jamapsychiatry.2014.1060

Lewczuk, P., Lelental, N., Spitzer, P., Maler, J. M., and Kornhuber, J. (2015). Amyloid-beta 42/40 cerebrospinal fluid concentration ratio in the diagnostics of Alzheimer's disease: validation of two novel assays. *J. Alzheimer's Dis.* 43, 183–191. doi: 10.3233/JAD-140771

Li, G., Sokal, I., Quinn, J. F., Leverenz, J. B., Brodey, M., Schellenberg, G. D., et al. (2007). CSF tau/Abeta42 ratio for increased risk of mild cognitive impairment: a follow-up study. *Neurology* 69, 631–639. doi: 10.1212/01.wnl.0000267428.62582.aa

Mann, D. M., Yates, P. O., and Marcyniuk, B. (1984). Alzheimer's presenile dementia, senile dementia of Alzheimer type and Down's syndrome in middle age form an age related continuum of pathological changes. *Neuropathol. Appl. Neurobiol.* 10, 185–207. doi: 10.1111/j.1365-2990.1984.tb00351.x

Masliah, E., Mallory, M., Alford, M., DeTeresa, R., Hansen, L. A., McKeel, D. W. Jr., et al. (2001). Altered expression of synaptic proteins occurs early during progression of Alzheimer's disease. *Neurology* 56, 127–129. doi: 10.1212/WNL.56.1.127

Mattsson, N., Andreasson, U., Persson, S., Carrillo, M. C., Collins, S., Chalbot, S., et al. (2013). CSF biomarker variability in the Alzheimer's Association quality control program. *Alzheimer's Demen.* 9, 251–261. doi: 10.1016/j.jalz.2013.01.010

Mattsson, N., Insel, P. S., Landau, S., Jagust, W., Donohue, M., Shaw, L. M., et al. (2014). Diagnostic accuracy of CSF Ab42 and florbetapir PET for Alzheimer's disease. *Ann. Clin. Trans. Neurol.* 1, 534–543. doi: 10.1002/acn3.81

Mattsson, N., Rosen, E., Hansson, O., Andreasen, N., Parnetti, L., Jonsson, M., et al. (2012). Age and diagnostic performance of Alzheimer disease CSF biomarkers. *Neurology* 78, 468–476. doi: 10.1212/WNL.0b013e3182477eed

Mattsson, N., Zetterberg, H., Hansson, O., Andreasen, N., Parnetti, L., Jonsson, M., et al. (2009). CSF biomarkers and incipient Alzheimer disease in patients with mild cognitive impairment. *JAMA* 302, 385–393. doi: 10.1001/jama.2009.1064

McKhann, G., Drachman, D., Folstein, M., Katzman, R., Price, D., and Stadlan, E. M. (1984). Clinical diagnosis of Alzheimer's disease: report of the NINCDS-ADRDA Work Group under the auspices of Department of Health and Human Services Task Force on Alzheimer's Disease. *Neurology* 34, 939–944. doi: 10.1212/WNL.34.7.939

McKhann, G. M., Knopman, D. S., Chertkow, H., Hyman, B. T., Jack, C. R. Jr., Kawas, C. H., et al. (2011). The diagnosis of dementia due to Alzheimer's disease: recommendations from the National Institute on Aging-Alzheimer's Association workgroups on diagnostic guidelines for Alzheimer's disease. *Alzheimer's Demen.* 7, 263–269. doi: 10.1016/j.jalz.2011.03.005

Motter, R., Vigo-Pelfrey, C., Kholodenko, D., Barbour, R., Johnson-Wood, K., Galasko, D., et al. (1995). Reduction of beta-amyloid peptide42 in the cerebrospinal fluid of patients with Alzheimer's disease. *Annal. Neurol.* 38, 643–648. doi: 10.1002/ana.410380413

Mountjoy, C. Q., Roth, M., Evans, N. J., and Evans, H. M. (1983). Cortical neuronal counts in normal elderly controls and demented patients. *Neurobiol. Aging* 4, 1–11. doi: 10.1016/0197-4580(83)90048-9

O'Bryant, S. E., Gupta, V., Henriksen, K., Edwards, M., Jeromin, A., Lista, S., et al. (2015). Guidelines for the standardization of preanalytic variables for blood-based biomarker studies in Alzheimer's disease research. *Alzheimer's Dement.* 11, 549–560. doi: 10.1016/j.jalz.2014.08.099

Petersen, R. C., Smith, G. E., Waring, S. C., Ivnik, R. J., Tangalos, E. G., and Kokmen, E. (1999). Mild cognitive impairment: clinical characterization and outcome. *Arch. Neurol.* 56, 303–308. doi: 10.1001/archneur.56.3.303

Pitschke, M., Prior, R., Haupt, M., and Riesner, D. (1998). Detection of single amyloid beta-protein aggregates in the cerebrospinal fluid of Alzheimer's patients by fluorescence correlation spectroscopy. *Nat. Med.* 4, 832–834. doi: 10.1038/nm0798-832

Portelius, E., Westman-Brinkmalm, A., Zetterberg, H., and Blennow, K. (2006). Determination of beta-amyloid peptide signatures in cerebrospinal fluid using immunoprecipitation-mass spectrometry. *J. Proteome Res.* 5, 1010–1016. doi: 10.1021/pr050475v

Pozueta, J., Lefort, R., and Shelanski, M. L. (2013). Synaptic changes in Alzheimer's disease and its models. *Neuroscience* 251, 51–65. doi: 10.1016/j.neuroscience.2012.05.050

Prince, J. A., Zetterberg, H., Andreasen, N., Marcusson, J., and Blennow, K. (2004). APOE epsilon4 allele is associated with reduced cerebrospinal fluid levels of Abeta42. *Neurology* 62, 2116–2118. doi: 10.1212/01.WNL.0000128088.08695.05

Reddy, P. H., Mani, G., Park, B. S., Jacques, J., Murdoch, G., Whetsell, W. Jr., et al. (2005). Differential loss of synaptic proteins in Alzheimer's disease: implications for synaptic dysfunction. *J. Alzheimer's Dis.* 7, 103–117; discussion 73–80.

Rembach, A., Faux, N. G., Watt, A. D., Pertile, K. K., Rumble, R. L., Trounson, B. O., et al. (2014). Changes in plasma amyloid beta in a longitudinal study of aging and Alzheimer's disease. *Alzheimer's Demen.* 10, 53–61. doi: 10.1016/j.jalz.2012.12.006

Sancesario, G. M., Cencioni, M. T., Esposito, Z., Borsellino, G., Nuccetelli, M., Martorana, A., et al. (2012). The load of amyloid-beta oligomers is decreased in the cerebrospinal fluid of Alzheimer's disease patients. *J. Alzheimer's Dis.* 31, 865–878. doi: 10.3233/JAD-2012-120211

Santos, A. N., Ewers, M., Minthon, L., Simm, A., Silber, R. E., Blennow, K., et al. (2012). Amyloid-beta oligomers in cerebrospinal fluid are associated with cognitive decline in patients with Alzheimer's disease. *J. Alzheimer's Dis.* 29, 171–176. doi: 10.3233/JAD-2012-111361

Savage, M. J., Kalinina, J., Wolfe, A., Tugusheva, K., Korn, R., Cash-Mason, T., et al. (2014). A sensitive abeta oligomer assay discriminates Alzheimer's and aged control cerebrospinal fluid. *J. Neurosci.* 34, 2884–2897. doi: 10.1523/JNEUROSCI.1675-13.2014

Scheff, S. W., Price, D. A., Schmitt, F. A., DeKosky, S. T., and Mufson, E. J. (2007). Synaptic alterations in CA1 in mild Alzheimer disease and mild cognitive impairment. *Neurology* 68, 1501–1508. doi: 10.1212/01.wnl.0000260698.46517.8f

Shaw, L. M., Vanderstichele, H., Knapik-Czajka, M., Clark, C. M., Aisen, P. S., Petersen, R. C., et al. (2009). Cerebrospinal fluid biomarker signature in Alzheimer's disease neuroimaging initiative subjects. *Ann. Neurol.* 65, 403–413. doi: 10.1002/ana.21610

Snider, B. J., Fagan, A. M., Roe, C., Shah, A. R., Grant, E. A., Xiong, C., et al. (2009). Cerebrospinal fluid biomarkers and rate of cognitive decline in very mild dementia of the Alzheimer type. *Arch. Neurol.* 66, 638–645. doi: 10.1001/archneurol.2009.55

Sze, C. I., Troncoso, J. C., Kawas, C., Mouton, P., Price, D. L., and Martin, L. J. (1997). Loss of the presynaptic vesicle protein synaptophysin in hippocampus correlates with cognitive decline in Alzheimer disease. *J. Neuropathol. Exp. Neurol.* 56, 933–944. doi: 10.1097/00005072-199708000-00011

Thorsell, A., Bjerke, M., Gobom, J., Brunhage, E., Vanmechelen, E., Andreasen, N., et al. (2010). Neurogranin in cerebrospinal fluid as a marker of synaptic degeneration in Alzheimer's disease. *Brain Res.* 1362, 13–22. doi: 10.1016/j.brainres.2010.09.073

van Rossum, I. A., Vos, S. J., Burns, L., Knol, D. L., Scheltens, P., Soininen, H., et al. (2012). Injury markers predict time to dementia in subjects with MCI and amyloid pathology. *Neurology* 79, 1809–1816. doi: 10.1212/WNL.0b013e3182704056

Verghese, P. B., Castellano, J. M., Garai, K., Wang, Y., Jiang, H., Shah, A., et al. (2013). ApoE influences amyloid-beta (Abeta) clearance despite minimal apoE/Abeta association in physiological conditions. *Proc. Natl. Acad. Sci. U.S.A.* 110, E1807–E1816. doi: 10.1073/pnas.1220484110

Visser, P. J., Verhey, F., Knol, D. L., Scheltens, P., Wahlund, L. O., Freund-Levi, Y., et al. (2009). Prevalence and prognostic value of CSF markers of Alzheimer's disease pathology in patients with subjective cognitive impairment or mild cognitive impairment in the DESCRIPA study: a prospective cohort study. *Lancet Neurol.* 8, 619–627. doi: 10.1016/S1474-4422(09)70139-5

Visser, P. J., Vos, S., van Rossum, I., and Scheltens, P. (2012). Comparison of International Working Group criteria and National Institute on Aging-Alzheimer's Association criteria for Alzheimer's disease. *Alzheimer's Demen.* 8, 560–563. doi: 10.1016/j.jalz.2011.10.008

Walsh, D. M., Klyubin, I., Fadeeva, J. V., Cullen, W. K., Anwyl, R., Wolfe, M. S., et al. (2002). Naturally secreted oligomers of amyloid beta protein potently inhibit hippocampal long-term potentiation *in vivo*. *Nature* 416, 535–539. doi: 10.1038/416535a

Wu, J., Li, J., Huang, K. P., and Huang, F. L. (2002). Attenuation of protein kinase C and cAMP-dependent protein kinase signal transduction in the neurogranin knockout mouse. *J. Biol. Chem.* 277, 19498–19505. doi: 10.1074/jbc.M109082200

Zhao, X., Lejnine, S., Spond, J., Zhang, C., Ramaraj, T. C., Holder, D. J., et al. (2015). A candidate plasma protein classifier to identify Alzheimer's disease. *J. Alzheimer's Dis.* 43, 549–563. doi: 10.3233/JAD-141149

8

Autosomal dominant Alzheimer disease: a unique resource to study CSF biomarker changes in preclinical AD

*Suzanne Elizabeth Schindler and Anne M. Fagan**

Department of Neurology, Knight Alzheimer's Disease Research Center, Hope Center for Neurological Disorders, Washington University School of Medicine, St. Louis, MO, USA

Edited by:
Sylvain Lehmann,
Montpellier University Hospital, France

Reviewed by:
Zhihui Yang,
University of Florida, USA
David Wallon,
CHU de Rouen, France

***Correspondence:**
Anne M. Fagan,
Department of Neurology,
Washington University School of Medicine, Campus Box 8111, 660 South Euclid Avenue, St. Louis, MO 63110, USA
fagana@neuro.wustl.edu

Our understanding of the pathogenesis of Alzheimer disease (AD) has been greatly influenced by investigation of rare families with autosomal dominant mutations that cause early onset AD. Mutations in the genes coding for amyloid precursor protein (*APP*), presenilin 1 (*PSEN-1*), and presenilin 2 (*PSEN-2*) cause over-production of the amyloid-β peptide (Aβ) leading to early deposition of Aβ in the brain, which in turn is hypothesized to initiate a cascade of processes, resulting in neuronal death, cognitive decline, and eventual dementia. Studies of cerebrospinal fluid (CSF) from individuals with the common form of AD, late-onset AD (LOAD), have revealed that low CSF Aβ42 and high CSF tau are associated with AD brain pathology. Herein, we review the literature on CSF biomarkers in autosomal dominant AD (ADAD), which has contributed to a detailed road map of AD pathogenesis, especially during the preclinical period, prior to the appearance of any cognitive symptoms. Current drug trials are also taking advantage of the unique characteristics of ADAD and utilizing CSF biomarkers to accelerate development of effective therapies for AD.

Keywords: cerebrospinal fluid, biomarkers, Alzheimer disease, autosomal dominant, familial

Introduction

In 1901, Dr. Alois Alzheimer began treating Auguste D., a 51-year-old woman with memory loss and hallucinations. Ms. D's dementia progressed and she died at the age of 56. Upon histopathological examination, Alzheimer found two types of abnormalities in the brain that were later termed amyloid plaques and neurofibrillary tangles (1). Over a century later, when patients die with a characteristic history of progressive cognitive decline and upon autopsy are found to have significant quantities of amyloid plaques and neurofibrillary tangles, they are assigned the neuropathological diagnosis of Alzheimer disease (AD). The vast majority of patients with AD develop dementia at age 65 or older. Genetic studies of patients like Ms. D, who develop cognitive decline before age 65, have revealed rare autosomal dominant mutations that cause AD (2). Recently, surviving samples from Ms. D were subjected to genetic analysis and found to have a genetic mutation in presenilin 1 (*PSEN-1*) (3), although there has been some controversy about this finding (4).

There is some concern that the pathogenesis of autosomal dominant AD (ADAD) may vary from the common late-onset AD (LOAD). However, while there are certainly some differences between ADAD and LOAD in terms of disease etiology, clinical features, and neuropathology, they share many characteristics including an abnormal pattern of cerebrospinal fluid (CSF) biomarkers (Table S1 in Supplementary Material). Although we cannot completely dismiss the notions that the pathogenesis of ADAD and LOAD are distinct and that findings from ADAD do not apply to LOAD, investigation of families with ADAD have contributed enormously to our understanding of AD. Finding mutations that cause ADAD identified key molecules in the disease process (5–9). Transgenic mice expressing human ADAD mutations revolutionized the field and have been used to examine almost every aspect of the disease (10). Recently, studies of CSF and brain imaging biomarkers have helped establish the time course of AD-related brain changes in individuals affected by ADAD, especially during the preclinical stage, prior to the appearance of cognitive symptoms (11, 12). Furthermore, after the failure of numerous drug trials to halt, slow, or reverse cognitive decline in symptomatic individuals with LOAD, clinical trials are now utilizing the unique nature of ADAD and the data derived from these families to design prevention trials for AD dementia in both ADAD mutation carriers (MCs) and individuals at risk for LOAD, while they are still asymptomatic (13, 14). Just as Ms. D's genetic misfortune benefited the entire field of AD research, it is likely that ADAD patients will lead us to better treatments for all people afflicted by this disease.

Epidemiology

Alzheimer disease is the most common cause of dementia and, in the United States, affects ~4.7 million individuals aged 65 and older (15). Less than five percent of AD patients develop symptoms before age 65 and are classified as having early onset Alzheimer disease (EOAD) (16). Even rarer are the <1% of AD patients who carry mutations that cause ADAD with 100% penetrance who are distributed world-wide. Carriers of ADAD mutations typically develop symptoms of dementia in their 30s to 60s, depending on their specific gene mutation and the age of onset within their family (17, 18). Much of our current knowledge about ADAD and biomarkers of ADAD comes from two large studies: the multi-center, international Dominantly Inherited Alzheimer Network (DIAN) cohort, and the Alzheimer's Prevention Initiative (API) cohort that studies a large pedigree living in the state of Antioquia in Colombia, South America. The DIAN cohort includes carriers and non-carrier (NC) family members with many different ADAD mutations, while the Colombian kindred is likely descended from a single individual (19) and carries the E280A mutation in the *PSEN-1* gene.

Clinical Features

Regardless of whether patients develop symptoms of AD before age 65 (EOAD) or after age 65 (LOAD), the typical first symptom of brain dysfunction is progressive episodic memory loss that slowly worsens over years (20). However, about 30–40% of patients with early symptom onset either from non-familial EOAD or ADAD have an increased frequency of atypical presentations, such as impairments in non-memory domains, including executive, behavioral, language, and visuospatial (21–23). *PSEN-1* MCs have been reported to be more likely to have headaches, myoclonus, gait abnormalities, pseudobulbar affect, and spastic paraparesis (24–26). Some mutations in the gene for amyloid precursor protein (*APP*) cause severe cerebral amyloid angiopathy (CAA), with resultant strokes and brain hemorrhages (27). These clinical features are rarely observed in LOAD.

Neuropathology

The hallmarks of AD, regardless of the age at dementia onset and its underlying cause (ADAD versus LOAD), are aggregation of the amyloid-β (Aβ) peptide into amyloid plaques and region-specific development of intraneuronal neurofibrillary tangles composed of hyperphosphorylated forms of the microtubule-associated protein, tau (28). AD-affected brains also demonstrate significant neuronal loss and associated neuroinflammation (29–31), although these features are not specific to AD.

In addition to these classic pathologies, some ADAD mutations have been associated with neuropathological abnormalities not typically seen in LOAD. For example, amyloid deposition has been observed in the cerebellum of *PSEN-1* E280A carriers (32), an area not typically affected in LOAD. "Cotton-wool" type plaques that are larger than typical plaques, lack congophilic cores and have few associated dystrophic neurites (33) are often seen in individuals carrying certain *PSEN-1* mutations (34). Some ADAD mutations (notably in *APP*) result in severe CAA, which appears histologically as deposition of Aβ40 in the blood vessel wall. The specific pattern of CAA distribution in the brain depends on the mutation (e.g., Dutch, Flemish, Arctic, Iowa, and Italian) (34).

Genetics and Pathogenesis

The genetics of ADAD have provided key insights into the molecular pathogenesis of AD. The observation in 1984 that older adults with Trisomy 21, also known as Down syndrome, develop the brain changes of AD suggested that a genetic locus on chromosome 21 might be involved in AD (35). Indeed, the first ADAD mutations were identified in the *APP* gene that resides on chromosome 21, thus implicating amyloid as a key player in AD pathogenesis (5–7, 36). We also now know that duplication of the *APP* locus results in ADAD (37, 38), likely because of amyloid over-production. Following the discovery of *APP* mutations, mutations in *PSEN-1* (8) and the gene for presenilin 2 (*PSEN-2*) (9) were identified and found to increase the amount of the more aggregation-prone Aβ42 compared to Aβ40 (39). Later, it was discovered that presenilin 1 is a critical component of the γ-secretase enzyme complex that cleaves APP to form Aβ (40). To date, 40 mutations in *APP*, 197 mutations in *PSEN-1*, and 25 mutations in *PSEN-2* have been identified that cause ADAD (2).

Since ADAD mutations either increase total Aβ or increase the ratio of Aβ42:Aβ42, amyloid has been hypothesized to be the initiator of AD, an idea described as the "Amyloid Hypothesis" (41). In further support of this hypothesis, a mutation was recently discovered in *APP* that decreases Aβ production and lowers the risk for AD (42). According to this hypothesis, initial deposition of Aβ into amyloid plaques leads to downstream tau-related neuronal pathology (tangles), neuronal injury, and subsequent neuronal death, which is then manifested as cognitive impairment, ultimately culminating in dementia at the end stage of the disease. Data from neuropathological, brain imaging, and CSF biomarker studies in LOAD are consistent with this hypothesis (43–49), but it has only been through study of ADAD that we have a more precise knowledge of the timing of these changes during the early, preclinical (presymptomatic) stage.

CSF Biomarkers in ADAD

Due to its high prevalence, the majority of AD biomarker studies to date have evaluated individuals with LOAD. CSF levels of Aβ42, tau, and phosphotau181 (ptau) (markers of amyloid, neuronal injury, and tangles, respectively) have stood the test of time in exhibiting both diagnostic and prognostic utility (50). Individuals diagnosed with very mild or mild AD dementia have low levels of CSF Aβ42 (51–54) that inversely correlate with the presence of amyloid as visualized by positron emission tomography (PET) (55–59). Concentrations of CSF tau and ptau are increased in AD and have been shown to positively correlate (albeit to differing degrees) with tangle load at autopsy (52, 53, 60) and regional brain atrophy as defined by magnetic resonance imaging (MRI) (61–64). When paired, the combination of low CSF Aβ42 and high tau/ptau has been shown to be a strong predictor of future cognitive decline in both early symptomatic (very mild dementia or mild cognitive impairment, MCI) and asymptomatic individuals (55, 65–68). However, while such analyses in individuals at risk for LOAD can estimate the risk for decline, they cannot provide the information that is most useful for clinical care – where an individual falls along the pathologic disease cascade or when an individual can expect to develop symptoms of dementia.

In contrast, ADAD provides a unique resource for characterizing changes in CSF biomarkers, especially those that occur long before the onset of dementia. With ADAD families, investigators know if and when an individual will develop dementia. Mutations have 100% penetrance, allowing investigators to know with certainty that an individual will develop AD. Furthermore, within a given family, the age of dementia onset remains fairly consistent, allowing researchers to calculate an estimated number of years until symptom onset (EYO). The EYO construct permits evaluation of biomarker concentrations as a function of where along the disease trajectory an individual falls, independent of the actual age of dementia onset of their parent (17). Using ADAD families, studies can examine biomarker levels in MCs and NCs at distinct time points throughout the course of the disease, including the preclinical AD interval many years prior to dementia onset. However, the low prevalence of ADAD has historically created difficulties in evaluating CSF biomarkers in these families. Most early studies analyzed CSF from fewer than 10 MCs (69–71) (**Table 1**), and with the exception of those evaluating the large Columbia kindred (*PSEN-1* E280A) (12, 72), most have pooled together carriers of

TABLE 1 | Studies examining CSF biomarkers in participants with autosomal dominant Alzheimer disease.

Study	Mutation(s)	Aβ42	Tau	pTau	Comments
Moonis et al. (69) 6 MC 6 Unrelated controls	*PSEN-1* C410Y, *PSEN-1* P242H, and R352H	↓	N.S.	Not tested	MC EYO −8 ± 3
Ringman et al. (74) 20 MC 9 NC	*PSEN-1* A431E, *PSEN-1* L235V, *PSEN-1* G206A, *APP* V717I	↓ (trend)	↑	↑	MC EYO ∼−12 NC EYO −9 ± 12
Fortea et al. (70) 8 MC 5 NC	*PSEN-1* L286P, *PSEN-1* M139T	↓ (trend)	N.S.	N.S.	MC EYO −6 ± 10 NC EYO −7 ± 9
Scholl et al. (71) 4 MC 7 Unrelated controls	*APP* KM670/671 NL, *APP* E693G, *PSEN-1* H163Y	↓	↑	↑	
Reiman et al. (72) 10 MC 10 NC	*PSEN-1* E280A (API)	↑	N.S.	N.S.	MC EYO ∼−25 NC EYO ∼−26
Ringman et al. (75) 13 MC 5 NC	*PSEN-1* A431E, *PSEN-1* L235V, *PSEN-1* S212Y, *APP* V717I	↓	↑	↑	MC EYO −12 ± 10 NC EYO −6 ± 14
Bateman et al. (11) 88 MC 40 NC	Many (DIAN)	↓ at EYO −10 and closer to EAO	↑ at EYO −15 and closer to EAO	Not shown	
Thordardottir et al. (76) 10 MC 12 NC	*APP* KM670/671 NL, *APP* E693G, *PSEN-1* H163Y, *PSEN-1* I143T	↓	↑	↑	MC EYO −7 ± 9 NC EYO −7 ± 12
Fleisher et al. (12) 32 MC 22 NC	*PSEN-1* E280A (API)	↓ at EYO −25 and closer to EAO	↑ at EYO −20 and closer to EAO	↑ at EYO −18 and closer to EAO	

API, Alzheimer's Prevention Initiative; APP, amyloid precursor protein; DIAN, Dominantly Inherited Alzheimer Network; EAO, estimated age of symptom onset; EYO, estimated years to symptom onset; MC, mutation carrier; NC, mutation non-carrier (typically first-degree relative of MC); N.S., not significant; PSEN-1; presenilin 1.
Numbers in parentheses refer to associated reference.

different mutations. Despite the relatively small sample sizes and potential heterogeneity caused by pooling together individuals with different mutations, the pattern of CSF biomarker changes seen in ADAD MCs is remarkably similar to that observed in LOAD, namely, reduced levels of CSF Aβ42 and elevated levels of tau and ptau (**Table 1**; Table S1 in Supplementary Material). The one exception is very young MCs (in their 20s, about 25 years prior to AD symptom onset), who have elevated CSF Aβ42 (72). This was hypothesized to reflect over-production of CSF Aβ42 in ADAD MCs, which has more recently been confirmed directly in kinetic studies (73).

The larger DIAN and API studies have permitted analysis of CSF and imaging biomarkers in greater numbers of both asymptomatic and symptomatic individuals that span a wide range of EYOs, thus allowing conclusions to be drawn regarding the timing of such biomarker changes during the preclinical period (**Figure 1**). Results from cross-sectional analyses demonstrate higher levels of CSF Aβ42 in MCs compared to NCs very early in the disease process (~20–30 years prior to estimated symptom onset, EYO −20 to −30), which then drop with disease progression, becoming significantly lower than NCs ~10–20 years prior to symptom onset (~EYO −10 to −20) (11, 12, 72, 77). These low levels then begin to plateau with the development of cognitive symptoms. After Aβ42 levels begin to drop, levels of tau and ptau in MCs become significantly higher than NCs (~EYO −15), and then continue to increase with disease progression. However, a recent study of within-person change in biomarkers in a small sub-cohort of DIAN participants with longitudinal biomarker data has shown that although levels of CSF tau and ptau increase in MCs during the preclinical (asymptomatic) phase, levels stabilize or decline over time in individuals who are symptomatic (77). Similar patterns were observed in levels of visinin-like protein 1 (VILIP-1) (77), a neuronal calcium sensor protein that is a marker of neuronal injury/death (78). Consistent with this pattern, a previous report of a single asymptomatic ADAD (*APP* V717I) MC showed substantial increases in tau and ptau over a 4- to 5-year period very early in the disease process (~EYO −19 to −14) (79), whereas a longitudinal decrease (or a lack of increase) in ptau was reported in a small Japanese cohort ($n = 4$) of symptomatic *PSEN1* MCs (80). Although not often discussed, results consistent with these changes in the trajectories of neuronal injury-related markers have been reported in LOAD (81–83).

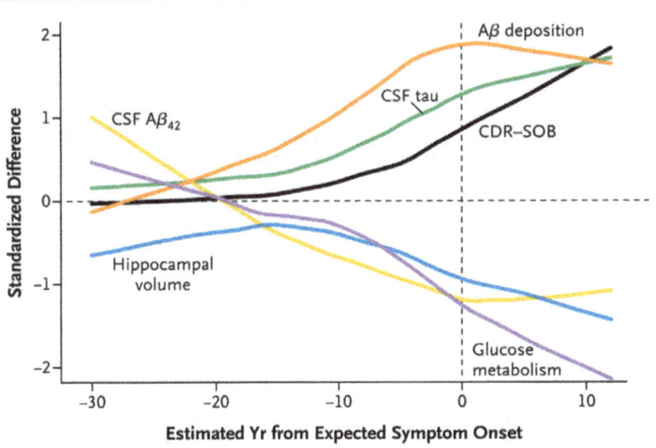

FIGURE 1 | A time course of changes in ADAD mutation carriers versus non-carriers. Cross-sectional data obtained in the DIAN cohort demonstrates that CSF Aβ42 (yellow) declines as Aβ deposition increases as shown by amyloid PET imaging (orange). CSF tau (green) increases as hippocampal volume (blue) and glucose metabolism as shown by FDG PET (purple) decreases. CDR-SOB (Clinical Dementia Rating-Sum of Boxes) (black), which quantifies clinical symptoms of dementia, increases (indicating worse performance) relatively late in the disease course. Reproduced with permission from Bateman et al. (11).

Although this general model is consistent with data obtained from cross-sectional studies in LOAD (49, 84–86) and suggests a common pathophysiology for AD due to mutations and the much more common "sporadic" form, the longitudinal data from DIAN supports a model that incorporates an eventual slowing down of the rate of neuronal injury and death as may be indicated by reductions in these markers. It is also possible that the later decreases during the symptomatic phase may reflect fewer neurons left to contribute to the pool of CSF tau/ptau/VILIP-1. If corroborated in additional cohorts, this reversing pattern of marker change will likely have an impact on the definition of a positive neurodegenerative biomarker outcome in clinical trials, especially during the symptomatic phase. For example, an effective therapy may only slow the rate of increase in injury markers in individuals who are in the preclinical phase, but stabilize or decrease the rate of change in injury markers later in the disease. Confirmation of such patterns awaits evaluation of biomarker trajectories in clinical trials.

Use of ADAD in Clinical Trial Design

Many clinical trials in symptomatic individuals with LOAD have failed to meet their clinical endpoints of delaying, halting, or reversing cognitive decline. One possibility proposed to explain this failure is that therapies must be delivered earlier, in individuals known to have underlying AD pathology, but before significant symptoms are manifest (87). However, there are several challenges associated with the design and implementation of such "prevention trials," including identifying asymptomatic participants with known underlying AD pathology and who are at a point in their disease trajectory when they are close to becoming symptomatic. Although CSF and imaging biomarkers are currently being used in clinical trials to confirm underlying amyloid pathology in individuals at risk for developing LOAD (http://www.nia.nih.gov/alzheimers/clinical-trials/), the onset of dementia in LOAD is characteristically difficult to predict, even in individuals who are biomarker-positive. As a result, large numbers of participants are required in order to provide adequate statistical power to show a potential drug effect. In contrast, since ADAD is fully penetrant and the time until onset of dementia symptoms in MCs can be predicted with relatively high precision, fewer trial participants are required to demonstrate treatment efficacy within a suitable timeframe. Two such prevention trials in ADAD are currently underway; the DIAN-Trials Unit (DIAN-TU) and API, both of which are testing monoclonal antibodies directed against various forms of Aβ (13, 14).

Another possibility to explain the failure of previous clinical trials in LOAD is that the drug did not engage its purported target. Given the compelling data from observational biomarker studies of ADAD (**Table 1**), biomarkers can serve as meaningful endpoints to verify target engagement even before the possible appearance of significant cognitive effects. To this end, the DIAN-TU has defined biomarkers as the primary endpoint [amyloid PET or CSF Aβ, with CSF tau(s) as downstream targets], with the trial design transitioning to a cognitive endpoint only for those drugs shown to have properly engaged their pathologic targets (14, 88, 89). CSF biomarkers are also being used as exploratory measures in the API trial (13) and the Anti-Amyloid Treatment in Asymptomatic Alzheimer's (A4) prevention trial in LOAD (90).

Conclusion

Although there are some differences in the pathology and clinical expression in ADAD compared to LOAD (Table S1 in Supplementary Material), studies of ADAD have provided critical insight that has propelled our knowledge and investigation of all forms of AD. Investigators have proposed the relative timing of biomarker changes in LOAD (48, 49), but these hypotheses cannot yet be empirically verified because we do not know *a priori* when individuals with LOAD will develop symptoms. Because the EYO is known in ADAD cases, data-based models of AD can be generated (**Figure 1**) (11, 12). Curves representing changes in CSF and imaging biomarkers over the disease course in ADAD can be superimposed on curves of cognitive function, resulting in a detailed road map of AD pathologic processes. These analyses confirm that AD brain changes begin to develop over two decades before the onset of dementia. Now, as researchers work to develop drugs that prevent dementia associated with AD pathology, they are using ADAD to accelerate clinical trials (13, 14). It would be appropriate if ADAD, which represents <1% of all AD but has provided so much insight into the disease, leads to a drug that ultimately prevents all forms of AD.

Author Contributions

SS and AF were involved in all aspects of preparing, writing, and editing the manuscript.

Acknowledgments

SS is supported by a NIH K career development award (5K12 HD001459-15). AF is supported by grants from the NIH (P01AG026276, PO1AG003991, 2UF1AG032438).

References

1. Alzheimer A, Stelzmann RA, Schnitzlein HN, Murtagh FR. An English translation of Alzheimer's 1907 paper, "uber eine eigenartige Erkankung der hirnrinde". *Clin Anat* (1995) **8**(6):429–31. doi:10.1002/ca.980080612
2. Chouraki V, Seshadri S. Genetics of Alzheimer's disease. *Adv Genet* (2014) **87**:245–94. doi:10.1016/B978-0-12-800149-3.00005-6
3. Muller U, Winter P, Graeber MB. A presenilin 1 mutation in the first case of Alzheimer's disease. *Lancet Neurol* (2013) **12**(2):129–30. doi:10.1016/S1474-4422(12)70307-1
4. Rupp C, Beyreuther K, Maurer K, Kins S. A presenilin 1 mutation in the first case of Alzheimer's disease: revisited. *Alzheimer Dement* (2014) **10**(6):869–72. doi:10.1016/j.jalz.2014.06.005
5. Goate A, Chartier-Harlin MC, Mullan M, Brown J, Crawford F, Fidani L, et al. Segregation of a missense mutation in the amyloid precursor protein gene with familial Alzheimer's disease. *Nature* (1991) **349**(6311):704–6. doi:10.1038/349704a0
6. Chartier-Harlin MC, Crawford F, Houlden H, Warren A, Hughes D, Fidani L, et al. Early-onset Alzheimer's disease caused by mutations at codon 717 of the beta-amyloid precursor protein gene. *Nature* (1991) **353**(6347):844–6. doi:10.1038/353844a0
7. Murrell J, Farlow M, Ghetti B, Benson MD. A mutation in the amyloid precursor protein associated with hereditary Alzheimer's disease. *Science* (1991) **254**(5028):97–9. doi:10.1126/science.1925564
8. Sherrington R, Rogaev EI, Liang Y, Rogaeva EA, Levesque G, Ikeda M, et al. Cloning of a gene bearing missense mutations in early-onset familial Alzheimer's disease. *Nature* (1995) **375**(6534):754–60. doi:10.1038/375754a0
9. Levy-Lahad E, Wijsman EM, Nemens E, Anderson L, Goddard KA, Weber JL, et al. A familial Alzheimer's disease locus on chromosome 1. *Science* (1995) **269**(5226):970–3. doi:10.1126/science.7638621
10. Hall AM, Roberson ED. Mouse models of Alzheimer's disease. *Brain Res Bull* (2012) **88**(1):3–12. doi:10.1016/j.brainresbull.2011.11.017
11. Bateman RJ, Xiong C, Benzinger TL, Fagan AM, Goate A, Fox NC, et al. Clinical and biomarker changes in dominantly inherited Alzheimer's disease. *N Engl J Med* (2012) **367**(9):795–804. doi:10.1056/NEJMoa1202753
12. Fleisher AS, Chen K, Quiroz YT, Jakimovich LJ, Gutierrez Gomez M, Langois CM, et al. Associations between biomarkers and age in the presenilin 1 E280a autosomal dominant Alzheimer disease kindred: a cross-sectional study. *JAMA Neurol* (2015) **72**(3):316–24. doi:10.1001/jamaneurol.2014.3314
13. Reiman EM, Langbaum JB, Fleisher AS, Caselli RJ, Chen K, Ayutyanont N, et al. Alzheimer's prevention initiative: a plan to accelerate the evaluation of presymptomatic treatments. *J Alzheimer Dis* (2011) **26**(Suppl 3):321–9. doi:10.3233/JAD-2011-0059
14. Mills SM, Mallmann J, Santacruz AM, Fuqua A, Carril M, Aisen PS, et al. Preclinical trials in autosomal dominant AD: implementation of the DIAN-TU trial. *Rev Neurol* (2013) **169**(10):737–43. doi:10.1016/j.neurol.2013.07.017
15. Hebert LE, Weuve J, Scherr PA, Evans DA. Alzheimer disease in the United States (2010-2050) estimated using the 2010 census. *Neurology* (2013) **80**(19):1778–83. doi:10.1212/WNL.0b013e31828726f5
16. Ferri CP, Prince M, Brayne C, Brodaty H, Fratiglioni L, Ganguli M, et al. Global prevalence of dementia: a Delphi consensus study. *Lancet* (2005) **366**(9503):2112–7. doi:10.1016/S0140-6736(05)67889-0
17. Ryman DC, Acosta-Baena N, Aisen PS, Bird T, Danek A, Fox NC, et al. Symptom onset in autosomal dominant Alzheimer disease: a systematic review and meta-analysis. *Neurology* (2014) **83**(3):253–60. doi:10.1212/WNL.0000000000000596
18. Wallon D, Rousseau S, Rovelet-Lecrux A, Quillard-Muraine M, Guyant-Marechal L, Martinaud O, et al. The French series of autosomal dominant early onset Alzheimer's disease cases: mutation spectrum and cerebrospinal fluid biomarkers. *J Alzheimers Dis* (2012) **30**(4):847–56. doi:10.3233/JAD-2012-120172
19. Lalli MA, Cox HC, Arcila ML, Cadavid L, Moreno S, Garcia G, et al. Origin of the PSEN1 E280A mutation causing early-onset Alzheimer's disease. *Alzheimer Dement* (2014) **10**(5 Suppl):S277–83. doi:10.1016/j.jalz.2013.09.005
20. McKhann GM, Knopman DS, Chertkow H, Hyman BT, Jack CR Jr, Kawas CH, et al. The diagnosis of dementia due to Alzheimer's disease: recommendations from the National Institute on Aging-Alzheimer's Association workgroups on diagnostic guidelines for Alzheimer's disease. *Alzheimer Dement* (2011) **7**(3):263–9. doi:10.1016/j.jalz.2011.03.005

21. Balasa M, Gelpi E, Antonell A, Rey MJ, Sanchez-Valle R, Molinuevo JL, et al. Clinical features and APOE genotype of pathologically proven early-onset Alzheimer disease. *Neurology* (2011) **76**(20):1720–5. doi:10.1212/WNL.0b013e31821a44dd
22. Koedam EL, Lauffer V, van der Vlies AE, van der Flier WM, Scheltens P, Pijnenburg YA. Early-versus late-onset Alzheimer's disease: more than age alone. *J Alzheimers Dis* (2010) **19**(4):1401–8. doi:10.3233/JAD-2010-1337
23. Mendez MF. Early-onset Alzheimer's disease: nonamnestic subtypes and type 2 AD. *Arch Med Res* (2012) **43**(8):677–85. doi:10.1016/j.arcmed.2012.11.009
24. Joshi A, Ringman JM, Lee AS, Juarez KO, Mendez MF. Comparison of clinical characteristics between familial and non-familial early onset Alzheimer's disease. *J Neurol* (2012) **259**(10):2182–8. doi:10.1007/s00415-012-6481-y
25. Houlden H, Baker M, McGowan E, Lewis P, Hutton M, Crook R, et al. Variant Alzheimer's disease with spastic paraparesis and cotton wool plaques is caused by PS-1 mutations that lead to exceptionally high amyloid-beta concentrations. *Ann Neurol* (2000) **48**(5):806–8. doi:10.1002/1531-8249(200011)48:5<806::AID-ANA18>3.3.CO;2-6
26. Lopera F, Ardilla A, Martinez A, Madrigal L, Arango-Viana JC, Lemere CA, et al. Clinical features of early-onset Alzheimer disease in a large kindred with an E280A presenilin-1 mutation. *JAMA* (1997) **277**(10):793–9. doi:10.1001/jama.277.10.793
27. Natte R, Maat-Schieman ML, Haan J, Bornebroek M, Roos RA, van Duinen SG. Dementia in hereditary cerebral hemorrhage with amyloidosis-Dutch type is associated with cerebral amyloid angiopathy but is independent of plaques and neurofibrillary tangles. *Ann Neurol* (2001) **50**(6):765–72. doi:10.1002/ana.10040
28. Holtzman DM, Morris JC, Goate AM. Alzheimer's disease: the challenge of the second century. *Sci Transl Med* (2011) **3**(77):77sr1. doi:10.1126/scitranslmed.3002369
29. Mouton PR, Martin LJ, Calhoun ME, Dal Forno G, Price DL. Cognitive decline strongly correlates with cortical atrophy in Alzheimer's dementia. *Neurobiol Aging* (1998) **19**(5):371–7. doi:10.1016/S0197-4580(98)00080-3
30. Price JL, Ko AI, Wade MJ, Tsou SK, McKeel DW, Morris JC. Neuron number in the entorhinal cortex and CA1 in preclinical Alzheimer disease. *Arch Neurol* (2001) **58**(9):1395–402. doi:10.1001/archneur.58.9.1395
31. Heneka MT, Carson MJ, Khoury JE, Landreth GE, Brosseron F, Feinstein DL, et al. Neuroinflammation in Alzheimer's disease. *Lancet Neurol* (2015) **14**(4):388–405. doi:10.1016/S1474-4422(15)70016-5
32. Lemere CA, Lopera F, Kosik KS, Lendon CL, Ossa J, Saido TC, et al. The E280A presenilin 1 Alzheimer mutation produces increased A beta 42 deposition and severe cerebellar pathology. *Nat Med* (1996) **2**(10):1146–50. doi:10.1038/nm1096-1146
33. Crook R, Verkkoniemi A, Perez-Tur J, Mehta N, Baker M, Houlden H, et al. A variant of Alzheimer's disease with spastic paraparesis and unusual plaques due to deletion of exon 9 of presenilin 1. *Nat Med* (1998) **4**(4):452–5. doi:10.1038/nm0498-452
34. Shepherd C, McCann H, Halliday GM. Variations in the neuropathology of familial Alzheimer's disease. *Acta Neuropathol* (2009) **118**(1):37–52. doi:10.1007/s00401-009-0521-4
35. Glenner GG, Wong CW. Alzheimer's disease and Down's syndrome: sharing of a unique cerebrovascular amyloid fibril protein. *Biochem Biophys Res Commun* (1984) **122**(3):1131–5. doi:10.1016/0006-291X(84)91209-9
36. Suzuki N, Cheung TT, Cai XD, Odaka A, Otvos L Jr, Eckman C, et al. An increased percentage of long amyloid beta protein secreted by familial amyloid beta protein precursor (beta APP717) mutants. *Science* (1994) **264**(5163):1336–40. doi:10.1126/science.8191290
37. Rovelet-Lecrux A, Hannequin D, Raux G, Le Meur N, Laquerriere A, Vital A, et al. APP locus duplication causes autosomal dominant early-onset Alzheimer disease with cerebral amyloid angiopathy. *Nat Genet* (2006) **38**(1):24–6. doi:10.1038/ng1718
38. Sleegers K, Brouwers N, Gijselinck I, Theuns J, Goossens D, Wauters J, et al. APP duplication is sufficient to cause early onset Alzheimer's dementia with cerebral amyloid angiopathy. *Brain* (2006) **129**(Pt 11):2977–83. doi:10.1093/brain/awl203
39. Scheuner D, Eckman C, Jensen M, Song X, Citron M, Suzuki N, et al. Secreted amyloid beta-protein similar to that in the senile plaques of Alzheimer's disease is increased in vivo by the presenilin 1 and 2 and APP mutations linked to familial Alzheimer's disease. *Nat Med* (1996) **2**(8):864–70. doi:10.1038/nm0896-864
40. De Strooper B. Aph-1, Pen-2, and nicastrin with presenilin generate an active gamma-secretase complex. *Neuron* (2003) **38**(1):9–12. doi:10.1016/S0896-6273(03)00205-8
41. Hardy J, Selkoe DJ. The amyloid hypothesis of Alzheimer's disease: progress and problems on the road to therapeutics. *Science* (2002) **297**(5580):353–6. doi:10.1126/science.1072994
42. Jonsson T, Atwal JK, Steinberg S, Snaedal J, Jonsson PV, Bjornsson S, et al. A mutation in APP protects against Alzheimer's disease and age-related cognitive decline. *Nature* (2012) **488**(7409):96–9. doi:10.1038/nature11283
43. Gomez-Isla T, Price J, McKeel D, Morris J, Growdon J, Hyman B. Profound loss of layer II entorhinal cortex neurons occurs in very mild Alzheimer's disease. *J Neursci* (1996) **16**:4491–500.
44. Morris J, Price J. Pathologic correlates of nondemented aging, mild cognitive impairment, and early stage Alzheimer's disease. *J Mol Neurosci* (2001) **17**:101–18. doi:10.1385/JMN:17:2:101
45. Hulette CM, Welsh-Bohmer KA, Murray MG, Saunders AM, Mash DC, McIntyre LM. Neuropathological and neuropsychological changes in "normal" aging: evidence for preclinical Alzheimer disease in cognitively normal individuals. *J Neuropathol Exp Neurol* (1998) **57**:1168–74. doi:10.1097/00005072-199812000-00009
46. Markesbery W, Schmitt F, Kryscio R, Davis D, Smith C, Wekstein D. Neuropathologic substrate of mild cognitive impairment. *Arch Neurol* (2006) **63**:38–46. doi:10.1001/archneur.63.1.38
47. Braak H, Braak E. Frequency of stages of Alzheimer-related lesions in different age categories. *Neurobiol Aging* (1997) **18**:351–7. doi:10.1016/S0197-4580(97)00056-0
48. Jack CR Jr, Knopman DS, Jagust WJ, Petersen RC, Weiner MW, Aisen PS, et al. Tracking pathophysiological processes in Alzheimer's disease: an updated hypothetical model of dynamic biomarkers. *Lancet Neurol* (2013) **12**(2):207–16. doi:10.1016/S1474-4422(12)70291-0
49. Jack CR Jr, Knopman DS, Jagust WJ, Shaw LM, Aisen PS, Weiner MW, et al. Hypothetical model of dynamic biomarkers of the Alzheimer's pathological cascade. *Lancet Neurol* (2010) **9**(1):119–28. doi:10.1016/S1474-4422(09)70299-6
50. Blennow K, Hampel H, Weiner M, Zetterberg H. Cerebrospinal fluid and plasma biomarkers in Alzheimer disease. *Nat Rev Neurol* (2010) **6**(3):131–44. doi:10.1038/nrneurol.2010.4
51. Jagust WJ, Landau SM, Shaw LM, Trojanowski JQ, Koeppe RA, Reiman EM, et al. Relationships between biomarkers in aging and dementia. *Neurology* (2009) **73**(15):1193–9. doi:10.1212/WNL.0b013e3181bc010c
52. Tapiola T, Alafuzoff I, Herukka SK, Parkkinen L, Hartikainen P, Soininen H, et al. Cerebrospinal fluid {beta}-amyloid 42 and tau proteins as biomarkers of Alzheimer-type pathologic changes in the brain. *Arch Neurol* (2009) **66**(3):382–9. doi:10.1001/archneurol.2008.596
53. Clark CM, Xie S, Chittams J, Ewbank D, Peskind E, Galasko D, et al. Cerebrospinal fluid tau and beta-amyloid: how well do these biomarkers reflect autopsy-confirmed dementia diagnoses? *Arch Neurol* (2003) **60**(12):1696–702. doi:10.1001/archneur.60.12.1696
54. Strozyk D, Blennow K, White LR, Launer LJ. CSF Abeta 42 levels correlate with amyloid-neuropathology in a population-based autopsy study. *Neurology* (2003) **60**(4):652–6. doi:10.1212/01.WNL.0000046581.81650.D0
55. Fagan AM, Roe CM, Xiong C, Mintun MA, Morris JC, Holtzman DM. Cerebrospinal fluid tau/beta-amyloid(42) ratio as a prediction of cognitive decline in nondemented older adults. *Arch Neurol* (2007) **64**(3):343–9. doi:10.1001/archneur.64.3.noc60123
56. Forsberg A, Engler H, Almkvist O, Blomquist G, Hagman G, Wall A, et al. PET imaging of amyloid deposition in patients with mild cognitive impairment. *Neurobiol Aging* (2008) **29**(10):1456–65. doi:10.1016/j.neurobiolaging.2007.03.029
57. Tolboom N, van der Flier WM, Yaqub M, Boellaard R, Verwey NA, Blankenstein MA, et al. Relationship of cerebrospinal fluid markers to 11C-PiB and 18F-FDDNP binding. *J Nucl Med* (2009) **50**(9):1464–70. doi:10.2967/jnumed.109.064360
58. Fagan AM, Mintun MA, Mach RH, Lee SY, Dence CS, Shah AR, et al. Inverse relation between in vivo amyloid imaging load and cerebrospinal fluid Abeta42 in humans. *Ann Neurol* (2006) **59**(3):512–9. doi:10.1002/ana.20730
59. Grimmer T, Riemenschneider M, Forstl H, Henriksen G, Klunk WE, Mathis CA, et al. Beta amyloid in Alzheimer's disease: increased deposition in brain is reflected in reduced concentration in cerebrospinal fluid. *Biol Psychiatry* (2009) **65**(11):927–34. doi:10.1016/j.biopsych.2009.01.027

60. Buerger K, Ewers M, Pirttila T, Zinkowski R, Alafuzoff I, Teipel SJ, et al. CSF phosphorylated tau protein correlates with neocortical neurofibrillary pathology in Alzheimer's disease. *Brain* (2006) **129**(Pt 11):3035–41. doi:10.1093/brain/awl269
61. de Souza LC, Chupin M, Lamari F, Jardel C, Leclercq D, Colliot O, et al. CSF tau markers are correlated with hippocampal volume in Alzheimer's disease. *Neurobiol Aging* (2012) **33**(7):1253–7. doi:10.1016/j.neurobiolaging.2011.02.022
62. Stricker NH, Dodge HH, Dowling NM, Han SD, Erosheva EA, Jagust WJ, et al. CSF biomarker associations with change in hippocampal volume and precuneus thickness: implications for the Alzheimer's pathological cascade. *Brain Imaging Behav* (2012) **6**(4):599–609. doi:10.1007/s11682-012-9171-6
63. Fagan AM, Head D, Shah AR, Marcus D, Mintun M, Morris JC, et al. Decreased cerebrospinal fluid Abeta(42) correlates with brain atrophy in cognitively normal elderly. *Ann Neurol* (2009) **65**(2):176–83. doi:10.1002/ana.21559
64. Fjell AM, Walhovd KB, Fennema-Notestine C, McEvoy LK, Hagler DJ, Holland D, et al. CSF biomarkers in prediction of cerebral and clinical change in mild cognitive impairment and Alzheimer's disease. *J Neursci* (2010) **30**(6):2088–101. doi:10.1523/JNEUROSCI.3785-09.2010
65. Hansson O, Zetterberg H, Buchhave P, Londos E, Blennow K, Minthon L. Association between CSF biomarkers and incipient Alzheimer's disease in patients with mild cognitive impairment: a follow-up study. *Lancet Neurol* (2006) **5**(3):228–34. doi:10.1016/S1474-4422(06)70355-6
66. Li G, Sokal I, Quinn JF, Leverenz JB, Brodey M, Schellenberg GD, et al. CSF tau/Abeta42 ratio for increased risk of mild cognitive impairment: a follow-up study. *Neurology* (2007) **69**(7):631–9. doi:10.1212/01.wnl.0000267428.62582.aa
67. Roe CM, Fagan AM, Grant EA, Hassenstab J, Moulder KL, Maue Dreyfus D, et al. Amyloid imaging and CSF biomarkers in predicting cognitive impairment up to 7.5 years later. *Neurology* (2013) **80**(19):1784–91. doi:10.1212/WNL.0b013e3182918ca6
68. Snider BJ, Fagan AM, Roe C, Shah AR, Grant EA, Xiong C, et al. Cerebrospinal fluid biomarkers and rate of cognitive decline in very mild dementia of the Alzheimer type. *Arch Neurol* (2009) **66**(5):638–45. doi:10.1001/archneurol.2009.55
69. Moonis M, Swearer JM, Dayaw MP, St George-Hyslop P, Rogaeva E, Kawarai T, et al. Familial Alzheimer disease: decreases in CSF Abeta42 levels precede cognitive decline. *Neurology* (2005) **65**(2):323–5. doi:10.1212/01.wnl.0000171397.32851.bc
70. Fortea J, Llado A, Bosch B, Antonell A, Oliva R, Molinuevo JL, et al. Cerebrospinal fluid biomarkers in Alzheimer's disease families with PSEN1 mutations. *Neurodegener Dis* (2011) **8**(4):202–7. doi:10.1159/000322229
71. Scholl M, Wall A, Thordardottir S, Ferreira D, Bogdanovic N, Langstrom B, et al. Low PiB PET retention in presence of pathologic CSF biomarkers in arctic APP mutation carriers. *Neurology* (2012) **79**(3):229–36. doi:10.1212/WNL.0b013e31825fdf18
72. Reiman EM, Quiroz YT, Fleisher AS, Chen K, Velez-Pardo C, Jimenez-Del-Rio M, et al. Brain imaging and fluid biomarker analysis in young adults at genetic risk for autosomal dominant Alzheimer's disease in the presenilin 1 E280A kindred: a case-control study. *Lancet Neurol* (2012) **11**(12):1048–56. doi:10.1016/S1474-4422(12)70228-4
73. Potter R, Patterson BW, Elbert DL, Ovod V, Kasten T, Sigurdson W, et al. Increased in vivo amyloid-beta42 production, exchange, and loss in presenilin mutation carriers. *Sci Transl Med* (2013) **5**(189):189ra77. doi:10.1126/scitranslmed.3005615
74. Ringman JM, Younkin SG, Pratico D, Seltzer W, Cole GM, Geschwind DH, et al. Biochemical markers in persons with preclinical familial Alzheimer disease. *Neurology* (2008) **71**(2):85–92. doi:10.1212/01.wnl.0000303973.71803.81
75. Ringman JM, Coppola G, Elashoff D, Rodriguez-Agudelo Y, Medina LD, Gylys K, et al. Cerebrospinal fluid biomarkers and proximity to diagnosis in preclinical familial Alzheimer's disease. *Dement Geriatr Cogn Disord* (2012) **33**(1):1–5. doi:10.1159/000335729
76. Thordardottir S, Stahlbom AK, Ferreira D, Almkvist O, Westman E, Zetterberg H, et al. Preclinical cerebrospinal fluid and volumetric magnetic resonance imaging biomarkers in Swedish familial Alzheimer's disease. *J Alzheimer Dis* (2015) **43**(4):1393–402. doi:10.3233/JAD-140339
77. Fagan AM, Xiong C, Jasielec MS, Bateman RJ, Goate AM, Benzinger TL, et al. Longitudinal change in CSF biomarkers in autosomal-dominant Alzheimer's disease. *Sci Transl Med* (2014) **6**(226):226ra30. doi:10.1126/scitranslmed.3007901
78. Schnurra I, Bernstein HG, Riederer P, Braunewell KH. The neuronal calcium sensor protein VILIP-1 is associated with amyloid plaques and extracellular tangles in Alzheimer's disease and promotes cell death and tau phosphorylation in vitro: a link between calcium sensors and Alzheimer's disease? *Neurobiol Dis* (2001) **8**(5):900–9. doi:10.1006/nbdi.2001.0432
79. Ringman JM, Taylor K, Teng E, Coppola G, Gylys K. Longitudinal change in CSF biomarkers in a presymptomatic carrier of an APP mutation. *Neurology* (2011) **76**(24):2124–5. doi:10.1212/WNL.0b013e31821f4488
80. Ikeda M, Yonemura K, Kakuda S, Tashiro Y, Fujita Y, Takai E, et al. Cerebrospinal fluid levels of phosphorylated tau and Abeta1-38/Abeta1-40/Abeta1-42 in Alzheimer's disease with PS1 mutations. *Amyloid* (2013) **20**(2):107–12. doi:10.3109/13506129.2013.790810
81. Kanai M, Matsubara E, Isoe K, Urakami K, Nakashima K, Arai H, et al. Longitudinal study of cerebrospinal fluid levels of tau, Ab1-40, and Ab1-42(43) in Alzheimer's disease: a study in Japan. *Ann Neurol* (1998) **44**:17–26. doi:10.1002/ana.410440108
82. Sunderland T, Wolozin B, Galasko D, Levy J, Dukoff R, Bahro M, et al. Longitudinal stability of CSF tau levels in Alzheimer patients. *Biol Psychiatry* (1999) **46**(6):750–5. doi:10.1016/S0006-3223(99)00143-2
83. Tapiola T, Pirttila T, Mikkonen M, Mehta PD, Alafuzoff I, Koivisto K, et al. Three-year follow-up of cerebrospinal fluid tau, beta-amyloid 42 and 40 concentrations in Alzheimer's disease. *Neurosci Lett* (2000) **280**(2):119–22. doi:10.1016/S0304-3940(00)00767-9
84. Perrin R, Fagan A, Holtzman D. Multi-modal techniques for diagnosis and prognosis of Alzheimer's disease. *Nature* (2009) **461**:916–22. doi:10.1016/j.neurobiolaging.2008.08.013
85. Jack C, Vemuri P, Wiste H, Weigand S, Aisen P, Trojanowski J, et al. Evidence for ordering of Alzheimer disease biomarkers. *Arch Neurol* (2011) **68**:1526–35. doi:10.1001/archneurol.2011.183
86. Sperling R, Aisen P, Beckett L, Bennett D, Craft S, Fagan A, et al. Toward defining the preclinical stages of Alzheimer's disease: recommendations from the National Institute on Aging-Alzheimer's Association workgroups on diagnostic guidelines for Alzheimer's disease. *Alzheimer Dement* (2011) **7**:280–92. doi:10.1016/j.jalz.2011.03.003
87. Kozauer N, Katz R. Regulatory innovation and drug development for early-stage Alzheimer's disease. *N Engl J Med* (2013) **368**(13):1169–71. doi:10.1056/NEJMp1302513
88. Bateman RJ, Aisen PS, De Strooper B, Fox NC, Lemere CA, Ringman JM, et al. Autosomal-dominant Alzheimer's disease: a review and proposal for the prevention of Alzheimer's disease. *Alzheimers Res Ther* (2011) **3**(1):1. doi:10.1186/alzrt59
89. Moulder KL, Snider BJ, Mills SL, Buckles VD, Santacruz AM, Bateman RJ, et al. Dominantly inherited Alzheimer network: facilitating research and clinical trials. *Alzheimers Res Ther* (2013) **5**(5):48. doi:10.1186/alzrt213
90. Sperling RA, Rentz DM, Johnson KA, Karlawish J, Donohue M, Salmon DP, et al. The A4 study: stopping AD before symptoms begin? *Sci Transl Med* (2014) **6**(228):228fs13. doi:10.1126/scitranslmed.3007941

9

The central biobank and virtual biobank of BIOMARKAPD: a resource for studies on neurodegenerative diseases

Babette L. R. Reijs[1], Charlotte E. Teunissen[2], Nikolai Goncharenko[3], Fay Betsou[3], Kaj Blennow[4], Inês Baldeiras[5], Frederic Brosseron[6], Enrica Cavedo[7], Tormod Fladby[8,9], Lutz Froelich[10], Tomasz Gabryelewicz[11], Hakan Gurvit[12], Elisabeth Kapaki[13], Peter Koson[14,15], Luka Kulic[16], Sylvain Lehmann[17], Piotr Lewczuk[18,19], Alberto Lleó[20,21], Walter Maetzler[22,23], Alexandre de Mendonça[24], Anne-Marie Miller[25], José L. Molinuevo[26], Brit Mollenhauer[27,28], Lucilla Parnetti[29], Uros Rot[30], Anja Schneider[31], Anja Hviid Simonsen[32], Fabrizio Tagliavini[33], Magda Tsolaki[34], Marcel M. Verbeek[35,36], Frans R. J. Verhey[1], Marzena Zboch[37], Bengt Winblad[38], Philip Scheltens[39], Henrik Zetterberg[40,41] and Pieter Jelle Visser[1,39]**

[1] Department of Psychiatry and Neuropsychology, School for Mental Health and Neuroscience, Alzheimer Center Limburg, Maastricht University Medical Center, Maastricht, Netherlands, [2] Neurochemistry Laboratory and Biobank, Department of Clinical Chemistry, VU University Medical Center, Amsterdam, Netherlands, [3] Integrated Biobank of Luxembourg, Luxembourg, Luxembourg, [4] Clinical Neurochemistry Laboratory, Department of Neuroscience and Physiology, Sahlgrenska University Hospital, The Sahlgrenska Academy at University of Gothenburg, Mölndal, Sweden, [5] Center for Neuroscience and Cell Biology, Institute for Biomedical Imaging and Life Sciences, Faculty of Medicine, University of Coimbra, Coimbra, Portugal, [6] German Center for Neurodegenerative Diseases (DZNE) e.V. Clinical Neuroscience and Biomarkers, Bonn, Germany, [7] Laboratory of Alzheimer's Neuroimaging and Epidemiology, IRCCS Fatebenefratelli, Brescia, Italy, [8] Department of Neurology, Akershus University Hospital, Lørenskog, Norway, [9] Institute of Clinical Medicine, University of Oslo, Oslo, Norway, [10] Department of Geriatric Psychiatry, Central Institute of Mental Health, Medical Faculty Mannheim, University of Heidelberg, Mannheim, Germany, [11] Department of Neurodegenerative Disorders, Mossakowski Medical Research Centre, Polish Academy of Sciences, Warsaw, Poland, [12] Behavioural Neurology and Movement Disorders Unit, Department of Neurology, Istanbul Faculty of Medicine, Istanbul University, Istanbul, Turkey, [13] Neurochemistry Unit, Division of Cognitive and Movement Disorders, 1st Department of Neurology, National and Kapodistrian University of Athens, Athens, Greece, [14] Department of Neurology, Slovak Medical University, University Hospital Bratislava, Bratislava, Slovakia, [15] Institute of Neuroimmunology, Slovak Academy of Sciences, Bratislava, Slovakia, [16] Division of Psychiatry Research, University of Zurich, Schlieren, Switzerland, [17] Laboratoire de Biochimie Protéomique Clinique, INSERM U1183, Institut de Médecine Régénérative et Biothérapies, CHRU de Montpellier, Université de Montpellier, Montpellier, France, [18] Department of Psychiatry and Psychotherapy, Universitätsklinikum Erlangen and Friedrich-Alexander Universität Erlangen-Nürnberg, Erlangen, Germany, [19] Department of Neurodegeneration Diagnostics, Medical University of Bialystok, Bialystok, Poland, [20] Memory Unit, Department of Neurology, Hospital de la Santa Creu i Sant Pau-Biomedical Research Institute Sant Pau, Barcelona, Spain, [21] Centro de Investigación Biomédica en Red de Enfermedades Neurodegenerativas (CIBERNED), Madrid, Spain, [22] Department of Neurodegeneration, Hertie Institute for Clinical Brain Research, University of Tübingen, Tübingen, Germany, [23] German Center for Neurodegenerative Diseases (DZNE), University of Tübingen, Tübingen, Germany, [24] Faculty of Medicine, University of Lisbon, Lisbon, Portugal, [25] Medical Gerontology, School of Medicine, Trinity College Dublin, Dublin, Ireland, [26] ICN Hospital Clinic i Universitari, Institut d'Investigacions Biomèdiques August Pi i Sunyer, Barcelona, Spain, [27] Paracelsus-Elena-Klinik, Kassel, Germany, [28] Department of Neurosurgery and Institute of Neuropathology, University Medical Center Göttingen, Göttingen, Germany, [29] Section of Neurology, Centre for Memory Disturbances, University of Perugia, Perugia, Italy, [30] Laboratory for CSF Diagnostics, Department of Neurology, University Medical Centre, Ljubljana, Slovenia, [31] Department of Psychiatry and Psychotherapy, University Medical Center Göttingen and Translational Dementia Research Group, German Center for Neurodegenerative Diseases (DZNE), Göttingen, Germany, [32] Danish Dementia Research Centre, Rigshospitalet, Copenhagen University Hospital, Copenhagen, Denmark, [33] Unit of Neuropathology, Department of Diagnostics and Technology, IRCCS Foundation "Carlo Besta" Neurological Institute, Milan, Italy, [34] 3rd Department of Neurology, Aristotle University of Thessaloniki, Thessaloniki, Greece, [35] Department of Neurology, Radboud Alzheimer Centre, Donders Institute for Brain, Cognition and Behaviour, Radboud University Medical Centre, Nijmegen, Netherlands, [36] Department of Laboratory Medicine, Radboud Alzheimer Centre, Donders Institute for Brain, Cognition and Behaviour, Radboud University Medical Centre, Nijmegen, Netherlands, [37] Research-Scientific-Didactic Centre of Dementia-Related Diseases, Wrocław Medical University, Scinawa, Poland, [38] Division of Neurogeriatrics, Center for Alzheimer Research, Department of Neurobiology, Care Sciences and Society, Karolinska Institutet, Huddinge, Sweden, [39] Department of Neurology, Alzheimer Center, VU University Medical Center, Amsterdam, Netherlands, [40] Department of Psychiatry and Neurochemistry, Institute of Neuroscience and Physiology, The Sahlgrenska Academy at the University of Gothenburg, Mölndal, Sweden, [41] UCL Institute of Neurology, London, UK

Edited by:
Ritchie Williamson, University of Bradford, UK

Reviewed by:
Roland Brandt, University of Osnabrück, Germany
Jason Eriksen, University of Houston, USA

***Correspondence:**
Babette L. R. Reijs
babette.reijs@maastrichtuniversity.nl;
Pieter Jelle Visser
pj.visser@maastrichtuniversity.nl

Biobanks are important resources for biomarker discovery and assay development. Biomarkers for Alzheimer's and Parkinson's disease (BIOMARKAPD) is a European multicenter study, funded by the EU Joint Programme-Neurodegenerative Disease Research, which aims to improve the clinical use of body fluid markers for the diagnosis and prognosis of Alzheimer's disease (AD) and Parkinson's disease (PD). The objective was to standardize the assessment of existing assays and to validate novel fluid biomarkers for AD and PD. To support the validation of novel biomarkers and assays, a central and a virtual biobank for body fluids and associated data from subjects with neurodegenerative diseases have been established. In the central biobank, cerebrospinal fluid (CSF) and blood samples were collected according to the BIOMARKAPD standardized pre-analytical procedures and stored at Integrated BioBank of Luxembourg. The virtual biobank provides an overview of available CSF, plasma, serum, and DNA samples at each site. Currently, at the central biobank of BIOMARKAPD samples are available from over 400 subjects with normal cognition, mild cognitive impairment (MCI), AD, frontotemporal dementia (FTD), vascular dementia, multiple system atrophy, progressive supranuclear palsy, PD, PD with dementia, and dementia with Lewy bodies. The virtual biobank contains information on over 8,600 subjects with varying diagnoses from 21 local biobanks. A website has been launched to enable sample requests from the central biobank and virtual biobank.

Keywords: biobank, cerebrospinal fluid, dementia, Alzheimer's disease, Parkinson's disease, neurodegenerative disorders, body fluids

Introduction

There is an urgent need for biomarkers facilitating diagnosis of Alzheimer's disease (AD) and Parkinson's disease (PD) at an early stage in the disease course before the onset of clinical symptoms and to predict disease progression. For AD, the 42 amino acid form of β-amyloid (Aβ42) reflecting Aβ deposition in plaques, total tau (T-tau) reflecting the intensity of neuroaxonal degeneration, and phosphorylated tau (P-tau) reflecting the amount of brain tangle pathology are promising cerebrospinal fluid (CSF) biomarkers for early detection (1), but they do not cover all the neurodegenerative processes involved. For PD and dementia with Lewy bodies (DLB), no diagnostic or prognostic CSF or blood biomarkers exist, except for α-synuclein in CSF (2). The use of Aβ42, tau proteins, and α-synuclein for the diagnosis and prognosis of AD and PD is challenged by the high intra- and inter-center variability in biomarker concentration measurements (3–5). The variability in measurements is likely caused by differences in pre-analytical and analytical protocols for sample collection, sample handling, and local assay handling (3, 6–10), as well as by inconsistencies in kit production with batch-to-batch and even within-plate variation (11, 12).

Biomarkers for Alzheimer's and Parkinson's Disease (BIOMARKAPD) was a European multicenter study, funded by EU Joint Programme-Neurodegenerative Disease Research (JPND), designed to standardize the assessment of existing assays and to validate novel fluid biomarkers for AD and PD. To support these objectives, BIOMARKAPD has established a central biobank and a virtual biobank for neurodegenerative diseases. Samples for the central biobank have been collected and handled according to standardized operating procedures (13). The virtual biobank provides an overview of the local sample stock at each site. In this article, we will give an overview of clinical data, availability of samples, and the methods for sample collection and processing. Finally, we will explain the procedures for requesting samples.

Materials and Methods

Central Biobank

Study Population

Inclusion criteria for subjects in the central biobank of BIOMARKAPD were a diagnosis of normal cognition, mild cognitive impairment (MCI), AD, PD, dementia with Lewy bodies (DLB), frontotemporal dementia (FTD), vascular dementia (VaD), progressive supranuclear palsy (PSP), multiple system atrophy (MSA), or another type of dementia. Subjects were required to be at least 55 years old (in the MCI group) or at least 40 years old (in all other diagnostic groups). Subjects with normal cognition were clinically evaluated and were required to score above the 10th percentile on the age and education corrected mini-mental state examination (MMSE) (14). MCI was defined as referral to a memory clinic because of cognitive complaints in the absence of dementia. MCI subtypes could be defined *post hoc* based on neuropsychological test performance or CDR score. Subjects with PD were clinically diagnosed according to the UKPDBB criteria (15) or Gelb criteria (16). Subjects with dementia had a minimum score of 18 on the MMSE and were clinically diagnosed according to the NINCDS-ADRDA criteria for probable or possible AD (17), Neary criteria for FTD (18), NINDS-AIREN criteria for VaD (19), and McKeith criteria for DLB (20). Exclusion criteria for all subjects were contra-indications for lumbar puncture and other obvious causes of cognitive impairment such as strokes, severe depression, or endocrine disorders.

Clinical Data

The central biobank collected information on age, gender, education, clinical history [e.g., diagnosis, medication use, a selection of co-morbid disorders (cardiovascular, cerebrovascular, neurological, endocrine, somatic, and psychiatric disorders)], smoking habits and alcohol intake, physical examination [i.e., blood pressure, height, weight, and body mass index (BMI)], general cognition (CDR and MMSE), neuropsychological test performance for the domains of memory, fluency, visuospatial construction, attention, and executive functioning (expressed as raw scores and as *z*-scores according to local norms corrected for age, gender, and education), procedures for sample collection and processing, and the availability of imaging data (e.g., MRI, PET). Clinical data were collected within a timeframe of 6 months around blood/CSF collection.

Standardized Operating Procedures

Samples for the central biobank were collected according to defined biobanking pre-analytical standard operating procedures (SOPs) of the BIOMARKAPD project. For CSF collection, processing, and storage, we adhered to the BIOMARKAPD SOP published by del Campo et al. (13). For plasma and serum samples, we adhered to the biobanking guidelines published by Teunissen et al. (21). In addition, we recommended a 60 min minimum clotting time for blood for serum samples in accordance with the instructions of the tube manufacturer. For blood for DNA samples, we recommended storage at maximal −20°C consistent with the guidelines by Teunissen et al. (22). Centers were asked to report deviations from the SOP.

Sample Collection, Processing, and Storage

Tubes for sample collection and storage were distributed by Integrated BioBank of Luxembourg (IBBL). Blood samples were collected in the following polypropylene tubes: 10 mL EDTA [Becton, Dickinson and Company (BD), ref. 367525] for plasma, 4 mL EDTA (BD, ref. 368861) for whole blood, and 10 mL clot activator tubes (CAT) (BD, ref. 367896) for serum. CSF was collected in 10 mL polypropylene tubes (Sarstedt, ref. 62.610.018). Blood samples for DNA were not centrifuged and stored at maximal −20°C. All other samples were centrifuged at room temperature at 2,000 × *g* (min 1,800 × *g*, max 2,200 × *g*) and stored at −80°C. A maximum of 2 h was allowed between collection and freezing. A more detailed description of the SOP used for the collection of samples for the central biobank can be found elsewhere (13). For every subject 2 mL CSF, 2 mL serum, and 2 mL plasma were stored in 0.5 aliquots (in 0.5 mL Matrix 2D Thermo tubes) and 4 mL blood was stored for DNA isolation. Primary specimens and samples derivatives were coded with a three-letter center code and a subject number. Samples were at first stored locally, and then shipped on dry ice to IBBL for long-term storage. DNA extraction was performed at the IBBL. Samples and associated data were processed and stored at IBBL in compliance with ISO 9001:2008, NF S96-900: 2011, and ISO 17025:2005 standards and the ISBER Best Practices.

Virtual Biobank

The virtual biobank provides an estimation of the number of samples, and clinical (i.e., age, gender, education, CDR scores, MMSE scores, Parkinson scales, neuropsychological test results, information on medication use, and co-morbid disorders) and other biomarker data (i.e., MRI data, amyloid PET, dopamine SPECT) available at each center of subjects with normal cognition, MCI, AD, PD, PD with dementia, DLB, FTD, VaD, PSP, MSA, and other types of dementia. Retrospectively collected samples had been collected according to the center's own SOPs. Centers that changed to the standardized BIOMARKAPD SOP during the project reported the transition date. All samples remained stored on site.

Ethics

Centers received approval from their local Ethical Committee and all subjects provided informed consent. All human research was conducted in accordance with the principles of the Declaration of Helsinki.

Results

Central Biobank

Sample collection for the central biobank was performed in the period October 2013–December 2015. A total of 14 European centers have contributed samples and data to the central biobank. Currently, the central biobank database contains clinical information on 419 subjects, of which 49 had normal cognition, 117 MCI, 164 AD, 24 FTD, 3 VaD, 11 DLB, 25 PD, 5 PD with dementia, 3 PSP, 1 MSA, and 18 other types of dementia (i.e., either unknown or mixed pathology). From almost all subjects CSF samples ($n = 410$), plasma samples ($n = 413$ subjects), serum samples ($n = 414$), and DNA samples ($n = 414$) are available at the central biobank. At the local sites, MRI imaging data are available from 299 subjects, SPECT from 6 subjects, amyloid PET from 14 subjects, and FDG-PET from 28 subjects. **Table 1** lists demographic information, neuropsychological tests results, and available imaging data according to diagnostic group. At least 1 neuropsychological test result was available from 307 subjects. The deviations reported from the SOP are shown in **Table 2**. The most common deviation (82%) was the use of a different needle than the 25G atraumatic needle. For most lumbar punctures,

TABLE 1 | Central biobank subject characteristics, *z*-scores on neuropsychological tests, and biomarker data available according to diagnostic group.

	Total (*n* = 419)	Normal cognition (*n* = 49)	MCI (*n* = 117)	AD (*n* = 164)	FTD (*n* = 24)	VaD (*n* = 3)	DLB (*n* = 11)	PD (*n* = 25)	PD with dementia (*n* = 5)	PSP (*n* = 3)	MSA (*n* = 1)	Other dementia (*n* = 18)
Demographics, *n*	419	49	117	164	24	3	11	25	5	3	1	18
Age, mean (SD)	68.0 (9.3)	62.5 (9.9)	67.1 (9.2)	70.6 (8.5)	63.8 (7.4)	72.3 (5.5)	75.6 (8.9)	68.0 (7.5)	72.2 (5.9)	54.7 (5.9)	80.0 (0)	65.8 (10.1)
Male, % (*n*)	49 (205)	61 (30)	53 (62)	37 (60)	63 (15)	67 (2)	73 (8)	60 (15)	60 (3)	67 (2)	0 (0)	44 (8)
Education, mean years (SD)	9.9 (3.7)	12.2 (2.9)	10.3 (3.4)	9.6 (3.8)	7.9 (3.4)	7.3 (3.1)	8.3 (3.5)	8.9 (3.3)	11.0 (2.8)	14.0 (3.5)	5.0 (0)	8.9 (3.8)
MMSE, *n*	386	49	109	150	23	3	11	17	5	3	1	15
Mean (SD)	23.9 (5.3)	27.6 (2.6)	27.0 (2.2)	21.1 (5.1)	22.9 (5.6)	25.3 (1.5)	21.1 (6.6)	26.3 (5.5)	22.6 (5.9)	22.3 (3.8)	23.0 (0)	19.1 (7.7)
CDR overall, *n*	283	44	82	113	16	2	4	3	1	3	0	15
Mean (SD)	0.8 (0.5)	0.2 (0.3)	0.5 (0.1)	1.1 (0.4)	1.1 (0.6)	1.0 (0)	0.8 (0.3)	1.7 (1.2)	0.5 (0)	1.0 (0)	–	1.2 (0.7)
NPA (at least 1z-score), *n*	307	45	100	108	17	3	7	10	3	3	0	11
Word list immediate recall	−1.8 (1.5)	−0.3 (1.1)	−1.5 (1.3)	−2.8 (1.2)	−2.8 (1.9)	−1.8 (0.4)	−2.3 (1.2)	−0.4 (2.2)	–	−1.8 (2.0)	–	−2.2 (0.5)
Word list delayed recall	−1.7 (1.4)	−0.7 (0.9)	−1.5 (1.4)	−2.5 (1.1)	−1.7 (1.0)	−2.2 (0.6)	−2.1 (1.7)	0.4 (0.4)	–	−1.4 (1.6)	–	−2.4 (0.6)
Story immediate recall	−1.2 (1.7)	0 (0.9)	−1.3 (2.0)	−2.4 (0.8)	−2.7 (0)	–	–	−3.9 (0)	–	–	–	−2.1 (0.4)
Story delayed recall	−0.8 (1.9)	−0.1 (0.9)	−1.7 (2.0)	−0.2 (3.6)	–	–	–	−4.8 (0)	–	–	–	−2.4 (0)
Fluency	−1.0 (1.4)	−0.5 (1.1)	−0.8 (1.5)	−1.5 (1.2)	−1.6 (1.2)	−1.3 (1.4)	0 (1.4)	−0.9 (0.9)	–	1.0 (2.8)	–	−1.1 (1.2)
Copy figures	−0.7 (1.4)	−1.4 (0.9)	−0.4 (1.4)	−0.9 (1.4)	−1.4 (1.6)	0.8 (0.5)	−0.7 (1.5)	0.4 (1.1)	–	−0.9 (2.2)	–	−1.2 (1.2)
TMTA	−1.2 (1.4)	−0.8 (1.4)	−0.9 (1.3)	−1.6 (1.2)	−1.9 (1.6)	−1.5 (0.6)	−0.2 (1.7)	−0.3 (0.8)	–	1.6 (3.7)	–	−2.5 (0.8)
TMTB	−1.5 (1.7)	−1.0 (1.4)	−1.2 (1.7)	−2.1 (1.6)	−2.4 (1.6)	−2.0 (1.6)	−2.1 (1.3)	1.3 (0.1)	–	1.8 (3.5)	–	−2.0 (1.3)
Fasted, % (*n*)	35.0 (140)	4.4. (2)	39.8 (45)	30.7 (47)	54.2 (13)	66.7 (2)	36.4 (4)	72.0 (18)	40.0 (2)	0	100 (1)	35.3 (6)
Erythrocyte count >500/µL, % (*n*)	5.0 (20)	8.9 (4)	3.5 (4)	7.0 (11)	0	0	0	0	0	0	0	5.9 (1)
MRI, *n*[a]	299	45	90	110	21	2	3	5	3	3	1	16
SPECT, *n*[a]	6	0	0	1	0	0	2	1	2	0	0	0
Amyloid PET, *n*[a]	14	2	1	8	1	0	0	0	0	1	0	1
FDG-PET, *n*[a]	28	1	6	11	4	0	0	0	0	1	0	5

MMSE, mini-mental state examination; CDR, Clinical dementia Rating; NPA, neuropsychological assessment; TMT, Trail Making Test; MCI, mild cognitive impairment; AD, Alzheimer's disease; FTD, frontotemporal dementia; VaD, vascular dementia; DLB, dementia with Lewy bodies; PD, Parkinson's disease; PSP, progressive supranuclear palsy; MSA, multiple system atrophy.

Data are mean (SD), count or valid percent.

[a]Not in central biobank, but available at local sites.

TABLE 2 | Deviations from the SOP reported for samples in the central biobank.

SOP recommendation	Number of deviations	Reason (number of subjects)
CSF collection		
Withdrawal of 10 mL CSF (+2 mL for clinical purposes)	14	Slow flow/flow stopped (2); unknown (7); difficulty with positioning (1); patient did not want to continue (2); impossible, no reason specified (2)
25G atraumatic needle	336	Neurologist preferred traumatic needle (79); atraumatic used, but different diameter: 25G not available (238), impossible with 25G (19)
LP location: intervertebral space L3-L5	0	–
Polypropylene tubes	0	–
Erythrocyte count <500/μL	20	Unknown (20)
CSF processing		
Centrifuge at 2,000 × *g* (or between 1,800 and 2,200 × *g*) for 10 min at RT	5	2,000 × *g* centrifuge not available (centrifuged at 1,120 × *g*) (5)
Maximum 2 h between collection and freezing (or temporarily store at 4°C)	1	Delay in sample delivery (1)
Freeze at −80°C	0	–
Maximum of 2 freeze and thaw cycles	0[a]	–
Blood for plasma, processing		
Centrifuge at 2,000 × *g* (or between 1,800 and 2,200 × *g*) for 10 min at RT	5	2,000 × *g* centrifuge not available (centrifuged at 1,120 × *g*) (5)
Maximum 2 h between collection and freezing (or temporarily store at 4°C	13	Delay in sample delivery (1); unknown (12)
Freeze at −80°C	0	–
Limit freeze and thaw cycles	0[a]	–
Blood for serum, processing		
Centrifuge at 2,000 × *g* (or between 1,800 and 2,200 × *g*) for 10 min at RT	5	2,000 × *g* centrifuge not available (centrifuged at 1,120 × *g*) (5)
Maximum 2 h between collection and freezing (or temporarily store at 4°C)	13	Delay in sample delivery (1); unknown (12)
At least 30 min (but preferably >60 min) between collection and centrifugation	10[b]	Mistake <30 min (10)
Freeze at −80°C	0	–
Limit freeze and thaw cycles	0[a]	–
Whole blood for DNA, processing		
Freeze below −20°C	0	–

SOP, standardized operating procedures; LP, lumbar puncture; RT, room temperature. Data are number of subjects in which a deviation of the SOP occurred.[a]One cycle: CSF (50), plasma (5) and serum (55).
[b]Clotting time: between 30 and 50 min (23) and between 50 and 59 min (35).

this needle was unavailable ($n = 239$), it was impossible to collect CSF with this needle ($n = 19$) or the neurologist preferred a traumatic needle ($n = 79$). None of the samples had more than the maximum of two freeze and thaw cycles, while 12% of the CSF samples, 1% of the plasma samples, and 13% of the serum samples underwent one freeze and thaw cycle. If the deviation related to needle use and number of freeze and thaw cycles was not taken into account, adherence to the BIOMARKAPD SOP was 91% for CSF collection and centrifugation, 96% for plasma collection and centrifugation, 93% for serum collection and centrifugation, and 100% for DNA collection and processing.

Virtual Biobank

Currently, 21 centers have contributed data to the virtual biobank of BIOMARKAPD. The virtual biobank contains information on CSF samples from 7,550 subjects, EDTA plasma samples from 8,676 subjects, and serum samples from 8,141 subjects. So far, 11 centers have reported that they followed, or changed to, the BIOMARKAPD SOP for sample collection and processing. **Table 3** lists the number of subjects per diagnostic group with CSF, EDTA plasma, and serum samples available.

Discussion

As part of BIOMARKAPD, a large central and virtual biobank with body fluids were established from over 9,000 subjects with neurodegenerative disorders. The central biobank contains samples from more than 400 subjects of which nearly 40% have AD. Adherence to the BIOMARKAPD SOP was high (>91%) for the collection and processing of CSF, plasma, and serum and blood samples. The virtual biobank contains CSF samples from over 7,500 subjects, plasma samples from over 8,600 subjects, and serum samples from over 8,100 subjects. Samples for the virtual biobank have been collected according to varying local SOPs.

TABLE 3 | Number of subjects in virtual biobank with CSF, EDTA plasma, and serum samples available according to diagnostic group.

	CSF	EDTA plasma	Serum
Normal cognition, *n*	890	1,831	1,316
MCI, *n*	1,969	1,894	2,066
AD, *n*	2,420	2,440	2,349
FTD, *n*	612	621	647
VaD, *n*	156	187	151
DLB, *n*	277	282	279
PD	439	720	748
PD with dementia, *n*	157	243	219
PSP, *n*	148	146	115
MSA, *n*	68	57	38
Other dementia, *n*	414	255	213
Total	7,550	8,676	8,141

CSF, cerebrospinal fluid; MCI, mild cognitive impairment; AD, Alzheimer's disease; FTD, frontotemporal dementia; VaD, vascular dementia; DLB, dementia with Lewy bodies; PD, Parkinson's disease; PSP, progressive supranuclear palsy; MSA, multiple system atrophy.
Data are number of subjects with CSF, EDTA plasma, or serum samples available.

However, so far more than half of the centers have reported adopting the BIOMARKAPD SOP in the course of the project.

Requesting Samples from the Central or Virtual Biobank

Researchers in the field of neurodegenerative disorders interested in requesting samples from the central biobank or from the virtual biobank of BIOMARKAPD are invited to consult the following website: http://jpnd.arone.com/. Requests should meet the objectives of BIOMARKAPD project, i.e., to standardize the assessment of existing assays and to validate novel fluid biomarkers for AD and PD. Sample requests will be evaluated by the Analysis Advisory Board (AAB). Approval from the AAB will depend on scientific quality, whether the sample request meets the objectives of BIOMARKAPD, and sample availability. Furthermore, the sample request must meet the following three criteria. First, the researcher must demonstrate that the analysis complies with local medical ethical standards, for example, by showing regulatory approval of a medical ethical committee (MEC), institutional review board (IRB), or equivalent. Second, technical characteristics of assays such as linearity, recovery, specificity, imprecision, sensitivity, and lot-to-lot variability have already been established and of sufficient performance. Third, prior to the request, the diagnostic or prognostic value of the assay should have been already demonstrated in at least 20 controls and 20 diseased subjects. For the central biobank, fees will apply to cover the costs for sample and data collection, processing, and sample storage. Before shipment a material transfer agreement (MTA) needs to be signed.

For the virtual biobank, individual centers can decide on a case-to-case basis whether or not they would like to provide samples and which conditions will apply. When requesting samples from the virtual biobank, contact details will be provided of centers that are interested in meeting the sample request. Centers may use the MTA from the central biobank for the shipment of samples. Detailed information on the methodology of sample preparation and handling, and available clinical information should be requested directly from the center.

Conclusion

The central and virtual biobanks of BIOMARKAPD provide access to a large repository of CSF and blood samples for researchers in the field of neurodegenerative disorders, enabling progress in the clinical use of biomarkers for the diagnosis and prognosis of neurodegenerative disorders.

Acknowledgments

This work is part of the BIOMARKAPD project within the EU Joint Programme for Neurodegenerative Diseases Research (JPND). This project is supported through the following funding organizations under the aegis of JPND – www.jpnd.eu

Funding organizations.

Country	Funding organization
Belgium	IWT
Canada	Fonds de la Recherche en Santé du Québec FRSQ
Denmark	Danish Strategic Research Council
Finland	The Academy of Finland AoF
France	French National Research Agency
Germany	German Bundesministerium für Bildung und Forschung (BMBF); LF received funding by BMBF/DLR (01ED1203J), PL received funding by BMBF (01ED1203D)
Greece	Ministry of Education, Life Long Learning and Religious Affairs, General Secretariat for Research and Technology
Ireland	Health Research Board
Italy	Ministero della Salute
Luxembourg	Fonds National de la Recherche, Luxembourg
The Netherlands	ZonMW- The Netherlands Organisation for Health Research and Development grant number 629000002
Norway	The Research Council of Norway
Poland	National Centre for Research and Development
Portugal	Fundação para a Ciência e a Tecnologia (FCT)
Slovakia	Ministry of Education, Science, Research and Sports of the Slovak Republic
Slovenia	Javna agencija za raziskovalno dejavnost Republike Slovenije
Spain	Instituto de Salud Carlos III (ISCII)
Sweden	Swedish Research Council (SRC)
Switzerland	Swiss National Science Foundation (SNSF)
Turkey	Türkiye Bilimsel ve Teknolojik Araştırma Kurumu
United Kingdom	Medical Research Council

We thank EU JPND and all national funding organizations involved for the BIOMARKAPD funding, and we thank IBBL for their various contributions in kind to the project, in particular for the provision of the IT infrastructure for the central and virtual biobanks, and for continuing storage of samples after the project.

References

1. Blennow K, Hampel H, Weiner M, Zetterberg H. Cerebrospinal fluid and plasma biomarkers in Alzheimer disease. *Nat Rev Neurol* (2010) **6**(3):131–44. doi:10.1038/nrneurol.2010.4
2. Mollenhauer B, Locascio JJ, Schulz-Schaeffer W, Sixel-Doring F, Trenkwalder C, Schlossmacher MG. alpha-Synuclein and tau concentrations in cerebrospinal fluid of patients presenting with parkinsonism: a cohort study. *Lancet Neurol* (2011) **10**(3):230–40. doi:10.1016/S1474-4422(11)70014-X
3. Mattsson N, Andreasson U, Persson S, Arai H, Batish SD, Bernardini S, et al. The Alzheimer's association external quality control program for cerebrospinal fluid biomarkers. *Alzheimers Dement* (2011) 7(4):386–395e386. doi:10.1016/j.jalz.2011.05.2243
4. Mollenhauer B, El-Agnaf OM, Marcus K, Trenkwalder C, Schlossmacher MG. Quantification of alpha-synuclein in cerebrospinal fluid as a biomarker candidate: review of the literature and considerations for future studies. *Biomark Med* (2010) **4**(5):683–99. doi:10.2217/bmm.10.90
5. Verwey NA, van der Flier WM, Blennow K, Clark C, Sokolow S, De Deyn PP, et al. A worldwide multicentre comparison of assays for cerebrospinal fluid biomarkers in Alzheimer's disease. *Ann Clin Biochem* (2009) **46**(Pt 3):235–40. doi:10.1258/acb.2009.008232
6. Bibl M, Esselmann H, Otto M, Lewczuk P, Cepek L, Ruther E, et al. Cerebrospinal fluid amyloid beta peptide patterns in Alzheimer's disease patients and nondemented controls depend on sample pretreatment: indication of carrier-mediated epitope masking of amyloid beta peptides. *Electrophoresis* (2004) **25**(17):2912–8. doi:10.1002/elps.200305992
7. Bjerke M, Portelius E, Minthon L, Wallin A, Anckarsater H, Anckarsater R, et al. Confounding factors influencing amyloid Beta concentration in cerebrospinal fluid. *Int J Alzheimers Dis* (2010) **2010**:11. doi:10.4061/2010/986310
8. Lewczuk P, Beck G, Esselmann H, Bruckmoser R, Zimmermann R, Fiszer M, et al. Effect of sample collection tubes on cerebrospinal fluid concentrations of tau proteins and amyloid beta peptides. *Clin Chem* (2006) **52**(2):332–4. doi:10.1373/clinchem.2005.058776
9. Schoonenboom NS, Mulder C, Vanderstichele H, Pijnenburg YA, Van Kamp GJ, Scheltens P, et al. Differences and similarities between two frequently used assays for amyloid beta 42 in cerebrospinal fluid. *Clin Chem* (2005) **51**(6):1057–60. doi:10.1373/clinchem.2005.048629
10. Teunissen CE, Verwey NA, Kester MI, van Uffelen K, Blankenstein MA. Standardization of assay procedures for analysis of the CSF biomarkers amyloid beta((1-42)), Tau, and phosphorylated Tau in Alzheimer's disease: report of an international workshop. *Int J Alzheimers Dis* (2010) **2010**:6. doi:10.4061/2010/635053
11. Mattsson N, Zegers I, Andreasson U, Bjerke M, Blankenstein MA, Bowser R, et al. Reference measurement procedures for Alzheimer's disease cerebrospinal fluid biomarkers: definitions and approaches with focus on amyloid beta42. *Biomark Med* (2012) **6**(4):409–17. doi:10.2217/bmm.12.39
12. Vos SJ, Visser PJ, Verhey F, Aalten P, Knol D, Ramakers I, et al. Variability of CSF Alzheimer's disease biomarkers: implications for clinical practice. *PLoS One* (2014) **9**(6):e100784. doi:10.1371/journal.pone.0100784
13. del Campo M, Mollenhauer B, Bertolotto A, Engelborghs S, Hampel H, Simonsen AH, et al. Recommendations to standardize preanalytical confounding factors in Alzheimer's and Parkinson's disease cerebrospinal fluid biomarkers: an update. *Biomark Med* (2012) **6**(4):419–30. doi:10.2217/bmm.12.46
14. Folstein MF, Folstein SE, McHugh PR. "Mini-mental state". A practical method for grading the cognitive state of patients for the clinician. *J Psychiatr Res* (1975) **12**(3):189–98. doi:10.1016/0022-3956(75)90026-6
15. Hughes AJ, Daniel SE, Kilford L, Lees AJ. Accuracy of clinical diagnosis of idiopathic Parkinson's disease: a clinico-pathological study of 100 cases. *J Neurol Neurosurg Psychiatry* (1992) **55**(3):181–4. doi:10.1136/jnnp.55.3.181
16. Gelb DJ, Oliver E, Gilman S. Diagnostic criteria for Parkinson disease. *Arch Neurol* (1999) **56**(1):33–9. doi:10.1001/archneur.56.1.33
17. McKhann G, Drachman D, Folstein M, Katzman R, Price D, Stadlan EM. Clinical diagnosis of Alzheimer's disease: report of the NINCDS-ADRDA Work Group under the auspices of Department of Health and Human Services Task Force on Alzheimer's disease. *Neurology* (1984) **34**(7):939–44. doi:10.1212/WNL.34.7.939
18. Neary D, Snowden JS, Northen B, Goulding P. Dementia of frontal lobe type. *J Neurol Neurosurg Psychiatry* (1988) **51**(3):353–61. doi:10.1136/jnnp.51.3.353
19. Roman GC, Tatemichi TK, Erkinjuntti T, Cummings JL, Masdeu JC, Garcia JH, et al. Vascular dementia: diagnostic criteria for research studies. Report of the NINDS-AIREN International Workshop. *Neurology* (1993) **43**(2):250–60. doi:10.1212/WNL.43.10.2160
20. McKeith IG, Galasko D, Kosaka K, Perry EK, Dickson DW, Hansen LA, et al. Consensus guidelines for the clinical and pathologic diagnosis of dementia with Lewy bodies (DLB): report of the consortium on DLB international workshop. *Neurology* (1996) **47**(5):1113–24. doi:10.1212/WNL.47.5.1113
21. Teunissen CE, Tumani H, Engelborghs S, Mollenhauer B. Biobanking of CSF: international standardization to optimize biomarker development. *Clin Biochem* (2014) **47**(4–5):288–92. doi:10.1016/j.clinbiochem.2013.12.024
22. Teunissen CE, Petzold A, Bennett JL, Berven FS, Brundin L, Comabella M, et al. A consensus protocol for the standardization of cerebrospinal fluid collection and biobanking. *Neurology* (2009) **73**(22):1914–22. doi:10.1212/WNL.0b013e3181c47cc2

10

Chasing the effects of pre-analytical confounders – a multicenter study on CSF-AD biomarkers

*Maria João Leitão[1], Inês Baldeiras[1,2,3], Sanna-Kaisa Herukka[4], Maria Pikkarainen[4], Ville Leinonen[5], Anja Hviid Simonsen[6], Armand Perret-Liaudet[7,8,9], Anthony Fourier[7,8], Isabelle Quadrio[7,8], Pedro Mota Veiga[10] and Catarina Resende de Oliveira[1,2,3]**

[1] Center for Neuroscience and Cell Biology (CNC), University of Coimbra, Coimbra, Portugal, [2] Neurochemistry Laboratory, Neurology Department, Coimbra University Hospital, Coimbra, Portugal, [3] Faculty of Medicine, University of Coimbra, Coimbra, Portugal, [4] Neurology Department, Institute of Clinical Medicine, Kuopio University Hospital, University of Eastern Finland, Kuopio, Finland, [5] Neurosurgery of NeuroCenter, Kuopio University Hospital, Kuopio, Finland, [6] Danish Dementia Research Centre, Copenhagen University Hospital Rigshospitalet, Copenhagen, Denmark, [7] Neurobiology, Biochemistry and Molecular Biology Department, University Hospital of Lyon, Lyon, France, [8] UMR5292, BioRan, CNRS, INSERM U1028, University of Lyon 1, Lyon, France, [9] Société Française de Biologie Clinique (SFBC), Alzheimer Biomarkers Group Co-Coordination, Lyon, France, [10] Statistics and Research – Curva de Gauss, Training and Consulting, Canas de Senhorim, Portugal

Edited by:
Sylvain Lehmann,
Montpellier University Hospital, France

Reviewed by:
Zhihui Yang,
University of Florida, USA
Sun Ah Park,
Soonchunhyang University Bucheon Hospital, South Korea

***Correspondence:**
Catarina Resende de Oliveira,
Neurochemistry Laboratory,
Neurology Department, Faculty of Medicine, Center for Neuroscience and Cell Biology, University Hospital Coimbra, Praceta Mota Pinto, Coimbra 3000-075, Portugal
catarina.n.oliveira@gmail.com

Introduction: Core cerebrospinal fluid (CSF) biomarkers – Aβ42, Tau, and phosphorylated Tau (pTau) – have been recently incorporated in the revised criteria for Alzheimer's disease (AD). However, their widespread clinical application lacks standardization. Pre-analytical sample handling and storage play an important role in the reliable measurement of these biomarkers across laboratories.

Aim: In this study, we aim to surpass the efforts from previous studies, by employing a multicenter approach to assess the impact of less studied CSF pre-analytical confounders in AD-biomarkers quantification.

Methods: Four different centers participated in this study and followed the same established protocol. CSF samples were analyzed for three biomarkers (Aβ42, Tau, and pTau) and tested for different spinning conditions [temperature: room temperature (RT) vs. 4°C; speed: 500 vs. 2000 vs. 3000 g], storage volume variations (25, 50, and 75% of tube total volume), as well as freezing-thaw cycles (up to five cycles). The influence of sample routine parameters, inter-center variability, and relative value of each biomarker (reported as normal/abnormal) was analyzed.

Results: Centrifugation conditions did not influence biomarkers levels, except for samples with a high CSF total protein content, where either non-centrifugation or centrifugation at RT, compared to 4°C, led to higher Aβ42 levels. Reducing CSF storage volume from 75 to 50% of total tube capacity decreased Aβ42 concentration (within analytical CV of the assay), whereas no change in Tau or pTau was observed. Moreover, the concentration of Tau and pTau appears to be stable up to five freeze–thaw cycles, whereas Aβ42 levels decrease if CSF is freeze-thawed more than three times.

Conclusion: This systematic study reinforces the need for CSF centrifugation at 4°C prior to storage and highlights the influence of storage conditions in Aβ42 levels. This study contributes to the establishment of harmonized standard operating procedures that will help reducing inter-lab variability of CSF-AD biomarkers evaluation.

Keywords: Alzheimer's disease, cerebrospinal fluid, biomarkers, BIOMARKAPD, standardized operating procedures, β-amyloid, tau protein, phosphorylated tau protein

Introduction

Cerebrospinal fluid (CSF) biomarkers, Aβ42, Tau protein, and phosphorylated Tau (pTau), are frequently assessed for their proven value as hallmarks of initial and coursing neuropathological events in Alzheimer's disease (AD) (1, 2). Studies over the years have shown a 250–300% increase of CSF Tau and pTau and a decrease of about 50% in CSF Aβ42 in AD patients compared to normal aging (3). The high sensitivity and specificity of these markers have been shown to be useful in discriminating AD from other dementias, as well as to identify AD before onset of dementia (the stage known as mild cognitive impairment - MCI), both in single-center and large-scale multicenter studies (4–7). Therefore, biomarkers have recently been incorporated in the new proposed revised criteria for AD (8). The development and application of revised diagnostic criteria, which include biomarkers, will substantially improve the diagnostic accuracy for AD toward other forms of dementia and can help anticipate the rate of progression and early disablement in AD (9, 10). Besides giving clues to pathogenic mechanisms of the disease, biomarkers can also favor therapeutics development by signaling desired effects of drugs in phase I–II clinical trials, allowing inclusion of early cases to longitudinal studies and even identifying sub-groups of patients in order to tailor treatment (11, 12).

However, in recent years, international scientific evaluation studies regarding neurochemical diagnosis of neurodegenerative diseases have shown that the inter-laboratory precision of those biomarkers measurements requires optimization (13). Cut-offs differ greatly between studies, and the widespread clinical application of revised criteria for early AD is hampered by lack of standardization of biomarkers (2, 8). These variations in biomarkers performance can be the result of several pre-analytical and analytical factors. Pre-analytical factors include lumbar puncture (LP), CSF handling, and storage procedures, while analytical factors are more assay-related, for instance to differences among centers in training of technicians, operating procedures, or batch-to-batch variations of kits (14, 15). Analytical outcome can also be influenced by biological variables intrinsic to study participants, such as genetic variations or relation between CSF and brain volume (16).

Several international standardization initiatives are already ongoing. The most extensive is the global Alzheimer's Association external quality control program for CSF measurements led by K. Blennow (17, 18), involving more than 80 laboratories worldwide. However, it is still purely descriptive and does not provide any active interventions to tackle variations. Among interested and connected centers for harmonization of AD biomarkers, there have been attempts to reach a consensus concerning CSF collection, handling, and storage, and to create uniformized standard operating procedures (USOPs) (19, 20). Reasonable amount of evidence already exists regarding how CSF biomarkers levels are influenced by certain pre-analytical conditions. For instance, it has been well-established that polypropylene (PP) tubes and pipet tips should be used for CSF collection, handling, and storage, since lipophilic proteins like Aβ peptides bind in a non-specific manner to non-PP tubes (21, 22). Several laboratories have also reported on the stability of CSF proteins between collection and storage (13, 23, 24), and it is a common consensus that they are stable for at least 5 days at 4°C (20). Moreover, some studies have analyzed the influence of freeze/thaw cycles on CSF-AD biomarkers and most have found a decrease in Aβ42 concentration as a result of freeze/thaw cycles, but different results were found in the number of cycles that led to this decrease.

However, all of these studies were done in a single center and employing a limited number of samples, generally no more than 10 samples per experimental condition. Also, most of them only address the effect of pre-analytical conditions on CSF Aβ42 and Tau levels or just in Aβ42, with only a few studies looking at the effect on pTau levels (13, 25). Therefore, a standardized protocol for handling CSF is still needed to allow for multicenter studies and data comparisons in a near future (18).

In 2011, a new consortium was launched under the scope of Joint Program for Neurodegenerative Diseases (JPND), the BIOMARKAPD, expected to exceed all ongoing initiatives as it involved a real European effort to solve standardization issues. The main aim of the project is to develop evidence-based guidelines for measurement and use of biomarkers in AD and Parkinson's disease (PD) in clinical practice, within 48 sites from 21 European countries and also Canada. The present multicenter study is part of this transnational project and its main aim is to assess CSF pre-analytical confounding factors, which have been less studied so far, that can possibly affect assay performance and biomarkers measurements across laboratories. We intend to test a large number of samples, for all three biomarkers, the effect of different spinning CSF conditions (temperature and speed) and of storing different CSF volumes per total tube volume into aliquots. We will also extend the study of the impact of the number of freeze–thaw cycles (up to five cycles) to pTau. By this, we expect to contribute to the development of new feasible, CSF handling USOPs that will help reducing interlaboratory variability of CSF-AD biomarkers.

Materials and Methods

Participants

Four centers (Neurochemistry Laboratory, Coimbra University Hospital, Portugal; Institute of Clinical Medicine-Neurology, Kuopio University Hospital, Finland; Danish Dementia Research

TABLE 1 | Participating centers and their sample contribution for the evaluation of CSF pre-analytical conditions (temperature and speed of centrifugation, CSF%/tube volume, and number of freeze/thaw cycles) on Aβ42, Tau, and pTau levels.

	Centrifugation		%CSF/tube vol.	Freeze–thaw cycles
	Temperature	Speed		
Coimbra (Portugal) Ctr = 0%; AD = 25.8%; MCI = 12.1% OD = 28.8%; OT = 33.3%	27	22	30	27
Copenhagen (Denmark) OT = 100%	8	8	–	–
Kuopio (Finland) Ctr = 10%; AD = 2.5%; MCI = 2.5% OD = 5%; OT = 80%	10	–	10	10
Lyon (France) Ctr = 4.5%; AD = 18.2%; MCI = 4.5% OD = 36.4%; OT = 13.6%	10	10	10	3
TOTAL = 136	55	40	50	40

Ctr, healthy controls; AD, Alzheimer's disease; MCI, mild cognitive impairment; OD, other dementias; OT, other.

Centre, Copenhagen University Hospital Rigshospitalet, Copenhagen, Denmark; Neurobiologie, University of Lyon, Lyon, France) participated in this study. All laboratories handled CSF samples in a standardized way, through the same previously established protocol. Contributions in terms of number of samples were variable (see **Table 1**). This study has been approved by the Ethical board of Coimbra's University Hospital, by local Ethical committee of French Ministry of Research and Higher Education, Ethical committee from the Capital Region of Denmark, and by Research Ethics Committee Hospital District of Northern Savo.

CSF Collection

The study was performed with freshly collected CSF samples, obtained by LP in the L3/L4 or L4/L5 intervertebral space by clinicians in the Neurology Departments of each center, using a 20 or 25 G needle and collected to 10 mL standardized PP tubes (Sarstedt 62.610.201). A total of 136 samples were collected from patients with different diagnoses, five of them not classified (healthy controls - 3.7%; MCI - 7.4%; AD - 16.2%; other dementia - 21.3%; other diagnosis - 47.8%). A small amount of CSF was used for routine analysis including cytological (white and red cell count) and chemical analysis (total protein and glucose content). From a total of 133 patients with this information, 50.7% had normal RBC count and 47.1% abnormal count; for CSF total protein, 69.1% had normal ($n = 88$; 32.2 ± 6.9 mg/dL; 15–44 mg/dL) content and 27.9% abnormal ($n = 44$; 61.2 ± 14.3, 45–99 mg/dL). The remaining CSF was processed according to the different pre-analytical conditions to be tested further on. In all cases, samples were handled at room temperature (RT) (18–25°C), and exposure to light and time between CSF collection and storage did not exceed 2 h.

Tested Pre-Analytical Conditions

Centrifugation

For each sample, CSF was first aliquoted (380 μL) into five PP tubes of 500 μL (Sarstedt ref. 72.730.006). Tube C1 was not spinned at all and was left standing at RT without spinning until other tubes were ready (kept into an intermediate tube until transfer to final aliquot in order to keep the same procedure compared to other centrifuged conditions); Tube C2 was centrifuged for 10 min, 2000 × g at RT; Tube C3 was centrifuged for 10 min, 2000 × g but at 4°C (standard condition used for routine processing at all four centers); Tube C4 and C5 underwent spinning for 10 min at RT, the former at 500 × g and the latter at 3000 × g. Tubes C2 and C3 were used to test the effect of temperature during centrifugation and Tubes C2, C4, and C5 to test for speed. We also compared Tubes C1 (no spinning) and C3 (routine protocol). The supernatant of centrifuged CSF, as well as the non-centrifuged CSF, was then immediately transferred from spinning tubes to final set of tubes (500 μL Sarstedt ref. 72.730.006) and frozen at −80°C until analysis.

To test the impact of RBC count in CSF, five different samples were spiked with blood at 1/1000 (3.6 μL in 3.5 mL of CSF) to reach a final number of 5000 RBC/μL (±10%). The spiked CSF was aliquoted and treated as described above.

CSF%/Tube Volume

For each sample, CSF was first centrifuged for 10 min, 2000 × g at 4°C, and then aliquoted into tubes, as described above, in order to fill different percentages of total tube volume - V1 (25%; i.e., 500 μL in a 2 mL tube; Sarstedt ref. 72.694.007); V2 (50%; 250 μL in a 500 μL tube; this volume represents the minimum amount required to perform the assays for Aβ42, Tau, and pTau); V3 (75%, our baseline condition, i.e., 380 μL in a 500 μL tube). The aliquoted CSF was then immediately stored at −80°C until analysis.

Freeze/Thaw Cycles

To test this condition, we aliquoted the same volume (380 μL) of centrifuged CSF (10 min, 2000 × g at 4°C) into three 500 μL tubes and stored them at −80°C. One of them (F1, baseline condition) was left frozen until the moment of analysis; for tube F2, we forced two freeze–thaw cycles (left on the benchtop for 2 h at RT to mimick assay time on two consecutive days after collection) prior to analysis, which would account for a total of three cycles; for tube F3, four freeze/thaw cycles were done prior to the day of analysis, therefore reaching a total of five freeze/thaw cycles.

CSF Analysis

All samples were quantified within 1 month of storage at −80°C. CSF levels of Aβ42, total Tau, and pTau 181P were determined using commercially available single-analyte ELISA kits [INNOTEST® β-AMYLOID (1-42), INNOTEST® hTAU-Ag, and INNOTEST® PHOSPHO-TAU (181P), Fujirebio, Spain], according to the manufacturer's instructions and consensus practices from within BIOMARKAPD consortium. All samples were run in duplicate and all conditions tested for the same sample were run simultaneously on the same ELISA plate. Concentrations were extrapolated from a four-parameter Sigmoidal Curve. If the CV of duplicates was >20%, samples were excluded from the study to avoid additional confounding factors. If concentrations were below the limit of detection of the method, the value was set equal to the lowest standard of the calibration curve. None of the samples were above the concentration of the highest standard for each of the assays. Results were expressed in picogram per milliliter and as a relative percentage of the baseline conditions. All the participants in the study were asked to classify each sample as "normal" or "abnormal," according to their own cut-off levels for Aβ42, Tau, and pTau.

Statistical Analysis

The statistical analysis was accomplished with SPSS for Windows version 22.0 and Graph Pad Prism 6.0. The following variables were tested for each protein assay (Aβ42, Tau, and pTau): centrifugation temperatures – "2000 × *g*/4°C" vs. "2000 × *g*/RT"; centrifugation speeds – "RT/500" vs. "RT/2000" vs. "RT/3000 × *g*," and also "no spinning" vs. protocol (2000 × *g*/4°C); percentage of CSF per total tube volume – "25" vs. "50" vs. "75%"; for freeze/thaw cycles – "1" vs. "3 " vs. "5 cycles". *t*-test was used for pairwise comparisons. Repeated measures were first performed for multiple comparisons and also adding the following co-variates: "Center," "Clinical Group," "Biomarker classification" as normal or abnormal according to laboratory cut-offs, "CSF Total Protein," and "RBC count" either as scale or ordinal variable. *Post hoc* tests (Bonferroni's) were applied to repeated measures testing, when multiple comparisons were significant. Correlations between variables were performed using Pearson's correlation coefficient. As only five samples were used for studying the effect of blood spiking in CSF, non-parametric tests for pairwise comparisons were used as Friedman and Wilcoxon.

Results

Influence of Centrifugation Parameters

We first analyzed the results obtained from non-centrifuged aliquots comparing to those centrifuged under protocol conditions (2000 × *g* at 4°C for 10 min). We observed no significant difference between protein concentrations and found that the absence of centrifugation seemed not to affect the outcome. Next, we looked for variations within spinning temperatures, 4°C (routine protocol) and RT. No significant difference was observed for any of the three biomarkers. When testing centrifugation speeds (500, 2000, and 3000 × *g*), still no statistically significant change was seen in any of the biomarkers (**Table 2**).

Data were reanalyzed, testing the influence of the following co-variates: "Center," "Clinical Group," "CSF Total Protein," and "RBC count" (both scale and dichotomized in normal/abnormal), "Biomarker Classification" in normal or abnormal for each protein according to each laboratory cut-offs. "CSF Total protein (TP)," dichotomized as normal/abnormal, influenced the effect of centrifugation conditions on Aβ42 levels (**Figure 1A**; $p = 0.029$). Samples with high TP (>44 mg/dL) had increased levels of Aβ42 if centrifuged at RT (571.5 ± 261.8) compared to 4°C (549.4 ± 238.0), whereas samples with normal TP had higher Aβ42 levels when centrifuged at 4°C (527.2 ± 226.2, 4°C vs. 498.4 ± 237.2, RT). Moreover, in samples with high TP content, which were not centrifuged, Aβ42 levels tended to increase in relation to centrifugation under baseline conditions (**Figure 1B**; $p = 0.176$). Other covariates had no impact concerning centrifugation conditions for the three markers.

TABLE 2 | Concentration of each biomarker (picogram/milliliter) according to the three different pre-analytical confounders.

Confounders	Biomarkers (pg/mL)		
	Aβ42	Tau	Phospho-Tau
Centrifugation			
Non-centrifuged	548.6 ± 233.9 (*n* = 55)	315.2 ± 194.8 (*n* = 55)	47.0 ± 25.0 (*n* = 55)
4°C	537.9 ± 224.7 (*n* = 55)	321.4 ± 197.4 (*n* = 55)	46.8 ± 25.1 (*n* = 55)
RT	524.3 ± 241.0 (*n* = 55)	316.1 ± 191.0 (*n* = 55)	47.3 ± 25.6 (*n* = 55)
500 × *g*	556.3 ± 230.1 (*n* = 40)	330.4 ± 211.6 (*n* = 40)	49.4 ± 27.9 (*n* = 40)
2000 × *g*	558.6 ± 239.7 (*n* = 40)	330.6 ± 209.0 (*n* = 40)	49.0 ± 27.6 (*n* = 40)
3000 × *g*	554.7 ± 234.0 (*n* = 40)	335.1 ± 216.2 (*n* = 40)	48.3 ± 26.4 (*n* = 40)
% CSF/tube vol.			
25	651.9 ± 337.1 (*n* = 50)	320.0 ± 214.9 (*n* = 50)	48.0 ± 26.9 (*n* = 50)
50	636.7 ± 352.0 (*n* = 50)*	323.4 ± 232. 3 (*n* = 50)	47.6 ± 25.8 (*n* = 50)
75	657.6 ± 334.4 (*n* = 50)	323.8 ± 230.1 (*n* = 50)	48.1 ± 26.1 (*n* = 50)
Freeze–thaw cycles			
1 time	597.9 ± 237.0 (*n* = 40)	353.9 ± 243.4 (*n* = 40)	47.5 ± 30.1 (*n* = 40)
3 times	597.5 ± 243.2 (*n* = 40)	358.2 ± 245.2 (*n* = 40)	47.5 ± 30.3 (*n* = 40)
5 times	569.8 ± 220.4 (*n* = 40)^{‡,ϱ}	358.5 ± 247.1 (*n* = 40)	47.8 ± 30.5 (*n* = 40)

Results are expressed in mean ± SD (95% CI).
RT, room temperature; tube vol., tube volume.
*Aβ42 %CSF/Tube vol: *$p < 0.05$ vs. 75%; Aβ42 Freeze/Thaw cycles: $^{ϱ}p = 0.072$ vs. three times; $^{‡}p < 0.05$ vs. one time.*
Centrifugation: N = 55-Ctr = 7.3%; AD = 18.2; MCI = 7.3%; OD = 23.6%; OT = 41.8%; N = 40-AD = 15%; MCI = 7.5%; OD = 30%; OT = 45%; %CSF/Tube Vol.: Ctr = 2.0%; AD = 18%; MCI = 10%; OD = 26%; OT = 36%; freeze–thaw cycles: AD = 25%; MCI = 10%; OD = 20%; OT = 45%.

Regarding experiments with blood spiked CSF, as we have tested only a limited number of samples, results are only indicative and could be used to define a more precise protocol. We observed no significant difference between protein concentrations using variations in spinning temperatures, 4°C (routine protocol) and RT. No significant difference was observed for any of the three biomarkers. When testing centrifugation speeds (500, 2000, and 3000 × *g*), again no statistically significant change was seen in any of the biomarkers. However, when we compared data obtained after centrifugation (routine protocol) and no centrifugation, we found a statistical increase of mean levels of Aβ42 and pTau in no centrifuged spiked samples by 6 and 11% ($p < 0.05$), whereas Tau levels were not impacted by the absence of centrifugation (data not shown).

Influence of CSF Percentage Per Total Tube Volume

We hypothesized that the amount of CSF aliquoted in relation with total tube volume would have impact on protein concentration

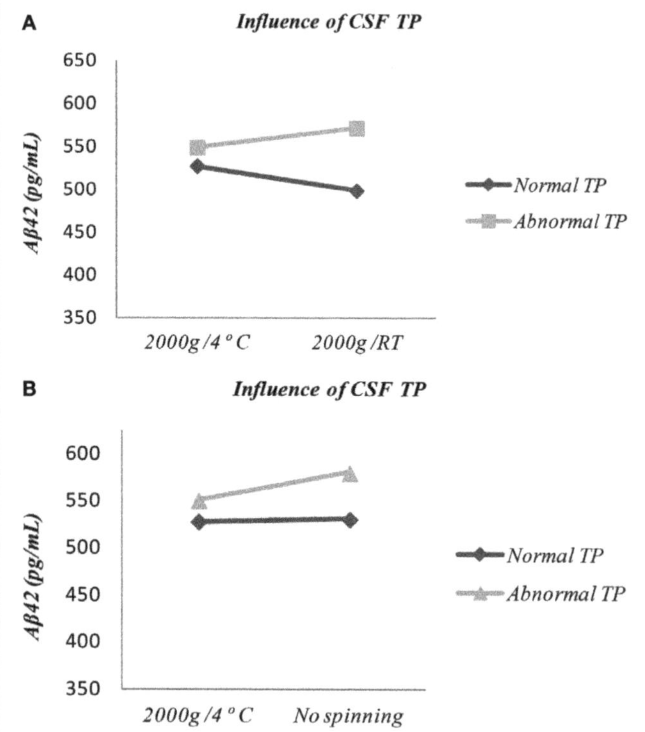

FIGURE 1 | (A) Significant influence of covariate "CSF Total protein content" (dichotomized in normal/abnormal facing reference values) in the comparison between Aβ42 levels after centrifugation at 4°C vs. room temperature ($p = 0.029$) (TP, total protein; RT, room temperature). **(B)** Discrete influence of covariate "CSF Total protein content" (dichotomized in normal/abnormal facing reference values) in the comparison between Aβ42 levels after centrifugation at 2000 × g/4°C vs. no spinning at all ($p = 0.176$). TP, total protein; Absolute values – no spinning: normal TP – 529.7 ± 234.2, abnormal TP – 579.2 ± 249.2); 4°C: normal TP – 498.4 ± 237.2, abnormal TP – 549.4 ± 238.0.

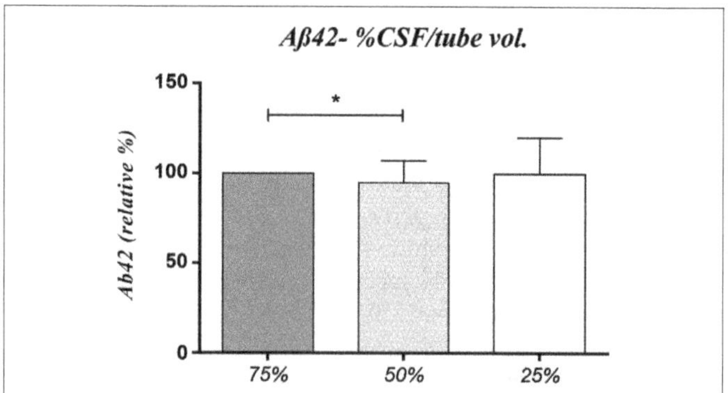

FIGURE 2 | Observed differences in Aβ42 levels between aliquots with 25 vs. 50 vs. 75% of total tube volume (75 vs. 50%, $p = 0.03$). Results expressed in relative percentage, facing the baseline condition (75% of tube volume representing 100%). Absolute concentration levels (mean ± SD): 25% – 651.9 ± 337.1; 50% – 636.7 ± 351.9; 75% – 657.6 ± 334.4.

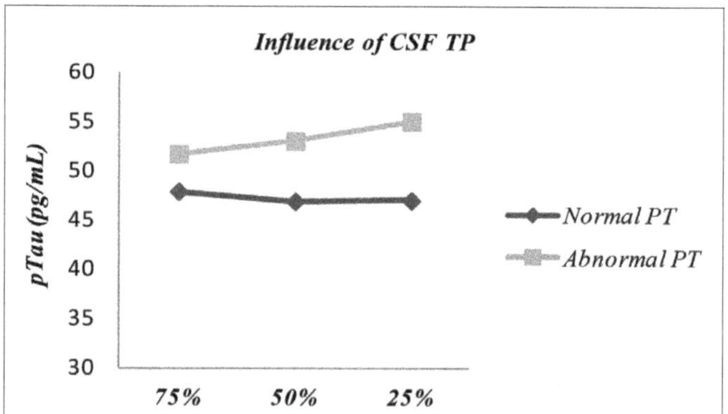

FIGURE 3 | Influence of covariate "CSF Total protein" (dichotomized in normal/abnormal facing reference values) in the comparison between pTau levels after aliquoting with different percentages of CSF per tube volume – 25 vs. 50 vs. 75% ($p = 0.027$). TP, total protein.

mainly because of the adhesive ability of Aβ42 and possibly Tau to tube walls, even though PP vials were always used throughout the study. Thus, different CSF volume percentages were tested in final aliquots and we found that decreasing the percentage of tube filling from 75% (baseline condition) to 50% resulted in a small but significant reduction of 3.7% in Aβ42 concentration ($p = 0.03$). This effect was indistinguishable from the analytical coefficient of variation of the assay. Moreover, when further decreasing the percentage of tube filling to 25%, Aβ42 levels increased to levels similar to the ones observed under baseline conditions (**Figure 2**). Neither Tau nor pTau proteins levels were influenced by the amount of CSF aliquoted in relation with total tube volume. Adding covariates to our tests showed influence of "CSF Total protein" (dichotomized as normal/abnormal) on pTau levels ($p = 0.027$), particularly in 25% filling volume aliquots presenting abnormal TP content (54.6 ± 30.5) vs. normal TP (47.1 ± 26.8) (**Figure 3**). Other covariates had no impact in any of the three biomarkers.

Influence of Number of Freeze–Thaw Cycles

In this section, we tried to simulate the frequent real-life need of defrosting a sample for other purposes, prior to biomarker measurements. Therefore, we compared the results of a regular procedure, where the sample is just thawed for biomarker assessment (one cycle), with other possible situations (thawed for two and four times prior to protein assay).

We observed that while Tau and pTau remain stable for up to the five freeze/thaw cycles, the same is not true for Aβ42. Although thawing the CSF sample three times did not change the measured Aβ42 levels, a statistical significant reduction of 5.0% in Aβ42 levels was observed when the number of freeze–thaw cycles was increased to 5 (**Figure 4**; $p = 0.028$). However, this decrease remained in the analytical coefficient of variation of the assay. Covariate inclusion had no impact, concerning the effect of the number of freeze/thaw cycles, for the three markers.

As the presence of increased total CSF proteins was the only covariate influencing the results, we studied the correlation between the levels of each biomarker and CSF protein content. We found significant correlations ($p < 0.05$, data not shown) between pTau levels and CSF TP in both non-centrifuged and centrifuged samples under protocol conditions (2000 × g, 4°C).

Discussion

There have been a few studies exploring potential CSF pre-analytical confounders, but a systematic analysis of some

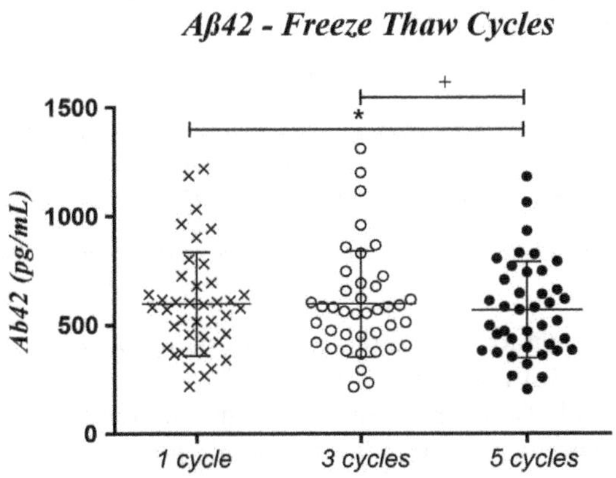

FIGURE 4 | Observed differences in Aβ42 levels between samples freeze/thawed three and five times prior to the moment of analysis (1 cycle) (1 vs. 5 cycles, $^{*}p = 0.028$; 3 vs. 5 cycles, $^{+}p = 0.072$). Absolute concentration levels (mean ± SD): one time – 597.9 ± 237.0; three times – 597.5 ± 243.2; five times – 569.7 ± 220.4.

conditions, such as centrifugation, storage volumes, and freeze/thawing cycles, is still missing. To the best of our knowledge, our study has so far the largest number of samples (over 40 samples for each condition) testing systematically these three potential major sources of variability. This study includes samples from different cohorts of patients with several clinical diagnosis, validating our results for a broad range of biomarkers quantitative values. Furthermore, the influence of multiple co-variates was evaluated, and all other variables related to CSF collection were strictly controlled (19, 26). In this study, all LPs were performed in the morning, as although no clear diurnal pattern in Aβ42 levels has been observed, a 1.5- to 4-fold variation in AD biomarkers during a 36 h period has been reported (20). Moreover, fasting, as well as possible adsorption to lumbar catheter walls during LP, was also suspected to influence Aβ42 levels, but so far such effects could not be demonstrated (27). Current guidelines regarding collection and storage tubes (14) were also strictly followed and CSF was processed and frozen within a maximum of 2 h after collection. According to some reports, Aβ42 content is altered if CSF is not immediately frozen (to avoid protein oxidation), while Tau proteins are stable and can be kept at room temperature up to 24 h (25) or even 4 days (13). The use of different types of tube materials (polycarbonate, polystyrene, PP, and other copolymers) has also been tested. In several studies comparing PP against others plastics, authors never tested the variability among the different PP tubes, therefore remaining a potential confounder (22, 27). A few studies compared several PP tubes and concluded that PP is not a warranty against adsorption and only specific tubes reported to avoid adsorption could be recommended (21, 28, 29). A very recent study has shown that even using only PP tubes, Aβ42 levels are reduced up to 25% simply through multiple tube transferences which, therefore, should be minimized (28).

Speed and temperature of CSF centrifugation vary considerably between laboratories. Therefore, in this study, we tested both the influence of spinning temperature (RT and 4°C) and speed (500, 2000, and 3000 × *g*) on biomarkers levels. Overall, neither of these conditions were found to influence the concentration of any of the biomarkers. A previous study has looked for the influence of CSF centrifugation protocols on Aβ42 levels (27) and observed a significant decrease in Aβ42 concentration in centrifuged samples (10 min, 2000 × *g*, either at RT or 4°C) compared to non-centrifuged samples. It has also been found that no difference occurred in Aβ42 and Tau levels in CSF samples stored at 4°C and centrifuged after 1, 4, 48, or 72 h (30). Furthermore, no differences were found comparing centrifuged samples immediately frozen and those left for 4 days at 4°C without spinning (30). Centrifugation speed has been reported not to have an effect on biomarkers levels, but the centrifugation of hemorrhagic samples at 2000 × *g*, RT, within 2 h after collection, in order to avoid cell lysis, is recommended (26).

The inclusion of covariates in our analysis showed that, in samples with a high total protein content, an increase in Aβ42 concentration upon centrifugation at RT occurs. It can be hypothesized that Aβ42 can bind to excess protein, thus preventing the adhesion to tube walls, and this interaction may be disrupted by freeze/thawing. In contrast, in samples with normal or low TP content, centrifugation at RT may promote the adhesion of Aβ42 to tube walls, leading to lower measured levels of the peptide. As the largest discrepancy in Aβ42 levels between samples with normal/abnormal TP is seen when centrifugation is done at RT, spinning at 4°C should be applied routinely. In line with a previous study, we also observed that no spinning increases the measured levels of Aβ42 in samples with a high CSF total protein content (27). We cannot neglect another hypothesis, consistent with a competition between proteins present in high amounts to adsorb onto the walls of tubes decreasing, therefore, the possibility of less concentrated proteins, as amyloids, to stick to the plastic. This characteristic is commonly used in ELISA test by saturating the plastic wells with albumin, gelatin, or milk proteins after coating the capture antibody. Currently, when 1 h at 37°C is enough to saturate non-specific residual sites, it takes overnight at 4°C, what is absolutely consistent with the recommendation we did, to spin at low temperature.

Despite the generalized use of atraumatic needles, the influence of blood contamination is still relevant, and controversial results have been reported. Bjerke et al. observed that up to 5000 RBC/μL of CSF had no effect on Aβ42 levels (27). However, Zimmermann et al. showed that approximately 1 g/L of CSF protein levels (that can happen after traumatic tap or in patients with disrupted blood brain barrier) could have an impact on AD biomarkers (13). In our study, the inclusion of RBC count as a co-variate had no effect on biomarkers levels. However, the majority of our samples had low or just above threshold RBC counts, thus the influence of CSF contamination with RBC could not be ruled out. Spiking blood in CSF was tested for few samples, the final concentration of RBC being 5000/μL of CSF. Even if, they need to be confirmed, as the increase of levels was found under or close to the analytical CV of duplicates of 10%, our preliminary data are consistent with current guidelines in which it is recommended to centrifuge samples to avoid blood contamination. Further studies should be made with spiked CSF to clarify the influence of high RBC content on biomarkers quantification, using at least different amounts of spike, for example, in a range of RBC 5000–10,000/μL.

Aliquot storage volume is another potential pre-analytical confounder that has not been often assessed. We addressed this potential source of variation by storing three different ratios (25, 50, and 75%) of CSF volume per total tube capacity. The tube filling volume did not influence CSF levels of Tau and pTau. Concerning Aβ42 levels, they decreased when CSF storage volume decreased from 75 to 50% and amazingly, they slightly increased in 25% filled tubes, as compared to 50% filling. The variations were found lower than the accepted analytical intra-assay range-to-average of duplicates (<20%), so in our study using aliquots in tubes of 500 μL, the filling tube is not a strong confounder. It can be hypothesized that decreasing the ratio of CSF volume to surface area of storage tube would lead to an increased analyte adsorption to the internal walls of the tube, lowering its levels in solution. Our results are in accordance with a recent study testing the influence of a wide range of CSF volumes (2.5–75% of CSF per total tube volume) in Aβ42, Tau, and pTau measurements (31). While Tau and pTau remained stable with the increase in storage volume percentage, they found that a volume increase of 10 μL caused an Aβ42 increase of 1 pg/mL, which is absolutely consistent with the increase of 3.7% between 250 and 380 μL (13 pg/mL) that we have found. In the studies by Toombs and colleagues (28, 31), the addition of 0.05% Tween 20 to the aliquots resulted in considerably higher concentrations of Aβ42, suggesting that in the presence of detergent a higher proportion of Aβ42 molecules were free in solution, thus supporting the hypothesis of protein adsorption to the tube walls, as previously reported (27). This is consistent with the fact that Tween 20 is used as a blocking agent in ELISA plates, avoiding further adsorption of proteins.

The influence of freeze/thaw cycles (one, three, and five) during CSF storage, before protein measurements, was also investigated. We observed that Tau and pTau levels were not altered, but Aβ42 levels decreased slightly (5%) with repeated freeze/thawing, especially above three cycles, but as reported for filling tube study, this decrease was under the accepted analytical intra-assay range-to-average of duplicates (<20%); so, in our study, using three freeze/thaw cycles has no strong effect onto the CSF levels of biomarkers. Our data are consistent with those of Zimmerman et al. (13) reporting the stability for up to three freeze/thaw cycles for the three biomarkers and partially with those of Simonsen et al. (24) reporting stable levels for Aβ42 but increased levels for pTau without inhibitors of protease. Our data are mainly different with those obtained in the study of Schoonenboom et al. (30), in which they showed that after three freeze–thaw cycles (for 2 h) Aβ42 levels decreased by 20%, mainly after the first cycle whereas Tau protein was not altered by six freeze–thaw cycles. In this last study, the exact reference of PP tubes used for the study was not done, whereas in study of Simonsen et al., the tubes were exactly the same that those we selected as tubes known to present a minimal adsorption of amyloid. So, the difference between data concluding absence of strong effect onto amyloid levels and those showing large decrease of amyloid levels could be explained by a larger synergistic effect of adsorption and freeze/thaw process in studies in which the reference of tubes was not given and the adsorption of amyloid onto tubes was not checked (30). Therefore, most of the data obtained before the standardization of tubes must be interpreted with caution.

TABLE 3 | Recommendations for CSF pre-analytical handling prior to evaluation of AD biomarkers.

Confounder	Recommendation
Spinning	Right after collection (within 2 h max); at 2000 × *g* 4°C – avoid multiple tube transfers
Storage volume	Tubes should be filled up close to total tube capacity to keep constant the relation surface area/tube walls
Freeze–thaw cycles	Avoid more than three cycles to prevent protein degradation

It should also be emphasized that, in our study, all measurements were carried out within 1 month storage and it cannot be ruled out that in samples kept for longer storage periods, different results could be obtained. We wanted to know to what extent the analysis of each condition would change after 1 and 2 years of storage. This was not performed after all, since it would surpass the length of the project. However, we would be reasonably comfortable to perform this analysis since there have been a few studies addressing the long-term stability of CSF biomarkers, concluding that Aβ42 and Tau proteins remain stable up to 6 years (if stored at −80°C immediately after collection and processing) (23), supporting the feasibility of biobanking over a large period of time. Thus, having this factor controlled, it would be possible to test variations within pre-analytical conditions.

In recent years, a strong effort has been done to develop and implement USOPs for CSF analysis, and this is also a major goal of the JPND-BIOMARKAPD Consortium. However, overall variability remains too high to allow assignment of universal biomarker cut-off values and is still compromising AD-like scores across laboratories (32–34). Taking this into account, our findings reinforce the existing guidelines and support new recommendations for CSF pre-analytical SOPs (**Table 3**).

We propose that centrifugation should be performed as fast as possible after CSF collection, at 4°C, the speed conditions being not a major factor (500, 2000, or 3000 × *g*); multiple tube transfer of CSF should be avoided and kept to a minimum. Storage aliquots should be filled up close to the maximum tube capacity in order to keep a constant surface area and avoid sublimation. It is preferable that samples should not be submitted to more than three freeze–thaw cycles to prevent protein degradation.

We strongly believe that this work will contribute to the establishment of core and broadly used feasible guidelines that will enable decisive AD large scale studies.

Acknowledgments

This study was done under the scope of an EU Joint Programme–Neurodegenerative Disease Research (JPND)–BIOMARKAPD project. The project is supported through the following funding organizations under the aegis of JPND – www.jpnd.eu: The Portuguese Science Foundation (FCT-JPND/0005/2011 project), Portugal; Innovation Fund Denmark grant number: 0603-00470B; Academy of Finland, Research Council for Health, decision n 263193; ANR grant number: 12-JPND-001-16. The authors also thank the patients and their families for informed consent.

References

1. Blennow K. Cerebrospinal fluid protein biomarkers for Alzheimer's disease. *NeuroRx* (2004) **1**:213–25. doi:10.1602/neurorx.1.2.213
2. Rosén C, Hansson O, Blennow K, Zetterberg H. Fluid biomarkers in Alzheimer's disease – current concepts. *Mol Neurodegener* (2013) **8**:20. doi:10.1186/1750-1326-8-20
3. Buchhave P, Blennow K, Zetterberg H, Stomrud E, Londos E, Andreasen N, et al. Longitudinal study of CSF biomarkers in patients with Alzheimer's disease. *PLoS One* (2009) **25**(4):583–94. doi:10.1371/journal.pone.0006294
4. Baldeiras I, Santana I, Santiago B, Correia H, Ribeiro MH, Lemos R, et al. Cerebrospinal fluid biomarkers in frontotemporal lobar degeneration. *J Neurol* (2011) **258**:S183–4.
5. Baldeiras I, Santana I, Ribeiro MH, Pascoal R, Lemos R, Santiago B, et al. Utility of cerebrospinal fluid markers in mild cognitive impairment. *Neurodegener Dis* (2011) **8**(S1–11):486.
6. Herukka S-K, Hallikainen M, Soininen H, Pirttilä T. CSF Abeta42 and tau or phosphorylated tau and prediction of progressive mild cognitive impairment. *Neurology* (2005) **64**(7):1294–7. doi:10.1212/01.WNL.0000156914.16988.56
7. Shaw LM, Soares H, Dean RA, Lilly E. Quantification of the analytical and clinical performance of CSF biomarker analyses in ADNI. *Acta Neuropathol* (2011) **121**(5):597–609. doi:10.1007/s00401-011-0808-0
8. Hort J, Bartos A, Pirttilä T, Scheltens P. Use of cerebrospinal fluid biomarkers in diagnosis of dementia across Europe. *Eur J Neurol* (2010) **17**(1):90–6. doi:10.1111/j.1468-1331.2009.02753.x
9. Hölttä M, Hansson O, Andreasson U, Hertze J, Minthon L, Nägga K, et al. Evaluating amyloid-β oligomers in cerebrospinal fluid as a biomarker for Alzheimer's disease. *PLoS One* (2013) **8**(6):e66381. doi:10.1371/journal.pone.0066381
10. Anoop A, Singh PK, Jacob RS, Maji SK. CSF biomarkers for Alzheimer's disease diagnosis. *Int J Alzheimers Dis* (2010) **2010**:606802. doi:10.4061/2010/606802
11. Blennow K, Zetterberg H, Minthon L, Lannfelt L, Strid S, Annas P, et al. Longitudinal stability of CSF biomarkers in Alzheimer's disease. *Neurosci Lett* (2007) **419**(1):18–22. doi:10.1016/j.neulet.2007.03.064
12. Höglund K, Bogstedt A, Fabre S, Aziz A, Annas P, Basun H, et al. Longitudinal stability evaluation of biomarkers and their correlation in cerebrospinal fluid and plasma from patients with Alzheimer's disease. *J Alzheimers Dis* (2012) **32**(4):939–47. doi:10.3233/JAD-2012-120976
13. Zimmermann R, Lelental N, Ganslandt O, Maler JM, Kornhuber J, Lewczuk P. Preanalytical sample handling and sample stability testing for the neurochemical dementia diagnostics. *J Alzheimers Dis* (2011) **25**(4):739–45. doi:10.3233/JAD-2011-110212
14. Teunissen CE, Verwey NA, Kester MI, van Uffelen K, Blankenstein MA. Standardization of assay procedures for analysis of the CSF biomarkers amyloid β((1-42)), tau, and phosphorylated tau in Alzheimer's disease: report of an international workshop. *Int J Alzheimers Dis* (2010) **2010**:635053. doi:10.4061/2010/635053
15. Lewczuk P, Beck G, Ganslandt O, Esselmann H, Deisenhammer F, Regeniter A, et al. International quality control survey of neurochemical dementia diagnostics. *Neurosci Lett* (2006) **409**(1):1–4. doi:10.1016/j.neulet.2006.07.009
16. Lewczuk P, Wiltfang J. Neurochemical dementia diagnostics: state of the art and research perspectives. *Proteomics* (2008) **8**(6):1292–301. doi:10.1002/pmic.200700703
17. Mattsson N. *CSF Biomarker Variability in the Alzheimer's Association Quality Control Program* (2013). Available from: http://www.alzheimersanddementia.com/article/S1552-5260(13)00042-3/pdf
18. Mattsson N, Andreasson U, Persson S, Arai H, Batish SD, Bernardini S, et al. The Alzheimer's association external quality control program for cerebrospinal fluid biomarkers. *Alzheimers Dement* (2011) **7**(4):386.e–95.e. doi:10.1016/j.jalz.2011.05.2243
19. Vanderstichele H, Bibl M, Engelborghs S, Le Bastard N, Lewczuk P, Molinuevo JL, et al. Standardization of preanalytical aspects of cerebrospinal fluid biomarker testing for Alzheimer's disease diagnosis: a consensus paper from the Alzheimer's biomarkers standardization initiative. *Alzheimers Dement* (2012) **8**(1):65–73. doi:10.1016/j.jalz.2011.07.004
20. Bateman RJ, Wen G, Morris JC, Holtzman DM. Fluctuations of CSF amyloid-beta levels: implications for a diagnostic and therapeutic biomarker. *Neurology* (2007) **68**:666–9. doi:10.1212/01.wnl.0000256043.50901.e3
21. Perret-Liaudet A, Pelpel M, Tholance Y, Dumont B, Vanderstichele H, Zorzi W, et al. Risk of Alzheimer's disease biological misdiagnosis linked to cerebrospinal collection tubes. *J Alzheimers Dis* (2012) **31**:13–20. doi:10.3233/JAD-2012-120361
22. Lewczuk P, Beck G, Esselmann H, Bruckmoser R, Zimmermann R, Fiszer M, et al. Effect of sample collection tubes on cerebrospinal fluid concentrations of tau proteins and amyloid beta peptides. *Clin Chem* (2006) **52**(2):332–4. doi:10.1373/clinchem.2005.058776
23. Schipke CG, Jessen F, Teipel S, Luckhaus C, Wiltfang J, Esselmann H, et al. Long-term stability of Alzheimer's disease biomarker proteins in cerebrospinal fluid. *J Alzheimers Dis* (2011) **26**:255–62. doi:10.3233/JAD-2011-110329
24. Simonsen AH, Bahl JMC, Danborg PB, Lindstrom V, Larsen SO, Grubb A, et al. Pre-analytical factors influencing the stability of cerebrospinal fluid proteins. *J Neurosci Methods* (2013) **215**:234–40. doi:10.1016/j.jneumeth.2013.03.011
25. Kaiser E, Schönknecht P, Thomann PA, Hunt A, Schröder J. Influence of delayed CSF storage on concentrations of phospho-tau protein (181), total tau protein and beta-amyloid (1-42). *Neurosci Lett* (2007) **417**(2):193–5. doi:10.1016/j.neulet.2007.02.045
26. Del Campo M, Mollenhauer B, Bertolotto A, Engelborghs S, Hampel H, Simonsen AH, et al. Recommendations to standardize preanalytical confounding factors in Alzheimer's and Parkinson's disease cerebrospinal fluid biomarkers: an update. *Biomark Med* (2012) **6**:419–30. doi:10.2217/bmm.12.46
27. Bjerke M, Portelius E, Minthon L, Wallin A, Anckarsäter H, Anckarsäter R, et al. Confounding factors influencing amyloid beta concentration in cerebrospinal fluid. *Int J Alzheimers Dis* (2010) **2010**:986310. doi:10.4061/2010/986310
28. Toombs J, Paterson RW, Schott JM, Zetterberg H. Amyloid-beta 42 adsorption following serial tube transfer. *Alzheimers Res Ther* (2014) **6**:5. doi:10.1186/alzrt236
29. Pica-Mendez AM, Tanen M, Dallob A, Tanaka W, Laterza OF. Nonspecific binding of Aβ42 to polypropylene tubes and the effect of tween-20. *Clin Chim Acta* (2010) **411**(21–22):1833. doi:10.1016/j.cca.2010.07.019
30. Schoonenboom NSM, Mulder C, Vanderstichele H, Van Elk E-J, Kok A, Van Kamp GJ, et al. Effects of processing and storage conditions on amyloid beta (1-42) and tau concentrations in cerebrospinal fluid: implications for use in clinical practice. *Clin Chem* (2005) **51**(1):189–95. doi:10.1373/clinchem.2004.039735
31. Toombs J, Paterson RW, Lunn MP, Nicholas JM, Fox NC, Chapman MD, et al. Identification of an important potential confound in CSF AD studies: aliquot volume. *Clin Chem Lab Med* (2013) **51**:2311–7. doi:10.1515/cclm-2013-0293
32. Mattsson N, Blennow K, Zetterberg H. *Inter-Laboratory Variation in Cerebrospinal Fluid Biomarkers for Alzheimer's Disease: United We Stand, Divided We Fall.* Clinical Chemistry and Laboratory Medicine (2010). p. 603–7.
33. Vos SJB, Visser PJ, Verhey F, Aalten P, Knol D, Ramakers I, et al. Variability of CSF Alzheimer's disease biomarkers: implications for clinical practice. *PLoS One* (2014) **9**(6):e100784. doi:10.1371/journal.pone.0100784
34. Teunissen CE, Tumani H, Engelborghs S, Mollenhauer B. Biobanking of CSF: international standardization to optimize biomarker development. *Clin Biochem* (2014) **47**(4–5):288–92. doi:10.1016/j.clinbiochem.2013.12.024

11

Preanalytical confounding factors in the analysis of cerebrospinal fluid biomarkers for Alzheimer's disease: the issue of diurnal variation

Claudia Cicognola, Davide Chiasserini and Lucilla Parnetti *

Section of Neurology, Department of Medicine, Centre for Memory Disturbances, University of Perugia, Perugia, Italy

Edited by:
Sylvain Lehmann,
Montpellier University Hospital, France

Reviewed by:
Zhihui Yang,
University of Florida, USA
Jurgen Claassen,
Radboud University Medical Center, Netherlands

***Correspondence:**
Lucilla Parnetti,
Centro Disturbi della Memoria, Clinica Neurologica, Ospedale S. Maria della Misericordia, S. Andrea delle Fratte, Perugia 06132, Italy
lucilla.parnetti@unipg.it

Given the growing use of cerebrospinal fluid (CSF) beta-amyloid (Aβ) and tau as biomarkers for early diagnosis of Alzheimer's disease (AD), it is essential that the diagnostic procedures are standardized and the results comparable across different laboratories. Preanalytical factors are reported to be the cause of at least 50% of the total variability. Among them, diurnal variability is a key issue and may have an impact on the comparability of the values obtained. The available studies on this issue are not conclusive so far. Fluctuations of CSF biomarkers in young healthy volunteers have been previously reported, while subsequent studies have not confirmed those observations in older subjects, the ones most likely to receive this test. The observed differences in circadian rhythms need to be further assessed not only in classical CSF biomarkers but also in novel forthcoming biomarkers. In this review, the existing data on the issue of diurnal variations of CSF classical biomarkers for AD will be analyzed, also evaluating the available data on new possible biomarkers.

Keywords: cerebrospinal fluid, biomarkers, diurnal variability, circadian rhythm, confounding factors, Alzheimer's disease

Relevance of CSF Biomarkers in Clinical Practice

In the past few years, the diagnostic criteria for Alzheimer's disease (AD) have gone through several rearrangements. According to the International Working Group (IWG) for New Research Criteria for the Diagnosis of Alzheimer's Disease, both cerebrospinal fluid (CSF) and imaging biomarkers have been recognized as mandatory for detection of AD predementia phases. The same priority has been considered in the National Institute on Aging–Alzheimer's Association (NIA–AA) criteria (1, 2). IWG criteria subdivide clinically manifest AD in *prodromal AD* and *AD dementia*, based on whether episodic memory loss or other cognitive symptoms prevent the subject from accomplishing the instrumental activities of daily living (IADL) or not. If any AD biomarker (CSF or imaging) is abnormal, this is sufficient to fulfill the biomarker criterion for AD. The NIA-AA criteria make a distinction between amyloid markers and neuronal injury markers (tau): the likelihood of preclinical stage and MCI diagnosis is dependent on how many of the markers are positive, where amyloid is the earliest to become positive. The IWG and NIA-AA criteria share the concept of a preclinical stage of the disease, which can be recognized before dementia onset, and highlight the need of AD biomarkers both for diagnosing the disease in early stages and for supporting the diagnosis in clinically overt pathology (**Table 1**).

TABLE 1 | Differences between IWG and NIA-AA criteria for AD.

Stages		Cognitive criteria		Biomarker criteria	
IWG	**NIA-AA**	**IWG**	**NIA-AA**	**IWG**	**NIA-AA**
Prodromal AD	MCI due to AD	Memory impairment	MCI	Any amyloid or injury marker	Likelihood: • High: amyloid and injury marker both + • Intermediate: one marker +, unknown the other • Uninformative: one marker +, - the other
AD dementia	Dementia due to AD	Memory impairment	Dementia	Any amyloid or injury marker	

The diagnostic value of biomarkers has been even more strengthened in the IWG-2 criteria (3). In these criteria, a simplified diagnostic algorithm based on CSF molecular AD phenotype or amyloid imaging was proposed. The algorithm consisted of decreased Aβ levels together with increased t-tau or p-tau concentrations, or an increased retention on amyloid PET tracer. CSF pathophysiological markers for AD include the beta-amyloid peptide 1–42 (Aβ42), which shows lower CSF levels the more the brain carries amyloid burden, total tau (t-tau), which directly reflects the intensity of neuronal degeneration, and phosphorylated tau (p-tau), which is believed to be a direct marker of tangle pathology (4). In an autopsy cohort, low CSF Aβ42 concentrations had a sensitivity of 96.4% for AD detection (5) and CSF markers significantly increased the diagnostic accuracy in clinically uncertain cases (6). However, low CSF levels of Aβ42 are not specific enough to diagnose AD, since they can also be found in non-AD dementias (Lewy body disease or vascular dementia) (7). A valuable tool for increasing the diagnostic performance of Aβ42 is the Aβ42/40 ratio, which proved to be more reliable than Aβ42 alone in providing comprehensive information on the total Aβ load in the brain. A marked reduction in CSF Aβ42 and in the Aβ42/Aβ40 ratio has consistently been found in patients at different stages of AD (4, 8, 9), and it can help in differentiating AD from non-AD forms, where the combination of the three classical biomarkers is of limited diagnostic value (10).

Several studies have shown that the combination of CSF biomarkers may improve their global diagnostic accuracy (11–15). Data so far indicate that the combination of Aβ42 with either t-tau or p-tau has the best specificity. Additionally, the combined analysis of the CSF biomarkers provides a more accurate differential diagnosis between AD and other degenerative dementias. Aβ42 and tau (t-tau or p-tau) should be used in combination, and the simultaneous presence of low Aβ42 and high t-tau or p-tau concentrations strongly suggests an AD diagnosis even at a prodromal stage, with a sensitivity of 90–95% and a specificity of about 90% (16–20).

The importance to have reliable CSF biomarkers relies in the need to validate the clinical diagnosis with a biological correlate. Unfortunately, the results obtained in research studies are not yet totally supported by significant outcomes in routine clinical use of CSF biomarkers. Additional testing, including CSF analysis, has still little diagnostic impact in the diagnostic work-up on patients suspected to suffer AD-dementia, being rather more useful in patients with an initial non-AD dementia diagnosis (21). Reliable biomarkers are needed not only to confirm a clinical suspect but also to allow an early diagnosis, which is vital in order to prevent severe clinical manifestations by starting, as soon as possible, the disease-modifying therapies that are being developed and will be hopefully available in a near future. To this purpose, the new algorithm proposed by Lewczuk et al. (22) for diagnosing preclinical patients has further validated the diagnostic value of CSF biomarkers. The algorithm introduced the concept of "border zones" by taking into account not only the mere alteration of the biomarkers but also the extent of the alteration, from slight to clearly pathologic. This may allow the subdivision of subjects into different groups according to the CSF pattern: no evidence for CNS disease, AD improbable, AD possible, and AD probable. The results obtained with this classification may allow a better coding of the CSF patterns not clearly pathologic when classified using IWG and NIA-AA criteria. This means that the CSF profile is a valuable diagnostic tool, even in the absence of clinical symptoms.

The Issue of Standardization of CSF AD Biomarkers for Routine Clinical Use

Even if the strong correlation between positive CSF AD biomarkers and AD pathology has been widely demonstrated, defining which patients are candidates to undergo lumbar puncture and AD CSF biomarkers analysis is a critical step for several reasons. Most of the AD patients are diagnosed using only clinical criteria, but a high number of patients do not ultimately have underlying AD pathology. The proportion of misdiagnosed patients is even higher in cases of early onset AD, atypical presentations, or dementia with mixed etiologies. It is also necessary to optimize the diagnosis of non-amnestic presentations and differentiate AD pathology from other neurodegenerative disorders, i.e., dementia with Lewy bodies, fronto-temporal dementia, vascular dementia, psychiatric conditions etc. The last consensus (2014) from the Alzheimer's Biomarkers Standardization Initiative (ABSI) (23) focused on the issues regarding clinical use of CSF biomarkers, and stated that patients in whom AD is part of the differential diagnosis may be candidates for lumbar puncture and CSF biomarkers analysis to increase specificity and minimize diagnostic errors. Given also the importance of early diagnosis, any patient with minimal but objective symptoms suggestive of AD is an appropriate candidate. CSF biomarkers analysis should be considered in all patients with early onset dementia, minimal or mild cognitive impairment, and atypical clinical presentation or complex differential diagnosis.

With these premises, it is clear that there is a major need for standardization in the CSF analysis procedures. Standardized protocols for biobanking are a prerequisite to guarantee that biomarker studies will not be influenced by preanalytical and analytical factors. One of the most important implications of biomarker standardization is to find univocal cut-off values for CSF biomarkers between and within laboratories, given that, even when using the same assay, significant variability has been found in the absolute concentrations of AD biomarkers (24). In 2009, the Alzheimer's Association started an international quality control (QC) program for CSF biomarkers (25). The aim of the program is to monitor, in a large network of laboratories all around the world, total analytical variability of CSF Aβ and tau, in order to identify the sources of variation and improve the standardization of the assays. All sources of variability (within-assay run, within/between-laboratory, within/between-assay kit lot) were considered, along with the variability coming from bias, systematic deviation from a reference value, imprecision and random deviation from a value. The overall variability was generally around 20–30%, with a small contribution of within-run variability (5%–10%). Within-laboratory longitudinal variability was higher, with a coefficient of variation (CV) of 5–19%. The main cause of the overall variability in the analysis of variance was the between-laboratory variability (19–28%). Even when the laboratory protocols and checklists were strictly followed, not a single factor was identified as the main source of variability. This led to the conclusion that laboratories can only be more accurate in following published guidelines (26). Moreover, it is critically important that kit manufacturers minimize lot-to-lot variations, to allow a broader use of these assays in the clinical setting. For now, the overall variability is still too high to allow the definition of univocal biomarker cut-off values; therefore, each laboratory should have internally qualified cut-off levels to guarantee optimal reproducibility over time.

Preanalytical Confounding Factors of CSF Biomarkers

Preanalytical factors are one of the main concerns in biochemical analysis, since they are responsible for about 40–60% of total laboratory variability (27). In previous meetings of the aforementioned ABSI, the preanalytical issues affecting Aβ and tau in CSF were discussed, and they came up with guidelines for CSF collection, storage, and analysis. Some aspects were identified as key issues for samples collection and analysis, for example, a possible CSF concentration gradient of the biomarkers. Brain-derived proteins often show a decreasing rostro-caudal gradient, implying that the volume of CSF withdrawn can alter the concentration of the proteins analyzed. Studies showed that AD CSF biomarkers concentrations are not significantly influenced by fractionated sampling, therefore gradient effect does not represent an issue in this circumstance (28). Other biomarkers can be affected, such as α-synuclein (29); therefore, a standardized volume of CSF collection (12 ml) is recommended (30). CSF for diagnostic purposes is usually obtained by lumbar puncture between the L3/L4 and L4/L5 intervertebral space, and a 22G atraumatic needle should be preferred to lower the risk of post-lumbar puncture headache (30). Moreover, a traumatic lumbar puncture increases the risk of blood contamination of the CSF sample; therefore, it is recommended to discard the first 1–2 ml to avoid any effect due to hemolysis and immediately centrifuge the sample before freezing (31). Some CSF analytes (for example, glucose) can be affected by meal consumption, making fasting a prerequisite for sampling, but this can be a problematic request in elderly patients with an AD suspect. Aβ levels in plasma proved to be stable and not influenced by the patient's food intake (32); therefore, there is no clear evidence that meal consumption affects CSF biomarker levels and so fasting is not a requirement for the analysis. Other preanalytical confounding factors concern laboratory procedures regarding collection and storage of the samples. Aβ peptides can bind non-specifically to non-polypropylene (PP) collection tubes, leading to lower values in measured concentrations. Therefore, PP tubes are the recommended standard for CSF samples collection and testing in routine clinical practice; each laboratory should always use the same PP tube, since different tubes may have a different adsorption level for the analytes (28). Vanderstichele et al. also recommended to aliquot the samples in small volumes (0.25 or 0.5 ml tube) and fill the tube up to 75%, to minimize the risk of adsorption and evaporation (28). However, a recent study by Willemse et al. showed no evaporation of CSF stored in biobanking tubes at –80°C or –20°C over a time span of 2 years (33). As mentioned, centrifugation of CSF samples is often performed, especially in the case of hemorrhagic lumbar punctures. However, the guidelines of Vanderstichele et al. pointed out no differences in classic biomarkers levels between centrifuged versus non-centrifuged samples (29). Nevertheless, the speed and temperature of centrifugation may be considerably different across laboratories; therefore, the consensus paper by Teunissen et al. recommended to centrifuge the hemorrhagic samples at a speed of 2000 $\times g$ for 10 min at room temperature (26). Time and temperature of storage may have a remarkable influence on the biomarkers levels, given their effects on serum and plasma proteins showed in proteomics studies (34). Vanderstichele et al. reported no significant effects on Aβ42, t-tau, and p-tau levels when the samples are left at room temperature for 5 days after CSF collection with respect to samples frozen immediately after collection (28). The recommendation is to keep the samples at 4°C for no longer than 5 days to avoid alterations of the final biochemical results (28). Different methods of freezing and storage do not cause significant variability in the results (32), but the freezing temperature of –80°C should be preferred for long-term storage (28). Few studies have been published regarding the stability of Aβ42, t-tau, and p-tau in CSF when stored frozen at –20°C or –80°C for many years, but this is an important issue in view of longitudinal studies. Vanderstichele et al. did not observe changes in stability for up to 10 years at –80°C, but the recommendation is not to go beyond 2 months of storage at –20°C, as this is considered a sufficiently long time to run the analysis (28). The number of freeze/thaw cycles is a matter of concern since it can affect CSF biomarkers and lead to significant losses in Aβ concentrations (35). Recent studies, however, showed no significant alteration in the level of Aβ42 when CSF underwent more than one freeze/thaw cycle (32). However, freeze/thaw cycles should not be more than two and CSF must be aliquoted in small volumes; every change in the number of the freeze/thaw cycles must be accurately documented (28). The recommendations for CSF collection and storage are summarized in **Table 2**.

Circadian Rhythm

Among all the preanalytical confounding factors mentioned before, diurnal variation may play an important role as a source of variability. Circadian rhythm is involved in several physiologic processes, so it is reasonable to hypothesize its influence even in CSF biomarkers metabolism. Diurnal variation physiology must be analyzed more deeply, beginning from a review on the

TABLE 2 | Summary of recommendations for preanalytical aspects of AD biomarker testing in CSF.

Possible variability factor	Recommendation
CSF gradient	No gradient observed
Lumbar puncture	L3–L4 or L4–L5 22G atraumatic needle to reduce the risk of blood contamination
Fasting	Not required
Tubes	PP (polypropylene)
Aliquotation	Aliquot the samples in small volumes (0.25 or 0.5 ml tube) Fill the tube up to 75%
Centrifugation	2000 × *g* for 10 min at room temperature
Time before storage	Up to 5 days
Temperature before storage	4°C
Freezing	−80°C −20°C for no longer than 2 months
Freeze/thaw cycles	No more than 1–2

anatomy of this "inner clock" that controls a large number of bodily functions.

Physiological Aspects

The suprachiasmatic nucleus (SCN) has a central role in the circadian rhythm system, together with its three primary afferent connections (36); the most important is the retino-hypothalamic projection through which information coming from rod/cone photoreceptors and retinal ganglion cells reaches the "inner clock." The other two afferent connections consist of the median raphe serotonergic pathway and the geniculohypothalamic (GHT) pathway from the thalamic intergeniculate leaflet (IGL). Though this network might seem elementary, the several interconnections between the pathways make it complex and convoluted. When SCN is destroyed, a wide range of bodily functions loses its daily rhythms: sleep–wake, locomotor activity, feeding, drinking, body temperature, and secretion of hormones (37). These observations were confirmed by SCN transplantation studies in which the transplant restored the lost daily rhythms (38).

One of the best-known circadian pathways is the adrenal gland axis, as glucocorticoids proved to be a humoral entraining signal for peripheral clocks (39). Rhythmic glucocorticoids release is controlled peripherally by sympathetic stimuli and centrally by the SNC, through the secretion of corticotropin releasing hormone (CRH) and ACTH (40). Behavioral processes are also under the control of the SCN, such as locomotor activity and feeding. These behaviors can be entraining factors for the "inner clock," therefore influencing endocrine function and body temperature.

Dysfunction of circadian rhythms has been shown to have a pathogenic role in several diseases, such as cancer and autoimmune diseases. Circadian rhythm disruption may play a role not only in the etiology but also in the progression of the clinical picture. This could be a consequence of the reciprocal relationship between the neuroendocrine system and proinflammatory cytokines involved in the pathological process (41, 42). Moreover, this imbalance can act much earlier in the natural history of the disease; in fact, alterations in sleeping and eating patterns in humans were found to be a source of predisposition to metabolic and cardiovascular diseases (41). A diurnal variation of the symptoms is also typical of many diseases with an immune or inflammatory component. For example, in rheumatoid arthritis, patients refer more joint pain and stiffness in the morning hours, whereas patients with osteoarthritis refer a pain that increases through the day (41).

Circadian Rhythms in AD

Many of the physiological bodily functions described become impaired in AD, but also in other neurodegenerative disorders such as Parkinson's disease and Huntington's disease. In these conditions, several brain areas are affected by neurodegenerative processes, including the nuclei involved in circadian regulation. Neurodegenerative disorders are associated with several sleep–wake rhythm disturbances, such as insomnia/hypersomnia, parasomnia, excessive nocturnal motor activity (for example, restless legs syndrome), and sleep apnea. In AD, sleep is often irregular and disturbed by multiple awakenings and, along with disease duration and progression to advanced stage, a phase shift of the sleep period is observed, often leading to a complete reversal of the day/night pattern (43). These signs and symptoms not only contribute to morbidity, poor quality of life, and institutionalization of individuals with AD (44) but could also be involved in the etiology of the pathological process (45).

Changes in rest-activity patterns correlate with the severity of dementia and could be a preclinical marker, in healthy subjects, of predisposition and possible future development of cognitive impairment and AD (46). A prospective actigraphy study led in a cohort of 1282 healthy women showed higher incidence of MCI and dementia in women with decreased circadian activity rhythm amplitude at follow up (approximately 5 years later). Reductions in total melatonin (the molecule that controls night-day cycle) levels are more profound in AD than in normally aging individuals, as showed in a post-mortem study (47–49). Melatonin showed protective anti-amyloidogenic effects *in vitro* and, interestingly, was found to be decreased in early (even preclinical) stages of the disease, both in total levels and width of the circadian oscillations (49, 50). These findings were supported by the observation of a decrease in the number of melatonin receptor-carrying neurons in the SCN in late-stage AD, alongside with a decrease of volume and total cell count in the whole SCN itself (51, 52). Moreover, the expression of "clock genes" is altered in the brain of AD patients, reflecting the disruption of the master control by the SCN (53). These alterations in circadian rhythms were demonstrated in animal models transgenic for AD-associated mutations (54).

Circadian disruption can be both a consequence of AD as well as worsening factor in AD pathological cascade, suggesting a biunivocal relationship between the two (55). On one hand, AD pathology can lead to day/night sleep pattern disturbances and subsequent poor quality of life; on the other hand, the same disturbances can influence the course of AD pathology. Sleep deprivation results in increased concentration and accumulation of Aβ, in contrast to sleep extension that has the opposite effect. The accumulation of Aβ results in increased wakefulness and altered sleep pattern, as observed in sleep-restricted animals that showed greater Aβ plaque deposition compared to controls (56). Studies on orexin, also known as hypocretin, (a molecule that regulates wakefulness, strongly implicated in sleep disorders) showed that its release from hypothalamic neurons and the pattern of Aβ in CSF have a comparable diurnal fluctuation, and that orexin itself shows a circadian rhythm in both AD patients and controls (56, 57). Aβ levels are also increased during orexin infusion and decreased with an orexin receptor antagonist, indicating a role of orexin and sleep-wake cycle disruption in the pathogenesis of AD (52). Low CSF Aβ42 levels have been found to be related to lower levels of orexin, further suggesting a relationship between AD pathology and orexin disturbance (57, 58). A clinical trial on a population of healthy middle-aged men confirmed these observations, showing a decrease of 6% in the CSF Aβ42 levels after one night of unrestricted sleep and a difference of 75.8 pg/ml between the CSF Aβ42 levels of the unrestricted sleep and sleep deprived group (59).

Diurnal Variation of CSF AD Biomarkers: State of the Art

As previously reported, diurnal variation can be a critical factor while studying molecules that can be influenced by circadian rhythms, making sampling time a matter of concern. Focusing on AD CSF biomarkers, Bateman et al. showed that human CSF Aβ levels varied significantly (1.5- to 4-fold) over 36 h (60). The Aβ levels showed no significant differences between the hours during the daytime period, but an increase during a 36-h period. All participants were screened to be in good general health and without neurologic diseases. Participants older than 65 were non-demented controls, and had a Clinical Dementia Rating of 0. Six milliliters of CSF were obtained each hour for 12, 24, or 36 h. CSF aliquots were frozen at –80°C immediately after collection in 1 ml PP tubes. One milliliter of CSF from each collection hour was thawed and Aβ40 and Aβ42 were measured by ELISA. A sinusoidal pattern of Aβ levels was observed across participants, supposed to be due to time of day, activity, or dynamic changes in the production or clearance rate of Aβ in the CNS. The study by Bateman was the first to arise the issue of a possible diurnal variation of CSF biomarkers that could represent a significant obstacle to an accurate diagnosis. However, a previous study by Andreasen et al. showed no significant fluctuations of Aβ42 on repeated lumbar puncture in subjects with AD (61). It may be that CSF Aβ variability is decreased in patients with AD pathology and amyloid plaques, but has higher fluctuations in individuals without plaques. Bjerke et al. also found no diurnal variation in 14 psychiatrically and neurologically healthy subjects carrying lumbar catheters due to knee surgery (32); CSF was serially collected by lumbar puncture at baseline, after 4–6 h and after 24 h. The samples were immediately stored at –80°C. Data showed more stable levels with a slight but significant decrease in CSF Aβ42 after 4–6 h, which tended to return to baseline levels after 24 h. A possible reason for these results is that, as opposed to Bateman et al., a smaller CSF volume was taken; this could have led to a minor impact on the CSF dynamics. Slats et al. also found no diurnal variation in CSF dynamics during a 36-h sampling (6 ml per hour) (62). They investigated the within-subject variability over 36 h in CSF Aβ and tau proteins, in older subjects, and AD patients. Six patients with mild stage AD [59–85 years, mini mental state examination (MMSE) 16–26 range] and six healthy older volunteers (64–77 years) underwent insertion of an intrathecal catheter from which 6 ml of CSF were collected each hour for 36 h. Variability of CSF Aβ40, Aβ42, t-tau, and p-tau concentrations was lower than expected and the diurnal variation was not as wide as in the younger subjects in Bateman's study. The most recent study was led by Moghekar et al. in a cohort of older mildly symptomatic individuals to determine whether CSF biomarkers of AD fluctuate significantly over time (63). Ten patients suspected of having idiopathic normal pressure hydrocephalus or pseudotumor cerebri were recruited. Intracranial pressure monitoring and CSF drainage represented part of their routine clinical care. Most of the patients had relatively modest cognitive problems associated with their suspected diagnosis (MMSE score range 20–30). Clinical diagnoses of dementia and MCI were based on informant history as well as cognitive testing, without knowledge of AD biomarker levels. All patients underwent insertion of a catheter into the lumbar subarachnoid space on the first day of hospitalization. After monitoring of intracranial pressure for 18 h, drainage of CSF was initiated at noon the following day. Collection of CSF for analysis started at 6 p.m. on the first day of drainage (the second hospital day). Forty milliliters of CSF were withdrawn from the lumbar catheter every 6 h for 24 or 36 consecutive hours and then stored at –80°C until further analysis. The levels of Aβ42, Aβ40, total tau, and p-tau, although significantly different between the patients, did not fluctuate appreciably over time. Significant fluctuations in Aβ did not occur in the patients with the highest CSF Aβ levels as well as in those with the lowest CSF Aβ levels. This study and the one from Bateman et al. have two major differences: age and health status of the population and sampling frequency. Population was significantly older and with ongoing neurological abnormalities, opposed to the young healthy subjects of Bateman's study; still, the role of age is uncertain, since no great differences were found in the fluctuations of Aβ42 between the youngest and oldest patients in the cohort. The samples were collected every 6 h instead of each hour as in Bateman's study; however, since the peak-to-peak variability for Aβ followed a 12-h cycle in the prior study, a significant level of variability would have been apparent in the latter study. All the results are summarized in **Table 3**.

Amyloid metabolism is characterized by several critical steps, which can cause variability in its CSF levels: production from cleavage of amyloid precursor protein (APP), degradation by proteases and microglia, and clearance by systemic circulation or lymphatics (64). However, up to now, none of these steps justifies the diurnal fluctuations of Aβ reported by Bateman, except for the diurnal variation in transcription, translation of APP, and regulation of the two secretases (beta or gamma secretase) that cleave APP to produce Aβ (65). In CNS, APP can be cleaved by either the β-secretase pathway or the α-secretase pathway: the first is amyloidogenic and generates soluble APP-β (sAPPβ) and Aβ; the second one is non-amyloidogenic and causes the release of soluble APP-α (sAPPα). In 2014, Dobrowolska et al. measured APP proteolytic products over 36 h in the CSF of cognitively normal and AD individuals, in order to clarify the role of APP metabolism in α- and β- pathway balance and, consequently, in Aβ diurnal pattern. Diurnal fluctuations were found in sAPPα, sAPPβ, Aβ40, and Aβ42, diminishing

TABLE 3 | Summary of the effects of diurnal variation on CSF AD biomarkers levels.

Reference #	Demographics	Population size	Samples collection	Assay	Effects of diurnal variation
(60)	Non-demented subjects: 23–78 years old	15	6 ml CSF from lumbar catheter Each hour for 12, 24, or 36 h CSF frozen at −80°C after collection in polypropylene tubes	Aβ determined with ELISA	Aβ varied significantly, showing an increase over a 36 h period
(32)	Healthy subjects undergoing knee surgery	14	10–12 ml CSF from lumbar puncture Baseline, after 4–6 h, after 24 h CSF frozen at −80°C after collection in polypropylene tubes	Aβ42 determined with xMAP-based assay	No significant diurnal variation, slight decrease in Aβ42 levels that tended to return to baseline after 24 h
(62)	Mild stage AD patients: 59–85 years old; healthy volunteers: 64–77 years old	6 + 6	6 ml CSF from intrathecal catheter During 36 h, each hour CSF frozen at −80°C after collection in polypropylene tubes	Aβ42, t-tau, and p-tau determined with xMAP-based assay. Aβ40 determined with ELISA	No significant diurnal variation, less pronounced circadian pattern compared with the one in younger subjects
(63)	Patients suspected of having idiopathic normal pressure hydrocephalus (n = 9) or pseudotumor cerebri (n = 1)	10	40 ml CSF from lumbar catheter Every 6 h for 24 or 36 consecutive hours CSF frozen at −80°C after collection in polypropylene tubes	Aβ42, total tau, and p-tau181 determined with xMAP-based assay. Aβ40 determined with ELISA	No significant diurnal variation

with increased age; these findings support the hypothesis that APP undergoes a circadian rhythm regulated in the central nervous system and thus results in Aβ diurnal fluctuations. Moreover, it was found that the ratio of sAPPβ to sAPPα was significantly higher in participants with cerebral Aβ deposits compared to those without deposits, therefore making sAPPβ/sAPPα ratio a valuable biomarker for cerebral amyloidosis (65). Time-dependent fluctuations were also observed in CSF Apolipoprotein E (apoE) (66, 67). ApoE is the probably the most important and acknowledged genetic risk factor for Alzheimer's disease and even for some other neurological disorders. ApoE has several isoforms; the most common are represented by ApoE2 and E4, each associated with a different effect on AD predisposition, with ApoE4 increasing and ApoE2 decreasing the risk of AD. Their role in modulating AD pathology is due to both the isoform and amount of ApoE in the brain, which directly reflects the extent of Aβ peptide deposition. Therefore, quantifying ApoE isoforms, especially ApoE4, could be a useful biological correlate in the study of AD pathology from preclinical to clinical stages. The main obstacle to the use of ApoE4 as a biomarker is that CNS and peripheral ApoE isoform turnover rates differ substantially, probably because the ApoE metabolism pathways are different in the CNS and the periphery, as observed in a study by Wildsmith et al. (67). The study also showed different turnover rates for each isoform of ApoE and a slower turnover rate for CSF ApoE than the Aβ one. Further *in vivo* studies are needed to determine if the fluctuations in ApoE metabolism are a limiting factor for its use as biomarker.

Conclusion

Classical AD CSF biomarkers show a promising diagnostic value, especially in research studies; current and future research should be devoted to the standardization of the collection and analysis procedures to increase the statistical power of the results and the comparability among laboratories. Univocal cut-off values for biomarkers should be available, along with standard operating procedures for preanalytical factors. The aim is to allow a more widespread use of CSF biomarkers and lumbar puncture in clinical routine for early AD diagnosis.

It must also be taken into account that most studies on diurnal variation focus only on Aβ and do not consider other neuronal injury markers. Up to now there are very few studies focusing on tau-related biomarkers and their possible fluctuations during the daytime period (62, 63). When speaking of accuracy of CSF diagnostics, further studies need to be performed before ruling out diurnal variation as a variability factor. Nevertheless, data so far are reassuring, since no significant diurnal fluctuations have been consistently found.

In case of novel biomarkers, the suggestion is that diurnal variation always needs to be analyzed as a variability factor; the recommendation is to record withdrawal time information to identify the possible diurnal variation of the new analyte. In conclusion, taking into account that CSF withdrawal is usually performed during daytime and that no significant changes have been found in the levels of classic AD CSF biomarkers at different times of day, there is no need to standardize a specific time interval during the day for CSF collection.

References

1. Dubois B, Feldman HH, Jacova C, Dekosky ST, Barberger-Gateau P, Cummings J, et al. Research criteria for the diagnosis of Alzheimer's disease: revising the NINCDS-ADRDA criteria. *Lancet Neurol* (2007) **6**:734–46. doi:10.1016/S1474-4422(07)70178-3
2. Jack CR Jr, Albert MS, Knopman DS, McKhann GM, Sperling RA, Carrillo MC, et al. Introduction to the recommendations from the National Institute on Aging- Alzheimer's Association workgroups on diagnostic guidelines for Alzheimers disease. *Alzheimers Dement* (2011) **7**:257–62. doi:10.1016/j.jalz.2011.03.004
3. Dubois B, Feldman HH, Jacova C, Hampel H, Molinuevo JL, Blennow K, et al. Advancing research diagnostic criteria for Alzheimer's disease: the IWG-2 criteria. *Lancet Neurol* (2014) **13**:614–29. doi:10.1016/S1474-4422(14)70090-0
4. Blennow K, Hampel H, Weiner M, Zetterberg H. Cerebrospinal fluid and plasma biomarkers in Alzheimer disease. *Nat Rev Neurol* (2010) **6**:131–44. doi:10.1038/nrneurol.2010.4

5. Buerger K, Ewers M, Pirttilä T, Zinkowski R, Alafuzoff I, Teipel SJ, et al. CSF phosphorylated tau protein correlates with neocortical neurofibrillary pathology in Alzheimer's disease. *Brain* (2006) **129**:3035–41. doi:10.1093/brain/awl269
6. Le Bastard N, Martin JJ, Vanmechelen E, Vanderstichele H, De Deyn PP, Engelborghs S. Added diagnostic value of CSF biomarkers in differential dementia diagnosis. *Neurobiol Aging* (2010) **31**:1867–76. doi:10.1016/j.neurobiolaging.2008.10.017
7. Slaets S, Le Bastard N, Theuns J, Sleegers K, Verstraeten A, De Leenheir E, et al. Amyloid pathology influences abeta1-42 cerebrospinal fluid levels in dementia with lewy bodies. *J Alzheimers Dis* (2013) **35**:137–46. doi:10.3233/JAD-122176
8. Blennow K, Hampel H. CSF markers for incipient Alzheimer's disease. *Lancet Neurol* (2003) **2**:605–13. doi:10.1016/S1474-4422(03)00530-1
9. Parnetti L, Chiasserini D, Eusebi P, Giannandrea D, Bellomo G, De Carlo C, et al. Performance of aβ1-40, aβ1-42, total tau, and phosphorylated tau as predictors of dementia in a cohort of patients with mild cognitive impairment. *J Alzheimers Dis* (2012) **29**(1):229–38. doi:10.3233/JAD-2011-111349
10. Spies PE, Slats D, Sjögren JM, Kremer BP, Verhey FR, Rikkert MG. The cerebrospinal fluid amyloid beta42/40 ratio in the differentiation of Alzheimer's disease from non-Alzheimer's dementia. *Curr Alzheimer Res* (2010) **7**(5):470–6. doi:10.2174/156720510791383796
11. Fagan AM, Roe CM, Xiong C, Mintun MA, Morris JC, Holtzman DM. Cerebrospinal fluid tau/beta-amyloid(42) ratio as a prediction of cognitive decline in nondemented older adults. *Arch Neurol* (2007) **64**:343–9. doi:10.1001/archneur.64.3.noc60123
12. Hampel H, Teipel SJ, Fuchsberger T, Andreasen N, Wiltfang J, Otto M, et al. Value of CSF beta-amyloid1-42 and tau as predictors of Alzheimer's disease in patients with mild cognitive impairment. *Mol Psychiatry* (2004) **9**:705–10. doi:10.1038/sj.mp.4001473
13. Hulstaert F, Blennow K, Ivanoiu A, Schoonderwaldt HC, Riemenschneider M, De Deyn PP, et al. Improved discrimination of AD patients using beta-amyloid(1-42) and tau levels in CSF. *Neurology* (1999) **52**:1555–62. doi:10.1212/WNL.52.8.1555
14. Smach MA, Charfeddine B, Ben Othman L, Lammouchi T, Dridi H, Nafati S, et al. Evaluation of cerebrospinal fluid tau/beta-amyloid(42) ratio as diagnostic markers for Alzheimer disease. *Eur Neurol* (2009) **62**:349–55. doi:10.1159/000241881
15. Vos SJ, Verhey F, Frölich L, Kornhuber J, Wiltfang J, Maier W, et al. Prevalence and prognosis of Alzheimer's disease at the mild cognitive impairment stage. *Brain* (2015) **138**(Pt 5):1327–38. doi:10.1093/brain/awv029
16. de Souza LC, Lamari F, Belliard S, Jardel C, Houillier C, De Paz R, et al. Cerebrospinal fluid biomarkers in the differential diagnosis of Alzheimer's disease from other cortical dementias. *J Neurol Neurosurg Psychiatry* (2011) **82**:240–6. doi:10.1136/jnnp.2010.207183
17. Schoonenboom NS, Reesink FE, Verwey NA, Kester MI, Teunissen CE, van de Ven PM, et al. Cerebrospinal fluid markers for differential dementia diagnosis in a large memory clinic cohort. *Neurology* (2012) **78**:47–54. doi:10.1212/WNL.0b013e31823ed0f0
18. Brys M, Pirraglia E, Rich K, Rolstad S, Mosconi L, Switalski R, et al. Prediction and longitudinal study of CSF biomarkers in mild cognitive impairment. *Neurobiol Aging* (2009) **30**:682–90. doi:10.1016/j.neurobiolaging.2007.08.010
19. Li G, Sokal I, Quinn JF, Leverenz JB, Brodey M, Schellenberg GD, et al. CSF tau/Abeta42 ratio for increased risk of mild cognitive impairment: a follow-up study. *Neurology* (2007) **69**:631–9. doi:10.1212/01.wnl.0000267428.62582.aa
20. Snider BJ, Fagan AM, Roe C, Shah AR, Grant EA, Xiong C, et al. Cerebrospinal fluid biomarkers and rate of cognitive decline in very mild dementia of the Alzheimer type. *Arch Neurol* (2009) **66**:638–45. doi:10.1001/archneurol.2009.55
21. Meijs AP, Claassen JA, Rikkert MG, Schalk BW, Meulenbroek O, Kessels RP, et al. How does additional diagnostic testing influence the initial diagnosis in patients with cognitive complaints in a memory clinic setting? *Age Ageing* (2015) **44**(1):72–7. doi:10.1093/ageing/afu053
22. Lewczuk P, Zimmermann R, Wiltfang J, Kornhuber J. Neurochemical dementia diagnostics: a simple algorithm for interpretation of the CSF biomarkers. *J Neural Transm* (2009) **116**(9):1163–7. doi:10.1007/s00702-009-0277-y
23. Molinuevo JL, Blennow K, Dubois B, Engelborghs S, Lewczuk P, Perret-Liaudet A, et al. The clinical use of cerebrospinal fluid biomarker testing for Alzheimer's disease diagnosis: a consensus paper from the Alzheimer's biomarkers standardization initiative. *Alzheimers Dement* (2014) **10**(6):808–17. doi:10.1016/j.jalz.2014.03.003
24. Mattsson N, Andreasson U, Persson S, Carrillo MC, Collins S, Chalbot S, et al. CSF biomarker variability in the Alzheimer's association quality control program. *Alzheimers Dement* (2013) **9**(3):251–61. doi:10.1016/j.jalz.2013.01.010
25. Mattsson N, Andreasson U, Persson S, Arai H, Batish SD, Bernardini S, et al. The Alzheimer's association external quality control program for cerebrospinal fluid biomarkers. *Alzheimers Dement* (2011) **7**:386–95. doi:10.1016/j.jalz.2011.05.2243
26. Teunissen CE, Petzold A, Bennett JL, Berven FS, Brundin L, Comabella M, et al. A consensus protocol for the standardization of cerebrospinal fluid collection and biobanking. *Neurology* (2009) **73**(22):1914–22. doi:10.1212/WNL.0b013e3181c47cc2
27. Plebani M. Errors in clinical laboratories or errors in laboratory medicine? *Clin Chem Lab Med* (2006) **44**:750–9. doi:10.1515/CCLM.2006.123
28. Vanderstichele H, Bibl M, Engelborghs S, Le Bastard N, Lewczuk P, Molinuevo JL, et al. Standardization of preanalytical aspects of cerebrospinal fluid biomarker testing for Alzheimer's disease diagnosis: a consensus paper from the Alzheimer's biomarkers standardization initiative. *Alzheimers Dement* (2012) **8**(1):65–73. doi:10.1016/j.jalz.2011.07.004
29. Mollenhauer B, Trautmann E, Otte B, Ng J, Spreer A, Lange P, et al. α-Synuclein in human cerebrospinal fluid is principally derived from neurons of the central nervous system. *J Neural Transm* (2012) **119**(7):739–46. doi:10.1007/s00702-012-0784-0
30. Del Campo M, Mollenhauer B, Bertolotto A, Engelborghs S, Hampel H, Simonsen AH, et al. Recommendations to standardize preanalytical confounding factors in Alzheimer's and Parkinson's disease cerebrospinal fluid biomarkers: an update. *Biomark Med* (2012) **6**(4):419–30. doi:10.2217/bmm.12.46
31. Berven FS, Kroksveen AC, Berle M, Rajalahti T, Flikka K, Arneberg R, et al. Pre-analytical influence on the low molecular weight cerebrospinal fluid proteome. *Proteomics Clin Appl* (2007) **1**(7):699–711. doi:10.1002/prca.200700126
32. Bjerke M, Portelius E, Minthon L, Wallin A, Anckarsäter H, Anckarsäter R, et al. Confounding factors influencing amyloid beta concentration in cerebrospinal fluid. *Int J Alzheimers Dis* (2010) **5**:2010. doi:10.4061/2010/986310
33. Willemse EA, Koel-Simmelink MJ, Durieux-Lu S, van der Flier WM, Teunissen CE. Standard biobanking conditions prevent evaporation of body fluid samples. *Clin Chim Acta* (2015) **442**:141–5. doi:10.1016/j.cca.2015.01.036
34. Greco V, Pieragostino D, Piras C, Aebersold R, Wiltfang J, Caltagirone C, et al. Direct analytical sample quality assessment for biomarker investigation: qualifying cerebrospinal fluid samples. *Proteomics* (2014) **14**(17–18):1954–62. doi:10.1002/pmic.201300565
35. Schoonenboom NS, Mulder C, Vanderstichele H, Van Elk EJ, Kok A, Van Kamp GJ, et al. Effects of processing and storage conditions on amyloid beta (1-42) and tau concentrations in cerebrospinal fluid: implications for use in clinical practice. *Clin Chem* (2005) **51**:189–95. doi:10.1373/clinchem.2004.039735
36. Morin LP. Neuroanatomy of the extended circadian rhythm system. *Exp Neurol* (2013) **243**:4–20. doi:10.1016/j.expneurol.2012.06.026
37. Tahara Y, Kuroda H, Saito K, Nakajima Y, Kubo Y, Ohnishi N, et al. In vivo monitoring of peripheral circadian clocks in the mouse. *Curr Biol* (2012) **22**(11):1029–34. doi:10.1016/j.cub.2012.04.009
38. Cho S, Yujnovsky I, Doi M, Sassone-Corsi P. Transplantation of mouse embryo fibroblasts: an approach to study the physiological pathways linking the suprachiasmatic nucleus and peripheral clocks. *Methods Enzymol* (2005) **393**:469–78. doi:10.1016/S0076-6879(05)93023-1
39. Mohawk JA, Green CB, Takahashi JS. Central and peripheral circadian clocks in mammals. *Annu Rev Neurosci* (2012) **35**:445–62. doi:10.1146/annurev-neuro-060909-153128
40. Kaneko M, Kaneko K, Shinsako J, Dallman MF. Adrenal sensitivity to adrenocorticotropin varies diurnally. *Endocrinology* (1981) **109**:70–5. doi:10.1210/endo-109-1-70
41. Arjona A, Silver AC, Walker WE, Fikrig E. Immunity's fourth dimension: approaching the circadian-immune connection. *Trends Immunol* (2012) **33**(12):607–12. doi:10.1016/j.it.2012.08.007
42. Narasimamurthy R, Hatori M, Nayak SK, Liu F, Panda S, Verma IM. Circadian clock protein cryptochrome regulates the expression of proinflammatory cytokines. *Proc Natl Acad Sci U S A* (2012) **109**(31):12662–7. doi:10.1073/pnas.1209965109
43. Harper DG, Stopa EG, McKee AC, Satlin A, Fish D, Volicer L. Dementia severity and Lewy bodies affect circadian rhythms in Alzheimer disease. *Neurobiol Aging* (2004) **25**:771–81. doi:10.1016/j.neurobiolaging.2003.04.009
44. Bianchetti A, Scuratti A, Zanetti O, Binetti G, Frisoni GB, Magni E, et al. Predictors of mortality and institutionalization in Alzheimer disease patients 1 year after discharge from an Alzheimer dementia unit. *Dementia* (1995) **6**:108–12.

45. Videnovic A, Lazar AS, Barker RA, Overeem S. 'The clocks that time us' – circadian rhythms in neurodegenerative disorders. *Nat Rev Neurol* (2014) **10**(12):683–93. doi:10.1038/nrneurol.2014.206
46. Tranah GJ, Blackwell T, Stone KL, Ancoli-Israel S, Paudel ML, Ensrud KE, et al. Circadian activity rhythms and risk of incident dementia and mild cognitive impairment in older women. *Ann Neurol* (2011) **70**:722–32. doi:10.1002/ana.22468
47. Skene DJ, Swaab DF. Melatonin rhythmicity: effect of age and Alzheimer's disease. *Exp Gerontol* (2003) **38**:199–206. doi:10.1016/S0531-5565(02)00198-5
48. Lin L, Huang QX, Yang SS, Chu J, Wang JZ, Tian Q. Melatonin in Alzheimer's disease. *Int J Mol Sci* (2013) **14**:14575–93. doi:10.3390/ijms140714575
49. Zhou JN, Liu RY, Kamphorst W, Hofman MA, Swaab DF. Early neuropathological Alzheimer's changes in aged individuals are accompanied by decreased cerebrospinal fluid melatonin levels. *J Pineal Res* (2003) **35**:125–30. doi:10.1034/j.1600-079X.2003.00065.x
50. Wu YH, Feenstra MG, Zhou JN, Liu RY, Toranõ JS, Van Kan HJ, et al. Molecular changes underlying reduced pineal melatonin levels in Alzheimer disease: alterations in preclinical and clinical stages. *J Clin Endocrinol Metab* (2003) **88**:5898–906. doi:10.1210/jc.2003-030833
51. Swaab DF, Fliers E, Partiman TS. The suprachiasmatic nucleus of the human brain in relation to sex, age and senile dementia. *Brain Res* (1985) **342**:37–44. doi:10.1016/0006-8993(85)91350-2
52. Wu YH, Zhou JN, Van Heerikhuize J, Jockers R, Swaab DF. Decreased MT1 melatonin receptor expression in the suprachiasmatic nucleus in aging and Alzheimer's disease. *Neurobiol Aging* (2007) **28**:1239–47. doi:10.1016/j.neurobiolaging.2006.06.002
53. Wu YH, Fischer DF, Kalsbeek A, Garidou-Boof ML, van der Vliet J, van Heijningen C, et al. Pineal clock gene oscillation is disturbed in Alzheimer's disease, due to functional disconnection from the "master clock". *FASEB J* (2006) **20**:1874–6. doi:10.1096/fj.05-4446fje
54. Sterniczuk R, Dyck RH, Laferla FM, Antle MC. Characterization of the 3xTg-AD mouse model of Alzheimer's disease: part 1. Circadian changes. *Brain Res* (2010) **1348**:139–48. doi:10.1016/j.brainres.2010.05.013
55. Ju YE, Lucey BP, Holtzman DM. Sleep and Alzheimer disease pathology – a bidirectional relationship. *Nat Rev Neurol* (2014) **10**:115–9. doi:10.1038/nrneurol.2013.269
56. Kang JE, Lim MM, Bateman RJ, Lee JJ, Smyth LP, Cirrito JR, et al. Amyloid-β dynamics are regulated by orexin and the sleep–wake cycle. *Science* (2009) **326**:1005–7. doi:10.1126/science.1180962
57. Slats D, Claassen JA, Lammers GJ, Melis RJ, Verbeek MM, Overeem S. Association between hypocretin-1 and amyloid-β42 cerebrospinal fluid levels in Alzheimer's disease and healthy controls. *Curr Alzheimer Res* (2012) **9**(10):1119–25. doi:10.2174/156720512804142840
58. Slats D, Claassen JA, Verbeek MM, Overeem S. Reciprocal interactions between sleep, circadian rhythms and Alzheimer's disease: focus on the role of hypocretin and melatonin. *Ageing Res Rev* (2013) **12**(1):188–200. doi:10.1016/j.arr.2012.04.003
59. Ooms S, Overeem S, Besse K, Rikkert MO, Verbeek M, Claassen JA. Effect of 1 night of total sleep deprivation on cerebrospinal fluid β-amyloid 42 in healthy middle-aged men: a randomized clinical trial. *JAMA Neurol* (2014) **71**(8):971–7. doi:10.1001/jamaneurol.2014.1173
60. Bateman RJ, Wen G, Morris JC, Holtzman DM. Fluctuations of CSF amyloid-beta levels: implications for a diagnostic and therapeutic biomarker. *Neurology* (2007) **68**(9):666–9. doi:10.1212/01.wnl.0000256043.50901.e3
61. Andreasen N, Hesse C, Davidsson P, Minthon L, Wallin A, Winblad B, et al. Cerebrospinal fluid beta-amyloid(1-42) in Alzheimer disease: differences between early- and late-onset Alzheimer disease and stability during the course of disease. *Arch Neurol* (1999) **56**(6):673–80. doi:10.1001/archneur.56.6.673
62. Slats D, Claassen JA, Spies PE, Borm G, Besse KT, van Aalst W, et al. Hourly variability of cerebrospinal fluid biomarkers in Alzheimer's disease subjects and healthy older volunteers. *Neurobiol Aging* (2012) **33**(4):e1–9. doi:10.1016/j.neurobiolaging.2011.07.008
63. Moghekar A, Goh J, Li M, Albert M, O'Brien RJ. Cerebrospinal fluid Aβ and tau level fluctuation in an older clinical cohort. *Arch Neurol* (2012) **69**(2):246–50. doi:10.1001/archneurol.2011.732
64. Spies PE, Verbeek MM, van Groen T, Claassen JA. Reviewing reasons for the decreased CSF Abeta42 concentration in Alzheimer disease. *Front Biosci* (2012) **17**:2024–34. doi:10.2741/4035
65. Dobrowolska JA, Kasten T, Huang Y, Benzinger TL, Sigurdson W, Ovod V, et al. Diurnal patterns of soluble amyloid precursor protein metabolites in the human central nervous system. *PLoS One* (2014) **9**(3):e89998. doi:10.1371/journal.pone.0089998
66. Yamauchi K, Tozuka M, Nakabayashi T, Sugano M, Hidaka H, Kondo Y, et al. Apolipoprotein E in cerebrospinal fluid: relation to phenotype and plasma apolipoprotein E concentrations. *Clin Chem* (1999) **45**(4):497–504.
67. Wildsmith KR, Basak JM, Patterson BW, Pyatkivskyy Y, Kim J, Yarasheski KE, et al. In vivo human apolipoprotein E isoform fractional turnover rates in the CNS. *PLoS One* (2012) 7(6):e38013. doi:10.1371/journal.pone.0038013

12

microRNA-based biomarkers and the diagnosis of Alzheimer's disease

*Yuhai Zhao[1,2], Surjyadipta Bhattacharjee[1], Prerna Dua[3], Peter N. Alexandrov[4] and Walter J. Lukiw[1,5,6]**

[1] LSU Neuroscience Center Louisiana State University Health Science Center, New Orleans, LA, USA, [2] Department of Cell Biology and Anatomy, LSU Neuroscience Center Louisiana State University Health Science Center, New Orleans, LA, USA, [3] Department of Health Information Management, Louisiana State University, Ruston, LA, USA, [4] Russian Academy of Medical Sciences, Moscow, Russia, [5] Department of Ophthalmology, LSU Neuroscience Center Louisiana State University Health Science Center, New Orleans, LA, USA, [6] Department of Neurology, LSU Neuroscience Center Louisiana State University Health Science Center, New Orleans, LA, USA

Edited by:
Charlotte Elisabeth Teunissen, VU University Medical Center Amsterdam, Netherlands

Reviewed by:
Cees Oudejans, VU University Medical Center Amsterdam, Netherlands
Argonde Corien Van Harten, VU University Medical Center Amsterdam, Netherlands

***Correspondence:**
Walter J. Lukiw
wlukiw@lsuhsc.edu

Keywords: aging, Alzheimer's disease, diagnostic panel, heterogeneity, human biochemical individuality, inflammation, microRNA, prion disease

Alzheimer's disease (AD) is characterized as a complex, age-related neurological disorder of the human central nervous system (CNS) that involves the progressive mis-regulation of multiple biological pathways at multiple molecular, genetic, epigenetic, neurophysiological, cognitive, and behavioral levels. It has been about 8 years since the first reports of altered microRNA (miRNA) abundance and speciation: (i) in anatomical regions of the brain targeted by the AD process after post-mortem examination, (ii) in blood serum, and (iii) in cerebrospinal fluid (CSF) (1–3). Since then an in depth overview of the peer-reviewed literature has provided no general consensus of what miRNAs are up-or-down regulated in any tissue or biofluid compartment in thousands of AD patients. In this brief "Opinion" paper on "*Biomarkers of Alzheimer's disease: the present and the future*," we will highlight the extremely heterogeneous nature of miRNA expression in AD, based on very recent advances in the analysis of miRNA populations in various biofluid compartments compared to normally aging, neurologically normal controls. This work is based against a background of our laboratory's 24 years of research experience into the structure and function of small, non-coding RNAs in the aging human CNS in health and in age-related neurological disease (4).

First, it is important to appreciate that all forms of dementia due to AD are broadly classified as either early onset (EOAD, under 65 years of age), or late onset (LOAD, over 65 years of age) (5, 6). About ~5% of all AD cases have a genetic component (see below) while the remaining ~95% of all AD cases are of a sporadic (idiopathic) nature or are of unknown origin (5–8). The extremely heterogeneous nature of AD pervades all molecular, genetic, neuropathological and behavioral, mnemonic, and cognitive levels, including the clinical presentation of the disease (6–15). For example, the key *neuropathological markers* of AD include: (i) the progressive deposition of amyloid-beta (Aβ) peptides into dense, insoluble pro-inflammatory senile plaques (SP); (ii) the accumulation of hyperphosphorylated tau into neurofibrillary tangles (NFT); (iii) synaptic atrophy, "pruning" and loss, neuronal degeneration and neuronal cell death; (iv) alterations in the innate-immune response; and (v) the progressive inflammatory neurodegeneration and anatomical targeting of only specific anatomical regions of the brain (1–15). These highly interactive characteristics collectively suggest the participation of multiple pathogenic pathways, and the involvement of multiple deficits in the expression of CNS genes (1–15). Accordingly, this culminates in a remarkably heterogeneous neuropathological scaffold for AD, with significant variations in disease onset, progression, severity of neuropathology, extent of behavioral and cognitive deficits, and memory loss (4–12). To cite one very recent example, a relatively large epidemiological study of

Abbreviations: miRNA, microRNA.

AD patient data ($N = 7815$) (12) indicated significant heterogeneity in the first cognitive/behavioral symptomatic "indicator" experienced by AD patients (13–16). In other recent studies, two laboratories have independently reported significant variation in the miRNA-34a-mediated triggering receptor expressed in myeloid/microglial cells-2 (TREM2) down-regulation in an African-American population that further underscores (i) the importance of investigating different ethnic populations for AD epigenetic risk; (ii) intrinsic variance and human *biochemical and genetic individuality*; and (iii) allelic heterogeneity and potentially diverse pathogenic contributory mechanisms to the AD process (sufficient TREM2 is important in the clearance of excessive Aβ peptides from the brain) (9–16). Related to these observations are studies that over the last 15 years have indicated that gene expression patterns at the messenger RNA (mRNA) level, Aβ peptide load, SP and NFT densities and localization, and familial and clinical histories further underscore AD heterogeneity (8–12, 17–20). Indeed, there appears to be intrinsic limitations of useful AD biomarkers because just one biomarker cannot define the mechanism of AD, by nature are associative and/or correlative, and are unable to unequivocally prove disease causality (13–17, 21–23). For example current genome-wide association studies (GWAS), whole-exome and whole-genome sequencing have revealed mutations in excess of 20 genetic loci associated with AD risk (11, 19, 20, 24). Three main genes are involved in EOAD: *amyloid precursor protein* (*APP*), *presenilin 1* (*PSEN1*), and *presenilin 2* (*PSEN2*), while the *apolipoprotein E* (*ApoE*) E4 allele has been found to be a main risk factor for LOAD (1, 17–19, 23). Additionally, recent studies have discovered other genes that might be peripherally involved in AD, including *clusterin* (*CLU*), *complement receptor 1* (*CR1*), *phosphatidylinositol binding clathrin assembly protein* (*PICALM*), *sortilin-related receptor* (*SORL1*), complement factor H (CFH), the *triggering receptor expressed on myeloid/microglial cells 2* (*TREM2*), and the *cluster of differentiation 33* (*CD33*) gene loci; although not one single case of AD has yet been found to be associated with more than one of these aberrant genetic loci (11, 25). Indeed, most AD cases do not contain any of these mutant genetic "*biomarkers*" (11, 20, 24–26). Further, the persistence of mutations in these genes from birth and throughout life, in contrast to the general development of AD in old age, suggests that multiple age-associated gene regulatory mechanisms must come into play to initiate and drive development and propagation of the AD process, and miRNAs are excellent candidates for these diverse age-related, developmental, and regulatory roles (1–5, 9, 22).

Regarding the rate and variability of cognitive decline in AD, one large recent study did not find evidence supporting a substantial role of the mini-mental status examination (MMSE) as a stand-alone single-administration test in the identification of mild cognitively impaired patients who eventually develop AD, suggesting the need for additional neuropsychological testing and comprehensive biomarker analysis (21–23). Indeed, although AD is the most common form of senile dementia, it can often be challenging to distinguish this insidious and fatal disorder from other equally heterogeneous neurodegenerative disorders, such as frontal temporal dementia, human prion disease [including bovine spongiform encephalopathy (BSE; mad cow disease), Creutzfeldt–Jakob disease, Gerstmann–Sträussler–Scheinker syndrome, and other relatively rare human prion diseases], Huntington's disease, Lewy Body dementia, Parkinson's disease, cerebrovascular disease, or vascular (multiple infarct) dementia (16–18, 21–23). Indeed, the diagnostic accuracy of when brain-mediated cognitive deficits actually begin may require a dimensional rather than a categorical classification, and a lifespan rather than aging grouping, and it has been recently suggested that a multidimensional system-vulnerability approach rather than a simple "*hypothetical biomarker*" model of age-associated cognitive decline and dementia may be more useful diagnostically (12, 20). Put another way, AD might be classified not as a discrete disease entity but rather as a "*neurological disconnection syndrome*" (7, 8, 11, 15, 24). This "*neurological disconnection syndrome*" is more broadly defined as an abnormal condition characterized by an established group of variable neurological signs, symptoms, and molecular markers, including miRNA abundance and speciation, that individually possess only limited neuropathological and cognition/behavioral similarities from patient to patient (7–9, 11–18, 21–24).

Further to the concept of AD heterogeneity are the ideas that form the conceptual basis for "*human biochemical and genetic individuality*" (5, 9, 18). These include individual gene sequence variation, gene-based susceptibility to disease and heterogeneity in miRNA abundance and complexity, that may in part drive a general redundancy in gene expression in different human populations (5, 9, 16, 21, 22). Interestingly, these variations may directly impact the genetic evolution of the human species (4, 5, 18–20, 24–26). Much independently derived data support the concept that the genetics, epigenetics, and genome-wide regulatory networks of AD vary considerably among different human populations that possess different genetic and/or environmental backgrounds. Furthermore, despite the fact that genetic factors are inherited and fixed, non-genetic factors, such as (i) environmental or occupational exposures to pesticides, organic solvents, anesthetics, and/or food additives; (ii) pre-existing medical conditions such as cancer, cerebrovascular, and/or cardiovascular disease, depression, diabetes, dyslipidemia, hypertension, traumatic brain injury, older age, female gender, and ApoE status; and (iii) lifestyle factors such as alcohol and coffee consumption, salt, sugar, and cholesterol and fat intake, body mass index, cognitive activity, physical activity, and smoking, are life-style determined and these are known to impact the incidence, development and propagation of AD (18–20, 24–31). Interestingly, certain potentially pathogenic "*pro-inflammatory miRNAs*" of the host are significantly inducible by common microbial and environmental factors such as herpes simplex-1 virus (HSV-1) and naturally occurring elements of the biosphere (such as aluminum oxides that make up almost 9% of the earth's crust) (32–35).

To make another important point concerning the variable contribution of specific miRNAs to AD, we surveyed the most recently published papers on "*miRNA biomarkers for AD*" using the National Institutes of Health National Library of Medicine website MedLine (www.ncbi.nlm.nih.gov; using the keywords "*Alzheimer's disease,*" "*miRNA*" *and* "*2015*"). The most recent findings of 15 independent labs further support the contention of extremely high miRNA heterogeneity in AD tissue and biofluids (36–50). For example, the last 15 reports of diagnostic markers in AD CSF (36–39; involving miRNA-27a, miRNA-29a, miRNA-191, miRNA-384) and others, AD blood serum (38–46; involving miRNA-107, miRNA-125b, miRNA-128, miRNA-132, miRNA-191, miRNA-206, miRNA-384) and others; "*humanized*" AD cell models (47–50; involving miRNA-125b, miRNA-128, miRNA-138) and others, and several recent reviews (51–55) *provides no common or general consensus of any single miRNA that defines causality for the onset or duration of the AD process.* To further complicate these findings, recent molecular-genetic studies have also shown that even when derived from homogenous source populations, such as pluripotent stem cells, individual cells from those populations exhibit significant differences in gene expression, protein abundance and phenotypic output; here specific families of miRNAs appear to have a deterministic role in reconfiguring the "*pluripotency network*" of individual cells with important downstream functional consequences (47–49, 56, 57).

It is further important to point out exactly what an advanced analytical technique will tell us. For example, most AD researchers would agree that the production of Aβ42 peptides is involved in the AD process. Aβ42 peptides and fragments are generated by a variety of secretases (chiefly α-, β-, and γ-secretases), however, other secretase-like enzymes and enzyme modifiers appear to be involved (5, 8, 14, 25, 31, 58). While RNA-seq and other "next generation sequencing" (NGS) methods will tell us something about the levels of expression of these secretases they would give us no clue about the activity of these secretases in the brain, and their ability to generate Aβ42 or other AD-relevant peptides, which are affected by many other genetic, epigenetic, non-genetic, environmental, and host lifestyle factors. So it is unlikely that RNA-seq, NGS, or other "advanced sequencing methodologies" could give us the entire story of what is going on in AD, although most agree it would give us very valuable insight as to what is happening at the molecular-genetic level, and perhaps be of some value diagnostically.

Lastly, if high-density microarray- and advanced RNA-sequencing based profiles of AD brain or biofluid samples are any indication of AD variability then there are real and significant human population differences in AD onset, incidence, epidemiology, disease course and progression (9, 16, 21, 22, 25, 50, 57). It is unlikely that a single miRNA in the CSF, blood serum, urine, or any other biofluid compartments from multiple human populations will be predictive for AD at any stage of the disease. However, what might be particularly useful for significantly improved AD diagnostics would be a selective, high-density panel of a "*pathogenic and neurodegeneration-associated miRNA family*" that along with other gene expression-based biometrics could more accurately predict the onset of AD-type change. This highly interactive, "*personalized medicine*" approach – involving a comprehensive evaluation that scores multiple AD deficiencies including miRNA-, mRNA-, and protein-based gene expression alterations, AD-relevant DNA mutations, pro-inflammatory biomarkers (such as C-reactive protein or CRP), and Aβ40- and Aβ42-peptide load in the CSF and blood serum, combined with data from MRI- and PET-based brain imaging, and familial, clinical history, lifestyle, and other factors could be extremely useful in the improved diagnosis of AD susceptibility and development (52–58). These *highly integrated and multidimensional diagnostic approaches* certainly lie within the grasp of current medical technologies – it will just be a matter of improved application, data acquisition and integration of clinical research and healthcare resources to frame a more accurate diagnostic portrait of the "*alleged AD patient.*" Indeed, an equally wide variety of individualistic prevention and "*personalized*" treatment strategies would be required to more effectively address such age-related neurological disorders, including the implementation of combinatorial and/or customized anti-miRNA strategies that have as yet not been considered.

Acknowledgments

This work was presented in part at the Society for Neuroscience (SFN) Annual Meeting 15–19 November 2014, Washington, DC, USA and at the Association for Research in Vision and Ophthalmology (ARVO) Annual conference 3–7 May 2015 in Denver, CO, USA. Sincere thanks are extended to Drs. L. Carver, E. Head, W. Poon, H. LeBlanc, F. Culicchia, C. Eicken, and C. Hebel for short post-mortem interval (PMI) human brain and/or retinal tissues or extracts, miRNA array work and initial data interpretation, and to D. Guillot and A. I. Pogue for expert technical assistance. Thanks are also extended to the many neuropathologists, physicians, and researchers of Canada and the US, who have provided high quality, short PMI human CNS and retinal tissues or extracted total brain and retinal RNA for scientific study. Research on miRNA in the Lukiw laboratory involving the innate-immune response in AD, AMD, and in other forms of neurological or retinal disease, amyloidogenesis, and neuro-inflammation was supported through an unrestricted grant to the LSU Eye Center from Research to Prevent Blindness (RPB); the Louisiana Biotechnology Research Network (LBRN), and NIH grants NEI EY006311, NIA AG18031, and NIA AG038834.

References

1. Lukiw WJ. MiRNA speciation in fetal, adult and Alzheimer's disease hippocampus. *Neuroreport* (2007) **18**:297–300. doi:10.1097/WNR.0b013e3280148e8b
2. Schipper HM, Maes OC, Chertkow HM, Wang E. MicroRNA expression in Alzheimer blood mononuclear cells. *Gene Regul Syst Bio* (2007) **1**:263–74.
3. Cogswell JP, Ward J, Taylor IA, Waters M, Shi Y, Cannon B, et al. Identification of miRNA changes in Alzheimer's disease brain and CSF yields putative biomarkers and insights into disease pathways. *J Alzheimers Dis* (2008) **14**(1):27–41.
4. Lukiw WJ, Handley P, Wong L, Crapper McLachlan DR. BC200 RNA in normal human neocortex, non-Alzheimer dementia (NAD), and senile dementia of the Alzheimer type (AD). *Neurochem Res* (1992) **17**:591–7. doi:10.1007/BF00968788
5. Jiang T, Yu JT, Tian Y, Tan L. Epidemiology and etiology of Alzheimer's disease: from genetic to non-genetic factors. *Curr Alzheimer Res* (2013) **10**:852–67. doi:10.2174/15672050113109990155
6. Guerreiro RJ, Gustafson DR, Hardy J. The genetic architecture of Alzheimer's disease: beyond APP, PSENs and APOE. *Neurobiol Aging* (2012) **33**:437–56. doi:10.1016/j.neurobiolaging.2010.03.025

7. Canobbio I, Abubaker AA, Visconte C, Torti M, Pula G. Role of amyloid peptides in vascular dysfunction and platelet dysregulation in Alzheimer's disease. *Front Cell Neurosci* (2015) **9**:65. doi:10.3389/fncel.2015.00065
8. Kim DH, Yeo SH, Park JM, Choi JY, Lee TH, Park SY, et al. Genetic markers for diagnosis and pathogenesis of Alzheimer's disease. *Gene* (2014) **545**:185–93. doi:10.1016/j.gene.2014.05.031
9. Lukiw WJ. Variability in micro RNA (miRNA) abundance, speciation and complexity amongst different human populations and potential relevance to Alzheimer's disease (AD). *Front Cell Neurosci* (2013) **7**:133. doi:10.3389/fncel.2013.00133
10. Sherva R, Tripodis Y, Bennett DA, Chibnik LB, Crane PK, de Jager PL, et al. Genome-wide association study of the rate of cognitive decline in Alzheimer's disease. *Alzheimers Dement* (2014) **10**:45–52. doi:10.1016/j.jalz.2013.01.008
11. Jin SC, Carrasquillo MM, Benitez BA, Skorupa T, Carrell D, Patel D, et al. TREM2 is associated with increased risk for Alzheimer's disease in African Americans. *Mol Neurodegener* (2015) **10**:19–26. doi:10.1186/s13024-015-0016-9
12. Barnes J, Dickerson BC, Frost C, Jiskoot LC, Wolk D, van der Flier WM. Alzheimer's disease first symptoms are age dependent: evidence from the NACC dataset. *Alzheimers Dement* (2015). doi:10.1016/j.jalz.2014.12.007
13. Verhülsdonk S, Hellen F, Höft B, Supprian T, Lange-Asschenfeldt C. Attention and CERAD test performances in cognitively impaired elderly subjects. *Acta Neurol Scand* (2015) **131**:364–71. doi:10.1111/ane.12346
14. Praticò D. Alzheimer's disease and the quest for its biological measures. *J Alzheimers Dis* (2013) **33**:S237–41. doi:10.3233/JAD-2012-129023
15. Wang Z, Wang J, Zhang H, Mchugh R, Sun X, Li K, et al. Interhemispheric functional and structural disconnection in Alzheimer's disease: a combined resting-state fMRI and DTI Study. *PLoS One* (2015) **10**(5):e0126310. doi:10.1371/journal.pone.0126310
16. Walhovd KB, Fjell AM, Espeseth T. Cognitive decline and brain pathology in aging-need for a dimensional, lifespan and systems vulnerability view. *Scand J Psychol* (2014) **55**:244–54. doi:10.1111/sjop.12120
17. Kim MO, Geschwind MD. Clinical update of Jakob-Creutzfeldt disease. *Curr Opin Neurol* (2015) **28**:302–10. doi:10.1097/WCO.0000000000000197
18. Li JQ, Tan L, Wang HF, Tan MS, Tan L, Xu W, et al. Risk factors for predicting progression from mild cognitive impairment to Alzheimer's disease: a systematic review and meta-analysis of cohort studies. *J Neurol Neurosurg Psychiatry* (2015). doi:10.1136/jnnp-2014-310095
19. Colangelo V, Schurr J, Ball MJ, Pelaez RP, Bazan NG, Lukiw WJ. Gene expression profiling of 12633 genes in Alzheimer hippocampal CA1. *J Neurosci Res* (2002) **70**:462–73. doi:10.1002/jnr.10351
20. Loring JF, Wen X, Lee JM, Seilhamer J, Somogyi R. A gene expression profile of Alzheimer's disease. *DNA Cell Biol* (2002) **20**:683–95. doi:10.1089/10445490152717541
21. Arevalo-Rodriguez I, Smailagic N, Roqué I, Figuls M, Ciapponi A, Sanchez-Perez E, et al. Mini-Mental State Examination (MMSE) for the detection of Alzheimer's disease and other dementias in people with mild cognitive impairment (MCI). *Cochrane Database Syst Rev* (2015) **3**:CD010783. doi:10.1002/14651858.CD010783.pub2
22. Blennow K, Dubois B, Fagan AM, Lewczuk P, de Leon MJ, Hampel H. Clinical utility of cerebrospinal fluid biomarkers in the diagnosis of early Alzheimer's disease. *Alzheimers Dement* (2015) **11**(1):58–69. doi:10.1016/j.jalz.2014.02.004
23. Chitravas N, Jung RS, Kofskey DM, Blevins JE, Gambetti P, Leigh RJ, et al. Treatable neurological disorders misdiagnosed as Creutzfeldt-Jakob disease. *Ann Neurol* (2011) **70**(3):437–44. doi:10.1002/ana.22454
24. Counts SE, Alldred MJ, Che S, Ginsberg SD, Mufson EJ. Synaptic gene dysregulation within hippocampal CA1 pyramidal neurons in mild cognitive impairment. *Neuropharmacology* (2014) **79**:172–9. doi:10.1016/j.neuropharm.2013.10.018
25. Chouraki V, Seshadri S. Genetics of Alzheimer's disease. *Adv Genet* (2014) **87**:245–94. doi:10.1016/B978-0-12-800149-3.00005-6
26. Tan MS, Jiang T, Tan L, Yu JT. Genome-wide association studies in neurology. *Ann Transl Med* (2014) **2**:124. doi:10.3978/j.issn.2305-5839.2014.11.12
27. Tai LM, Ghura S, Koster KP, Liakaite V, Maienschein-Cline M, Kanabar P, et al. APOE-modulated Aβ-induced neuroinflammation in Alzheimer's disease. *J Neurochem* (2015) **133**:465–88. doi:10.1111/jnc.13072
28. Yaghmoor F, Noorsaeed A, Alsaggaf S, Aljohani W, Scholtzova H, Boutajangout A, et al. The role of TREM2 in Alzheimer's disease and other neurological disorders. *J Alzheimers Dis Parkinsonism* (2014) **4**(5):160. doi:10.4172/2161-0460.1000160
29. Cheng XJ, Gao Y, Zhao YW, Cheng XD. Sodium chloride increases Aβ Levels by suppressing Aβ clearance in cultured cells. *PLoS One* (2015) **10**:e0130432. doi:10.1371/journal.pone.0130432
30. Baumgart M, Snyder HM, Carrillo MC, Fazio S, Kim H, Johns H. Summary of the evidence on modifiable risk factors for cognitive decline and dementia: a population-based perspective. *Alzheimers Dement* (2015) **11**:718–26. doi:10.1016/j.jalz.2015.05.016
31. Østergaard SD, Mukherjee S, Sharp SJ, Proitsi P, Lotta LA, Day F, et al. Associations between potentially modifiable risk factors and Alzheimer disease. *PLoS Med* (2015) **12**:e1001841. doi:10.1371/journal.pmed.1001841
32. Bhela S, Mulik S, Reddy PB, Richardson RL, Gimenez F, Rajasagi NK, et al. Critical role of microRNA-155 in herpes simplex encephalitis. *J Immunol* (2014) **192**:2734–43. doi:10.4049/jimmunol.1302326
33. Hill JM, Clement C, Zhao Y, Lukiw WJ. Induction of the pro-inflammatory NF-kB-sensitive miRNA-146a by human neurotrophic viruses. *Front Microbiol* (2015) **6**:43. doi:10.3389/fmicb.2015.00043
34. Alexandrov PN, Zhao Y, Jones BM, Bhattacharjee S, Lukiw WJ. Expression of the phagocytosis-essential protein TREM2 is down-regulated by an aluminum-induced miRNA-34a in a murine microglial cell line. *J Inorg Biochem* (2013) **128**:267–9. doi:10.1016/j.jinorgbio.2013.05.010
35. Pogue AI, Percy ME, Cui JG, Li YY, Bhattacharjee S, Hill JM, et al. Up-regulation of NF-kB-sensitive miRNA-125b and miRNA-146a in metal sulfate-stressed human astroglial (HAG) primary cell cultures. *J Inorg Biochem* (2011) **105**:1434–7. doi:10.1016/j.jinorgbio.2011.05.012
36. Müller M, Jäkel L, Bruinsma IB, Claassen JA, Kuiperij HB, Verbeek MM. microRNA-29a is a candidate biomarker for Alzheimer's disease in cell-free cerebrospinal fluid. *Mol Neurobiol* (2015). doi:10.1007/s12035-015-9156-8
37. Sala Frigerio C, Lau P, Salta E, Tournoy J, Bossers K, Vandenberghe R, et al. Reduced expression of hsa-miR-27a-3p in CSF of patients with Alzheimer disease. *Neurology* (2013) **81**:2103–6. doi:10.1212/01.wnl.0000437306.37850.22
38. Liu CG, Wang JL, Li L, Wang PC. MicroRNA-384 regulates both amyloid precursor protein and β-secretase expression and is a potential biomarker for Alzheimer's disease. *Int J Mol Med* (2014) **34**:160–6. doi:10.3892/ijmm.2014.1780
39. Nagpal N, Kulshreshtha R. miR-191: an emerging player in disease biology. *Front Genet* (2014) **5**:99. doi:10.3389/fgene.2014.00099
40. Wang T, Chen K, Li H, Dong S, Su N, Liu Y, et al. The feasibility of utilizing plasma miRNA107 and BACE1 messenger RNA gene expression for clinical diagnosis of amnestic mild cognitive impairment. *J Clin Psychiatry* (2015) **76**:135–41. doi:10.4088/JCP.13m08812
41. Xie B, Zhou H, Zhang R, Song M, Yu L, Wang L, et al. Serum miR-206 and miR-132 as potential circulating biomarkers for mild cognitive impairment. *J Alzheimers Dis* (2015) **45**:721–31. doi:10.3233/JAD-142847
42. Tan L, Yu JT, Liu QY, Tan MS, Zhang W, Hu N, et al. Circulating miR-125b as a biomarker of Alzheimer's disease. *J Neurol Sci* (2014) **336**:52–6. doi:10.1016/j.jns.2013.10.002
43. Tiribuzi R, Crispoltoni L, Porcellati S, Di Lullo M, Florenzano F, Pirro M, et al. miR128 up-regulation correlates with impaired amyloid β(1-42) degradation in monocytes from patients with sporadic Alzheimer's disease. *Neurobiol Aging* (2014) **35**:345–56. doi:10.1016/j.neurobiolaging.2013.08.003
44. Leidinger P, Backes C, Deutscher S, Schmitt K, Mueller SC, Frese K, et al. A blood based 12-miRNA signature of Alzheimer disease patients. *Genome Biol* (2013) **14**:R78. doi:10.1186/gb-2013-14-7-r78
45. Satoh J, Kino Y, Niida S. MicroRNA-seq data analysis pipeline to identify blood biomarkers for Alzheimer's disease from public data. *Biomark Insights* (2015) **10**:21–31. doi:10.4137/BMI.S25132
46. Burgos K, Malenica I, Metpally R, Courtright A, Rakela B, Beach T, et al. Profiles of extracellular miRNA in CSF and serum from patients with Alzheimer's and Parkinson's diseases correlate with disease status and features of pathology. *PLoS One* (2014) **9**:e94839. doi:10.1371/journal.pone.0094839
47. Gstir R, Schafferer S, Scheideler M, Misslinger M, Griehl M, Daschil N, et al. Generation of a neurospecific microarray reveals novel differentially expressed noncoding RNAs in mouse models for neurodegenerative diseases. *RNA* (2014) **20**:1929–43. doi:10.1261/rna.047225.114
48. Kumar RM, Cahan P, Shalek AK, Satija R, Daley Keyser AJ, Li H, et al. Deconstructing transcriptional heterogeneity in pluripotent stem cells. *Nature* (2014) **516**:56–61. doi:10.1038/nature13920
49. Patel AP, Tirosh I, Trombetta JJ, Shalek AK, Gillespie SM, Wakimoto H, et al. Single-cell RNA-seq highlights intratumoral heterogeneity in primary glioblastoma. *Science* (2015) **344**:1396–401. doi:10.1126/science.1254257

50. Danborg PB, Simonsen AH, Waldemar G, Heegaard NH. The potential of miRNAs as biofluid markers of neuro-degenerative disease - a systematic review. *Biomarkers* (2014) **19**:259–68. doi:10.3109/1354750X.2014.904001
51. Wang X, Tan L, Lu Y, Peng J, Zhu Y, Zhang Y, et al. MicroRNA-138 promotes tau phosphorylation by targeting retinoic acid receptor alpha. *FEBS Lett* (2015) **589**:726–9. doi:10.1016/j.febslet.2015.02.001
52. Femminella GD, Ferrara N, Rengo G. The emerging role of microRNAs in Alzheimer's disease. *Front Physiol* (2015) **6**:40. doi:10.3389/fphys.2015.00040
53. Cheng L, Quek CY, Sun X, Bellingham SA, Hill AF. The detection of microRNA associated with Alzheimer's disease in biological fluids using next-generation sequencing technologies. *Front Genet* (2013) **4**:150. doi:10.3389/fgene.2013.00150
54. Koh W, Pan W, Gawad C, Fan HC, Kerchner GA, Wyss-Coray T, et al. Noninvasive in vivo monitoring of tissue-specific global gene expression in humans. *Proc Natl Acad Sci U S A* (2014) **111**:7361–6. doi:10.1073/pnas.1405528111
55. Grasso M, Piscopo P, Confaloni A, Denti MA. Circulating miRNAs as biomarkers for neurodegenerative disorders. *Molecules* (2014) **19**:6891–910. doi:10.3390/molecules19056891
56. Liu ZP. Reverse engineering of genome-wide gene regulatory networks from gene expression data. *Curr Genomics* (2015) **16**:3–22. doi:10.2174/1389202915666141110210634
57. Li Y, Zhang Z. Computational Biology in microRNA. *Wiley Interdiscip Rev RNA* (2015) **6**(4):435–52. doi:10.1002/wrna.1286
58. Michaud M, Balardy L, Moulis G, Gaudin C, Peyrot C, Vellas B, et al. Proinflammatory cytokines, aging, and age-related diseases. *J Am Med Dir Assoc* (2013) **14**:877–82. doi:10.1016/j.jamda.2013.05.009

13

Biochemical markers of physical exercise on mild cognitive impairment and dementia

Camilla Steen Jensen[1]*, *Steen Gregers Hasselbalch*[1,2], *Gunhild Waldemar*[1,2] *and Anja Hviid Simonsen*[1]

[1] *Department of Neurology, Danish Dementia Research Centre, Rigshospitalet – Copenhagen University Hospital, Copenhagen, Denmark,* [2] *Department of Clinical Medicine, University of Copenhagen, Copenhagen, Denmark*

Edited by:
Charlotte Elisabeth Teunissen, VU University Medical Center, Netherlands

Reviewed by:
Jason Eriksen, University of Houston, USA
Wiesje M. Van Der Flier, VU University Medical Center, Netherlands

Correspondence:
Camilla Steen Jensen, Department of Neurology, Danish Dementia Research Center, Copenhagen University Hospital Rigshospitalet, Blegdamsvej 9, Copenhagen DK-2100, Denmark camilla.steen.jensen@regionh.dk

Background: The cognitive effects of physical exercise in patients with dementia disorders or mild cognitive impairment have been examined in various studies; however the biochemical effects of exercise from intervention studies are largely unknown. The objective of this systematic review is to investigate the published results on biomarkers in physical exercise intervention studies in patients with MCI or dementia.

Methods: The PubMed database was searched for studies from 1976 to February 2015. We included intervention studies investigating the effect of physical exercise activity on biomarkers in patients with MCI or dementia.

Results: A total of eight studies were identified (n = 447 patients) evaluating exercise regimes with variable duration (single session–three sessions/week for 26 weeks) and intensity (light-resistance training–high-intensity aerobic exercise). Various biomarkers were measured before and after intervention. Seven of the eight studies found a significant effect on their selected biomarkers with a positive effect of exercise on brain-derived neurotrophic factor, cholesterol, testosterone, estradiol, dehydroepiadrosterone, and insulin in the intervention groups compared with controls.

Conclusion: Although few studies suggest a beneficial effect on selected biomarkers, we need more knowledge of the biochemical effect of physical exercise in dementia or MCI.

Keywords: dementia, MCI, exercise intervention, biomarkers, physical activity

Introduction

The prevalence of dementia is increasing, currently affecting more than 44 million people, and estimated affect 75 million people worldwide by 2030. Alzheimer's disease (AD) accounts for the majority of dementia cases (1–3). Currently there is no cure for these disorders, and there are currently no effective pharmacological interventions (4, 5). Attention has therefore turned toward non-pharmacological approaches, including exercise, to slow the cognitive decline associated with dementia (2, 6). Linking evidence from population-based cohorts or RCT studies with biochemical evidence will be crucial in order to understand how non-pharmacological interventions may potentially alter the course of the disease.

In epidemiological studies, retrospective cohort studies, and case–control studies, there is consensus that an active lifestyle in midlife decreases the risk of dementia in late adulthood (7, 8). The cognitive effects of physical exercise and an active lifestyle in healthy elderly subjects, and in those with MCI and dementia, have also been examined in various cross-sectional studies, intervention studies, and prospective studies, with conflicting results (9–21). Almost all studies in patients with mild cognitive impairment (MCI) show some effect on cognition, but recent systematic reviews call for caution when interpreting results in dementia due to limited evidence (22, 23). Lack of consensus could be due to differences in the study methodologies used, type of physical activity, or in the cognitive measures used.

Because some studies have identified a clinical effect of physical exercise, it is imperative to understand if and how exercise alters the pathophysiology of dementia. Such an understanding is necessary for the successful promotion and implementation of physical exercise as a part of the treatment for dementia. Our current knowledge comes largely from animal studies. Beta-Amyloid (Aβ) pathology can be altered in response to exercise in a mouse and rat model for AD (24, 25), and brain plasticity proteins, like brain-derived neurotrophic factor (BDNF), can be up-regulated in response to physical exercise (26). Also, long-term exercise treatment reduces oxidative stress (OX) in the hippocampus of aging rats (27). In a large study of healthy elderly subjects, lower plasma and brain Aβ was observed in those reporting higher levels of physical activity (21), and similar findings has been found in preclinical AD subjects (28), consistent with animal studies suggesting that physical activity may modulate specific AD pathology in humans as well. However, because observational and cross-sectional designs cannot establish causality, we need randomized controlled intervention trials to understand the biochemical effects of exercise.

Exercise-based interventions studies in various diseases have clarified some of the biochemical effects of physical activity, such as improved metabolic homeostasis in diabetes mellitus (29), reduced OX in obese subjects (30), and reduced low-grade inflammation in coronary artery disease (31). Thus, physical exercise may exert its effect through modulation of specific AD pathology and/or through pathological processes common to other diseases.

Therefore, the object of this study was to systematically review and evaluate the scientific literature regarding the biochemical effect of exercise in MCI and dementia disorders in intervention trials and furthermore to provide recommendations for future biochemical studies in this field. Based on the studies cited above, we hypothesized that physical exercise interventions would improve not only specific Aβ pathology, but also pathological processes downstream of Aβ accumulation.

Methods

This systematic review was performed according to the recommendation of the Cochrane collaboration (32) and the Preferred Reporting Items for Systematic Review and Meta-Analysis: the PRISMA statement (33).

Eligibility Criteria

Randomized controlled trials or clinical trials investigating the effect of physical exercise or activity on patients with MCI or dementia were selected to review. Studies must have obtained bio-fluid markers, regardless of whether the biomarkers were included as primary or secondary outcome.

Search Strategy

The following electronic database was searched: MEDLINE (accessed via PubMed). The database PubMed was selected because it contains more that 23 million citations from biomedical literature from MEDLINE, life science journals and online books.

The search conducted in February 2015 searched databases for the following MeSH terms and their English synonyms. Studies published from 1976 to 2015 were included.

Medline (Via Pubmed.org) was searched with the keywords and Boolean operators with the filter English and Human:

("Dementia"[Majr]) AND ("Exercise"[Majr])
("Mild Cognitive impairment"[Majr]) AND ("Exercise"[Majr])
("Dementia"[Majr]) AND ("physical fitness"[Majr])
("Mild Cognitive impairment"[Majr]) AND ("Physical fitness"[Majr])

The search was done by two authors separately (first and second) author. The search results are described in **Figure 1**.

Inclusion criteria included: original work (no review or meta-analysis), physical activity/exercise as intervention, only full-text publication, and English language.

Study Selection and Data Extraction

Studies were selected on the basis of the inclusion criteria listed above. The selected studies are listed in **Table 1** and Table S1 in Supplementary Material. Data extraction was done by the first author according to the data extraction form seen in Table S2 in Supplementary Material, in regards to author, endpoints measured, subjects, intervention, and results found.

Results

The initial search gave 228 publications, from which 187 were collected for further reading and 111 of which were excluded due to irrelevance or because they did not meet the inclusion criteria on the basis of their title or abstract. From the remaining 76 publications, 54 met inclusion and exclusion criteria and were selected for analysis. After a detailed analysis, publications were excluded if they did not include analysis of biomarkers. The excluded publications are listed in Table S1 in Supplementary Material. In total, eight publications remained for inclusion in the review. Publications included are listed in **Table 1**. **Figure 1** shows the flowchart of the data gathering process.

Sample Subjects

Although our MeSH term search covered all dementia diagnoses, the majority of identified publications studied patients

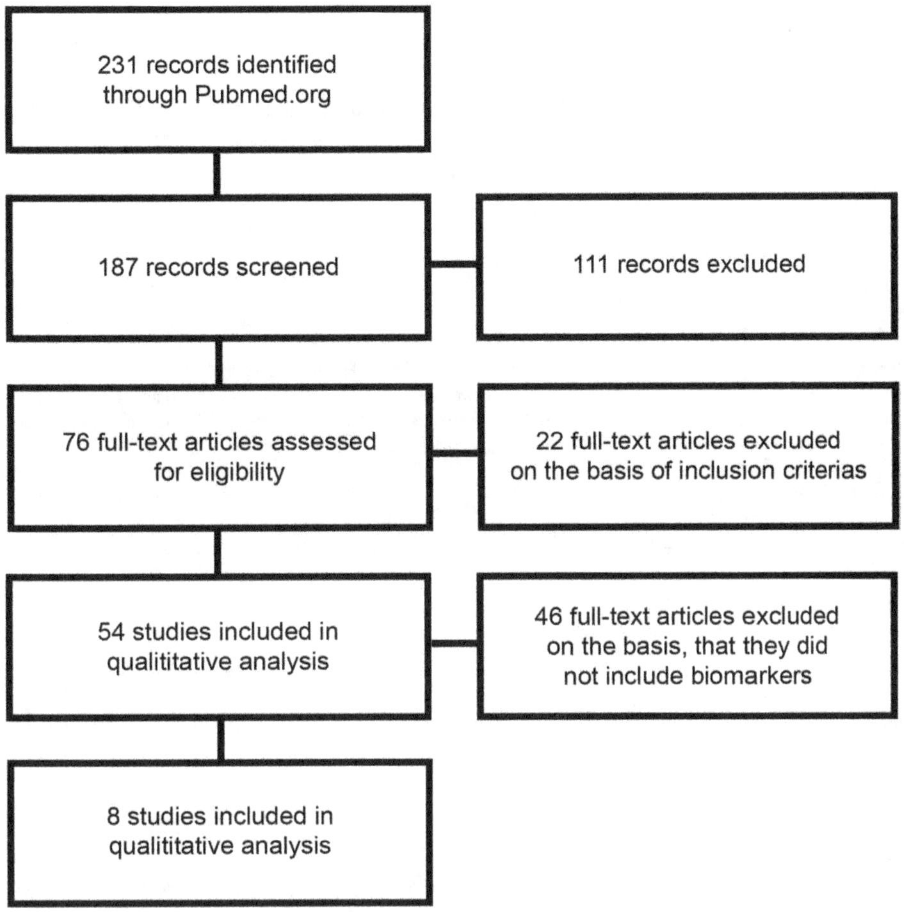

FIGURE 1 | Flowchart of the publication search and selection process.

with AD. Subjects were either from a nursing home-residing population (15, 35, 37) or a home-living population (34, 41, 42). Two studies did not describe living status (38, 41).

In **Table 1**, mean age and mean MMSE have been listed, giving a general indication of the sample subjects studied. The age range was from 66.4 to 85.4 years. The MMSE range was from 13.9 to 28.7. Only Baker et al. have a population with a MMSE above 21, which indicated that the majority of the studies have been on patients with moderate-to-severe dementia.

Sample Size

The numbers of subjects used in the selected studies range from 13 to 110 subjects. In general, the small sample sizes have generated little power for calculation of effect.

Exercise Protocol

Four studies implemented an aerobic training program with low-to-high intensity (34, 35, 37, 39), three studies investigated the effect of a single bout of high-intensity aerobic or resistance training exercise (38, 41, 42) and one study investigated the effect of light resistance training and stretching (15). Thus, most studies investigated aerobic training to investigate the effect on biochemical biomarkers. The studies reviewed applied very different training regimes, with regards to intensity, duration and frequency. Eggermont et al. (37) applied the lowest intensity with a walking program at a self-selected speed, and they did not report any significant results on any of their selected biomarkers. Cheng et al. applied a light exercise program and found that the exercise groups had a slower decline in their cognitive measures compared to controls. The three remaining aerobic exercise studies have applied a moderate-to-high-intensity exercise program, and they found a significant increase in levels of their selected biomarkers, and in the cognitive measures.

Exercise Supervision

Five of the eight selected studies had non-supervised training or supervision by caregivers. Three studies had supervision by trainers. Two studies reported use of heart rate monitors to ensure that the intended exercise intensity of the exercise was reached. In Baker et al. (34), only some of the training sessions were supervised.

Cognition

Six out of these eight studies also investigated cognitive performance (15, 34, 35, 37, 39, 41). Of these six studies, four reported

TABLE 1 | Studies chosen for review.

Publication	Endpoint	Subjects	Intervention	Results on cognition	Results biomarkers
Akishita et al. (15)	Cognitive markers ADL MMSE Blood markers: Estradiol Testosterone DHEA DHEA sulfate Sex hormone-binding globulin	13 ♀ AD[a] Nursing home residents Mean age: 84.5 ± 5 Mean MMSE: 13.9 ± 1.9	*N* = 13, resistance training (light) + stretching 30 min 2/week[c] + 5/week[b] × 12 weeks	No change in MMSE No change in ADL	↑ Testosterone ↑ Estradiol ↑ DHEA
Baker et al. (34)	Cognitive markers: Symbol-digit modalities Verbal fluency Trail B STROOP Task switching Story recall List-learning Blood markers: Insulin IGF-1 Cortisol BDNF Platelet factor 4 $A\beta_{42}$ Cholesterol Cardio markers: VO_2 peak	29 MCI[a] Home living Mean age Stretching 66 ± 6.0 Intervention 71 ± 7.5 Mean MMSE Stretching 28.8 ± 1.0 Intervention 28.6 ± 1.2	*n* = 10, stretching (<50% HRR) 45–60 min 4/week × 26 weeks[c] *n* = 19, aerobic exercise (75–85% HRR) 45–60 min 4/week × 26 weeks[c]	♀ Increased executive function Increased performance in STROOP Both Increased performance in trail B	Gender difference ♀ ↑ Insulin sensitivity ↑ Insulin ↑ Cortisol in control group ↑ BDNF ♂ ↓ Cortisol in controls group ↓ BDNF ↑ IGF-1 Both ↓ Body fat ↓ Total Cholesterol ↑ VO_2 peak
Cheng et al. (35)	Cognitive markers: MMSE Call-recall Categorical fluency Digit span Blood markers: Cholesterol HDL Tri-glycerides Glucose Genetic markers: ApoE genotype	110 dementia[a] Nursing home residents Mean age Control 80.8 ± 7.2 Mahjong 81.9 ± 6.2 Tai Chi 81.8 ± 7.4 Mean MMSE Control 18.8 ± 4.1 Mahjong 19.0 ± 3.2 Tai Chi 18.7 ± 3.9	*n* = 39, aerobic exercise (Tai Chi) 60 min 3/week × 12 weeks[b] *n* = 36, cognitive activity (Mahjong) 60 min 3/week × 12 weeks[b]	Tai Chi Slower decline in cognitive measures Mahjong Slower decline in cognitive measures	Non-reported
Coelho et al. (36)	Blood markers: BDNF	21 AD[a] 18 cognitive normal (used as controls) Home living Mean age AD 76.3 ± 6.2 Controls 74.5 ± 4.7 Mean MMSE AD 21.0 ± 3.9 Controls 28.0 ± 2.5	*n* = 39, acute aerobic exercise (85% HRR) 17–22 min once[c]	None studied	Both: ↑ BDNF
Eggermont et al. (37)	Cognitive markers MMSE Face recognition Picture recognition Delayed word call Digit span backwards Category fluency Letter fluency Genetic markers ApoE	97 dementia[a] Nursing home residents Mean age: 85.4 Mean MMSE: 17.7	*n* = 51, walking 30 min 5/week × 6 weeks[b]	No significant results reported	No significant results reported

(Continued)

TABLE 1 | Continued

Publication	Endpoint	Subjects	Intervention	Results on cognition	Results biomarkers
Mancuso et al. (38)	Blood markers: COX Lactate	18 AD[a] 20 cognitive normal No mention of living status Mean age AD 66.4 ± 8.9 Controls 63.4 ± 9.1 Mean MMSE AD 17.4 ± 4.9 Controls, not reported	*n* = 38, acute resistance training (increment 10–70% 1RM) once[b]	Not studied	↑ Lactate ↓ Lactate recovery after exercise ↓ COX activity
Nascimento et al. (39, 41)	Cognitive markers: MoCA Blood markers BDNF TNF-α IL-6	37 MCI[a] 30 cognitive normal Home living Mean age MCI used as controls 68.5 ± 5.9 MCI exercise 67.3 ± 5.3 Cognitive normal used as controls 68.1 ± 5.7 Cognitive normal exercise 66.6 ± 7.9 Median MoCA MCI used as controls 21 MCI exercise 20 Cognitive normal used as controls 27 Cognitive normal exercise 27	*n* = 35 (20 MCI, 15),aerobic exercise (60–80% HRR) 60 min 3/week × 16 weeks[c]	MCI: increased cognition	Both ↓ TNF ↓ IL
Segal et al. (41)	Cognitive marker: IAPS Saliva markers: alpha-amylase	23 aMCI[a] 31 cognitive normal No mentioning of home status Mean age aMCI 71.4 ± 2.4 Cognitive normal 69 ± 2 Mean MMSE aMCI, not reported Cognitive normal, not reported	*n* = 26 (11a MCI, 15 controls) acute aerobic exercise (70% VO_{2max}) 6 min once[b]	Both: increased picture recall	Both: ↑ saliva alpha-amylase

ADL, activities of daily living; DHEA, dehydroepiadrosterone; AD, Alzheimer's disease; aMCI, amnestic mild cognitive impairment; MCI, mild cognitive impairment; IGF-1, insulin-like growth factor 1; BDNF, brain-derived neurotrophic factor; $A\beta_{40+42}$, beta-amyloid isoform 40 and 42; VO_2 peak, peak oxygen uptake; HRR, heart rate reserve; ♀, women; ♂, men; MMSE, mini-mental state examination; HDL, high-density lipoprotein; COX, cytochrome c oxidase; MoCA, Montreal Cognitive Assessment; TNF-a, tumor necrosis factor alpha; IL-6, interleukin-6; IPAS; International Affective Picture Set.

[a]Diagnosed according to international guidelines.

[b]Supervised by caregiver, healthcare worker, or not mentioned.

[c]Supervised by trainer or physiotherapist.

any significant effect on the cognitive measures. Baker et al. (34) reported an improvement in several tests of executive function, but only in women, Cheng et al. (35) reported a reduced decline in MMSE, Nascimento et al. (39) found an improved cognition measured by the Montreal Cognitive Assessment (MoCA), and Segal et al. (41) found a significant improved picture recall after exercise.

Effect on Biomarkers

In total, eight studies that focused on biochemical markers were identified. Seven out of eight studies investigated protein biomarkers (15, 34, 35, 38–42), and two studies investigated the difference in the effect of exercise depending on the patients ApoE genotype (35, 37). One study also investigated markers of cardiovascular health (34). **Table 1** summarized the biochemical and cognitive findings.

In seven out of eight studies, a positive relationship was found between their selected biomarkers and the exercise intervention. Only one study did not find any significant results on any of their selected biomarkers (37).

Coelho et al. (36) and Segal et al. (41), found that exercise resulted in a significant up-regulation in the neuroplasticity protein BDNF. Baker et al. (34) also measured BDNF and found higher levels after exercise, however only in women. Nascimento et al. reported BDNF as one of their end points, however they did not report any findings. They did, however, report decreased Tumor necrosis factor alpha (TNF-α) and interleukin-6 (IL-6) levels after exercise.

Besides blood levels of BDNF, other biochemical compounds in blood including cholesterol and insulin were analyzed. Baker et al. (34) and Cheng et al. (35), measured plasma levels of insulin and cholesterol. Cheng et al. (35) also measured HDL, tri-glycerides, and glucose. Only Baker et al. (34) reported an effect of the intervention on these biomarkers, namely a significant decrease in cholesterol and an increase in insulin sensitivity.

On a different note besides neurological markers and metabolic markers, Akishita et al. (15) found that exercise had a significant up-regulating effect on selected sex hormones (testosterone, estradiol, and DEHA) in women. Segal et al. (41) found an increase in salivary alpha-amylase (sAA), an indirect measure of endogenous norepinephrine (NE), after a single session of high-intensity exercise (70% HRR). Mancuso et al. (38) found that lactate increased after exercise, and that platelet mitochondria COX activity was decreased.

We did not find any intervention studies that investigated the effect of exercise on established diagnostic markers for dementia disease, such as Aβ, tau, p-tau, and α-synuclein.

Discussion

Physical exercise as a non-pharmacological treatment for medical disease has proven beneficial for reducing the risk for many diseases including stroke, high blood pressure, and mental disorders like chronic stress and depression (43). However, compared to our understanding or physical exercise's impact on cardiovascular health and general fitness, our understanding of physical exercise's impact on cognitive health is still very much in its infancy. An impact of physical exercise on quality of life and activity of daily living in patients with dementia has been established; however evidence of the molecular effects is not clear.

The objective of this study was to conduct a systematic review to identify and evaluate the scientific literature published on the effect of an exercise intervention in dementia, in regards to relevant biomarkers.

Biochemical Evidence of the Effects of Exercise

Insulin and diabetes have been connected to an increased risk of developing AD and cognitive impairment (44, 45). Two of the reviewed studies measured insulin sensitivity or glucose control. Baker et al. (34) found increased insulin sensitivity and increased insulin in the exercise group, however only in women. Cheng et al. (35) measured blood glucose levels, but they did not find any significant result.

Mancuso et al. (38) investigated the reactive oxygen species (ROS) generation and OX, measured via COX activity and lactate production in platelets. ROS and OX are thought to be involved in AD through the neurotoxicity of amyloid build up, metabolic impairments and free-radical production in mitochondria (46, 47). To investigate the metabolic contribution of mitochondrial impairment, COX activity and lactate production was measured before and after an exercise intervention. At baseline, the AD groups displayed higher levels of lactate and significantly lower activity of COX, compared to aged match cognitive normal individuals. This increased level of lactate in AD patients was unchanged throughout the exercise intervention, indicating mitochondrial impairment in AD. The exercise intervention did not alter COX activity, indicating that exercise might not be able to influence the mitochondrial electron transport chain (ETC). However, since Mancuso et al. (38) did not find any correlation with cognitive elements, such as MMSE, mitochondrial impairment might be an angle to study the pathology of AD, and not so much a way to improve cognitive decline.

Nascimento et al. (39, 41) investigated the influence of exercise on inflammation markers in MCI and cognitively normal subjects and found decreased levels of the pro-inflammatory cytokines, TNF-α and IL-6. Inflammation is a known factor in neurodegenerative diseases (48–50). Both pro-inflammatory cytokines (e.g., IL-6) and anti-inflammatory cytokines (e.g., IL-10 and IL-18) have been found to be increased in AD (51), and wherein it is speculated that an increased inflammatory response negatively contributes to neurodegeneration in AD (50). Several studies have shown that inflammation is directly influenced by physical activity, which down-regulates pro-inflammatory reactions in the brain (52). For further insight into the pathology of neuroinflammation, it might be beneficial to measure a variety of factors, both pro-inflammatory and anti-inflammatory.

Three of eight identified studies have focused on BDNF, all of which found an increase in BDNF after exercise. Lower levels of brain tissue BDNF have been seen in patients with AD compared to healthy controls (26, 53). The exercise-induced BDNF increase seen in the studies in this review has also been reported in animal studies, where brain levels of BDNF were increased after exercise (26), and in an intervention study in young healthy men, where plasma BDNF was increased with exercise. In order to achieve a more precise measurement of neuronal BDNF without the systemic component, BDNF levels in CSF could be assessed.

Alongside BDNF, Akishita et al. (15) measured increased levels of female sex hormones after exercise. Lower levels of sex hormones have previously been shown to increase the risk of AD (54). Exercise has been found to increase sex hormones and sex hormone-binding globulin in post-menstrual women (55–57). One could therefore speculate that an increase in sex hormones is beneficial to the cognitive performance in patients already diagnosed with AD. In the study by Akishita et al. (15), there was no effect on ADL or cognition, and the up-regulating effect of exercise on sex hormones was lost after 3 months post-exercise.

Pharmacological evidence established that NE is involved in memory modulation, and can be regulated by exercise (58–60). This makes NE modulation by exercise an ideal target for memory modulation in patients with cognitive impairments. Segal et al. (41) studied this relationship with a single bout of high-intensity exercise in patients with aMCI. The cognitive performance was investigated with picture recall before and after exercise, and NE was measured indirectly via sAA. They found that performance in picture recall was significantly improved in the exercise cognitive normal control group as well in the exercise aMCI groups, and not in the corresponding non-exercise groups. Furthermore, sAA levels were equally increased in both exercise groups (cognitive normal and aMCI). When it comes to dementia diseases, like AD with more advanced neurodegeneration, it is unknown if exercise is able to up-regulate NE, so further studies are needed. In addition, the potential harms of recurring acute increases in NE need to be investigated.

None of the review studies in this review focused their attention on already previously established markers of neurodegenerative disease. Baker et al. (61) has studied the effect of a diet intervention with or without high-intensity physical activity, and its effect on CSF levels of the amyloidogenic peptide $A\beta_{42}$. The main outcome was that patients with MCI subjected to a modulated diet, and who had a high-intensity physically active lifestyle, had higher levels of CSF $A\beta_{42}$, than those without an active lifestyle. Furthermore, brain levels of $A\beta_{42}$ have been shown in animal studies to be reduced in response to physical exercise (62). $A\beta_{42}$ therefore appears to be a physiologically relevant biomarker that was not measured in any of the included studies likely due to difficulty of including CSF measures in study design, attributable to the discomfort of lumbar puncture.

Normal Aging

In previous studies on the effect of exercise in a population of healthy elderly individuals, a decrease in the metabolic biomarkers of cholesterol, HDL, and leptin (63) was described. Furthermore, the exercise group showed increased glucose sensitivity after intervention, compared to controls (63). Aging is connected with chronic low-grade inflammation, increased risk for disease, poor physical function and mortality (64). Exercise has been shown to decrease the levels of circulating inflammatory cytokines (65). The expected effects of exercise on biomarkers of metabolism and inflammation are similar between normal aging individuals and patients with dementia. In the study by Nascimento et al. (39, 41), where aged matched cognitive normal controls were studied, the effect of exercise on the inflammation biomarkers were not specific to either the dementia group or the control group. However, only the MCI group showed improved cognition. This could indicate a link between cognitive measures and alterations in the inflammation profile. One could speculate that the lack of effect on cognition seen in the control group could be due to the scale chosen for measuring cognition (MoCA). MoCA may not be sensitive enough to quantify cognition in a group that already performs well cognitively, as this group had high MoCA scores even before intervention, and thereby improvement in the controls group will not be detected.

BDNF has previously been investigated not only for its brain plasticity modulating effect in dementia patients, but also in subjects with depression (66) and in animal studies, high-intensity exercise has a modulating effect on BDNF (26). Studies have found that BDNF levels decline with age, and it has been shown to be associated with memory deficits (67). An up-regulation of BDNF would therefore be beneficial, and maybe act as a protecting factor against dementia and other memory deficiencies.

Genetic Risk Factors

The effect of the known risk factor for AD, ApoE (68), was found not to have an effect for the outcome on biomarkers after an exercise intervention. Previous studies have indicated that that outcome of an exercise intervention could be ApoE genotype dependent (69). However, neither Eggermont et al. (37) nor Cheng et al. (35), found any significant difference in effect according to ApoE genotype.

A possibility to further explore the ApoE effect on AD could be to investigate the gene product of ApoE, the protein apoE. A recent study has indicated that low levels of apoE increases risk of AD (70). Currently there are no plasma markers for AD, and perhaps apoE may have the potential to be a ground-breaking new risk factor for AD.

Exercise Intervention

In regards to the exercise protocol, most studies applied an aerobic training, like walking, to investigate the effect on biochemical markers. The studies reviewed have applied varying training regimes, durations, and frequencies. This makes a direct comparison difficult. However, most of the studies applying a moderate-to-high-intensity aerobic exercise protocol, have found a significant effect on biomarkers, while low-intensity protocols did not show significant effects. This could indicate that the level of intensity of the aerobic exercise is important for achieving an effect of an exercise intervention.

The level of supervision for protocol adherence and intensity varied greatly among the reviewed studies. Overall supervision is necessary to ensure general adherence to the program and that exercise intensity is maintained, especially when it comes to moderate-to-high-intensity exercise, where the physical demands on the patients are far greater. For example, supervised training sessions with professional trainers and equipment, such as a pulse watch, can be used.

Cognition

Another caveat worth considering is whether the effect of physical exercise on cognition is caused by measurable changes in biomarkers that reflect the pathophysiology of the disorder or whether exercise improves cognition through general improvement of brain function through other mechanisms. These could include up-regulation of neurotransmitters relevant for cognition, such as NE or increase in vascular endothelial growth factor (71). This remains to be determined.

Biomarkers are the main outcome assessed in this review article, but when studying dementias, cognitive measures have to be taken into account. It is unclear whether lack of cognitive assessment as a measured outcome is due to negative findings or that cognition went untested. Although a change in a biochemical markers with physical exercise does not imply a therapeutic effect on symptomatology, an objectively measurable effect on a relevant pathophysiological biochemical parameter will support the importance of an implementation of physical exercise as part of the treatment for dementia.

Recommendations for Sampling and Analysis

Of all the studies that have been conducted on exercise in patients with dementia disease or cognitive impairment, only eight studies have included biomarkers as a part of their assessment. However, the effect on functional activity and quality of life are relevant to the patient and caregiver, useful biochemical measures of these effects are still lacking.

Our recommendation for investigating the effect of physical exercise effect on dementia at a biochemical level is to (1) investigate whether any metabolic pathways that can be altered by increased physical activity could also be involved in dementia, (2) measure molecules from these pathways that have a neuronal contribution, and distinguishing their neuronal-specific contribution from systemic contribution, (3) investigate proteins and pathways that are involved not only in the generation and maintenance of neurons, but also relevant for cognitive function in general, and (4) measure an broad cytokine effect on neuroinflammation, since exercise has a putative anti-inflammatory effect (72).

Due to the fact that many established diagnostic markers for dementia disease are measured in CSF, including $A\beta_{42}$ (73), tau (74), p-tau (74), α-synuclein (75), and huntingtin (76), we would further recommend to include CSF assessment in future studies, as this better reflects cerebral biomarker levels.

In order to achieve valid biomarker measurements, the highest quality of samples for analysis are required, and we recommend that strict sampling processing and storage procedures are observed (77).

Conclusion

Eight out of fifty-four exercise studies in dementia or MCI have investigated biochemical markers of the effect of exercise on dementia and MCI. There is an overall trend of beneficial effect of exercise on the selected biomarkers. However, there were no studies that investigated specific Aβ pathology, or pathological processes downstream of Aβ accumulation.

Future studies with greater samples size, more thorough exercise supervision, educated trainers and well-defined intensity measures, as well as various sampling protocols (blood, CSF, etc.) are required. Such studies are in progress (78) and will hopefully help to understand the beneficial effect of physical exercise on dementia.

Author Contributions

Study conception and design: CJ, AS, and SH. Acquisition of data: CJ and SH. Analysis and interpretation of data: CJ, SH, GW, and AS. Drafting of manuscript: CJ, SH, GW, and AS. Critical revision: SH, GW, and AS.

Acknowledgments

The project was supported by the Innovation Fund Denmark. This study was performed under Neurodegenerative Disease Research (JPND) – Innovation fund Denmark (grant no. 0603-00470B).

References

1. Alzheimer's Disease International. *Policy Brief for Heads of Government: The Global Impact of Dementia*. London: Alzheimer's Disease International (2013). p. 2013–50.
2. Brookmeyer R, Johnson E, Ziegler-Graham K, Arrighi H. Forecasting the global burden of Alzheimer's disease. *Alzheimers Dement* (2007) **3**:186–9. doi:10.1016/j.jalz.2007.04.381
3. Thies W, Bleiler L. 2013 Alzheimer's disease facts and figures. *Alzheimers Dement* (2013) **9**:208–45. doi:10.1016/j.jalz.2013.02.003
4. Raina P, Santaguide P, Ismaila A, Patterson C, Cowan D, Levine M, et al. Effectiveness of cholinesterase inhibitor and memantine for treating dementia: evidence review for a clinical practive guideline. *Ann Intern Med* (2008) **148**:379–97. doi:10.7326/0003-4819-148-5-200803040-00009
5. Sink KM, Holden KF, Yaffe K. Pharmacological treatment of neuropsychiatric symptoms of dementia: a review of the evidence. *JAMA* (2005) **293**:596–608. doi:10.1001/jama.293.5.596
6. Mölsä P, Marttila R, Rinne U. Long-term survival and prediction of mortality in Alzheimer's disease and multi-infarct dementia. *Acta Neurol Scand* (1995) **91**:159–64. doi:10.1111/j.1600-0404.1995.tb00426.x
7. Andel R, Crowe M, Pedersen NL, Fratiglioni L, Johansson B, Gatz M. Physical exercise at midlife and risk of dementia three decades later: a population-based study of Swedish twins. *J Gerontol A Biol Sci Med Sci* (2008) **63**:62–6. doi:10.1093/gerona/63.1.62
8. Nyberg J, Åberg MAI, Schiöler L, Nilsson M, Wallin A, Torén K, et al. Cardiovascular and cognitive fitness at age 18 and risk of early-onset dementia. *Brain* (2014) **137**:1514–23. doi:10.1093/brain/awu041
9. Lytle ME, Vander Bilt J, Pandav RS, Dodge HH, Ganguli M. Exercise level and cognitive decline: the MoVIES Project. *Alzheimer Dis Assoc Disord* (2004) **18**:57–64. doi:10.1097/01.wad.0000126614.87955.79
10. Winchester J, DIck M, Gillen D, Reed B, Miller B, Tinklenberg J, et al. Walking stabilizes cognitive functioning in Alzheimer's disease (AD) across on year. *Arch Gerontol Geriatr* (2013) **56**:96–103. doi:10.1016/j.archger.2012.06.016
11. Bowen ME. A prospective examination of the relationship between physical activity and dementia risk in later life. *Am J Health Promot* (2012) **26**:333–40. doi:10.4278/ajhp.110311-QUAN-115
12. Middleton LE, Mitnitski A, Fallah N, Kirkland SA, Rockwood K. Changes in cognition and mortality in relation to exercise in late life: a population based study. *PLoS One* (2008) **3**:e3124. doi:10.1371/journal.pone.0003124
13. Barnes D, Santos-Modesitt W, Poelke G, Kramer A, Castro C, Middelton L, et al. The mental activity and exercise (MAX) trial: a randomized controlled trial to enhance cognitive function in older adults. *JAMA Intern Med* (2013) **173**:797–804. doi:10.1001/jamainternmed.2013.189
14. Chang S-H, Chen C-Y, Shen S-H, Chiou J-H. The effectiveness of an exercise programme for elders with dementia in a Taiwanese day-care centre. *Int J Nurs Pract* (2011) **17**:213–20. doi:10.1111/j.1440-172X.2011.01928.x
15. Akishita M, Yamada S, Nishiya H, Sonohara K, Nakai R, Toba K. Effects of physical exercise on plasma concentrations of sex hormones in elderly women with dementia. *J Am Geriatr Soc* (2005) **53**:1076–7. doi:10.1111/j.1532-5415.2005.53338_4.x
16. La Rue A, Felten K, Turkstra L. Intervention of multi-modal activities for older adults with dementia translation to rural communities. *Am J Alzheimers Dis Other Demen* (2015) **30**:468–77. doi:10.1177/1533317514568888
17. Hagerman PA, Thomas VS. Gait performance in dementia: the effects of a 6-week resistance training program in an adult day-care setting. *Int J Geriatr Psychiatry* (2002) **17**:329–34. doi:10.1002/gps.597
18. Uemura K, Shimada H, Makizako H, Doi T, Daisuke Y, Tsutsumimoto K, et al. Cognitive function affects trainability for physical performance in exercise intervention among older adults with mild cognitive impairment. *Clin Interv Aging* (2013) **8**:97–102. doi:10.2147/CIA.S39434
19. Yu F, Leon AS, Bliss D, Dysken M, Savik K, Wyman JF. Aerobic training for older men with Alzheimer's disease: individual examples of progression. *Res Gerontol Nurs* (2011) **4**:243–50. doi:10.3928/19404921-20110303-01
20. Ellis KA, Rainey-Smith SR, Rembach A, Macaulay SL, Villemagne VL. Enabling a multidisciplinary approach to the study of ageing and Alzheimer's disease: an update from the Australian Imaging Biomarkers and Lifestyle (AIBL) study. *Int Rev Psychiatry* (2013) **25**:699–710. doi:10.3109/09540261.2013.870136

21. Brown BM, Peiffer JJ, Taddei K, Lui JK, Laws SM, Gupta VB, et al. Physical activity and amyloid-β plasma and brain levels: results from the Australian imaging, biomarkers and lifestyle study of ageing. *Mol Psychiatry* (2013) **18**:875–81. doi:10.1038/mp.2012.107
22. Öhman H, Savikko N, Strandberg TE, Pitkälä KH. Effect of physical exercise on cognitive performance in older adults with mild cognitive impairment or dementia: a systematic review. *Dement Geriatr Cogn Disord* (2014) **38**:347–65. doi:10.1159/000365388
23. Forbes D, Thiessen EJ, Blake CM, Forbes SC, Forbes S. Exercise programs for people with dementia. *Cochrane Database Syst Rev* (2013) **12**:CD006489. doi:10.1002/14651858.CD006489.pub3
24. Kim B-K, Shin M-S, Kim C-J, Baek S-B, Ko Y-C, Kim Y-P. Treadmill exercise improves short-term memory by enhancing neurogenesis in amyloid beta-induced Alzheimer disease rats. *J Exerc Rehabil* (2014) **10**:2–8. doi:10.12965/jer.140086
25. Adlard PA, Perreau VM, Pop V, Cotman CW. Voluntary exercise decreases amyloid load in a transgenic model of Alzheimer's disease. *J Neurosci* (2005) **25**:4217–21. doi:10.1523/JNEUROSCI.0496-05.2005
26. Um H, Kang E, Leem Y, Cho I, Yang C, Chae K, et al. Exercise training acts as a therapeutic strategy for reduction of the pathogenic phenotypes for Alzheimer's disease in an NSE/APPsw-transgenic model. *Int J Mol Med* (2008) **4**:529–39. doi:10.3892/ijmm
27. Marosi K, Bori Z, Hart N, Sárga L, Koltai E, Radák Z, et al. Long-term exercise treatment reduces oxidative stress in the hippocampus of aging rats. *Neuroscience* (2012) **226**:21–8. doi:10.1016/j.neuroscience.2012.09.001
28. Okonkwo OC, Schultz SA, Oh JM, Larson J, Edwards D, Cook D, et al. Physical activity attenuates age-related biomarker alterations in preclinical AD. *Neurology* (2014) **83**:1753–60. doi:10.1212/WNL.0000000000000964
29. Hamman RF, Wing RR, Edelstein SL, Lachin JM, Bray GA, Delahanty L, et al. Effect of weight loss with lifestyle intervention on risk of diabetes. *Diabetes Care* (2006) **26**:2102–7. doi:10.2337/dc06-0560
30. Krause M, Rodrigues-Krause J, O'Hagan C, Medlow P, Davison G, Susta D, et al. The effects of aerobic exercise training at two different intensities in obesity and type 2 diabetes: implications for oxidative stress, low-grade inflammation and nitric oxide production. *Eur J Appl Physiol* (2014) **114**:251–60. doi:10.1007/s00421-013-2769-6
31. Adamopoulos S, Schmid J-P, Dendale P, Poerschke D, Hansen D, Dritsas A, et al. Combined aerobic/inspiratory muscle training vs. aerobic training in patients with chronic heart failure: the Vent-HeFT trial: a European prospective multicentre randomized trial. *Eur J Heart Fail* (2014) **16**:574–82. doi:10.1002/ejhf.70
32. Higgins JP, Green S. *Cochrane Handbook for Systematic Review of Intervention.* (2011).
33. Moher D, Liberati A, Tetzlaff J, Altman DG, The PRISMA Group. Perferred reporting items for systematic reviews and meta-analysis: the PRISMA statement. *PLoS Med* (2009) **6**. doi: 10.1371/journal.pmed.1000097
34. Baker LD, Frank LL, Foster-Schubert K, Green PS, Wilkinson CW, McTiernan A, et al. Effects of aerobic exercise on mild cognitive impairment: a controlled trial. *JAMA Neurol* (2010) **67**:71–9. doi:10.1001/archneurol.2009.307
35. Cheng S-T, Chow PK, Song Y-Q, Yu ECS, Chan ACM, Lee TMC, et al. Mental and physical activities delay cognitive decline in older persons with dementia. *Am J Geriatr Psychiatry* (2014) **22**:63–74. doi:10.1016/j.jagp.2013.01.060
36. Coelho FG, de M, Andrade LP, Pedroso RV, Santos-Galduroz RF, Gobbi S, et al. Multimodal exercise intervention improves frontal cognitive functions and gait in Alzheimer's disease: a controlled trial. *Geriatr Gerontol Int* (2013) **13**:198–203. doi:10.1111/j.1447-0594.2012.00887.x
37. Eggermont LHP, Swaab DF, Hol EM, Scherder EJ. Walking the line: a randomised trial on the effects of a short term walking programme on cognition in dementia. *J Neurol Neurosurg Psychiatry* (2009) **80**:802–4. doi:10.1136/jnnp.2008.158444
38. Mancuso M, Filosto M, Bosetti F, Ceravolo R, Rocchi A, Tognoni G, et al. Decreased platelet cytochrome c oxidase activity is accompanied by increased blood lactate concentration during exercise in patients with Alzheimer disease. *Exp Neurol* (2003) **182**:421–6. doi:10.1016/S0014-4886(03)00092-X
39. Nascimento CMC, Pereira JR, de Andrade LP, Garuffi M, Talib LL, Forlenza OV, et al. Physical exercise in MCI elderly promotes reduction of pro-inflammatory cytokines and improvements on cognition and BDNF peripheral levels. *Curr Alzheimer Res* (2014) **11**:799–805. doi:10.2174/156720501108140910122849
40. Nascimento C, Pereira J, Pires, de Andrade L, Garuffi M, Ayan C, et al. Physical exercise improves peripheral BDNF levels and cognitive fenctions in elderly mild cognitive impairment individuals with different BDNF Val166Met genotypes. *J Alzheimers Dis* (2015) **43**(1):81–91. doi:10.3233/JAD-140576
41. Segal SK, Cotman CW, Cahill LF. Exercise-induced noradrenergic activation enhances memory consolidation in both normal aging and patients with amnestic mild cognitive impairment. *J Alzheimers Dis* (2012) **32**:1011–8. doi:10.3233/JAD-2012-121078
42. Coelho FGDM, Vital TM, Stein AM, Arantes FJ, Rueda AV, Camarini R, et al. Acute aerobic exercise increases brain-derived neurotrophic factor levels in elderly with Alzheimer's disease. *J Alzheimers Dis* (2014) **39**:401–8. doi:10.3233/JAD-131073
43. Lee C, Do Folsom AR, Blair SN. Physical activity and stroke risk: a meta-analysis. *Stroke* (2003) **34**:2475–82. doi:10.1161/01.STR.0000091843.02517.9D
44. Ravona-Springer R, Lou X, Schmeidler J, Wysocki M, Lesser G, Rapp M, et al. Diabetes ia associated with increased rate of cognitive decline in questionably demented elderly. *Dement Geriatr Cogn Disord* (2010) **29**:68–74. doi:10.1159/000265552
45. Ravona-Springer R, Moshier E, Schmeidler J, Godbold J, Akrivos J, Rapp M, et al. Changes in glycemic control are associated with chnages in cognition in non-diabetic alderly. *J Alzheimers Dis* (2012) **30**:299–309. doi:10.3233/JAD-2012-120106.Changes
46. Casley CS, Canevari L, Land JM, Clark JB, Sharpe MA. Beta-amyloid inhibits integrated mitochondrial respiration and key enzyme activities. *J Neurochem* (2002) **80**:91–100. doi:10.1046/j.0022-3042.2001.00681.x
47. Raha S, Robinson BH. Mitochondria, oxygen free radicals, and apoptosis. *Am J Med Genet* (2001) **106**:62–70. doi:10.1002/ajmg.1398
48. AmorS,PuentesF,BakerD,vanderValkP.Inflammationinneurodegenerativediseases. *Immunology* (2010) **129**:154–69. doi:10.1111/j.1365-2567.2009.03225.x
49. Faria MC, Gonçalves GS, Rocha NP, Moraes EN, Bicalho MA, Gualberto Cintra MT, et al. Increased plasma levels of BDNF and inflammatory markers in Alzheimer's disease. *J Psychiatr Res* (2014) **53**:166–72. doi:10.1016/j.jpsychires.2014.01.019
50. McGeer EG, McGeer PL. Neuroinflammation in Alzheimer's disease and mild cognitive impairment: a field in its infancy. *J Alzheimers Dis* (2010) **19**:355–61. doi:10.3233/JAD-2010-1219
51. Brosseron F, Krauthausen M, Kummer M, Heneka MT. Body fluid cytokine levels in mild cognitive impairment and Alzheimer's disease: a comparative overview. *Mol Neurobiol* (2014) **50**:534–44. doi:10.1007/s12035-014-8657-1
52. Souza LC, Filho CB, Goes ATR, Fabbro L, Del, de Gomes MG, Savegnago L, et al. Neuroprotective effect of physical exercise in a mouse model of Alzheimer's disease induced by β-amyloid$_{1-40}$ peptide. *Neurotox Res* (2013) **24**:148–63. doi:10.1007/s12640-012-9373-0
53. Erickson K, Miller D, Roecklein K. The aging hippocampus:interactions between exercise, depression, and BDNF. *Neuroscientist* (2012) **18**:82–97. doi:10.1177/1073858410397054.The
54. Phung TK, Waltroft BL, Laursen TM, Settnes A, Kessing LV, Mortensen PB, et al. Hysterectomy, oophorectomy and risk of dementia: a nationwide historical cohort study. *Dement Geriatr Cogn Disord* (2010) **30**:43–50. doi:10.1159/000314681
55. Jurkowki JE, Jones NL, Ealker C, Younglai EV, Sutton JR. Ovarian hormonal responses to exercise. *J Appl Physiol Respir Env Exerc Physiol* (1978) **44**:109–14.
56. Bonen A, Ling W, MacIntyre K, Neil R, McGrail J, Belcastro A. Effects of exericse on the serum concentration of FSH, LH, progesterone, and esterdiol. *Eur J Appl Physiol Occup Physiol* (1979) **42**:15–23. doi:10.1007/BF00421100
57. Zmuda JM, Thompson PD, Winthers SJ. Exercise increases serum testosterone and sex hormone-binding globulin levels in older men. *Metabolism* (1996) **45**:935–9. doi:10.1016/S0026-0495(96)90258-9
58. Segal SK, Cahill L. Endogenous noradrenergic activation and memory for emotional material in men and women. *Psychoneuroendocrinology* (2009) **34**:1263–71. doi:10.1016/j.psyneuen.2009.04.020
59. McIntyre CK, Hatfield T, McGaugh JL. Amygdala norepinephrine levels after training predict inhibitory avoidance retention performance in rats. *Eur J Neurosci* (2002) **16**:1223–6. doi:10.1046/j.1460-9568.2002.02188.x
60. Galvez R, Mesches MH, McGaugh JL. Norepinephrine release in the amygdala in response to footshock stimulation. *Neurobiol Learn Mem* (1996) **66**:253–7. doi:10.1006/nlme.1996.0067
61. Baker LD, Bayer-Carter JL, Skinner J, Montine TJ, Cholerton BA, Callaghan M, et al. High-intensity physical activity modulates diet effects on cerebrospinal

amyloid-β levels in normal aging and mild cognitive impairment. *J Alzheimers Dis* (2012) **28**:137–46. doi:10.3233/JAD-2011-111076

62. Maesako M, Uemura K, Kubota M, Sasaki H, Hayashida N, Asada-Utsugi M, et al. Exercise is more effective than diet control in preventing high fat diet-induced beta-amyloid deposition and memory deficit in amyloid precursor protein transgenic mice. *J Biol* (2012) **287**:23024–33. doi:10.1074/jbc.M112.367011
63. Lin X, Zhang X, Guo J, Roberts C, McKenzie S, Wu W, et al. Effects of exercise training on cardiorespiratory fitness and biomarkers of cardimetabolic health: a systematic review and meta-analysis of randomized controlled trials. *J Am Hear Assoc* (2015) **4**(7). doi:10.1161/JAHA.115.002014
64. Brüünsgaard H, Pedersen B. Age-related inflammatory cytokines and disease. *Immunol Allergy Clin North Am* (2003) **23**:15–39. doi:10.1016/S0889-8561(02)00056-5
65. Woods JA, Wilund KR, Martin SA, Kistler BM. Exercise, inflammation and aging. *Aging Dis* (2012) **3**:130–40.
66. Yeh S, Lin L, Chuang Y, Liu C, Tsai F, Lee M, et al. Effects of music aerobic exercise on depression and brain-derived neurotrophic factor levels in community dwelling women. *Biomed Res Int* (2015) **2015**:135893. doi:10.1155/2015/135893
67. Erickson KI, Prakash RS, Voss MW, Chaddock L, Heo S, McLaren M, et al. Brain-derived neurotrophic factor is associated with age-related decline in hippocampal volume. *J Neurosci* (2010) **30**:5368–75. doi:10.1523/JNEUROSCI.6251-09.2010
68. Hauser PS, Ryan RO. Impact of Apolipoprotein E on Alzheimer's disease. *Curr Alzheimer Res* (2013) **10**:809–17. doi:10.2174/15672050113109990156
69. Nichol K, Deeny SP, Seif J, Camaclang K, Cotman CW. Exercise improves cognition and hippocampal plasticity in APOE e4 mice. *Alzheimers Dement* (2009) **5**:287–94. doi:10.1016/j.jalz.2009.02.006
70. Rasmussen KL, Tybjaerg-Hansen A, Nordestgaard BG, Frikke-Schmidt R. Plasma levels of apolipoprotein E and risk of dementia in the general population. *Ann Neurol* (2015) **77**:301–11. doi:10.1002/ana.24326
71. Hohman TJ, Bell SP, Jefferson AL. The role of vascular endothelial growth factor in neurodegeneration and cognitive decline: exploring interactions with biomarkers of Alzheimer disease. *JAMA Neurol* (2015) **72**:520–9. doi:10.1001/jamaneurol.2014.4761
72. Petersen AMW, Pedersen BK. The anti-inflammatory effect of exercise. *J Appl Physiol* (2005) **98**:1154–62. doi:10.1152/japplphysiol.00164.2004
73. Holtzman D. CSF biomarkers for Alzheimer's disease: current utility and potential future use. *Neurobiol Aging* (2011) **32**(Suppl 1):9. doi:10.1016/j.neurobiolaging.2011.09.003
74. Andreasen N, Minthon L, Davidsson P, Vanmechelen E, Vanderstichele H, Winblad B, et al. Evaluation of CSF-tau and CSF-amyloid beta42 as diagnostic markers for Alzheimer disease in clinical practice. *Arch Neurol* (2001) **58**:373–9. doi:10.1001/archneur.58.3.373
75. Gao L, Tang H, Nie K, Wnag L, Zhao J, Gan R, et al. Cerebrospinal fluid alpha-synuclein as a bioamrkers for Parkinson's disease diagnosis: a systematic review and meta-analysis. *Int J Neurosci* (2014) **125**(9):645–54. doi:10.3109/00207454.2014.961454
76. Wild E, Robertson N, Miller J, Traeger U, Haider S, Mcdonalds D, et al. Quantifying mutant huntingtin in Huntington's disease CSF. *J Neurol Neurosurg Psychiatry* (2014) **85**. doi: 10.1136/jnnp-2014-309236.23
77. del Campo M, Mollenhauer B, Bertolotto A, Engelborghs S, Hampel H, Simonsen AH, et al. Recommendations to standardize preanalytical confounding factors in Alzheimer's and Parkinson's disease cerebrospinal fluid biomarkers: an update. *Biomark Med* (2012) **6**:419–30. doi:10.2217/bmm.12.46
78. Hoffmann K, Frederiksen KS, Sobol NA, Beyer N, Vogel A, Simonsen AH, et al. Preserving cognition, quality of life, physical health and functional ability in Alzheimer's disease: the effect of physical exercise (ADEX trial): rationale and design. *Neuroepidemiology* (2013) **41**:198–207. doi:10.1159/000354632

14

Central nervous system and peripheral inflammatory processes in Alzheimer's disease: biomarker profiling approach

Constance Delaby[1], Audrey Gabelle[1,2], David Blum[3], Susanna Schraen-Maschke[3], Amandine Moulinier[1], Justine Boulanghien[1], Dany Séverac[4], Luc Buée[3], Thierry Rème[5] and Sylvain Lehmann[1]*

[1] Laboratoire de Biochimie-Protéomique Clinique, Institute for Regenerative Medicine and Biotherapy (IRMB), CHU de Montpellier and Université Montpellier, Montpellier, France, [2] Centre Mémoire Ressource Recherche Languedoc Roussillon, Hôpital Gui de Chauliac, CHU de Montpellier, Montpellier, France, [3] INSERM U837, CHU de Lille, Lille, France, [4] MGX-Montpellier GenomiX, Institut de Génomique Fonctionnelle, Montpellier, France, [5] INSERM U1040, CHU de Montpellier, Montpellier, France

Edited by:
Jesus Avila,
Centro de Biología Molecular Severo Ochoa, Spain

Reviewed by:
Michal Novak,
Slovak Academy of Sciences, Slovakia
Miguel Calero,
Instituto de Salud Carlos III, Spain

***Correspondence:**
Constance Delaby,
Laboratoire de Biochimie-Protéomique Clinique, CHU de Montpellier, 80 Avenue Augustin Fliche, 34295 Montpellier Cedex 5, France
c-delaby@chu-montpellier.fr

Brain inflammation is one of the hallmarks of Alzheimer disease (AD) and a current trend is that inflammatory mediators, particularly cytokines and chemokines, may represent valuable biomarkers for early screening and diagnosis of the disease. Various studies have reported differences in serum level of cytokines, chemokines, and growth factors in patients with mild cognitive impairment or AD. However, data were often inconsistent and the exact function of inflammation in neurodegeneration is still a matter of debate. In the present work, we measured the expression of 120 biomarkers (corresponding to cytokines, chemokines, growth factors, and related signaling proteins) in the serum of 49 patients with the following diagnosis distribution: 15 controls, 14 AD, and 20 MCI. In addition, we performed the same analysis in the cerebrospinal fluid (CSF) of 20 of these patients (10 AD and 10 controls). Among the biomarkers tested, none showed significant changes in the serum, but 13 were significantly modified in the CSF of AD patients. Interestingly, all of these biomarkers were implicated in neurogenesis or neural stem cells migration and differentiation. In the second part of the study, 10 of these putative biomarkers (plus 4 additional) were quantified using quantitative multiplex ELISA methods in the CSF and the serum of an enlarged cohort composed of 31 AD and 24 control patients. Our results confirm the potential diagnosis interest of previously published blood biomarkers, and proposes new ones (such as IL-8 and TNFR-I). Further studies will be needed to validate these biomarkers which could be used alone, combined, or in association with the classical amyloid and tau biomarkers.

Keywords: Alzheimer disease, biomarkers, inflammation, cerebrospinal fluid, serum

Background

Alzheimer disease (AD) is the most common neurodegenerative disorder worldwide. It is characterized by progressive memory loss and cognitive function deficit. Emerging evidences suggest that inflammation plays a central role in AD, and that the pathogenesis of the disease is not restricted to the neuronal compartment, but also involves immunological mechanisms. However, the exact function of inflammation in neurodegeneration is still matter of debate, and it probably has both beneficial and detrimental sides (1).

The chronic inflammatory response occurring in AD patients appears to be triggered by damaged neurons, amyloid beta (Aβ) peptides, and neurofibrillary tangles (2), which are neuropathogenic characteristics of the disease. Inflammation is present from pre-clinical to terminal stages of the disease, as reflected by activated microglia and reactive astrocytes that surround plaques. Microglia activation is a complex phenomenon, resulting in various phenotypes of the cells (secreting different types of cytokines), indicative of their interaction with the environment and allowing for either inflammatory or anti-inflammatory responses. The reactive astrocytes that accumulate around the plaques participate in the clearance of Aβ deposits and in cytokine secretion, thus enhancing the neuroinflammatory response initiated by microglia [for review, see Ref. (3)].

Diagnosis of AD relies on multidisciplinary approaches, requiring in particular expensive imaging procedures and invasive collection of cerebrospinal fluid (CSF) for biomarkers analysis (4): Aβ (in particular Aβ42), tau, and phospho-tau (p-tau) proteins. Anyway and because of the non-specificity of the symptoms characterizing the disease, its diagnosis is often delayed at a time when the injuries have progressed. The diagnosis of certitude is based on the presence of two neuropathologic processes: neurofibrillary tangles and amyloid senile plaques composed of accumulated tau proteins and Aβ peptides, respectively (5, 6). Despite intensive investigation, there is no cure currently available but only therapies that aim at slowing down the progression of neuronal injuries (4). These drugs are mostly effective at the earliest time course of the disease but are unfortunately administered later, at a time when the diagnosis is defined and injuries have progressed.

Because of the necessity of early diagnosis for optimal treatment and adequate handling of the patients, a reliable signature of specific biomarkers improving identification of pre-clinical AD would be of great interest. If CSF remains the most direct mean to study biochemical changes occurring in the brain, ideal biomarkers should be detectable and measurable in a fluid obtained through less invasive technique, such as the blood. Various groups have recently focused on the search of a plasma panel of AD biomarkers, thus opening promising perspectives in terms of diagnosis of the disease, including at prodromal stages (7–12). However, results were often controversial, because in particular of the heterogeneity of the population-based cohort used and/or the limitation in the sensitivity of the methods used. Thus no blood-based panel has been validated so far as an aid for the diagnosis of AD (13, 14).

Because of the inflammatory component of AD, one can hypothesize that pathological processes associated with this disorder would produce disease-specific molecular changes in the CSF and the blood, as a consequence of the inflammatory mechanisms. Thus, cytokines, chemokines, and growth factors could be expected to be modified, as these are the primary means of communication between cells. They could therefore represent valuable biomarkers for early screening and diagnosis of the disease. To test this hypothesis, we performed multiplex analysis of CSF and serum human samples and simultaneously evaluated the level of expression of 120 biomarkers (corresponding to cytokines, chemokines, growth factors, and related signaling proteins) in these fluids. We discuss our results in this paper, in light of previously published results.

Materials and Methods

Sample Collection and Handling

Blood was collected by venous puncture (BD vacutainer collection tube with clot activator, ref 368815), let it clot at room temperature (RT) for at least 30 min, centrifuged in the next 4 h at 1500 *g* at RT for 10 min. Serum supernatant was subsequently aliquoted by 0.5 mL in 1.5 mL eppendorf microtube (Eppendorf Protein LoBind, ref 0030 108.116) and stored at −80°C until analysis. CSF samples were collected by lumbar puncture in polypropylene tubes (Starstedt; 10 mL, ref 62.610.201), according to standard operating procedures (15), centrifuged at 1000 *g* at 4°C during 10 min, and the supernatant aliquoted and stored as for serum samples.

Patient Description and Samples

CSF and sera originated from a sample collection of patients who gave their informed consent from Montpellier neurological and Clinical Research Memory Centers (CMRR) for cognitive or behavioral disorders (officially registered collection DC-2008-417 of the certified NFS 96-900 biobank of the CHRU of Montpellier BB-0033-00031). This study was ethically approved under the number 12.128Ter by the "Comité consultatif sur le traitement de l'information en matière de recherche" (CCTIRS).

Patients were selected based for AD on the clinical criteria established in 1984 by the National Institute of Neurological and Communicative Disorders and Stroke (NINCDS) and the Alzheimer's Disease and Related Disorders Association (ADRDA) (16). MCI patients were selected following the Petersen MCI diagnosis criteria (17) with a concern regarding a change in cognition, impairment in one or more cognitive domains, preservation of independence in functional abilities without dementia. Mini-mental state examination (MMSE) values illustrating differences in cognition of the different clinical groups are provided in **Table 1**.

For the microarrays approach, a total of 49 serum samples were analyzed. Sera originated from control subjects ($n = 15$), AD ($n = 14$), or MCI ($n = 20$) patients. Among these MCI patients, 10 showed biological characteristics of AD. Of note, the time between the collection of the samples and their analysis was not significantly different between groups (**Table 1**).We also analyzed the CSF of 20 of these 49 patients (10 AD patients and 10 control subjects).

In the second step, and as a validation study, we selected 31 AD patients (9 of them belonging also to the initial cohort) with a PLM scale of 2 or 3 (18). We also selected 24 control patients (4 of them belonging also to the initial cohort) with a PLM scale of 0 or 1 (18) and the following diagnoses: amyotrophic lateral sclerosis ($n = 1$), Parkinson ($n = 2$), progressive supranuclear palsy ($n = 2$), vascular dementia ($n = 3$), normal pressure hydrocephalus ($n = 2$), Lewy body dementia ($n = 2$), peripheral neuropathy ($n = 1$), and subjective cognitive impairment ($n = 11$).

TABLE 1 | Demographic and CSF biomarkers in the population.

	Diagnosis						p (t-test)
	Control			AD			
	N	Mean	SD	*N*	Mean	SD	
Age	24	66.63	13.30	31	70.84	8.71	0.162
Sex	24	0.67	0.48	31	0.52	0.51	0.17 (Fischer's test)
IATI	24	1.91	0.72	31	0.95	0.65	<0.001
CSF Aβ42 (pg/mL)	24	1024.58	350.39	31	812.10	314.71	0.059
CSF p-Tau (pg/mL)	24	32.33	10.74	31	87.19	32.74	<0.0001
CSF Tau (pg/mL)	24	188.00	74.27	31	635.97	272.45	<0.0001
CSF protein (g/L)	22	0.49	0.15	29	0.51	0.20	0.397
Serum CRP (mg/L)	21	3.12	4.79	22	2.39	2.64	0.397
Mini-mental state examination (MMSE)/30	20	25.40	6.80	28	22.20	4.80	0.066

Demographic data, CSF biomarker levels (Aβ42, tau, and p-tau), IATI, CSF proteins, serum CRP (inflammation biomarker), and MMSE are shown for control and AD groups. Results are presented as mean and SD. t-test and Fischer exact test were computed.

Protein-Arrays Analysis

The relative abundance of 120 known signaling proteins (Table S1 in Supplementary Material) was measured in the 69 biological samples (49 sera and 20 CSF) using protein antibodies-based arrays (RayBio® Human Cytokine Antibody Array G-Series 1000, AAH-CYT-G1000-8). Antibodies used for detection of the 120 proteins are distributed on two slides (G6 and G7), each one allowing the semi-quantitation of 60 of the signaling proteins (see Table S1 in Supplementary Material for protein maps). Every sample tested was thereafter and simultaneously hybridized on two slides: G6 and G7.

One hundred microliters of native CSF or diluted serum (1:2.5) of each patient was hybridized on the slides, according to the provider's recommendations. As an internal quality control, a pool of five sera (originating from control patients) was prepared in our laboratory and hybridized on every slide, thus ensuring the control of the homogeneity of the results between the arrays. Slides were scanned at 532 nm (GenePix 4200AL, Axon instruments).

All the numeric data obtained following scan of the arrays were normalized according to the manufacturer's recommendations [using the normalization file provided with the kit (AAH-CYT-G1000-8, RayBio®)].

Quantitative Analysis Through ELISA and Electrochemiluminescence Assays

Quantitative multiplex or simplex methods were performed in both the CSF and serum of 55 patients (31 AD patients and 24 control subjects), using either electrochemiluminescence (MesoScaleDiscovery technology, MSD, Sector Imager 2400A) or ELISA method. Quantification of FABP3, TIMP-1, MIP-1beta, and RANTES was performed using simplex detection MSD kit, while GRO-alpha, IL-8, MCP-1, MIP-3beta, and sTNFR-I were simultaneously measured using MSD custom V-Plex detection (MSD MULTI-SPOT® 7 Spot Special Order Human 5Plex). Quantification of IGFBP-6, sIL-6R, IL-3, and MIP-1alpha was performed through simplex ELISA, purchased from Clinisciences. CSF samples were measured directly, without previous dilution. Depending on the cytokine measured, serum samples were diluted (1:2–1:50).

Statistical Analysis

For protein-arrays analysis, prediction analysis for microarrays (PAM) was performed with normalized array measurements of the 120 signaling proteins quantified in the training set (software R 3.1). To minimize the risk of overfitting, the PAM approach used as a training set 90% of the population, and as a validation the remaining 10%. This cross-validation was repeated 10 times. For exploitation of quantitative ELISA results, Student's *t*-test and area under ROC curves (AUC) analysis were performed using medCalc® software ver 15.2.2. The logistic regression was achieved with the same software with backward stepwise selection using a significance level of 0.10. Classification trees were obtained using a Microsoft Visual Studio routine (available upon request), which computed the sensitivity and specificity of all possible pair combination of biomarkers at the different cut-offs (corresponding to the values of the biomarkers in the population).

Results

Semi-Quantitative Analysis of 120 Proteins Through Protein-Arrays Approach

Forty-nine patients of clinically characterized diagnosis were included for the protein-array analysis: the cohort was composed of individuals with pre-symptomatic (MCI, mild cognitive impairment, $n = 20$) or late-stage AD ($n = 14$) patients and from control subjects ($n = 15$), **Figure 1A**. MMSE differed between the groups and was, as expected, significantly correlated with Aβ42, Tau or p-Tau ($p < 0.001$, "Spearman" rank correlation).

The serum of these 49 patients and the CSF of 20 of them (10 controls and 10 AD) were hybridized simultaneously on G6 and G7 slides, in order to evaluate the relative abundance of the 120 proteins detectable on the arrays (**Figures 1A,B**, left panel). Before proceeding to the analysis of the slides and to ensure for their homogeneity, an internal quality control (CQI) was hybridized on every array, in the very same conditions than biological samples included in that study. This CQI corresponds to a pool of sera (originated from control subjects) prepared in our laboratory and was used to compare and homogenize the slides, so that the fluorescence detected could be attributed to specific variation of expression of the proteins in a sample, rather

A

	diagnosis			
	Control (A)	Alzheimer disease. AD (B)	MCI	
			non AD profile (C)	AD profile (D)
N	15	14	10	10
men	7	10	7	6
women	8	4	3	4
Biological sample analysed	serum + CSF	serum + CSF	serum	serum
Time between collection of sample and analysis (months)	18.4 ± 7.1	20.8 ± 3.7	20.3 ± 4.5	18.2 ± 7.3
Mini-Mental State Examination (MMSE) /30	22.9 ± 5.8	21.8 ± 5.8	28.4 ± 1.1	24.7 ± 4.5

B

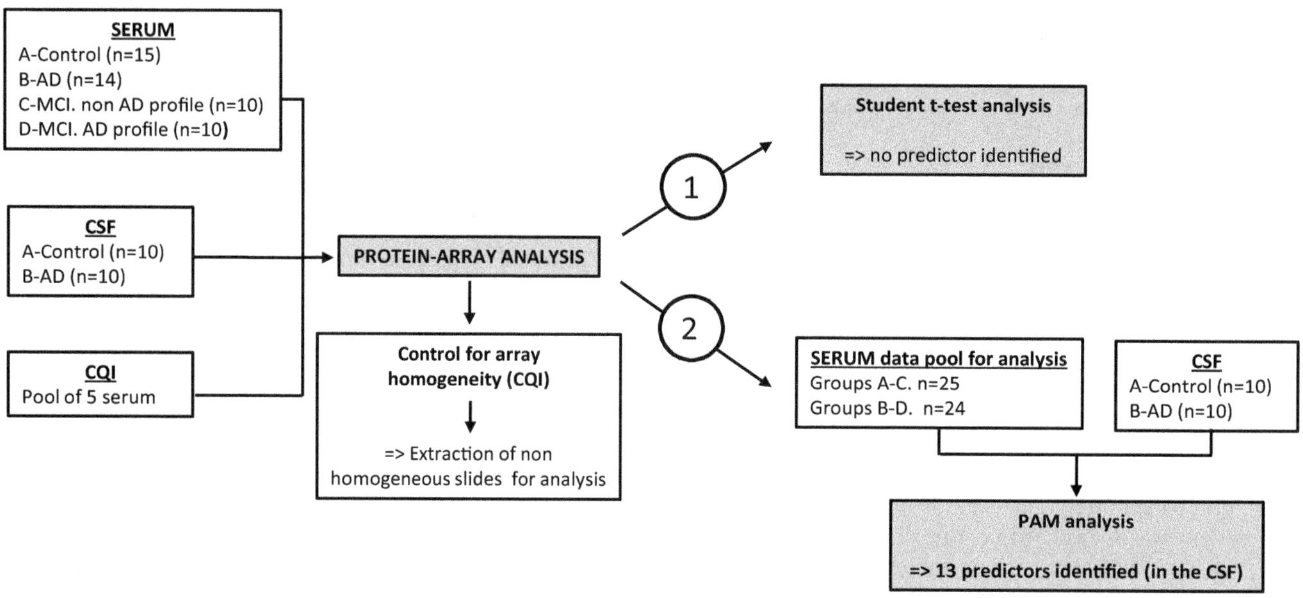

FIGURE 1 | Cohort patients and study outline. **(A)** A total of 49 patients were included in the preliminary study for protein-arrays analysis: 15 control subjects (A), 14 AD late-stage patients (B) and 20 MCI (mild cognitive impairment): 10 MCI with non-AD profile (C) and 10 MCI presenting AD profile (D). Serum was analyzed for every patient included; CSF was analyzed for 20 of them (10 patients from groups A and B). Time between collection of samples (serum and CSF) and their analysis is indicated (in months): results are mean ± SD. Mini-mental state examination (MMSE) is indicated (MMSE/30) as mean ± SD. **(B)** Sera, CSF, and our internal quality control (CQI, corresponding to a pool of five control sera) were hybridized on the protein arrays. Homogeneity of the slides was controlled thanks to the CQI: non-homogeneous slide identified was extracted before proceeding to the analysis of the arrays. Normalized array data of 120 serum signaling proteins were analyzed in the training set with statistical Student's *t*-test to discover differences in protein abundance between samples (strategy 1). As no predictor could be identified, serum data were pooled for groups A–C and B–D (strategy 2). To discover predictors for classification, the training set was analyzed through prediction analysis for microarrays (PAM) approach.

than a slide effect (**Figure 1B**, left and central panels and Data S1 in Supplementary Material). Our data show that CQI inter-slide are homogenous between G7 slides, which validated the subsequent analysis of numeric data obtained for the proteins studied on these arrays (Data S1 in Supplementary Material, left graph). On the other hand, analysis of CQI on G6 slides showed that one of these arrays gave non-homogenous results (Data S1, right graph, gray-highlighted results); the corresponding slide was thereafter extracted before proceeding to the subsequent analysis (**Figure 1B**, central panel).

Following this preliminary control of the slides, normalized data generated from the 49 sera and 20 CSF hybridized were analyzed through semi-quantitative protein-arrays approach: the relative abundance of 120 proteins of known function (cytokines, chemokines, and other signaling proteins) was simultaneously evaluated (**Figure 1B**, right panel).

The numeric and normalized data obtained from the protein arrays were first of all analyzed through Student's *t*-test, in order to identify a set of putative biomarkers in the serum that could participate to the discrimination of control, MCI, and late-stage AD patients (**Figure 1B**, right and up panel); however, this statistical analysis did not provide exploitable results, as no biomarker appeared to be significantly and specifically associated to one group more than another one (results not shown). Furthermore, we decided to pool together the data obtained with the serum of all the AD patients (MCI with AD profile and late-stage) and control patients (control and MCI no AD profile) and to focus on the discrimination between control and AD patients (**Figure 1B**, right panel strategy 2). Prediction analysis for microarrays (PAM) was thereafter performed with the normalized array measurements. In the serum, we were still unable to identify proteins significantly modified between the two groups. On the other hand, the same analysis in the CSF led to the discovery of a repeatedly optimal set of 13 predictors giving the lowest possible classification error between control and AD groups (**Figures 2A,B**). Results showed that all of them were decreased in AD group (negative *d*-score, **Figure 2B**).

Quantitative Analysis of Putative Biomarkers in the CSF and the Serum

Among the 13 putative proteins of interest identified in the CSF, 10 of them (plus 4 additional selected following literature) were subsequently analyzed through quantitative method in the CSF and the serum of AD and control patients. This quantification was performed on an enlarged cohort, composed of 55 individuals (31 AD patients and 24 control subjects), characterized clinically and biologically for CSF biomarkers: Aβ42, tau, and p-tau (**Table 1**; **Figure 3**). According to their clinical diagnosis, AD patients showed a decrease of CSF $A\beta_{1-42}$, together with an increase of CSF tau and p-tau ($p < 0.0001$). The ratio IATI [$A\beta_{1-42}/(240 + 1.18 \times \text{tau})$] was calculated for these patients and allowed for diagnostic discrimination of the two groups ($p < 0.001$, **Figure 3D**). Groups were homogeneous in terms of age, sex repartition, CRP, and CSF protein, and MMSE was decreased in AD group (**Table 1**).

We tested for normal distribution of the data concerning the 14 proteins measured and thereafter proceeded for *t*-student statistical test to evaluate significant difference between AD and control groups (**Table 2**). Results showed that in the CSF, among the 14 tested proteins, 3 biomarkers were significantly different between the two groups (**Table 2**, bolded and gray-highlighted results): sIL-6R, TIMP-1, and sTNFR-I. These three proteins were increased in the CSF of AD patients, compared to control subjects (**Figures 4A–C**). Furthermore, three of the 14 biomarkers quantified were undetectable in the CSF of patients (FABP3, GRO-gamma, and TGF-beta1). On the other side, all of the 14 biomarkers tested were detectable in the serum but none of them were detected at a level significantly different between AD and control patients (**Table 2; Figures 4D–F**).

A

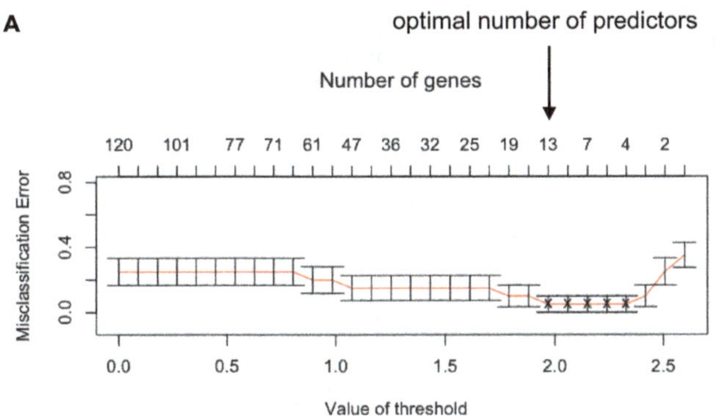

B

protein identification	control-score	AD-score
TIMP-1	0.1401	-0.1401
IL-11	0.137	-0.137
sTNF-RI	0.1187	-0.1187
MIP-3beta	0.1036	-0.1036
Thrombopoietin	0.0589	-0.0589
sIL-6R	0.0529	-0.0529
TGF-beta1	0.052	-0.052
MCP-1	0.0303	-0.0303
GRO	0.0303	-0.0303
IL.3	0.0165	-0.0165
IL.8	0.0125	-0.0125
IGFBP6	0.0113	-0.0113
GRO-alpha	0.0029	-0.0029

FIGURE 2 | Predictors discovery. (A) Predictor discovery by prediction analysis for microarrays (PAM) was performed with normalized array measurements of 120 signaling proteins in the training set. Internal cross-validation (redline) decreasing the centroid threshold (lower *x*-axis) resulted in an increase in the number of markers (inserted upper *x*-axis) that were used for classification and calculation of the classification error (*y*-axis). This led to the discovery of an optimal set of 13 predictors with lowest possible classification error. **(B)** The 13 predictors identified through PAM analysis are presented. Proteins are arranged in columns, with *d*-score corresponding in each group. Control group corresponded to control subjects and MCI non-AD patients (groups A–C defined for protein-arrays analysis); AD group corresponded to AD late-stage patients and MCI presenting AD profile (groups B–D defined for protein-arrays analysis). Positive *d*-score is indicative of increased expression and negative *d*-score reflects decrease in the expression of the proteins analyzed.

ROC Curves, Regression Analysis and Decision Trees of the Biomarkers in the Serum and the CSF

We compared the area under the ROC curves (AUC) of all the analytes measured in the serum and the CSF of the 55 patients (**Table 3**). CSF tau and p-tau appeared to be the most efficient analytes to discriminate AD patients and control subjects (AUC values = 0.942 and 0.946, respectively). Among the analytes tested, seven presented an AUC ≥ 0.655 (**Table 3**, bolded and highlighted results). To combine these CSF biomarkers, we tested a logistic regression model which retained three biomarkers with the following equation: $\text{sIL6R} \times 0.0034615 + \text{TIMP1} \times 0.000024458 + \text{TNFRI} \times 0.001016 - 9.2101$ (pg/mL). As illustrated in **Figure 5A**, this resulted in an important improvement of the AUC reaching 0.858 (corresponding at its best to a sensitivity of 74.2% and a specificity of 91.7%). The relevance of these biomarkers for AD was also supported by the fact that a significant "Spearman" rank correlation was observed between MMSE and CSF TIMP-1 ($p = 0.03950$) and between tau or p-tau and CSF sIL6R ($p < 0.001$). The low differences in expression of the biomarkers in the blood prevented their integration in the logistic regression model.

We also tested a simple classification tree model based on only two analytes (nodes) to minimize the risk of overfitting (**Figures 5B,C**). For the CSF biomarkers, this resulted in a classification involving IGFBP6 and MIP-3 beta, reaching on their own a sensitivity of 81% and a specificity of 92% (**Figure 5B**). Interestingly, the logistic regression and the classification tree resulted in a different biomarker selection and the patients selected with the two models were also different. Additional studies on larger cohort will be needed to reconcile and eventually combine these results. Applying the same approach for serum biomarkers, it resulted in a classification involving IL-8 and TNFR-1, reaching a sensitivity of 77% and a specificity of 75% (**Figure 5C**).

Of note, the control misclassified patients of the classification trees (**Figures 5B,C**) corresponded to various diagnoses (Lewy

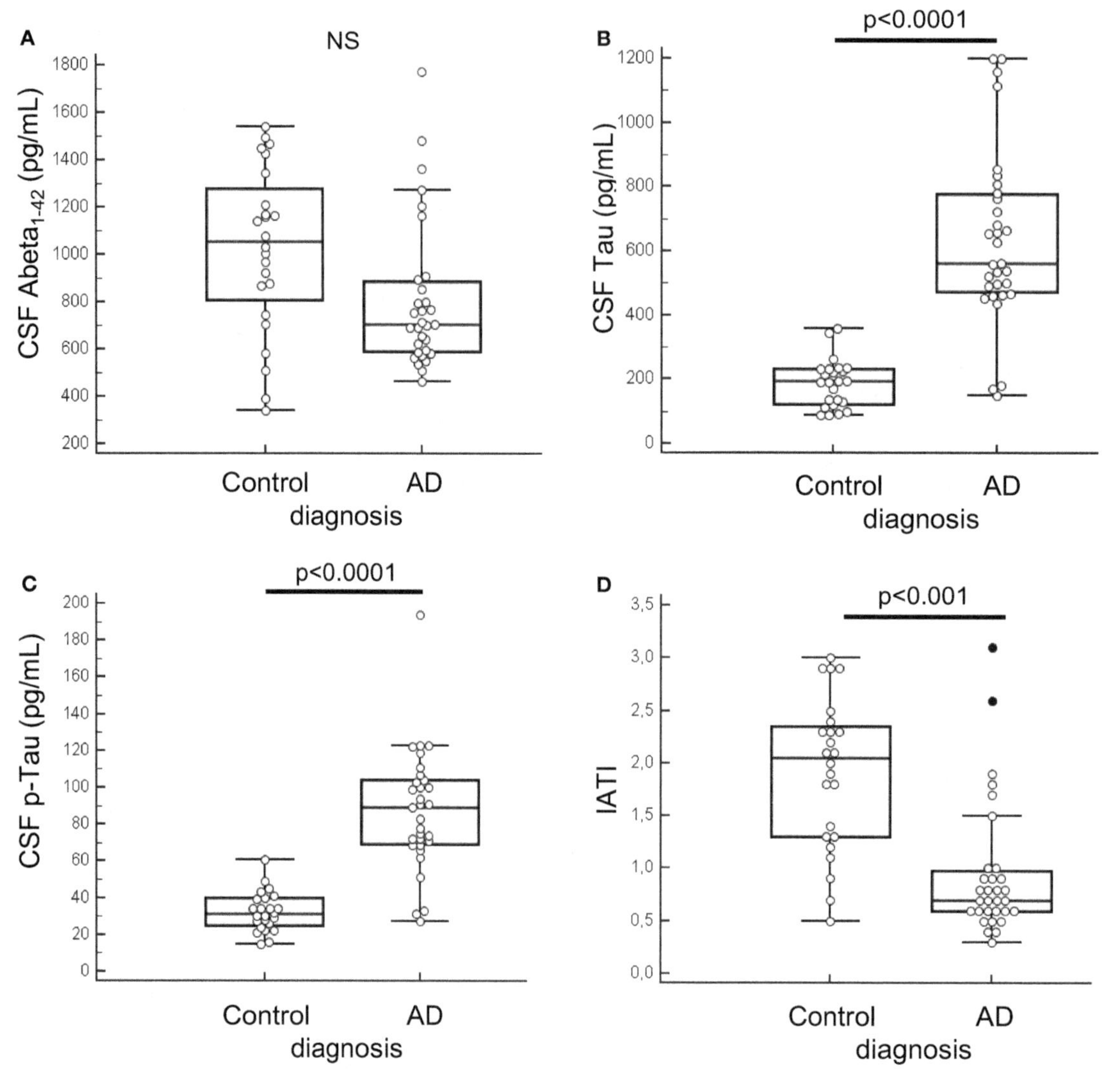

FIGURE 3 | Clinical biochemical characterization of patients. The 55 patients (AD, $n = 31$ and control subjects, $n = 24$) of the enlarged cohort used for the second part of the study were characterized clinically and quantified for CSF biomarkers: Aβ42, tau, and p-tau, using Fujirebio ELISA quantification kits **(A–C)**. IATI ratio [Aβ42/(240 + 1,18tau)] **(D)** was calculated for every subject of the cohort. Outliers are indicated with black circle. Outliers are defined as a value that is smaller than the lower quartile minus three times the interquartile range, or larger than the upper quartile plus three times the interquartile range.

body dementia, vascular dementia, and subjective cognitive impairment). Based on the available clinical and biological data, it was not apparent why these patients were misclassified.

Discussion

The 2011 revision of criteria for AD clinical diagnosis includes CSF biomarkers analysis: quantification of Aβ42 peptides, tau, and p-tau proteins; however and despite its utility, its use in routine clinical practice and for the follow-up of patient is limited because in particular of the invasive character of lumbar puncture.

The link between neuro-inflammation and AD has opened attractive perspectives for the early diagnosis and handling of patients. Indeed, the possibility to identify a blood-based panel of biomarkers to detect AD patients could allow for a systematic and early diagnosis of them, at the time of the first signs indicative of cognitive impairment, therefore optimizing their care and treatment. In addition, the perspective of feasibility of an early biochemical diagnosis of patients through minimally invasive technique (such as venous puncture) is quite seducing.

Various studies described such a signature in the blood: among them, Ray et al. identified 18 blood biomarkers, some of which were subsequently confirmed by ADNI (8, 19). The present work aimed at investigating the molecular mechanisms involved in inflammatory processes occurring in AD, intending to identify or confirm a profile of biomarkers characteristic of AD. To this end, the modification of various signaling proteins (chemokines and cytokines) in the CSF and the serum of AD patients were evaluated using multiplex strategies.

The protein-arrays approach used in the first place is very attractive because it offers the opportunity to evaluate, in a single test and through a reduced volume of biological sample,

TABLE 2 | CSF and serum quantification of predictors identified.

		Diagnosis						*p* (*t*-test)
		Control			AD			
		N	Mean	SD	*N*	Mean	SD	
CSF	FABP-3 (pg/mL)	24	ND	ND	31	ND	ND	–
	GRO-alpha (pg/mL)	24	22.79	12.28	31	29.97	18.63	0.101
	GRO-gamma (pg/mL)	24	ND	ND	27	ND	ND	–
	IGFBP6 (pg/mL)	24	76,4473.50	680,240.30	31	65,6967.45	317,572.10	0.440
	IL-3 (pg/mL)	24	71.08	55.42	31	81.94	141.47	0.721
	IL-8 (pg/mL)	24	2476.46	2164.15	31	3398.90	3307.04	0.242
	MCP-1 (pg/mL)	24	484.54	110.74	31	524.87	221.39	0.420
	MIP-1beta (pg/mL)	24	11.38	7.89	31	11.58	3.09	0.957
	MIP-3beta (pg/mL)	24	193.33	137.71	31	249.97	110.29	0.096
	RANTES (pg/mL)	24	4.25	8.36	31	9.81	20.49	0.210
	sIL6-R (pg/mL)	**24**	**1125.71**	**304.31**	**31**	**1455.42**	**384.44**	**0.001**
	TGF-beta1 (pg/mL)	24	ND	ND	31	ND	ND	–
	TIMP-1 (pg/mL)	**24**	**94,953.75**	**23,724.34**	**31**	**117,507.10**	**31,685.66**	**0.005**
	sTNFR-I (pg/mL)	**24**	**2058.88**	**700.90**	**31**	**2601.94**	**693.10**	**0.006**
Serum	FABP-3 (pg/mL)	24	7.13	2.47	31	6.36	2.44	0.247
	GRO-alpha (pg/mL)	23	106.50	64.10	31	111.10	56.08	0.777
	GRO-gamma (pg/mL)	24	98.91	231.92	27	128.44	258.91	0.676
	IGFBP6 (pg/mL)	24	887,849.71	565,626.11	31	717,297.23	325,456.73	0.306
	IL-3 (pg/mL)	24	2353.25	7191.47	31	1242.19	1409.37	0.372
	IL-8 (pg/mL)	24	21.42	17.54	31	17.36	16.77	0.392
	MCP-1 (pg/mL)	24	319.21	100.39	31	319.13	99.70	0.993
	MIP-1beta (pg/mL)	24	28.67	13.78	31	28.45	16.95	0.957
	MIP-3beta (pg/mL)	24	230.71	452.88	31	154.94	188.86	0.403
	RANTES (pg/mL)	24	189.58	93.68	31	216.16	117.38	0.368
	sIL6-R (pg/mL)	24	88,788.79	30,096.89	31	79,709.42	26,040.66	0.236
	TGF-beta1 (pg/mL)	24	1.13	0.34	31	1.26	0.44	0.677
	TIMP-1 (pg/mL)	24	65,6950	248,683.10	31	660,009.68	342,382.44	0.971
	sTNFR-I (pg/mL)	24	5139.29	1880.56	31	4424.97	1242.77	0.096

Ten predictors previously identified following PAM analysis and four supplemental ones (FABP3, GRO gamma, RANTES, and MIP-1beta) were quantified in the CSF and the serum of AD (n = 31) and control (n = 24) patients using quantitative ELISA and MSD approaches. Results are presented as mean and SD. The three bolded and gray-highlighted biomarkers present significant difference in the CSF between control and AD groups (Student's t-test). None of the proteins tested in the serum show significant difference between the two groups. ND corresponds to proteins undetectable in the CSF.

the simultaneous level of expression of numerous proteins. In the present study, the large screening of 120 signaling proteins in serum and CSF of AD patients seemed very promising but appeared unfortunately quite disappointing in the serum. Indeed, no putative biomarker could be identified through this approach. One cannot exclude the possibility that the protein-arrays approach might lack sensitivity and reproducibility to detect small and discrete differences in the level of expression of the proteins tested between the groups of our cohort. Anyway such observation remains quite intriguing because other studies, using similar approaches, described a blood-based panel of biomarkers discriminating control subjects and AD patients (8). However, a strict comparison of these works remains challenging because of the heterogeneity and the different size of the cohorts used, and also because of the nature of the samples used (serum versus plasma). On the other hand, the technique provided interesting results in the CSF, as 13 putative biomarkers potentially discriminating control subjects and AD patients could be identified. Although such method is very useful as a first-step and large screening of candidates, it remains semi-quantitative and poorly sensitive. Thus, the putative biomarkers identified in the CSF had to be subsequently tested for confirmation through quantitative and sensitive methods.

Among the 13 predictors identified, 10 were analyzed through such quantitative approaches, according to the availability of the existent kits: GRO-alpha, IGFBP6, IL-3, IL-8, MCP-1, MIP-3beta, sIL-6R, TGF-beta1, TIMP-1, and sTNF-RI. Because of their potential implication in inflammatory processes and AD, we also evaluated the abundance of four supplemental proteins present in our panels: GRO-gamma, RANTES, MIP-1beta, and FABP3, which were also described in the literature as putative AD biomarkers. These 14 proteins were quantified in both the CSF and the serum of an enlarged cohort of 55 subjects (AD patients and control individuals). Among these biomarkers, three presented significant increase in the CSF: sIL-6R, TIMP-1, and sTNFR-I, and could be combined in a logistic regression model. Interestingly, sIL-6R and sTNF-RI presented opposite way of variation in the serum, although not being significant in this fluid.

Microglia and astrocytes are the major sources of cytokines production in AD. Thus, Aβ42 accumulation has been suggested to be a strong inducer of the neuro-inflammatory response in AD, exposure of microglia to Aβ42 deposits increasing production of IL-6 and M-CSF (20). M-CSF was also described to be increased in the plasma and the CNS of patients at the dementia stage of AD compared to control or MCI age-matched patients (20, 21). Controversial results were obtained by Ray et al., describing a

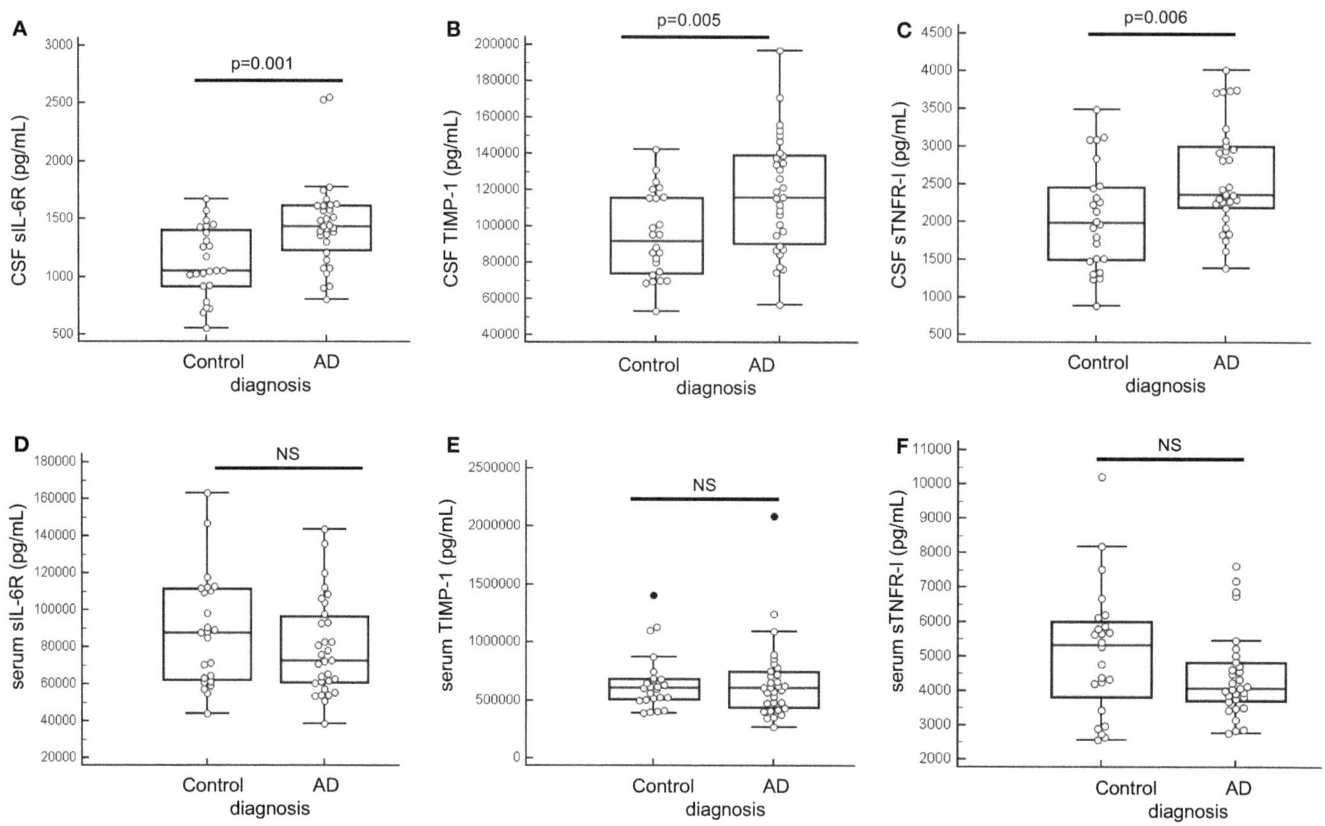

FIGURE 4 | Predictors quantification in the CSF and the serum. sIL-6R, TIMP-1, and sTNFR-I were quantified in the CSF **(A–C)** and in the serum **(D–F)** of 55 patients (AD, $n = 31$ and control subjects, $n = 24$). Outliers are indicated with black circle. Outliers are defined as a value that is smaller than the lower quartile minus three times the interquartile range, or larger than the upper quartile plus three times the interquartile range.

decrease of M-CSF in the plasma of AD patients (8). In our study, this cytokine presented a very low basal level and did not show any significant modification of level neither in the CSF or serum of our patients (protein-array results). In addition, IL-6 was barely detectable in the CSF and serum of our patients but as noticed above, its receptor (sIL-6R) was significantly increased in the CSF and showed a tendency to decrease in the serum of AD patients although not being significant. A CSF cytokine profile characterized by an increase of TNF-alpha associated with a decrease of TGF-beta could be a marker of the conversion of MCI to AD (22). In addition, TNF-alpha was reported to be decreased in the plasma of AD patients versus control (8). In our study anyway, we did not observe significant change in the CSF or the serum of TNF-alpha and TGF-beta level among the patients. Interestingly, the receptor of TNF-alpha (sTNFR-I) was significantly increased in the CSF of AD patients compared to control subjects and showed a tendency to decrease in the serum of AD patients. Of note, He et al. recently demonstrated that deletion of TNF-RI can inhibit Aβ generation and prevents cognitive deficits in AD mice (23), through the reduction of expression and activity of BACE1 mediated by NF-κB signaling. Thus, chronic overexpression of neuronal TNF-alpha has been described to enhance local inflammatory responses in transgenic AD mice (24). However, the pro-inflammatory cytokine TNF-alpha is also reported to present neuroprotective effects in the brain (25). In addition and very interestingly, analysis of AUC of ROC curves in our study shows that association of sTNF-RI was among the best biomarkers and that its combination with TIMP-1 and sILR-6 provides the most powerful combination for AD diagnosis. Such observation will have to be confirmed in another study through an enlarged cohort.

On the other side, IL-3 is described in the literature to be reduced in the plasma of AD patients, which was also observed in our cohort (although not being significant). In addition, IL-1beta is known to be secreted by activated microglia cells following Aβ42 stimulation *in vitro* (26). Thus this pro-inflammatory cytokine can be detected in microglial cells surrounding Aβ deposits and in the CSF of AD patients (26). Anyway, only very low level of this cytokine was detectable in the CSF and serum of our patients and no difference in its concentration could be noted among the patients. IGFBP6 is also described to be increased in the plasma of AD patients (8) but we did not detect significant changes of its level in our study. Interestingly, this molecule was retained in the classification tree model, which would need further validation in a larger cohort.

Chemio-attractive chemokines are known to participate in the inflammatory process of AD, through regulation of microglial cells migration at the site of inflammation (27). In particular, CCL4 (MIP-1beta) has been described in reactive astrocytes surrounding Aβ deposits (28) and CXCL8 (IL-8), CCL2 (MCP-1), and CCL3 (MIP-1alpha) are increased following Aβ42 exposition

TABLE 3 | Values of area under the ROC curves.

	Variable	AUC	SE	95% CI
CSF	IATI	0.788	0.0739	0.636–0.898
	Abeta 1–42	0.69	0.0789	0.550–0.807
	GRO-alpha	0.604	0.0794	0.463–0.733
	IGFBP6	0.511	0.0867	0.372–0.648
	IL-3	0.566	0.0748	0.425–0.699
	IL-8	0.614	0.0792	0.473–0.742
	MCP-1	0.503	0.0791	0.365–0.641
	MIP-1beta	**0.655**	**0.0776**	**0.514–0.778**
	MIP-3beta	**0.727**	**0.0787**	**0.590–0.839**
	p-Tau	**0.946**	**0.0315**	**0.849–0.989**
	RANTES	0.618	0.0748	0.477–0.745
	sIL6-R	**0.755**	**0.0659**	**0.620–0.861**
	Tau	**0.942**	**0.034**	**0.843–0.987**
	TIMP-1	**0.692**	**0.0756**	**0.544–0.816**
	sTNFR-I	**0.699**	**0.0771**	**0.551–0.821**
	CSF protein	0.514	0.0854	0.367–0.660
Serum	CRP	0.512	0.0924	0.355–0.667
	Fabp-3	0.646	0.0817	0.497–0.778
	GRO-alpha	0.57	0.0873	0.421–0.710
	GRO-gamma	0.579	0.076	0.430–0.719
	IGFBP6	0.586	0.0801	0.445–0.717
	IL-3	0.549	0.0797	0.409–0.684
	IL-8	0.599	0.081	0.459–0.729
	MCP-1	0.501	0.0806	0.363–0.639
	MIP-1beta	0.548	0.0821	0.408–0.683
	MIP-3beta	0.622	0.0761	0.481–0.750
	RANTES	0.556	0.079	0.416–0.690
	sIL6-R	0.595	0.0789	0.455–0.726
	TGF-beta1	0.567	0.0528	0.426–0.700
	TIMP-1	0.52	0.0795	0.381–0.657
	sTNFR-I	0.625	0.0838	0.484–0.752

Area under the ROC curve (AUC) for all the biochemical analytes quantified in the 55 patients (AD, n = 31 and control subjects, n = 24) of the study was evaluated. The seven biomarkers bolded and gray-highlighted analytes present AUC ≥ 0.650.

of astrocytes (29, 30). IL-8 has also previously been described to be increased in the plasma of AD patient (8). In our study, we detected increase of IL-8 and MCP-1 in the CSF of AD patients and no significant modification of MIP-1alpha or beta, neither in the CSF nor the serum.

On the other side, CCL5 (RANTES) was described to be down-regulated in the plasma of AD patients (8) and we noted no significant variation of this chemokine between the two groups of our study. GRO-alpha has also been reported to be a CSF biomarker of interest for AD diagnosis (31) but its level remained unchanged between our two groups. GRO-gamma (CXCL3) was undetectable in the CSF of our patients and remained unchanged in the serum among the patients.

In addition, matrix metalloproteinases (MMP) are believed to be involved in the pathologic processes of AD. TIMP-1 is the tissue inhibitor of MMP-9 and has been described to be increased in the CSF of AD and MCI patients (32). In our study, TIMP-1 was also significantly increased in the CSF of AD patients. Its level appeared stable in the serum of all populations of our cohort.

Finally, obesity, defined as a disorder in which excess fat accumulates in the body, also induces chronic inflammatory processes. Indeed, obesity has been associated with higher risk to develop AD (33). FABP3 is a member of the fatty acid binding proteins and has recently been described to be down-regulated in the brain of AD patients (34). However, FABP3 was not detectable in the CSF and presented no significant variation in the serum of our patients.

Identification of a molecular signature for AD diagnosis is very promising in terms of handling of patients and early diagnosis of AD, but remains quite challenging. Indeed, numerous studies have described panels of biomarkers of potential interest but at the time of their confirmation, results appeared to be largely

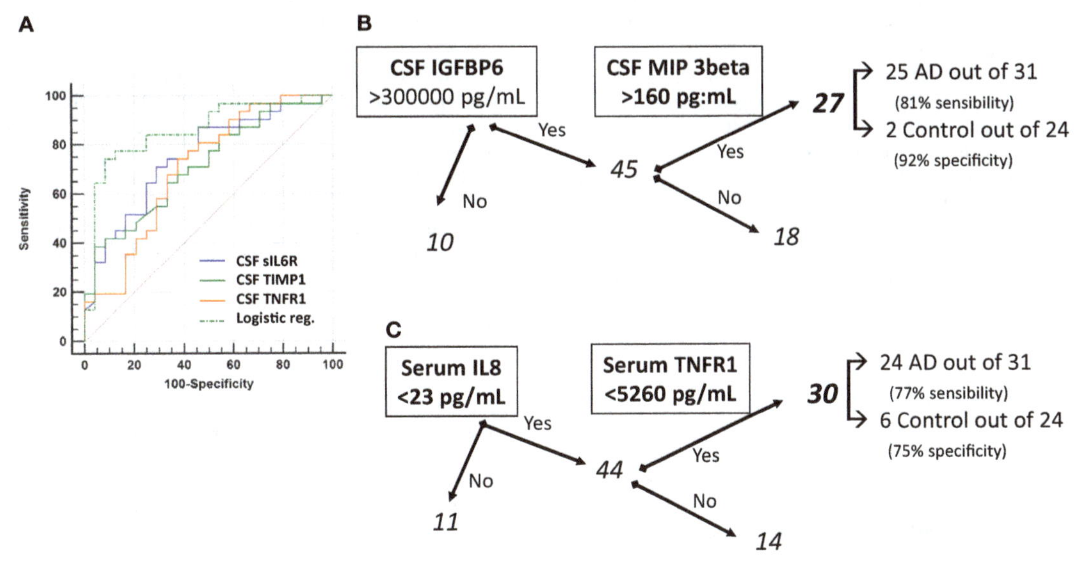

FIGURE 5 | Area under ROC curve (AUC) of Tau, p-Tau, and sTNFR-I. ROC curves **(A)** of the three most efficient biomarkers for AD diagnosis sIL-6R, TIMP-1, and sTNFR-I were plotted along with their combination (logistic regression, see text). The classification tree for CSF biomarkers **(B)** defined as AD samples those with IGFBP6 >300,000 pg/mL and MIP-3beta >160 pg/mL. Using serum biomarkers **(C)**, the criteria selected for AD diagnosis was: IL8 <23 pg/mL and TNFR-I <5260 pg/mL.

controversial [for review, see Ref. (3)]. Our study led us to identify three differential biomarkers in the CSF of AD patients (sIL-6R, TIMP-1, and sTNFR-I), which could be efficiently combined. They were, however, not differential in the serum. On the other hand, using classification trees, we could obtain notable results in both CSF and serum, involving, respectively, IGFBP6 and MIP-3 beta or IL-8, and TNFR-I. Upon confirmation, these results could represent interesting new means for the diagnostic of AD. These biomarkers, associated with the biochemical diagnostic tools currently used for AD diagnosis (such as CSF biomarkers Aβ, tau, and p-tau), could be of particular interest for early diagnosis of AD or for patients presenting ambiguous profiles.

In conclusion, this study confirms the potential diagnosis interest of previously published blood biomarkers, and proposes new ones (such as IL-8 and TNFR-I). Further studies will be needed to validate these biomarkers which could be used alone, combined, or in association with the classical CSF biomarkers.

Table S1 | Antibody array map of G6 and G7 slides. Each array allowed for the detection and semi-quantitation of 60 human cytokines. POS and NEG correspond to positive and negative control, respectively, and are used for normalization of fluorescence detected from the slides.

Data S1 | CQI homogeneity between arrays. CQI was hybridized on each array (G6 and G7) in the very same conditions than the biological samples studied. Non-homogenous slide (G6, gray-highlighted) was extracted before analysis of the normalized data generated.

References

1. Latta CH, Brothers HM, Wilcock DM. Neuroinflammation in Alzheimer's disease: a source of heterogeneity and target for personalized therapy. *Neuroscience* (2014) **302**:103–11. doi:10.1016/j.neuroscience.2014.09.061
2. Akiyama H. Inflammation and Alzheimer's disease. *Neurobiol Aging* (2000) **21**(3):383–421. doi:10.1016/S0197-4580(00)00124-X
3. Heneka MT, Carson MJ, El Khoury J, Landreth GE, Brosseron F, Feinstein DL, et al. Neuroinflammation in Alzheimer's disease. *Lancet Neurol* (2015) **14**(4):388–405. doi:10.1016/S1474-4422(15)70016-5
4. Blennow K, Hampel H, Weiner M, Zetterberg H. Cerebrospinal fluid and plasma biomarkers in Alzheimer disease. *Nat Rev Neurol* (2010) **6**(3):131–44. doi:10.1038/nrneurol.2010.4
5. Masters CL, Simms G, Weinman NA, Multhaup G, McDonald BL, Beyreuther K. Amyloid plaque core protein in Alzheimer disease and Down syndrome. *Proc Natl Acad Sci U S A* (1985) **82**(12):4245–9. doi:10.1073/pnas.82.12.4245
6. Grundke-Iqbal I, Iqbal K, Tung YC, Quinlan M, Wisniewski HM, Binder LI. Abnormal phosphorylation of the microtubule-associated protein tau (tau) in Alzheimer cytoskeletal pathology. *Proc Natl Acad Sci U S A* (1986) **83**(13):4913–7. doi:10.1073/pnas.83.13.4913
7. Doecke JD, Laws SM, Faux NG, Wilson W, Burnham SC, Lam CP, et al. Blood-based protein biomarkers for diagnosis of Alzheimer disease. *Arch Neurol* (2012) **69**(10):1318–25. doi:10.1001/archneurol.2012.1282
8. Ray S, Britschgi M, Herbert C, Takeda-Uchimura Y, Boxer A, Blennow K, et al. Classification and prediction of clinical Alzheimer's diagnosis based on plasma signaling proteins. *Nat Med* (2007) **13**(11):1359–62. doi:10.1038/nm1653
9. O'Bryant SE, Xiao G, Barber R, Huebinger R, Wilhelmsen K, Edwards M, et al. A blood-based screening tool for Alzheimer's disease that spans serum and plasma: findings from TARC and ADNI. *PLoS One* (2011) **6**(12):e28092. doi:10.1371/journal.pone.0028092
10. Llano DA, Laforet G, Devanarayan V. Derivation of a new ADAS-cog composite using tree-based multivariate analysis: prediction of conversion from mild cognitive impairment to Alzheimer disease. *Alzheimer Dis Assoc Disord* (2011) **25**(1):73–84. doi:10.1097/WAD.0b013e3181f5b8d8
11. Hye A, Riddoch-Contreras J, Baird AL, Ashton NJ, Bazenet C, Leung R, et al. Plasma proteins predict conversion to dementia from prodromal disease. *Alzheimers Dement* (2014) **10**(6):799e–807e. doi:10.1016/j.jalz.2014.05.1749
12. Hu WT, Holtzman DM, Fagan AM, Shaw LM, Perrin R, Arnold SE, et al. Plasma multianalyte profiling in mild cognitive impairment and Alzheimer disease. *Neurology* (2012) **79**(9):897–905. doi:10.1212/WNL.0b013e318266fa70
13. Thambisetty M, Lovestone S. Blood-based biomarkers of Alzheimer's disease: challenging but feasible. *Biomark Med* (2010) **4**(1):65–79. doi:10.2217/bmm.09.84
14. Galasko D, Golde TE. Biomarkers for Alzheimer's disease in plasma, serum and blood – conceptual and practical problems. *Alzheimers Res Ther* (2013) **5**(2):10. doi:10.1186/alzrt164
15. del Campo M, Mollenhauer B, Bertolotto A, Engelborghs S, Hampel H, Simonsen AH, et al. Recommendations to standardize preanalytical confounding factors in Alzheimer's and Parkinson's disease cerebrospinal fluid biomarkers: an update. *Biomark Med* (2012) **6**(4):419–30. doi:10.2217/bmm.12.46
16. McKhann G, Drachman D, Folstein M, Katzman R, Price D, Stadlan EM. Clinical diagnosis of Alzheimer's disease: report of the NINCDS-ADRDA Work Group under the auspices of Department of Health and Human Services Task Force on Alzheimer's Disease. *Neurology* (1984) **34**(7):939–44. doi:10.1212/WNL.34.7.939
17. Petersen RC, Smith GE, Waring SC, Ivnik RJ, Tangalos EG, Kokmen E. Mild cognitive impairment: clinical characterization and outcome. *Arch Neurol* (1999) **56**(3):303–8. doi:10.1001/archneur.56.3.303
18. Lehmann S, Dumurgier J, Schraen S, Wallon D, Blanc F, Magnin E, et al. A diagnostic scale for Alzheimer's disease based on cerebrospinal fluid biomarker profiles. *Alzheimers Res Ther* (2014) **6**(3):38. doi:10.1186/alzrt267
19. Johnstone D, Milward EA, Berretta R, Moscato P, Alzheimer's Disease Neuroimaging Initiative. Multivariate protein signatures of pre-clinical Alzheimer's disease in the Alzheimer's disease neuroimaging initiative (ADNI) plasma proteome dataset. *PLoS One* (2012) **7**(4):e34341. doi:10.1371/journal.pone.0034341
20. Lue LF, Rydel R, Brigham EF, Yang LB, Hampel H, Murphy GM Jr, et al. Inflammatory repertoire of Alzheimer's disease and nondemented elderly microglia in vitro. *Glia* (2001) **35**(1):72–9. doi:10.1002/glia.1072
21. Laske C, Stransky E, Hoffmann N, Maetzler W, Straten G, Eschweiler GW, et al. Macrophage colony-stimulating factor (M-CSF) in plasma and CSF of patients with mild cognitive impairment and Alzheimer's disease. *Curr Alzheimer Res* (2010) **7**(5):409–14. doi:10.2174/156720510791383813
22. Tarkowski E, Andreasen N, Tarkowski A, Blennow K. Intrathecal inflammation precedes development of Alzheimer's disease. *J Neurol Neurosurg Psychiatry* (2003) **74**(9):1200–5. doi:10.1136/jnnp.74.9.1200
23. He P, Zhong Z, Lindholm K, Berning L, Lee W, Lemere C, et al. Deletion of tumor necrosis factor death receptor inhibits amyloid beta generation and prevents learning and memory deficits in Alzheimer's mice. *J Cell Biol* (2007) **178**(5):829–41. doi:10.1083/jcb.200705042
24. Janelsins MC, Mastrangelo MA, Park KM, Sudol KL, Narrow WC, Oddo S, et al. Chronic neuron-specific tumor necrosis factor-alpha expression enhances the local inflammatory environment ultimately leading to neuronal death in 3xTg-AD mice. *Am J Pathol* (2008) **173**(6):1768–82. doi:10.2353/ajpath.2008.080528
25. Figiel I. Pro-inflammatory cytokine TNF-alpha as a neuroprotective agent in the brain. *Acta Neurobiol Exp (Wars)* (2008) **68**(4):526–34.
26. Akama KT, Van Eldik LJ. Beta-amyloid stimulation of inducible nitric-oxide synthase in astrocytes is interleukin-1beta- and tumor necrosis factor-alpha (TNFalpha)-dependent, and involves a TNFalpha receptor-associated factor- and NFkappaB-inducing kinase-dependent signaling mechanism. *J Biol Chem* (2000) **275**(11):7918–24.
27. Savarin-Vuaillat C, Ransohoff RM. Chemokines and chemokine receptors in neurological disease: raise, retain, or reduce? *Neurotherapeutics* (2007) **4**(4):590–601. doi:10.1016/j.nurt.2007.07.004
28. Xia MQ, Qin SX, Wu LJ, Mackay CR, Hyman BT. Immunohistochemical study of the beta-chemokine receptors CCR3 and CCR5 and their ligands in normal

and Alzheimer's disease brains. *Am J Pathol* (1998) **153**(1):31–7. doi:10.1016/S0002-9440(10)65542-3

29. Smits HA, Rijsmus A, van Loon JH, Wat JW, Verhoef J, Boven LA, et al. Amyloid-beta-induced chemokine production in primary human macrophages and astrocytes. *J Neuroimmunol* (2002) **127**(1–2):160–8. doi:10.1016/S0165-5728(02)00112-1
30. Stuart MJ, Baune BT. Chemokines and chemokine receptors in mood disorders, schizophrenia, and cognitive impairment: a systematic review of biomarker studies. *Neurosci Biobehav Rev* (2014) **42**:93–115. doi:10.1016/j.neubiorev.2014.02.001
31. Craig-Schapiro R, Kuhn M, Xiong C, Pickering EH, Liu J, Misko TP, et al. Multiplexed immunoassay panel identifies novel CSF biomarkers for Alzheimer's disease diagnosis and prognosis. *PLoS One* (2011) **6**(4):e18850. doi:10.1371/journal.pone.0018850
32. Hanzel CE, Iulita MF, Eyjolfsdottir H, Hjorth E, Schultzberg M, Eriksdotter M, et al. Analysis of matrix metallo-proteases and the plasminogen system in mild cognitive impairment and Alzheimer's disease cerebrospinal fluid. *J Alzheimers Dis* (2014) **40**(3):667–78. doi:10.3233/JAD-132282
33. Whitmer RA, Gustafson DR, Barrett-Connor E, Haan MN, Gunderson EP, Yaffe K. Central obesity and increased risk of dementia more than three decades later. *Neurology* (2008) **71**(14):1057–64. doi:10.1212/01.wnl.0000306313.89165.ef
34. Cheon MS, et al. Heart type fatty acid binding protein (H-FABP) is decreased in brains of patients with Down syndrome and Alzheimer's disease. *J Neural Transm Suppl* (2003) **67**:225–34.

A practical guide to immunoassay method validation

Ulf Andreasson[1], Armand Perret-Liaudet[2], Linda J. C. van Waalwijk van Doorn[3,4], Kaj Blennow[1], Davide Chiasserini[5], Sebastiaan Engelborghs[6,7], Tormod Fladby[8,9], Sermin Genc[10], Niels Kruse[11], H. Bea Kuiperij[3,4], Luka Kulic[12], Piotr Lewczuk[13], Brit Mollenhauer[14,15], Barbara Mroczko[16], Lucilla Parnetti[5], Eugeen Vanmechelen[17], Marcel M. Verbeek[3,4], Bengt Winblad[18], Henrik Zetterberg[1,19], Marleen Koel-Simmelink[20] and Charlotte E. Teunissen[20]*

[1] Clinical Neurochemistry Laboratory, Institute of Neuroscience and Physiology, The Sahlgrenska Academy, University of Gothenburg, Mölndal, Sweden, [2] Neurobiology Laboratory, Centre for Memory Resources and Research (CMRR), Groupement Hospitalier Est (GHE), Hôpitaux de Lyon, Université Lyon 1, CNRS UMR5292, INSERM U1028, Lyon, France, [3] Department of Neurology, Donders Institute for Brain, Cognition and Behaviour, Radboud University Medical Center, Nijmegen, Netherlands, [4] Department of Laboratory Medicine, Donders Institute for Brain, Cognition and Behaviour, Radboud Alzheimer Centre, Nijmegen, Netherlands, [5] Laboratory of Clinical Neurochemistry, Department of Medicine, Section of Neurology, University of Perugia, Perugia, Italy, [6] Reference Center for Biological Markers of Dementia (BIODEM), Institute Born-Bunge, University of Antwerp, Antwerp, Belgium, [7] Department of Neurology and Memory Clinic, Hospital Network Antwerp (ZNA) Middelheim and Hoge Beuken, Antwerp, Belgium, [8] University of Oslo, Oslo, Norway, [9] Department of Neurology, Akershus University Hospital, Lørenskog, Norway, [10] Department of Neuroscience, Institute of Health Science, Dokuz Eylul University, Izmir, Turkey, [11] Department of Neuropathology, University Medical Center, Göttingen, Germany, [12] Division of Psychiatry Research, University of Zurich, Schlieren, Switzerland, [13] Department of Psychiatry and Psychotherapy, Universitätsklinikum Erlangen, Friedrich-Alexander Universität Erlangen-Nürnberg, Erlangen, Germany, [14] Paracelsus-Elena Klinik, Kassel, Germany, [15] Department of Neuropathology, University Medical Center Göttingen, Göttingen, Germany, [16] Department of Neurodegeneration Diagnostics, Medical University of Białystok, Białystok, Poland, [17] ADx NeuroSciences, Ghent, Belgium, [18] Karolinska Institutet, Stockholm, Sweden, [19] Institute of Neurology, University College London, London, UK, [20] Neurochemistry Laboratory and Biobank, Department of Clinical Chemistry, Neurocampus Amsterdam, VU University Medical Center, Amsterdam, Netherlands

Edited by:
Wendy Noble,
King's College London, UK

Reviewed by:
Haung Yu,
Columbia University, USA
Selina Wray,
University College London, UK

Correspondence:
Ulf Andreasson,
Clinical Neurochemistry Laboratory, Institute of Neuroscience and Physiology, The Sahlgrenska Academy at the University of Gothenburg, Hus V3, Mölndal 43180, Sweden
ulf.andreasson@neuro.gu.se

Biochemical markers have a central position in the diagnosis and management of patients in clinical medicine, and also in clinical research and drug development, also for brain disorders, such as Alzheimer's disease. The enzyme-linked immunosorbent assay (ELISA) is frequently used for measurement of low-abundance biomarkers. However, the quality of ELISA methods varies, which may introduce both systematic and random errors. This urges the need for more rigorous control of assay performance, regardless of its use in a research setting, in clinical routine, or drug development. The aim of a method validation is to present objective evidence that a method fulfills the requirements for its intended use. Although much has been published on which parameters to investigate in a method validation, less is available on a detailed level on how to perform the corresponding experiments. To remedy this, standard operating procedures (SOPs) with step-by-step instructions for a number of different validation parameters is included in the present work together with a validation report template, which allow for a well-ordered presentation of the results. Even though the SOPs were developed with the intended use for immunochemical methods and to be used for multicenter evaluations, most of them are generic and can be used for other technologies as well.

Keywords: immunoassays, method validation, precision, limits of quantitation, robustness

Introduction

Biochemical markers (biomarkers) play a central role in the decision-making in clinical medicine. Examples include making a clinical diagnosis, initiating and monitoring treatment, predicting prognosis or disease recurrence after treatment. Among brain disorders, the Alzheimer's disease (AD) field is in the good situation that a panel of cerebrospinal fluid (CSF) biomarkers is at hand, including the 42 amino acid variant of β-amyloid (Aβ42), total tau (T-tau), and phosphorylated tau (P-tau), and have in numerous studies been shown to have high diagnostic accuracy for AD also in the early stage of the disease (1). Except for an increasing use in clinical routine, these biomarkers are also used in clinical trials, both as diagnostic and as theragnostic markers (2). Last, these CSF biomarkers are applied in clinical studies on disease pathogenesis, and many research reports present novel biomarker candidates. The vast majority of such fluid biomarkers are low-abundance proteins, for which antibody-based immunoassays, often in the enzyme-linked immunosorbent assay (ELISA) format, is needed to get enough analytical sensitivity. However, to get reliable and reproducible results, rigorous control of assay performance is essential, which also should be presented in a standardized format.

Validation of a method is the confirmation by examination and the provision of objective evidence that the particular requirements for a specific intended use are fulfilled (3). It is important as it defines whether it will produce reliable results in the context of its intended use. This last item is sometimes overlooked; the intended use of a method needs to be carefully specified before any time consuming and costly validation experiments are performed. This notion is generic to any method. However, this paper will now focus on the validation of methods used to determine analyte concentrations in biofluids. The intended use for such a method could be to use the outcome as a diagnostic marker and in this case some evidence should be in place showing that there is a disease-dependent change in the analyte concentration in a biological sample. Furthermore, the magnitude of the change should have an impact on the acceptable variability of the method, i.e., if the change is small the higher is the demand on the precision and on the analytical sensitivity and specificity.

Much has been published on the topic of method validation but a consensus protocol on how to perform the task is yet to be found. This could be partly due to the fact that different analytical technologies have different requirements on which validation parameters that need to be addressed or that local initiatives by national societies in the clinical chemistry field were not discussed and spread at international level (4). For example, carryover should be investigated in a chromatography-based method while it is not applicable in an ELISA. The aim of the present work was to present straightforward step-by-step standard operating procedures (SOPs) for the validation of methods in which an analyte is determined in a biofluid matrix; the SOPs have been developed with the intention that they should be possible to follow without any advanced prior training.

This work is the main deliverable of the sub-task "Development of assay qualification protocols" in the BIOMARKAPD project supported by the European Union initiative Joint Programme – Neurodegenerative Disease Research. The BIOMARKAPD project aims for standardization of biomarker measurements for AD and Parkinson's disease (PD), including pre-analytical and analytical procedures, assay validation, and development of reference measurement procedures (RMP) and certified reference materials (CRM) for harmonization of results across assay formats and laboratories. The work flow in the present project consisted of writing draft SOPs for each parameter relevant to validation of a method for determination of an analyte concentration in a biofluid. Task members were then asked to review and revise the SOPs, whereafter they were evaluated in at least three multicenter studies. End-users commented on the draft SOPs, and, after an additional round of reviews, final, consensus SOPs were produced which form the core of the current report. All members of the task were invited to critically revise the manuscript.

Full vs. Partial Validation

Standard operating procedures for 10 different validation parameters are presented. If a method is developed in-house, a full validation should be performed, meaning that all parameters should be investigated. As a consensus agreement in the group, it was decided that a partial validation of a commercial assay should include all parameters except for robustness, which should have been covered by the manufacturer during method development. Even more limited partial validations may be eligible under other circumstances. For example, if a validated *in vitro* diagnostic (IVD) method is transferred to another laboratory to be run on a different instrument by a different technician it might be sufficient to revalidate the precision and the limits of quantification since these variables are most sensitive to the changes, while more intrinsic properties for a method, e.g., dilution linearity and recovery, are not likely to be affected.

It is also advisable to have a dialog with the client/sponsor to agree to what extent the method should be validated. Unfortunately, the standard ISO 15189 (20), which is designed for clinical laboratories, does not provide much rigor by only stating that "The validations shall be as extensive as are necessary to meet the needs in the given application or field of application."

Validation Report

If a laboratory is, or plan to be, accredited to some international standard there is usually a high demand on documentation. For example, in order to comply with the standard ISO 15189 "The laboratory shall record the results obtained and the procedure used for the validation (20)." To facilitate this and at the same time allow for a well-ordered presentation of the results a validation report template can be found in Data Sheet S1 in Supplementary Material. The template has been adapted from a Swedish handbook on method validation (5), with the permission of the authors. Below an outline of the 10 validation parameters is given and a short definition of each are presented in **Table 1**. To aid in the extraction of information from measurement data the Data Sheet S2 in Supplementary Material can be used.

Robustness

Robustness or ruggedness is the ability of a method to remain unaffected by small variations in method parameters. If the instructions from the manufacturer of a commercially available

TABLE 1 | Short description of the validation parameters for which SOPs are presented.

	Parameter	Definition	Reference
1	Robustness	The ability of a method to remain unaffected by small variations in method parameters	(6)
2	Precision	The closeness of agreement between independent test results obtained under stipulated conditions	(7)
3	Trueness	The closeness of agreement between the average value obtained from a large series of test results and an accepted reference value	(7)
4	Uncertainty	A parameter associated with the result of a measurement, that characterizes the dispersion of the values could reasonably be attributed to the measurand	(8)
5	Limits of quantification	Highest and lowest concentrations of analyte that have been demonstrated to be measurable with acceptable levels of precision and accuracy	(6)
6	Dilutional linearity	Dilutional linearity is performed to demonstrate that a sample with a spiked concentration above the ULOQ can be diluted to a concentration within the working range and still give a reliable result	(6)
7	Parallelism	Relative accuracy from recovery tests on the biological matrix or diluted matrix against the calibrators in a substitute matrix	(6)
8	Recovery	The recovery of an anlayte in an assay is the detector response obtained from an amount of the analyte added to and extracted from the biological matrix, compared to the detector response obtained for the true concentration of the analyte in the solvent	(9)
9	Selectivity	The ability of the bioanalytical method to measure and differentiate the analytes in the presence of components that may be expected to be present	(9)
10	Sample stability	The chemical stability of an analyte in a given matrix under specific conditions for given time intervals	(9)

assay does not contain any information indicative of a robustness assessment the manufacturer should be contacted and asked to provide this information since it is likely that such data is available given that the method development was sound. In case of an in-house method, the robustness should be investigated as a part of the method development and the results should be reflected in the assay protocol before other validation parameters are investigated. The reason for this is that a validation is linked to an assay protocol and changes in the latter might demand a new validation to be performed.

Procedure

1. Identify critical parameters in the procedure, e.g., incubation times and temperatures.
2. Perform the assay with systematic changes in these parameters, one at the time, using the same set samples at each occasion.
3. If the measured concentrations do not depend on the changes, adjust the protocol by adding appropriate intervals, e.g., 30 ± 3 min or 23 ± 5°C, to the critical parameters.
4. If the changes systematically alter the measured concentrations, lower the magnitude of the changes until no dependence is observed. Incorporate the results into the protocol.

Note: if many critical steps are identified the number of experiments can be reduced using dedicated software, e.g., MODDE (Umetrics) or published methods (10).

Precision

Precision is defined as "The closeness of agreement between independent test results obtained under stipulated conditions" (7). There are three different types of precisions depending on the stipulated conditions and these are repeatability (r), intermediate precision (Rw), and reproducibility (R). Repeatability is the variability observed when as many factors as possible, e.g., laboratory, technician, days, instrument, reagent lot, are held constant and the time between the measurements is kept to a minimum as opposed to reproducibility conditions where all factors are varied and measurements are carried out over several days. For intermediate precision, all factors except laboratory are allowed to vary and for clarity the factors changed should be stated in the validation report. Repeatability is sometimes called within-run or within-day precision while intermediate precision is also known as between-run or between day repeatability.

Precision is difficult to quantify and it is therefore the inversely related imprecision that is commonly reported. As measures of the imprecision it is usual to report both the SD and coefficient of variation (%CV) for the different levels of the measurand investigated with the condition as a subscript, e.g., $\%CV_{Rw}$. Analysis of variance (ANOVA) is used in the estimation of the imprecision and to facilitate in the calculations an excel file (Data Sheet S3 in Supplementary Material) has been created using the formulas in ISO 5725-2 (11).

Procedure

1. Collect samples with known high and low concentrations of the measurand. Pool samples if necessary.
2. Make 25 aliquots of each sample and store at −80°C pending analysis.
3. At day 1–5 measure 5 replicates on each sample. Note: the days need not to be consecutive, only different.
4. Insert data, separate days on different rows, in the excel file Data Sheet S3 in Supplementary Material that calculates the mean value, SD, %CV for both the repeatability and intermediate precision.

Five samples with different levels have been suggested as a general rule to cover a wide measuring range (7). However, it can be argued that if the levels are chosen with care, for example, one above and one below the decision limit, two samples might be enough. In addition, it is not always possible to obtain samples covering a wide range, e.g., when levels in patients and controls do not differ much or when these levels are still to be defined. If large volumes of the samples are available, more aliquots than the ones needed for the precision measurements can be prepared for use as internal quality control samples when the method has been put in service.

Other experimental schemes than the one suggested under points 2–3 in the procedure are possible, e.g., 12 replicates on 1 day and 3 replicates on 4 different days, or as the Clinical and Laboratory Standards Institute recommends, 2 separate runs on 20 days (total 40 runs) (12). The latter scheme will allow for more different factors to be explored, which will give a better estimate of the variability. At the same time, it is very impractical and expensive if the method is, e.g., a commercial ELISA kit where the number of calibrator curves that can be constructed in each kit-package is usually very limited.

Trueness

Trueness is defined as "The closeness of agreement between the average value obtained from a large series of test results and an accepted reference value" (7). Ideally, the reference value is derived directly from a CRM or from materials that can be traced to the CRM. The quantity in which the trueness is measured is called bias (b), which is the systematic difference between the test result and the accepted reference value.

Procedure

1. Given that there exists a CRM, calculate the bias (b_{CRM}) using formula (1) where the measured mean value ($\overline{X}$) is calculated from five replicates and x_{ref} is the assigned reference value.
2. If there exists an external quality control (QC) program, but no CRM, the bias (b_{QC}) is calculated as the mean value of the deviations from the assigned QC values using formula (2). Note: the bias might be concentration-dependent and therefore b_{QC} should preferably be calculated using a longitudinal QC sample.

Formulas

$$b_{CRM} = \overline{X}\text{-}\, X_{ref} \tag{1}$$

$$b_{QC} = \frac{\sum_{i=1}^{n} (X_i - X_{QCi})}{n} \tag{2}$$

where n is the number of measurements, x_i is the value measured in the laboratory, and x_{QCi} is the value from the ith sample in the QC program.

Once the bias is determined, it can be used to compensate the measured concentration resulting in a method without systematic effects (8). If the bias is constant over the measurement interval the bias is simply subtracted from the measured value and if the bias is proportional to the measured concentration the correction is done by multiplication of a factor determined from bias evaluations at different concentrations. Alternatively, the calibrators can be assigned new values to compensate for the bias. The total bias is the sum of two components originating from the method and the laboratory, respectively. When a CRM is available, manufacturers are obliged to calibrate their method against materials traceable to the CRM and then the total bias should in principle be equal to the laboratory bias.

Uncertainty

The intermediate precision provides information about the dispersion characteristics of the results within a laboratory with no regard to the true value of a measurand in a sample. Therefore, in the absence of a CRM, the measurements rather deliver relative concentrations as opposed to absolute ones that can be achieved if the calibrators were traceable to a CRM. However, if different methods can be used for quantifying the same analyte and if a universal cutoff value is warranted there is a need for a CRM that can be used by the kit manufacturers to calibrate their methods against, in order to minimize the bias. This will also enable calculating absolute concentrations but the uncertainty in the results must then include not only the uncertainty from the method but also the uncertainty of the assigned value for the CRM.

Procedure

1. Given that there exists a CRM, calculate the combined uncertainty (u_c) from the standard uncertainty of the precision ($u_{precision}$) and the CRM (u_{CRM}) using formula (3). Note: both $u_{precision}$ and u_{CRM} have to be SDs. Note: this way of calculating the u_c assumes that the bias has been adjusted for as outlined in the trueness section above. Note: the results from the precision measurements can be used as an estimate of the uncertainty, e.g., $u_{precision} = s_{RW}$.
2. Calculate the expanded uncertainty (U) using formula (4). Note: the coverage factor (k) is set to 2 for a confidence interval of approximately 95%. Note: the coverage factor for a given confidence interval is dependent on the degrees of freedom. Details on this and coverage factors for other confidence intervals can be found elsewhere (8).

Formulas

$$u_c = \sqrt{(u_{precision})^2 + (u_{CRM})^2} \tag{3}$$

$$U = k \cdot u_c \tag{4}$$

Limits of Quantification

The working range for a method is defined by the lower and upper limits of quantification (LLOQ and ULOQ, respectively). At least for the LLOQ, there is more than one definition and these can be classified as either determined based on the signals from the instrument or the calculated concentrations from samples. For the former, a number of blank samples are analyzed and the average and SD of the signal are calculated (13).

Procedure

1. Run 16 blank samples (immunodepleted matrix or sample diluent)
2. Calculate the mean and SD of the signal.
3. Determine the concentration based on a signal of 10 SDs above the mean of the blank. Note: this procedure gives only the LLOQ but not the ULOQ.

To determine the concentration based on a signal the inverse of the calibration function must be used. The two most common models used in immunochemical calibrations are the four and five parametric logistic models. The four parametric function and its inverse are:

$$\text{Signal} = \frac{A-D}{1+\left(\frac{\text{Concentration}}{C}\right)^B} + D \Leftrightarrow \text{Concentration} = C\left(\frac{A-D}{\text{Signal}-D} - 1\right)^{\frac{1}{B}} \quad (5)$$

For the five-parameter logistic model the corresponding functions are:

$$\text{Signal} = \frac{A-D}{\left(1+\left(\frac{\text{Concentration}}{C}\right)^B\right)^E} + D \Leftrightarrow \text{Concentration} = C\left(\left(\frac{A-D}{\text{Signal}-D} - 1\right)^{\frac{1}{E}} - 1\right)^{\frac{1}{B}} \quad (6)$$

The parameters A–E should be available from the software used for data acquisition and analysis.

Based on the concentrations the LLOQ and ULOQ can be defined as the endpoints of an interval in which the %CV is under a specific level with the option of a higher %CV at the endpoints (9, 14).

Procedure

1. Analyze, in duplicates, samples with very low and very high concentrations of the measurand.
2. Calculate the average concentration and %CVs for the samples.
3. Make a scatter plot of the %CV as a function of concentration for all samples.
4. Determine the LLOQ by identifying the lowest mean level above which the %CV < 20% for the greater majority of the samples.
5. Determine the ULOQ by identifying the highest mean level below which the %CV < 20% for the greater majority of the samples.

Dilution Linearity

Dilution linearity is performed to demonstrate that a sample with a spiked concentration above the ULOQ can be diluted to a concentration within the working range and still give a reliable result. In other words, it determines to which extent the dose–response of the analyte is linear in a particular diluent within the range of the standard curve. Thereby dilution of samples should not affect the accuracy and precision. At the same time, the presence of a hook effect, i.e., suppression of signal at concentrations above the ULOQ, is investigated.

Procedure

1. Spike three samples (undiluted) with calibrator stock solution, as high as possible. Note: if possible, spike (undiluted) samples with 100- to 1000-fold the concentration at ULOQ using the calibrator stock solution. Biological samples can also be diluted less than the prescribed concentration, if an assay allows to.
2. Make serial dilutions of the spiked samples, using sample diluent in small vials until the theoretical concentration is below LLOQ. Note: the dilution should be performed using vials and not directly in the wells of the ELISA plate.
3. Analyze the serial dilutions in duplicates and compensate for the dilution factor.
4. Calculate for each sample the mean concentration for the dilutions that fall into the range of LLOQ and ULOQ. Moreover, calculate for each sample the %Recovery for the calculated concentration at each dilution. Note: the calculated concentration for a dilution that fall into the range of LLOQ and ULOQ should be within the acceptance criteria for the precision defined in the "SOP for fit-for-purpose" as should the calculated SD. Also, plot the signal against the dilution factor to investigate if the signal is suppressed at much higher concentrations than the ULOQ of the measurand ("hook effect").

Dilution linearity should not be confused with linearity of quantitative measurement procedures as defined by CLSI (15), which concerns the linearity of the calibration curve.

Parallelism

Conceptually parallelism and dilution linearity are similar. The major difference is that in the dilution linearity experiments the samples are spiked with the analyte to such a high concentration that after dilution the effect of the sample matrix is likely to be negligible. For parallelism, on the other hand, no spiking is allowed but only samples with high endogenous concentrations of the analyte must be used. However, the concentrations must be lower than the ULOQ. The goal of investigating the parallelism is to ascertain that the binding characteristic of the endogenous analyte to the antibodies is the same as for the calibrator.

Procedure

1. Identify four samples with high, but below ULOQ, endogenous concentration of the measurand.
2. Make at least three, two-fold serial dilutions using sample diluent in reaction vials until the calculated concentration is below LLOQ. Note: the dilution factor should be adjusted to obtain concentrations that are evenly spread over the standard curve. For example, dilution factor 10 if a standard curve includes values between 0.1 and 200 pg/ml.
3. Analyze the neat samples and the serial dilutions in duplicates, in the same run, and compensate for the dilution factor.
4. For each sample, calculate the %CV using results from neat sample and the dilutions.

There are different views on what the acceptance criteria for the %CV should be for showing the presence of parallelism. It has been suggested that %CV $\leq$ 30% for the samples in the dilution series is enough (14, 16) while others advocate a lower level of below 20% (17) or within the range 75–125% compared to the neat sample (18). None of these suggestions, however, relate the acceptance criteria to the precision of the method under investigation.

Recovery

The recovery of an analyte in an assay is the detector response obtained from an amount of the analyte added to and extracted from the biological matrix, compared to the detector response obtained for the true concentration of the analyte in solvent (9). A spike recovery test is conducted to investigate if the concentration–response relationship is similar in the calibration curve and the samples. A bad outcome of the test suggests that there are differences between the sample matrix and calibrator diluent that affects the response in signal. Data obtained from this study could help to find a diluent mimicking the biological sample in which the calibrator and the native protein give the comparable detector signals all along the measuring range.

Procedure

1. Collect five samples were the concentrations of the measurand have previously been determined and divide each sample into 4 aliquots.
2. Spike three of the aliquots, using calibrator stock solution, to expected concentrations that are evenly distributed over the linear range of the standard curve (low, medium, high). Note: all additions should be in the same volume, preferable <10% of the sample volume. The same volume of measurand-free calibrator diluent must also be added to the neat sample (fourth aliquot) to compensate for the dilution. Note: the theoretical concentration in the spiked samples should be lower than the ULOQ. Different spiking concentrations should be used to investigate possible dependency on the amount of added substance. The low spike should be slightly higher than the lowest reliable detectable concentration. Note: alternatively, samples can be spiked after dilution if there is limited availability of the calibrator and high working dilutions.
3. Analyze both the neat and spiked samples in the same run. Dilute each sample as advised for each assay to be used,
4. Calculate the recovery using formula (7). Note: acceptance range for the recovery is usually 80–120%.

$$\% \text{ Recovery} = \frac{\text{Measured concentration}_{\text{spiked sample}} - \text{Measuered concentration}_{\text{neat sample}}}{\text{Theoretical concentration}_{\text{spiked}}} \times 100 \quad (7)$$

Selectivity

Selectivity can be defined as "the ability of the bioanalytical method to measure and differentiate the analytes in the presence of components that may be expected to be present" (9). The terms "selectivity" and "specificity" are often used interchangeably while their significances are different. Selectivity is something that can be graded while specificity is an absolute characteristic. Specificity can be considered as the ultimate selectivity. For this reasons, selectivity should be preferred and is the recommended terminology. Of the different validation parameters the selectivity is in principle the only one for which a certain amount of knowledge about the analyte and related substances is demanded. For example, if the analyte is a peptide of a specific length do slightly longer or shorter peptides also give rise to a signal in the assay? Do metabolites of the analyte or post translational modifications of a protein analyte interfere with the assay?

Procedure

1. Identify substances that are physiochemically similar to the one that the assay is developed for.
2. Investigate to what degree the measurements are interfered by spiking samples with substances identified in step 1. Note: if information is available regarding the endogenous concentration of an investigated substance the spiking concentration should be at least two times the reference limit. Otherwise a titration is recommended.
3. For antibody-based methods, an epitope mapping should be performed.

Sample stability

Sample handling prior to analysis has the potential to dramatically influence the results of a measurement. For this reason, it is important to investigate if different storage conditions contribute to systematic errors in order to provide the clinicians with adequate sample collection and transport instructions. The information gathered will also be useful once the sample reaches the laboratory, i.e., how it should be stored until analysis or pending a possible need for a re-run. Examples of factors that potentially affect the results of an analysis, but are not included in the following procedure includes, sample tube, type of plasma anticoagulant, gradient effects (concerns CSF samples), centrifugation conditions, extended mixing, and diurnal variations. If data are not available on how these factors influence the measurement the sample instructions should be written in a way to prevent variations potentially induced by these.

Procedure

1. Repeat the following steps for three independent samples, preferably with different concentrations of the measurand (low, medium, high).
2. Divide the sample into nineteen aliquots with equal sample volume.
   Note: it is important that every aliquot contains the same sample volume and to use the same kind of reaction vials, since unequal sample volumes may affect the concentration of the measurand due to adsorption.
3. Place aliquots #1–6 at −80°C.
4. Thaw aliquots #2–6 and store again at −80°C.
   Note: thaw for 2 h at room temperature and next store the sample at least 12 h at −80°C for each freeze/thaw cycle.
5. Thaw aliquots #3–6 and store again at −80°C.
6. Thaw aliquots #4–6 and store again at −80°C.
7. Thaw aliquot #5–6 and store again at −80°C.
8. Thaw aliquot #5–6 and store again at −80°C.
9. Thaw aliquot #6 and store again at −80°C.
10. Thaw aliquot #6 and store again at −80°C.
11. At time point 0, store aliquots #7–12 at room temperature and another six aliquots #13–18 at 4°C.
12. At time points $t=1$ h, $t=2$ h, $t=4$ h, $t=24$ h, $t=72$ h, $t=168$ h, transfer one sample stored at each temperature, RT and 4°C, to −80°C.
13. Store aliquot #19 at −20°C during 1 month before transfer to −80°C.

14. Thaw all aliquots for a given sample simultaneously and analyze them in duplicates in the same run.
15. Insert raw data of aliquots #1–19 (replicates of observed concentrations) in the Excel file Data Sheet S4 in Supplementary Material. The file calculates the mean value, SD, and coefficient of variation (%CV) for both the observed concentration and normalized concentration. Note: the SD for the storage conditions and the freeze/thaw aliquots should be within the acceptance criteria for the precision defined in the fit-for-purpose.

The above conditions tested should only serve as an example and the can be modified to better suit the environment and different routine handling of samples at the individual laboratories.

Internal Quality Control Program

The experiments in a validation are usually performed within a month time and therefore the results represent a kind of snapshot of the performance characteristics of the method. To ascertain that the quality does not degrade over time an internal quality control program should be initiated before the assay is taken into service. The results from quality control samples should be used to determine if a run is accepted and the objective multi rules presented by Westgard should be used (19).

Summary

In the present study, we present SOPs for validation of assays for biochemical markers together with a template for validation reports. Although this study is part of a project on biomarkers for AD and PD, the SOPs and validation report is generalizable to biomarker assays in any field of clinical medicine. The main focus for the presented SOPs has been on validation parameters relevant to immunochemical methods such as ELISA and related techniques for determination of the concentration of an analyte in a biofluid. Still, many of the parameters are generic and the SOPs could be used outside the realm of immunochemistry. It should also be stressed that the procedures presented here are practical suggestions on how to collect the information needed to demonstrate that the requirements for a method are fulfilled. As such, they could be used also by persons with limited experience in the field of method validation. We believe that validation of biomarker assays before introduction in clinical routine or implementation in clinical trials is essential to get reliable and interpretable results. Information on assay validation is also important in research reports on novel biomarker candidates.

Acknowledgments

This publication was funded by the Italian Ministry of Health; the Bundesministerium für Bildung und Forschung, Germany; the Netherlands Organization for Health Research and Development (ZonMw); the Leading National Research Centre, Poland; the Scientific and Technological Research Council of Turkey; Norwegian Research Council; and the Swedish Research Council, and is a part of the BIOMARKAPD project in the JPND programme (www.jpnd.eu). SE was supported by the University of Antwerp Research Fund and the Alzheimer Research Foundation (SAO-FRA); the Agency for Innovation by Science and Technology (IWT: www.iwt.be); the Research Foundation Flanders (FWO: www.fwo.be); the Belgian Science Policy Office Interuniversity Attraction Poles (IAP) program (BELSPO: www.belspo.be); the Flemish Government initiated Methusalem excellence grant (EWI: www.ewi-vlaanderen.be); the Flanders Impulse Program on Networks for Dementia Research (VIND). PL received consultation or lecture honoraria from Innogenetics, Roche, Beckman Coulter, AJ Roboscreen, and IBL International, and holds a position of a visiting professor at the Medical University of Bialystok.

References

1. Blennow K, Hampel H, Weiner M, Zetterberg H. Cerebrospinal fluid and plasma biomarkers in Alzheimer disease. *Nat Rev Neurol* (2010) **6**:131–44. doi:10.1038/nrneurol.2010.4
2. Lleo A, Cavedo E, Parnetti L, Vanderstichele H, Herukka SK, Andreasen N, et al. Cerebrospinal fluid biomarkers in trials for Alzheimer and Parkinson diseases. *Nat Rev Neurol* (2015) **11**:41–55. doi:10.1038/nrneurol.2014.232
3. ISO/IEC 17025. *General Requirements for the Competence of Testing and Calibration Laboratories* (2005).
4. Vassault A, Hulin A, Chapuzet E, Arnaud J, Giroud C; Membres Du Sous-Groupe 2 Analytique De La SFBC. [Verification/validation of the performances of analytical method]. *Ann Biol Clin (Paris)* (2010) **68**(Spec No 1):247–94. doi:10.1684/abc.2011.0562
5. Magnusson B, Örnemark U. *Metodvalidering – Handbok för laboratoriet*. Borås: SP Sveriges Tekniska Forskningsinstitut (2012).
6. Lee JW, Devanarayan V, Barrett YC, Weiner R, Allinson J, Fountain S, et al. Fit-for-purpose method development and validation for successful biomarker measurement. *Pharm Res* (2006) **23**:312–28. doi:10.1007/s11095-005-9045-3
7. ISO 5725-1. *Accuracy (Trueness and Precision) of Measurement Methods and Results – Part 1: General Principles and Definitions* (1994).
8. JCGM 100:2008. *Evaluation of Measurement Data – Guide to the Expression of Uncertainty in Measurement* (2008).
9. Guidance for Industry. Bioanalytical method validation. *Fed Regist* (2001) **66**:28526–7.
10. Plackett RL, Burman JP. The design of optimum multifactorial experiments. *Biometrika* (1946) **33**:305–25. doi:10.1093/biomet/33.4.305
11. ISO 5725-2. *Accuracy (Trueness and Precision) of Measurement Methods and Results – Part 2: Basic Method for the Determination of Repeatability and Reproducibility of a Standard Measurement Method* (1994).
12. CLSI. Evaluation of precision performance of quantitative measurement. methods; approved guideline-second edition. In: Wilhelm DM, editor. *CLSI Document EP05-A2*. Wayne, PA: Clinical and Laboratory Standards Institute (2004). p. 1–39.
13. Long GL, Winefordner JD. Limit of detection: a closer look at the IUPAC definition. *Anal Chem* (1983) **55**:712A–24A. doi:10.1021/ac00258a001
14. EMA. *Guideline on Bioanalytical Method Validation* (2011).
15. CLSI. Evaluation of the linearity of quantitative measurement procedures: a statistical approach; approved guideline. In: Polgar PE, editor. *CLSI Document*

EP06-A. Wayne, PA: Clinical and Laboratory Standards Institute (2003). p. 1–47.

16. Desilva B, Smith W, Weiner R, Kelley M, Smolec J, Lee B, et al. Recommendations for the bioanalytical method validation of ligand-binding assays to support pharmacokinetic assessments of macromolecules. *Pharm Res* (2003) **20**:1885–900. doi:10.1023/B:PHAM.0000003390.51761.3d
17. Plikaytis BD, Holder PF, Pais LB, Maslanka SE, Gheesling LL, Carlone GM. Determination of parallelism and nonparallelism in bioassay dilution curves. *J Clin Microbiol* (1994) **32**:2441–7.
18. Valentin MA, Ma S, Zhao A, Legay F, Avrameas A. Validation of immunoassay for protein biomarkers: bioanalytical study plan implementation to support pre-clinical and clinical studies. *J Pharm Biomed Anal* (2011) **55**:869–77. doi:10.1016/j.jpba.2011.03.033
19. Westgard JO, Barry PL, Hunt MR, Groth T. A multi-rule Shewhart chart for quality control in clinical chemistry. *Clin Chem* (1981) **27**:493–501.
20. ISO 15189:2003. *Medical Laboratories – Particular Requirements for Quality and Competence* (2003).

16

Cerebrospinal fluid Aβ40 improves the interpretation of Aβ42 concentration for diagnosing Alzheimer's disease

Aline Dorey[1,2], Armand Perret-Liaudet[1,2,3], Yannick Tholance[2,4†], Anthony Fourier[2,3] and Isabelle Quadrio[2,3]*

[1] Center for Memory Resources and Research, Hospices Civils de Lyon, Charpennes Hospital, Lyon 1 University, Villeurbanne, France, [2] Neurochemistry Unit, Biochemistry Department, Hospices Civils de Lyon, Groupement Hospitalier Est, Bron, France, [3] BioRaN Team, Lyon Neuroscience Research Center, CNRS UMR 5292, INSERM U1028, Lyon 1 University, Bron, France, [4] WAKE Team, Lyon Neuroscience Research Center, CNRS UMR5292, INSERM U1028, Lyon 1 University, Lyon, France

Edited by:
Raymond Scott Turner, Georgetown University, USA

Reviewed by:
Benedict C. Albensi, University of Manitoba, Canada
Zhihui Yang, University of Florida, USA

***Correspondence:**
Armand Perret-Liaudet
armand.perret-liaudet@chu-lyon.fr

The combination of decreased amyloid β42 (Aβ42) and increased total tau proteins (T-Tau) and phosphorylated tau (P-Tau) in cerebrospinal fluid (CSF) has recently been considered as a biological diagnostic criterion of Alzheimer's disease (AD). Previous studies showed significant heterogeneity in CSF Aβ42 levels to discriminate AD from non-AD patients. It was also suggested that the CSF amyloid peptide β42/β40 ratio has better diagnostic performance than Aβ42 alone. The objective of the present study was to investigate the potential added value of determining CSF amyloid β40 peptide (Aβ40) for biological diagnosis of AD when CSF Aβ42 levels failed. CSF AD biomarkers were run in 2,171 samples from 1,499 AD and 672 non-AD patients. The following pathologic thresholds were used to define an AD-positive CSF biomarker profile: T-Tau $\geq$ 400 ng/L, P-Tau181 $\geq$ 60 ng/L, and Aβ42 $\leq$ 700 ng/L. CSF Aβ40 was assayed in AD patients with CSF Aβ42 levels above 700 ng/L and non-AD patients with CSF Aβ42 levels below 700 ng/L. CSF Aβ40 levels were higher in AD than non-AD patients. The receiver operator characteristic curves of CSF Aβ40 and the Aβ42/Aβ40 ratio defined AD cut-off values at 12,644 ng/L and 0.06, respectively. In AD patients with non-pathological CSF Aβ42, CSF Aβ40 concentration was able to correct 76.2% of cases when expressed as CSF Aβ42/Aβ40 ratio and 94.7% of cases when used alone. Using CSF Aβ42 and then CSF Aβ40, the percentage of misinterpreted AD patients fell to 1.0%. CSF Aβ40 concentration improved interpretation of Aβ42 level for the diagnosis of AD. CSF Aβ40 alone showed better diagnostic performance than the amyloid peptide Aβ42/Aβ40 ratio. The added value of determining CSF Aβ40 in AD diagnosis now needs confirming in a cohort of definite AD patients and to be completed with novel amyloid cascade biomarkers.

Keywords: dementia, Alzheimer, Aβ42, Aβ40, cerebrospinal fluid

INTRODUCTION

According to the revised criteria for Alzheimer's disease (AD), definite diagnosis is founded on neuropathology as gold standard, when patients meet the clinical and cognitive criteria for AD dementia (1). Diagnosis of AD onset during the patient's lifetime is said to be "possible" or "probable." Amyloid β42 (Aβ42), total Tau (T-Tau), and phosphorylated Tau proteins (P-Tau) assay in cerebrospinal fluid (CSF) is recommended to increase the level of diagnostic certainty for AD in atypical clinical phenotypes, for inclusion of patients in clinical trials and to improve AD diagnosis at the earliest stages of the disease (1–5). A positive AD CSF biomarker profile was defined as increased CSF Tau and/or P-Tau181 and decreased CSF Aβ42 concentrations (1, 6–8). However, researchers and clinicians continue to debate the sensitivity and specificity of various biomarkers, and especially CSF Aβ42. A recent meta-analysis highlighted significant heterogeneity in CSF Aβ42 values between different disease groups (9), reporting sensitivity and specificity ranging from 71 to 91% and 44 to 82%, respectively. Moreover, Rosen et al. showed that "normal" CSF Aβ42 levels were observed in AD patients, leading to misinterpretation of the AD CSF biomarker profile in 23.2% of AD patients (10).

One of the crucial challenges to improve screening in clinical trials is to identify an accurate CSF biomarker reflecting amyloid pathology. There is now strong evidence that CSF Aβ42 levels depend not only on impaired brain clearance in Alzheimer's pathophysiology, but also on the total load of amyloid peptides, which shows large interindividual variability (11–14). Gamma-secretase cleaves amyloid precursor protein (APP) at several sites, resulting in different C-terminally truncated Aβ variants: amyloid β40 (Aβ40) is the most abundant amyloid peptide in CSF (15), while Aβ42 accounts for only about 10% of the total Aβ peptide population (12, 16–18). Total Aβ concentration was found not to vary significantly between various dementia disorders (11, 18, 19), and Aβ40 concentration did not differ between AD (or presymptomatic AD) patients, healthy controls, and non-AD dementia patients (19–23). CSF Aβ40 concentration could, therefore, be considered to most closely reflect total Aβ load in the brain (13). Previous studies showed that the Aβ42/Aβ40 ratio in CSF is reduced in AD patients, and its assessment improves AD diagnostic accuracy (21–25). More recently, a few studies demonstrated added value for CSF Aβ40 or CSF Aβ42/Aβ40 ratio for differential diagnosis of AD using CSF P-Tau181 levels or in ambiguous AD CSF biomarker profiles (26–28). Therefore, the objective of the present study was to investigate whether determining CSF Aβ40 level and CSF Aβ42/Aβ40 ratio could improve diagnosis in AD patients without low CSF Aβ42 levels.

MATERIALS AND METHODS

Cerebrospinal fluid samples were collected between October 2010 and January 2013 from 2,171 patients who underwent lumbar puncture (LP) for routine clinical diagnosis of AD in the Neurochemistry Unit and Biochemistry Department of the University Hospital of Lyon (France). Patients were included in a multicenter memory clinic and had at least 2 years' follow-up. They were classified into two groups: 1,499 AD and 672 non-AD patients. The non-AD group consisted of 259 patients with probable frontotemporal lobar degeneration (FTLD), 119 with probable dementia with Lewy bodies (DLB), 159 with normal pressure hydrocephalus (NPH), and 135 with psychiatric disorders.

The patients' age, gender, and mini mental state evaluation (MMSE) score were recorded when the LP was performed. At that time, initial diagnosis was based on medical history, caregiver interviews, neurologic examination, neuropsychological battery evaluation, and brain imaging. Clinical diagnosis was made in multidisciplinary team meeting, comprising neurologists, neuropsychologists, and radiologists, and confirmed on follow-up. Dementia was defined according to DSM IV-TR criteria (29), and all AD patients were classified as having AD dementia with evidence of the AD pathophysiological process (1). Patients with mild cognitive impairment were excluded. The non-AD patients diagnosed with FTLD and DLB met the international criteria (30, 31). The non-AD patients with psychiatric disorders or NPH with cognitive complaints unrelated to AD or other degenerative disease were age matched with AD patients, and showed no progression of cognitive impairment within 2 years after CSF analysis.

This study, based on routine biological analyses, was not considered as "biomedical research" under French regulations, and therefore did not require informed consent. Samples were, however, stored in a biobank with authorization from the French Ministry of Health (Declaration number DC-2008-304). Authorization for handling personal data was granted by the French data protection commission [*Commission Nationale de l'Informatique et des Libertés* (CNIL)].

All patients underwent LP to collect CSF using a standard procedure. CSF collection, sampling, and storage were performed according to the international consensus (32, 33). All CSF samples were collected in Sarstedt polypropylene tubes (ref. 62.610.201) showing low adsorption of amyloid peptides (7). CSF biomarker analyses were performed, blind to clinical diagnosis, in the Neurochemistry Unit and Biochemistry Department of the University Hospital of Lyon. This department is involved in two external quality control schemes, one at French national level (working group of the French Society of Clinical Biology: *Société Française de Biologie Clinique*) and the other with the Alzheimer's Association QC program (34). CSF concentrations of Aβ42, T-Tau, and P-Tau181 were measured using the standardized commercially available sandwich ELISA kit (INNOTEST®) according to the manufacturer's procedures (Fujirebio, Ghent, Belgium).

For each CSF sample, Aβ42, T-Tau, and P-Tau181 biomarkers were simultaneously analyzed. As previously described (7), the cut-off values defining positive AD CSF biomarker profile were: T-Tau $\geq$ 400 ng/L, P-Tau181 $\geq$ 60 ng/L, and Aβ42 $\leq$ 700 ng/L.

Aβ40 level in CSF was quantified using ELISA tests [Human Amyloid b (1–40) (N) Assay kit, IBL, Japan] in AD patients with CSF Aβ42 levels above 700 ng/L and in non-AD patients with CSF Aβ42 levels below 700 ng/L.

Statistical Analysis

Chi-square test, Mann–Whitney *U* test, Kruskal–Wallis test, and receiver operator characteristic (ROC) analyses were performed using MedCalc version 11.3.1.0 (http://www.medcalc.be). Differences were considered statistically significant at $p < 0.05$. ROC curves were applied to define optimal biomarker cut-off values to discriminate between AD and non-AD groups. The cut-off value was defined as the value corresponding to the highest average for sensitivity and specificity. Accuracy was calculated as the sum of true positives and true negatives in the total number of patients (35).

RESULTS

Cerebrospinal fluid data according to diagnostic group are summarized in **Table 1** and **Figure 1**.

About 81.3% of AD patients (1,218/1,499) fulfilled the pathological CSF Aβ42 criteria; the remaining 18.7% (281/1,499) presented CSF Aβ42 levels above cut-off (>700 ng/L). 63.7% of non-AD patients (428/672) presented CSF Aβ42 levels above 700 ng/L; 36.3% (244/672) had CSF Aβ42 levels below 700 ng/L (**Figure 2**). CSF Aβ40 levels were then determined in these 525 patients: 281 AD patients (>700 ng/L) and 244 non-AD patients (≤700 ng/L).

The ROC curves of CSF Aβ40 level and the Aβ42/Aβ40 ratio determined AD cut-off values of ≥12,644 ng/L and ≤0.06, respectively (**Figure 3**).

TABLE 1 | Demographic, pathologic, and biological parameters of study populations.

		AD	Non-AD
Gender	*n*	1,499	672
	M/F	643/856	358/314
Age (years)	*n*	1,499	672
	Mean	71.6	70.0
	SD	9.5	10.6
MMSE score (/30)	*n*	1,093	488
	Mean	20.2	21.6
	SD	5.6	5.5
T-Tau (ng/L)	*n*	1,499	672
	Median	650	230
	25th–75th P	487–913	168–311
P-Tau_{181} (ng/L)	*n*	1,499	672
	Median	83	38
	25th–75th P	68–109	30–48
Aβ42 (ng/L)	*n*	1,499	672
	Median	539	807
	25th–75th P	443–663	570–1,056
Aβ40 (ng/L)	*n*	281	244
	Median	19,198	7,112
	25th–75th P	15,162–22,409	5,643–9,636
Aβ42/Aβ40 ratio	*n*	281	244
	Median	0.053	0.066
	25th–75th P	0.041–0.059	0.049–0.084

AD, Alzheimer's disease; MMSE, mini mental state evaluation; M, male; F, female; SD, standard deviation; P, percentile.

In the overall population, the percentage of patients in whom amyloid pathology was misinterpreted fell from 24.2% (525/2,171) using CSF Aβ42 alone to 7.8% (169/2,171) when it was followed by CSF Aβ42/Aβ40 ratio, and to 1.7% (37/2,171) when followed by CSF Aβ40 (**Figure 2**). In patients in whom CSF Aβ40 level was determined ($n = 525$), sensitivity and specificity for AD diagnosis were 76.2 and 58.2%, respectively (accuracy, 0.678) using the CSF Aβ42/Aβ40 ratio, and 94.7 and 91.0%, respectively (accuracy, 0.930) using CSF Aβ40 determination.

About 58.2% of the 244 non-AD patients with CSF Aβ42 levels below 700 ng/L (142/244) had CSF Aβ42/Aβ40 ratios higher than 0.06 and 91.0% (222/244) had CSF Aβ40 levels below 12,644 ng/L.

About 76.2% of AD patients (214/281) had CSF Aβ42/Aβ40 ratios below 0.06 and 94.7% (266/281) had CSF Aβ40 levels higher than 12,644 ng/L. In the overall AD population, percentage misinterpretation fell from 18.7% (281/1,499) with CSF Aβ42 alone to 4.5% (67/1,499) using CSF Aβ42 and then CSF Aβ42/Aβ40 ratio and 1.0% (15/1,499) using CSF Aβ42 and then CSF Aβ40 (**Figure 2**).

DISCUSSION

We investigated the potential added value of CSF Aβ40 assay to improve the interpretation of Aβ42 level. The main finding was that CSF Aβ40 appeared to be an interesting complementary biomarker. CSF Aβ40 levels were higher in AD than non-AD patients. Thus, determining CSF Aβ40 concentrations corrected biological diagnosis in AD patients with non-pathological CSF Aβ42 levels in 76.2% of cases using the CSF Aβ42/Aβ40 ratio and in 94.7% using CSF Aβ40 alone; using CSF Aβ42 and then CSF Aβ40, percentage misinterpretation fell to 1.0%.

Cerebrospinal fluid Aβ42 concentrations led to misinterpretation of the AD CSF biomarker profile in 24.2% of our total population and notably in 18.7% of AD patients. This low performance of CSF Aβ42 is in perfect agreement with previous reports (7, 10, 18, 20, 36, 37). The presence of CSF Aβ42 concentrations ≤700 ng/L in non-AD patients could reflect low total CSF amyloid load, while CSF Aβ42 >700 ng/L in AD patients could result from high amyloid load. This concept justifies CSF Aβ40 assay to complete amyloid pathway interpretation.

As reported in various studies (20, 26, 27, 36), the CSF Aβ42/Aβ40 ratio showed better diagnostic performance than CSF Aβ42 alone. The CSF Aβ42/Aβ40 ratio cut-off value at 0.06 was identical to that reported by Lewczuk et al. (36). The discrepancy with Hansson et al.'s (20) 0.095 cut-off might be due to the Genetics Company ELISA kit halving the range of CSF Aβ40 levels. We found an increase in the rate of correct interpretation from 75.8% with CSF Aβ42 alone to 92.2% when CSF Aβ42 assay was followed by determining the CSF Aβ42/Aβ40 ratio, similarly to other reports (20, 28, 36).

The type of sampling and storage tubes is an important source of variability because of amyloid adsorption (33, 37, 38). CSF sample selection from biological banks should, therefore, be performed rigorously. There is parallel adsorption of CSF Aβ42 and Aβ40 onto the sampling tube surface, regardless of the type of plastic (personal data). Systematic use of the CSF

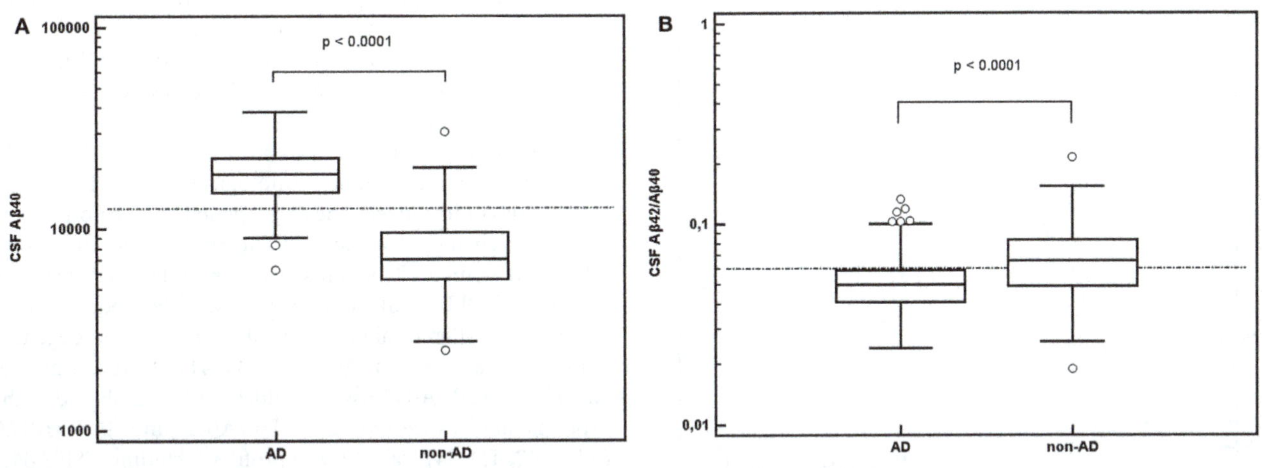

FIGURE 1 | CSF Aβ42/Aβ40 ratio (A) and CSF Aβ40 concentrations in nanograms per liter (B) in AD and non-AD populations. Abbreviation: AD: Alzheimer's disease.

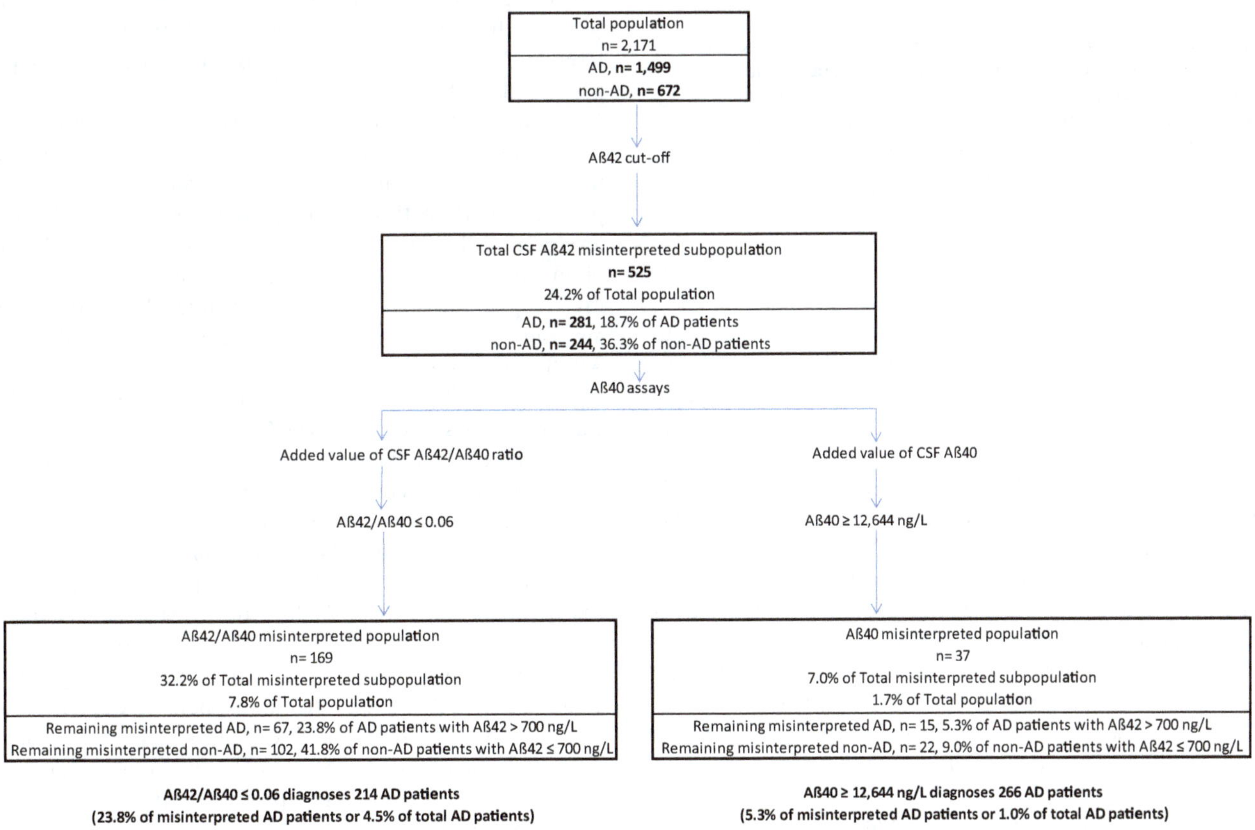

FIGURE 2 | Patient classification based on the determination of cerebrospinal fluid (CSF) amyloid peptides. First, according to CSF Aβ42 levels, we obtained a percentage of misinterpreted patients with discordant results regarding clinical diagnosis. The CSF Aβ40 assay was performed in this subpopulation. Performance in accurately classifying patients was tested for CSF Aβ42/Aβ40 ratio and for CSF Aβ40 alone. Both CSF Aβ42/Aβ40 ratio and CSF Aβ40 could reclassify a high percentage of patients. CSF Aβ40 provided the best correct classification rate. Abbreviation: AD: Alzheimer's disease.

Aβ42/Aβ40 ratio would provide complete interpretation of CSF amyloid biomarker results, integrating the impact of plastic tube type. In the present study, however, samples were analyzed sequentially, leading to higher between-run imprecision for the CSF Aβ42/Aβ40 ratio than for CSF Aβ42 alone [coefficient of variation (CV), 13.3 and 10.2%, respectively]. One solution

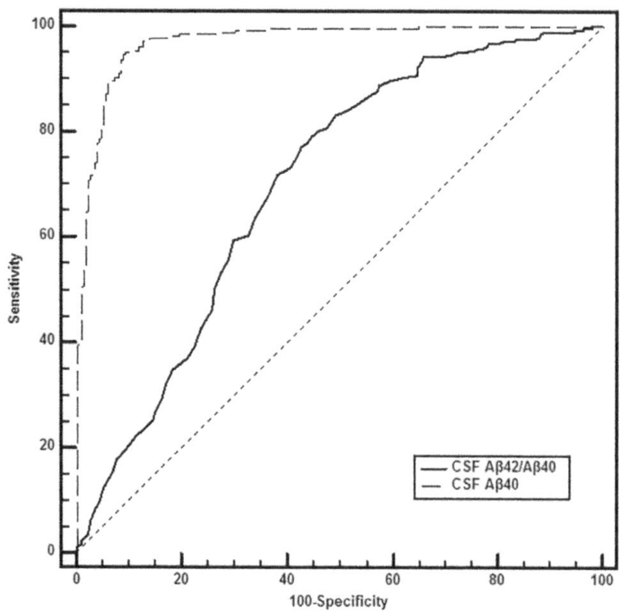

FIGURE 3 | Receiver operating characteristic curve comparison for AD diagnosis in the "discordant CSF Aβ42 values" subpopulation. DeLong et al.'s (1988) method was used to compare the values of the area under the curve (AUC). In the 525 selected patients, accuracy of diagnostic performance was significantly higher for CSF Aβ40 compared to CSF Aβ42/Aβ40 ratio, with 94.7% sensitivity and 91.0% specificity for CSF Aβ40 ≥12,644 ng/L (AUC, 0.969) compared to 76.2 and 58.2%, respectively for CSF Aβ42/Aβ40 ratio ≤0.06 (AUC, 0.700).

to decrease the CV of the CSF Aβ42/Aβ40 ratio would be to use multiplex assays to analyze both amyloid peptides simultaneously. Unfortunately, at the moment, there is no analytical validation available for CSF Aβ42 and CSF Aβ40 in multiplex assays for *in vitro* diagnostic use.

In the present study, CSF Aβ40 was determined only in AD patients with CSF Aβ42 levels above 700 ng/L and in non-AD patients with levels below 700 ng/L. CSF Aβ40 concentrations were significantly higher in AD than non-AD patients. The optimal CSF Aβ40 cut-off value was 12,644 ng/L. To our knowledge, there is currently no effective CSF Aβ40 cut-off value to discriminate AD from non-AD patients reported in the literature; only a slight increase in CSF Aβ40 was found in two other studies (20, 24), and a recent study focusing on AD-MCI patients found a significant increase in CSF Aβ40 values compared to a control group (36). However, the present data contrasted with those reported in another study (26) including AD and non-AD dementia. Selection of the non-AD patient population to compare with the AD population was probably one of the major differences. Another difference may be the biological factor used for the patients' initial classification, CSF P-Tau181 concentrations in intermediate levels (26). Similarly, Sauvee et al. suggested using the CSF Aβ42/Aβ40 ratio when data for CSF Aβ42 combined to CSF P-Tau181 are inconclusive (27). In these particular cases, adding the CSF Aβ42/Aβ40 ratio improved their proportion of interpretable biological profiles from 68 to 89% (27). Moreover, in confirmation of our sequential approach, Sauvee et al. showed that adding CSF Aβ40 peptide concentration and CSF Aβ42/Aβ40 ratio did not change their conclusions when CSF Aβ42 and CSF P-Tau181 were concordant.

In the present study, it was also interesting that 36.3% of non-AD patients presented pathological CSF Aβ42 levels. One hypothesis could concern the heterogeneity of the non-AD population, which included patients with psychiatric disorders and NPH and demented patients with neurodegenerative diseases (FTLD and DLB). CSF Aβ42 was previously reported to be less effective for differential diagnosis of the main neurodegenerative dementia than CSF Tau proteins (39–41). To discriminate AD and FTLD, CSF Aβ42 assay could then be combined with Tau proteins and expressed as T-Tau/Aβ42 and P-Tau181/Aβ42 ratios (42, 43). Typical CSF AD profiles including CSF Aβ42 and Tau proteins were reported in 47% of patients meeting clinical diagnostic criteria for DLB and in 30% of FTLD patients (41), suggesting coexisting pathologies, as strongly highlighted by postmortem studies (44, 45). NPH patients also have lower CSF amyloid peptide and Tau protein concentrations than controls (46, 47). To validate our hypothesis and strategy regarding differential diagnosis, postmortem confirmation on autopsy-proven patients should be carried out.

The diagnostic performance of CSF Aβ42 is increasingly questioned. It should be noted that biological diagnosis as performed in specialized memory clinics is also founded on the second pathway of AD pathophysiology, reflected by CSF Tau protein levels. Nevertheless, a more accurate evaluation of CSF amyloid biomarkers is important to include patients in therapeutic trials involving the amyloid cascade, using added Aβ peptides or other amyloid cascade biomarkers. For example, the soluble peptide APPβ (sAPPβ) and CSF Aβ40 come from the same enzymatic digestion of APP, and it would be interesting to assess sAPPβ to complete this study. Increased CSF sAPPβ levels were already reported in AD patients as compared to non-AD demented patients (48) and FTD patients (49).

In conclusion, the present study offers an improvement in biological diagnosis of AD focusing on the amyloid pathway. In the misinterpretation using CSF Aβ42 levels, classification based on the CSF Aβ42/Aβ40 ratio gives good results. More interestingly, CSF Aβ40 assay alone also provides better results: the misinterpretation rate using CSF Aβ42 and then CSF Aβ40 alone falls to 1.7%. Sequential assessment of CSF Aβ40 would also provide a better cost-effectiveness ratio than systematic determination of the CSF Aβ42/Aβ40 ratio. Finally, these results need to be confirmed in a prospective study including autopsy-proven AD patients, and completed with novel amyloid cascade biomarkers.

ACKNOWLEDGMENTS

This study was conducted under the EU Joint Program – Neurodegenerative Disease Research (JPND) – BIOMARKAPD JPND 0005/2011 project. The authors thank the patients and their families for their participation.

REFERENCES

1. McKhann GM, Knopman DS, Chertkow H, Hyman BT, Jack CR Jr, Kawas CH, et al. The diagnosis of dementia due to Alzheimer's disease: recommendations from the National Institute on Aging-Alzheimer's Association workgroups on diagnostic guidelines for Alzheimer's disease. *Alzheimers Dement* (2011) 7(3):263–9. doi:10.1016/j.jalz.2011.03.005
2. Dubois B, Feldman HH, Jacova C, Hampel H, Molinuevo JL, Blennow K, et al. Advancing research diagnostic criteria for Alzheimer's disease: the IWG-2 criteria. *Lancet Neurol* (2014) **13**(6):614–29. doi:10.1016/S1474-4422(14)70090-0
3. Hort J, O'Brien JT, Gainotti G, Pirttila T, Popescu BO, Rektorova I, et al. EFNS guidelines for the diagnosis and management of Alzheimer's disease. *Eur J Neurol* (2010) **17**(10):1236–48. doi:10.1111/j.1468-1331.2010.03040.x
4. Dubois B, Feldman HH, Jacova C, Cummings JL, Dekosky ST, Barberger-Gateau P, et al. Revising the definition of Alzheimer's disease: a new lexicon. *Lancet Neurol* (2010) **9**(11):1118–27. doi:10.1016/S1474-4422(10)70223-4
5. Albert MS, DeKosky ST, Dickson D, Dubois B, Feldman HH, Fox NC, et al. The diagnosis of mild cognitive impairment due to Alzheimer's disease: recommendations from the National Institute on Aging-Alzheimer's Association workgroups on diagnostic guidelines for Alzheimer's disease. *Alzheimers Dement* (2011) **7**(3):270–9. doi:10.1016/j.jalz.2011.03.008
6. Seguin J, Formaglio M, Perret-Liaudet A, Quadrio I, Tholance Y, Rouaud O, et al. CSF biomarkers in posterior cortical atrophy. *Neurology* (2011) **76**(21):1782–8. doi:10.1212/WNL.0b013e31821ccc98
7. Lehmann S, Schraen S, Quadrio I, Paquet C, Bombois S, Delaby C, et al. Impact of harmonization of collection tubes on Alzheimer's disease diagnosis. *Alzheimers Dement* (2013) **10**(5 Suppl):S390–4. doi:10.1016/j.jalz.2013.06.008
8. Molinuevo JL, Blennow K, Dubois B, Engelborghs S, Lewczuk P, Perret-Liaudet A, et al. The clinical use of cerebrospinal fluid biomarker testing for Alzheimer's disease diagnosis: a consensus paper from the Alzheimer's Biomarkers Standardization Initiative. *Alzheimers Dement* (2014) **10**(6):808–17. doi:10.1016/j.jalz.2014.03.003
9. Mo JA, Lim JH, Sul AR, Lee M, Youn YC, Kim HJ. Cerebrospinal fluid beta-amyloid1-42 levels in the differential diagnosis of Alzheimer's disease – systematic review and meta-analysis. *PLoS One* (2015) **10**(2):e0116802. doi:10.1371/journal.pone.0116802
10. Rosen C, Farahmand B, Skillback T, Nagga K, Mattsson N, Kilander L, et al. Benchmarking biomarker-based criteria for Alzheimer's disease: data from the Swedish Dementia Registry, SveDem. *Alzheimers Dement* (2015). doi:10.1016/j.jalz.2015.04.007
11. Wiltfang J, Esselmann H, Bibl M, Hull M, Hampel H, Kessler H, et al. Amyloid beta peptide ratio 42/40 but not A beta 42 correlates with phospho-Tau in patients with low- and high-CSF A beta 40 load. *J Neurochem* (2007) **101**(4):1053–9. doi:10.1111/j.1471-4159.2006.04404.x
12. Wiltfang J, Esselmann H, Bibl M, Smirnov A, Otto M, Paul S, et al. Highly conserved and disease-specific patterns of carboxyterminally truncated Abeta peptides 1-37/38/39 in addition to 1-40/42 in Alzheimer's disease and in patients with chronic neuroinflammation. *J Neurochem* (2002) **81**(3):481–96. doi:10.1046/j.1471-4159.2002.00818.x
13. Spies PE, Slats D, Sjogren JM, Kremer BP, Verhey FR, Rikkert MG, et al. The cerebrospinal fluid amyloid beta42/40 ratio in the differentiation of Alzheimer's disease from non-Alzheimer's dementia. *Curr Alzheimer Res* (2010) **7**(5):470–6. doi:10.2174/156720510791383796
14. Lewczuk P, Kamrowski-Kruck H, Peters O, Heuser I, Jessen F, Popp J, et al. Soluble amyloid precursor proteins in the cerebrospinal fluid as novel potential biomarkers of Alzheimer's disease: a multicenter study. *Mol Psychiatry* (2010) **15**(2):138–45. doi:10.1038/mp.2008.84
15. Portelius E, Westman-Brinkmalm A, Zetterberg H, Blennow K. Determination of beta-amyloid peptide signatures in cerebrospinal fluid using immunoprecipitation-mass spectrometry. *J Proteome Res* (2006) **5**(4):1010–6. doi:10.1021/pr050475v
16. Otto M, Lewczuk P, Wiltfang J. Neurochemical approaches of cerebrospinal fluid diagnostics in neurodegenerative diseases. *Methods* (2008) **44**(4):289–98. doi:10.1016/j.ymeth.2007.06.012
17. Gravina SA, Ho L, Eckman CB, Long KE, Otvos L Jr, Younkin LH, et al. Amyloid beta protein (A beta) in Alzheimer's disease brain. Biochemical and immunocytochemical analysis with antibodies specific for forms ending at A beta 40 or A beta 42(43). *J Biol Chem* (1995) **270**(13):7013–6.
18. Lewczuk P, Wiltfang J. Neurochemical dementia diagnostics: state of the art and research perspectives. *Proteomics* (2008) **8**(6):1292–301. doi:10.1002/pmic.200700703
19. Verbeek MM, De Jong D, Kremer HP. Brain-specific proteins in cerebrospinal fluid for the diagnosis of neurodegenerative diseases. *Ann Clin Biochem* (2003) **40**(Pt 1):25–40. doi:10.1258/000456303321016141
20. Hansson O, Zetterberg H, Buchhave P, Andreasson U, Londos E, Minthon L, et al. Prediction of Alzheimer's disease using the CSF Abeta42/Abeta40 ratio in patients with mild cognitive impairment. *Dement Geriatr Cogn Disord* (2007) **23**(5):316–20. doi:10.1159/000100926
21. Mehta PD, Pirttila T, Mehta SP, Sersen EA, Aisen PS, Wisniewski HM. Plasma and cerebrospinal fluid levels of amyloid beta proteins 1-40 and 1-42 in Alzheimer disease. *Arch Neurol* (2000) **57**(1):100–5. doi:10.1001/archneur.57.1.100
22. Shoji M, Matsubara E, Kanai M, Watanabe M, Nakamura T, Tomidokoro Y, et al. Combination assay of CSF tau, A beta 1-40 and A beta 1-42(43) as a biochemical marker of Alzheimer's disease. *J Neurol Sci* (1998) **158**(2):134–40. doi:10.1016/S0022-510X(98)00122-1
23. Kanai M, Matsubara E, Isoe K, Urakami K, Nakashima K, Arai H, et al. Longitudinal study of cerebrospinal fluid levels of tau, A beta1-40, and A beta1-42(43) in Alzheimer's disease: a study in Japan. *Ann Neurol* (1998) **44**(1):17–26. doi:10.1002/ana.410440108
24. Fukuyama R, Mizuno T, Mori S, Nakajima K, Fushiki S, Yanagisawa K. Age-dependent change in the levels of Abeta40 and Abeta42 in cerebrospinal fluid from control subjects, and a decrease in the ratio of Abeta42 to Abeta40 level in cerebrospinal fluid from Alzheimer's disease patients. *Eur Neurol* (2000) **43**(3):155–60. doi:10.1159/000008157
25. Schoonenboom NS, Mulder C, Van Kamp GJ, Mehta SP, Scheltens P, Blankenstein MA, et al. Amyloid beta 38, 40, and 42 species in cerebrospinal fluid: more of the same? *Ann Neurol* (2005) **58**(1):139–42. doi:10.1002/ana.20508
26. Slaets S, Le Bastard N, Martin JJ, Sleegers K, Van Broeckhoven C, De Deyn PP, et al. Cerebrospinal fluid Abeta1-40 improves differential dementia diagnosis in patients with intermediate P-tau181P levels. *J Alzheimers Dis* (2013) **36**(4):759–67. doi:10.3233/JAD-130107
27. Sauvee M, DidierLaurent G, Latarche C, Escanye MC, Olivier JL, Malaplate-Armand C. Additional use of Abeta(4)(2)/Abeta(4)(0) ratio with cerebrospinal fluid biomarkers P-tau and Abeta(4)(2) increases the level of evidence of Alzheimer's disease pathophysiological process in routine practice. *J Alzheimers Dis* (2014) **41**(2):377–86. doi:10.3233/JAD-131838
28. Dumurgier J, Schraen S, Gabelle A, Vercruysse O, Bombois S, Laplanche JL, et al. Cerebrospinal fluid amyloid-beta 42/40 ratio in clinical setting of memory centers: a multicentric study. *Alzheimers Res Ther* (2015) **7**(1):30. doi:10.1186/s13195-015-0114-5
29. American-Psychiatric-Association. *Diagnostic and Statistical Manual of Mental Disorders (IV-TR)*. 4th ed. Washington, DC: American-Psychiatric-Association (2000).
30. McKeith IG, Dickson DW, Lowe J, Emre M, O'Brien JT, Feldman H, et al. Diagnosis and management of dementia with Lewy bodies: third report of the DLB Consortium. *Neurology* (2005) **65**(12):1863–72. doi:10.1212/01.wnl.0000187889.17253.b1
31. Rascovsky K, Hodges JR, Knopman D, Mendez MF, Kramer JH, Neuhaus J, et al. Sensitivity of revised diagnostic criteria for the behavioural variant of frontotemporal dementia. *Brain* (2011) **134**(Pt 9):2456–77. doi:10.1093/brain/awr179
32. Vanderstichele H, Bibl M, Engelborghs S, Le Bastard N, Lewczuk P, Molinuevo JL, et al. Standardization of preanalytical aspects of cerebrospinal fluid biomarker testing for Alzheimer's disease diagnosis: a consensus paper from the Alzheimer's Biomarkers Standardization Initiative. *Alzheimers Dement* (2012) **8**(1):65–73. doi:10.1016/j.jalz.2011.07.004
33. del Campo M, Mollenhauer B, Bertolotto A, Engelborghs S, Hampel H, Simonsen AH, et al. Recommendations to standardize preanalytical confounding factors in Alzheimer's and Parkinson's disease cerebrospinal fluid biomarkers: an update. *Biomark Med* (2012) **6**(4):419–30. doi:10.2217/bmm.12.46
34. Mattsson N, Andreasson U, Persson S, Carrillo MC, Collins S, Chalbot S, et al. CSF biomarker variability in the Alzheimer's Association quality control program. *Alzheimers Dement* (2013) **9**(3):251–61. doi:10.1016/j.jalz.2013.01.010

35. Metz CE. Basic principles of ROC analysis. *Semin Nucl Med* (1978) **8**(4):283–98. doi:10.1016/S0001-2998(78)80014-2
36. Lewczuk P, Lelental N, Spitzer P, Maler JM, Kornhuber J. Amyloid-beta 42/40 cerebrospinal fluid concentration ratio in the diagnostics of Alzheimer's disease: validation of two novel assays. *J Alzheimers Dis* (2015) **43**(1):183–91. doi:10.3233/JAD-140771
37. Lewczuk P, Beck G, Esselmann H, Bruckmoser R, Zimmermann R, Fiszer M, et al. Effect of sample collection tubes on cerebrospinal fluid concentrations of tau proteins and amyloid beta peptides. *Clin Chem* (2006) **52**(2):332–4. doi:10.1373/clinchem.2005.058776
38. Fourier A, Portelius E, Zetterberg H, Blennow K, Quadrio I, Perret-Liaudet A. Pre-analytical and analytical factors influencing Alzheimer's disease cerebrospinal fluid biomarkers variability. *Clin Chim Acta* (2015) **449**:9–15. doi:10.1016/j.cca.2015.05.024
39. Grossman M, Farmer J, Leight S, Work M, Moore P, Van Deerlin V, et al. Cerebrospinal fluid profile in frontotemporal dementia and Alzheimer's disease. *Ann Neurol* (2005) **57**(5):721–9. doi:10.1002/ana.20477
40. Koopman K, Le Bastard N, Martin JJ, Nagels G, De Deyn PP, Engelborghs S. Improved discrimination of autopsy-confirmed Alzheimer's disease (AD) from non-AD dementias using CSF P-tau(181P). *Neurochem Int* (2009) **55**(4):214–8. doi:10.1016/j.neuint.2009.02.017
41. Schoonenboom NS, Reesink FE, Verwey NA, Kester MI, Teunissen CE, van de Ven PM, et al. Cerebrospinal fluid markers for differential dementia diagnosis in a large memory clinic cohort. *Neurology* (2012) **78**(1):47–54. doi:10.1212/WNL.0b013e31823ed0f0
42. de Souza LC, Lamari F, Belliard S, Jardel C, Houillier C, De Paz R, et al. Cerebrospinal fluid biomarkers in the differential diagnosis of Alzheimer's disease from other cortical dementias. *J Neurol Neurosurg Psychiatry* (2011) **82**(3):240–6. doi:10.1136/jnnp.2010.207183
43. Toledo JB, Brettschneider J, Grossman M, Arnold SE, Hu WT, Xie SX, et al. CSF biomarkers cutoffs: the importance of coincident neuropathological diseases. *Acta Neuropathol* (2012) **124**(1):23–35. doi:10.1007/s00401-012-0983-7
44. Kovacs GG, Milenkovic I, Wohrer A, Hoftberger R, Gelpi E, Haberler C, et al. Non-Alzheimer neurodegenerative pathologies and their combinations are more frequent than commonly believed in the elderly brain: a community-based autopsy series. *Acta Neuropathol* (2013) **126**(3):365–84. doi:10.1007/s00401-013-1157-y
45. Rahimi J, Kovacs GG. Prevalence of mixed pathologies in the aging brain. *Alzheimers Res Ther* (2014) **6**(9):82. doi:10.1186/s13195-014-0082-1
46. Graff-Radford NR. Alzheimer CSF biomarkers may be misleading in normal-pressure hydrocephalus. *Neurology* (2014) **83**(17):1573–5. doi:10.1212/WNL.0000000000000916
47. Jeppsson A, Zetterberg H, Blennow K, Wikkelso C. Idiopathic normal-pressure hydrocephalus: pathophysiology and diagnosis by CSF biomarkers. *Neurology* (2013) **80**(15):1385–92. doi:10.1212/WNL.0b013e31828c2fda
48. Gabelle A, Roche S, Geny C, Bennys K, Labauge P, Tholance Y, et al. Correlations between soluble alpha/beta forms of amyloid precursor protein and Abeta38, 40 and 42 in human cerebrospinal fluid. *Brain Res* (2010) **1357**:175–83. doi:10.1016/j.brainres.2010.08.022
49. Gabelle A, Roche S, Geny C, Bennys K, Labauge P, Tholance Y, et al. Decreased sAbetaPPbeta, Abeta38, and Abeta40 cerebrospinal fluid levels in frontotemporal dementia. *J Alzheimers Dis* (2011) **26**(3):553–63. doi:10.3233/JAD-2011-110515

17

Facilitating the validation of novel protein biomarkers for dementia: an optimal workflow for the development of sandwich immunoassays

Marta del Campo[1,2], Wesley Jongbloed[2], Harry A. M. Twaalfhoven[1,2], Robert Veerhuis[1,3], Marinus A. Blankenstein[2] and Charlotte E. Teunissen[1,2]*

[1] Neurochemistry Laboratory, VU University Medical Center, Amsterdam, Netherlands, [2] Department of Clinical Chemistry, VU University Medical Center, Amsterdam, Netherlands, [3] Department of Psychiatry, VU University Medical Center, Amsterdam, Netherlands

Edited by:
Jesus Avila,
Centro de Biología Molecular Severo Ochoa, CSIC-UAM, Spain

Reviewed by:
Jason Eriksen,
University of Houston, USA
Olga Calero,
CIBERNED-Instituto de Salud Carlos III, Spain

***Correspondence:**
Marta del Campo,
Neurochemistry Laboratory, Department of Clinical Chemistry, VU University Medical Center, PK1 Br016, De Boelelaan 1117, Amsterdam 1081 HV, Netherlands
m.delcampomilan@vumc.nl

Different neurodegenerative disorders, such as Alzheimer's disease (AD) and frontotemporal dementia (FTD), lead to dementia syndromes. Dementia will pose a huge impact on society and thus it is essential to develop novel tools that are able to detect the earliest, most sensitive, discriminative, and dynamic biomarkers for each of the disorders. To date, the most common assays used in large-scale protein biomarker analysis are enzyme-linked immunosorbent assays (ELISA), such as the sandwich immunoassays, which are sensitive, practical, and easily implemented. However, due to the novelty of many candidate biomarkers identified during proteomics screening, such assays or the antibodies that specifically recognize the desired marker are often not available. The development and optimization of a new ELISA should be carried out with considerable caution since a poor planning can be costly, ineffective, time consuming, and it may lead to a misinterpretation of the findings. Previous guidelines described either the overall biomarker development in more general terms (i.e., the process from biomarker discovery to validation) or the specific steps of performing an ELISA procedure. However, a workflow describing and guiding the main issues in the development of a novel ELISA is missing. Here, we describe a specific and detailed workflow to develop and validate new ELISA for a successful and reliable validation of novel dementia biomarkers. The proposed workflow highlights the main issues in the development of an ELISA and covers several critical aspects, including production, screening, and selection of specific antibodies until optimal fine-tuning of the assay. Although these recommendations are designed to analyze novel biomarkers for dementia in cerebrospinal fluid, they are generally applicable for the development of immunoassays for biomarkers in other human body fluids or tissues. This workflow is designed to maximize the quality of the developed ELISA using a time- and cost-efficient strategy. This will facilitate the validation of the dementia biomarker candidates ultimately allowing accurate diagnostic conclusions.

Keywords: novel biomarkers, dementia, CSF, ELISA, workflow, guidelines, AD, FTD

Introduction

Advancing age is the greatest risk factor of dementias, such as Alzheimer's disease (AD), dementia with Lewy bodies (DLB), and frontotemporal dementia (FTD). As life span increases, dementia will impose a huge social and economic burden with more than 100 million of individuals predicted to suffer from dementia by 2050 worldwide (1). Up to now, there are no adequate treatment options to halt progression of the various types of neurodegenerative diseases leading to dementia. To be able to tailor treatment, it is important to determine the underlying pathological processes and the stage of progression of these processes at the individual level, before irreversible damage is done. Thus, there is a great interest in developing specific, sensitive, and practical tools to differentially diagnose and discriminate the different types of dementia in their earliest possible phase (i.e., AD, FTD, DLB, vascular dementia, etc.). Although the currently available cerebrospinal fluid (CSF) biomarkers for AD [i.e., amyloid β (Aβ), total Tau (t-Tau), and phosphorylated Tau (p-Tau) (2, 3)] have a high sensitivity and specificity for AD, there is still no test to effectively predict the development of AD in a pre-symptomatic stage (4). In addition, there are no biomarkers available for the diagnosis of other types of dementia, such as FTD or DLB (5). This can be partially attributed to the limited knowledge about the etiological factors underlying the neuropathology of the different disorders. Thus, there is an urgent need to unravel novel pathways and proteins in order to find new biomarkers reflecting the pathogenesis of the different dementia syndromes (i.e., AD, DLB, FTD), which will likely promote the development of novel alternative diagnostic and therapeutic strategies.

Global protein profiling by mass spectrometry (MS)-based proteomics has evolved as a new hypothesis-free (unbiased) avenue to optimally unravel new candidate protein biomarkers involved in different diseases, including neurodegenerative disorders (6). The sensitivity, speed, and the practicability of the different proteomics approaches has improved rapidly over the years (7, 8), leading to the discovery of an enormous number of biomarker candidates (9, 10). Most of the identified biomarker candidates have not yet been validated, which hampers their implementation in clinical practice (8). In order to facilitate the validation process, a coherent pipeline has been suggested for the development of novel biomarkers, which divides the overall process into four phases: discovery, qualification, verification, and validation (**Figure 1**) (11). Due to the high number of candidates identified in the discovery phase by unbiased proteomics [ranging between twenty and several hundred (10)], and the costs of assay development and validation, a prioritize selection of the discovered biomarker candidates should be performed (12) based on (i) the fold-change between control and disease cases, (ii) the possible relationship of the candidate with the pathological mechanisms, (iii) supporting literature, and/or (iv) the availability of the reagents to detect a specific target.

Noteworthy, unbiased-MS can only analyze a limited number of samples which, together with the extensive sample preparation required, leads to high false positive rate (13). Thus, the subsequent qualification phase serves to identify the potential false positive candidates and to confirm the differential abundance of the selected proteins using an alternative targeted methodology (11). During verification, prioritized markers are specifically analyzed in a larger cohort of samples. Among all the different technologies that are able to detect a specific protein in the qualification and verification phases, targeted proteomics [i.e., multiple reaction monitoring (MRM)] is a compelling option due to the higher accuracy and sensitivity compared to unbiased MS-approaches (10, 14). However, those techniques may not be readily available. Alternatively, antibody-based techniques [i.e., Western blotting, immunohistochemistry, enzyme-linked immunosorbent assays (ELISA)] can be used for qualification and verification. Due to the unbiased nature of the discovery phase, however, the specific reagents needed may not be commercially available, which will be the next critical issue during the validation phase. During validation, the reliability of the corresponding molecule as a biomarker is tested with the use of a highly specific assay that allows high throughput screening of samples.

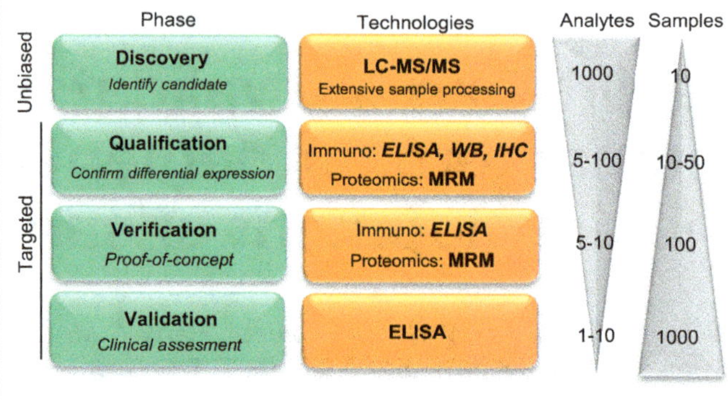

FIGURE 1 | Pipeline reflecting the development on novel protein biomarker candidates. Biomarker development pipeline is divided into four main phases. Biomarker development starts with a low throughput screening of samples in the unbiased phase to a high throughput analysis in the latest clinical validation stage, where hundreds to thousands of samples are evaluated for the clinical assessment of the biomarker candidate. "Analytes" and "Samples" refer to the number of different protein targets or samples, respectively, that are evaluated in each phase. LC-MS/MS, liquid chromatography tandem mass spectrometry; MRM, multiple reaction monitoring; IHC, immunohistochemistry; WB, Western blotting. Figure adapted from Rifai et al. (11).

To date, the most accepted assay for biomarker validation is ELISA since it can measure numerous samples simultaneously with low variation (11). In addition, its use does not require highly qualified expertise or technology, allowing its implementation in every laboratory (14). Though different immunoassay formats are available, sandwich ELISA is the most common assay used in biomarker analysis due to its high specificity and sensitivity (15). In this format, the target protein will be detected using two different antibodies (capture and detection antibodies). For many of the candidate biomarkers, a commercially available assay will not exist and specific antibodies against the target of interest and/or the corresponding ELISA need to be developed. The development and optimization of an ELISA requires a careful design since a wide range of variables, ranging from the antibody specificity to the concentration and composition of the different reagents, can affect the final result and therefore the validity of the biomarker candidate. Thus, a careful design can reduce the development costs and ineffectiveness, and will probably lead to more accurate analytical outcomes. Previous guidelines described either the overall biomarker development in more general terms (i.e., the process from biomarker discovery to validation) (11) or how to perform the ELISA procedure itself (15), but not the main issues regarding the development of optimal ELISA for novel protein biomarker candidates in CSF. Here, we suggest a step-by-step workflow (**Figure 2**) to facilitate the development of new ELISA's and the validation of novel biomarker candidates based on the literature available and our own best practice. In each step, different key issues need to be tested (**Table 1**). An estimated time-line for every step is also provided.

Antibody Design, Production, and Selection

Antibody Design

The specificity and sensitivity of the antibody are the critical determinants defining the quality of an ELISA (16). It is essential that the antibodies used in the ELISA recognize the native protein or protein fragments in order to avoid sample processing and minimize variation of the final outcome. Noteworthy, the samples used to discover biomarker candidates are denatured, reduced, and trypsinized prior to analysis for the proteomics workup. Thus, the results of the unbiased approach provide information about unique peptides derived from proteins that are differently regulated between clinical groups. It is therefore important to have information about the protein characteristics, such as its 3D structure, hydrophobicity, post-translational modifications, and/or binding sites. For instance, an antibody developed against an epitope detected in the proteomics study that belongs to a highly hydrophobic or glycosylated part of the protein may not be suitable for ELISA since the corresponding epitope is masked under native conditions (17) (**Figure 3A**). Protein characteristics are accessible in different databases, such as the Universal Protein Resource (UniProt) or the protein data bank (PDB) (18, 19), but are also provided by companies specialized in antibody production. In addition, a novel online platform named Protter is very useful to get an overall representation of the target protein in which different annotations, including previous proteomics results or

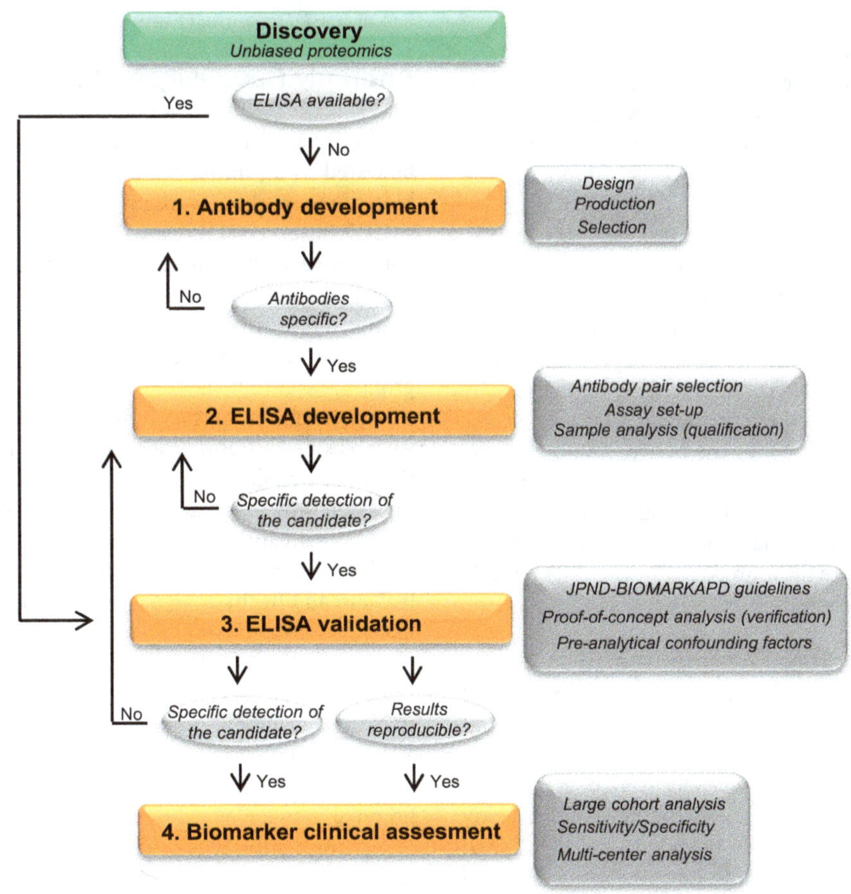

FIGURE 2 | Recommended workflow for the development of a novel ELISA. Workflow to facilitate the development and analytical validation of assays for the validation of novel biomarker candidates. The process is divided into four different steps (orange rectangles). In each step, different analyses are performed (dark gray rectangles) and specific questions are addressed before moving into the next phase (light gray circles). When the different criteria in a specific phase cannot be reached, changes should be performed one phase back. If a specific ELISA is already available, it should undergo a validation process for the targeted matrix (step 3). JPND-BIOMARKAPD guidelines are published in this special issue by Andreasson and colleagues.

TABLE 1 | Critical issues of biomarker immunoassays.

Workflow step	Key issue
1. Antibody production	Antibody design: optimal epitope selection Antibody production: polyclonal antibodies using peptides Internal control sample preparation Antibody selection: specificity tests
2. ELISA development	Optimal antibody pair selection (titration checkerboard) Assay set-up: concentrations, blocking buffers, etc. Biomarker candidate qualification
3. ELISA validation	JPND-BIOMARKAPD guidelines Pre-analytical confounding factors
4. Biomarker clinical assessment	Large cohort analysis: power analysis Biomarker sensitivity/specificity: AUC, ROC Reproducible results: multi-center studies

CSF, cerebrospinal fluid; LOD, limit of detection, LOQ, limit of quantitation, AUC, area under the curve, ROC, receiver operating characteristic. JPND-BIOMARKAPD guidelines published in this special issue by Andreasson and colleagues.

the known protein characteristics (binding and transmembrane domains, post-translational modifications, or cleavage sites) are presented (**Figure 3B**) (20).

Immunogen Selection

Based on the need to detect the native protein or protein fragments during the analysis to avoid sample processing, the optimal immunogen for antibody production should be the purified or recombinant full-length protein (21). However, the production and purification of full-length proteins is usually time consuming, costly and challenging from a technical perspective [i.e., aberrant protein folding, cells stress, solubility issues, etc. (22)]. In addition, the epitope recognized by the developed antibody might ultimately not be specific for the targeted native protein but rather to a general conformational state (17). Thus, it may be more effective to start antibody production using highly specific peptides. During peptide selection one should always consider: (i) the location of the peptide within the native protein and the post-translational modifications of the different epitopes within the protein to increase the chance that antibodies will detect the native protein and (ii) consider the peptide-ranges identified in the unbiased approach, since those are known to be differentially expressed in the clinical groups.

Polyclonal vs. Monoclonal Antibodies

It is important to decide whether to use and produce polyclonal or monoclonal antibodies, which have their own advantages and disadvantages (23). Monoclonal antibodies are usually used in ELISA since, unlike polyclonals, they benefit from being derived from an indefinite source to produce exactly the same antibody (i.e., hybridoma cells), which significantly reduces batch-to-batch variation. Moreover, monoclonal antibodies are considered to be more specific than polyclonal since they recognize a single epitope. Nevertheless, if a small peptide is used for animal immunization (i.e., 15 amino acid), the different epitopes that the polyclonal antibodies can recognize are limited, equating the specificity between monoclonal and polyclonal antibodies. In addition, the time and thus the costs needed to produce monoclonal antibodies are considerably higher than those for polyclonal antibodies, which are therefore often chosen in early development stages. Rabbits are commonly used for polyclonal antibody production if there is no identified need for a specific animal species (i.e., remarkably large amounts of antibody needed) due to its easy handling, size, high titer, and high-affinity antiserum (24). Thus, we suggest starting with the production of polyclonal antibodies recognizing at least five different epitopes (one epitope per animal) within the protein. The affinity purification of the produced antibodies will remarkably increase the chances of obtaining specific signals. Large-scale production of monoclonal antibodies can start once the most reactive antibody to the targeted biomarker in the desired matrix is defined and the optimal antibody pairs for ELISA are identified.

Whenever available, it is recommended to select commercial antibodies based on a demonstrated high specificity (by, e.g., Western Blot of CSF or brain tissue) and described suitability for ELISA. In this respect, several initiatives that provide information about the antibodies available and their validation procedure are currently ongoing, such as the Antibody initiative of the Human Proteome Organization (25) or the Swedish Human Proteome Resource Program (26). Production of polyclonal antibodies may last at least 2 months (**Figure 3C**).

Antibody Reactivity and Specificity

The specificity and reactivity of the different affinity-purified antibodies in different matrices (i.e., immunogen, CSF, tissue) can be tested using simple techniques, such as dot blot and Western blot. Some antibodies might be already excluded when no reactivity is observed (**Figure 4A**). In order to optimally compare the data between the different experiments, it is recommended to define and select a specific set of samples to be used continuously as internal controls (positive control sample) (27). For instance, individual CSF samples can be pooled into the different clinical groups (i.e., controls and AD) and aliquoted in order to have a large number of the same sample available. Pre-analytical variables (i.e., freeze/thaw cycles, storage temperature) affect the measurements of the CSF biomarkers (28–30) and thus the final outcome of the analyses. It is therefore important to follow specific guidelines for storage and handling of the CSF samples used in order to minimize the effect of possible pre-analytical bias already in this stage of development (31, 32). Since CSF is likely reflecting the biochemical alterations ongoing in the brain (33), it is conceivable to find changes of the identified proteins in brain tissue as well. Thus, when available, it is recommended to include also post-mortem brain tissue homogenates as it usually shows highly reactive bands. Noteworthy, our experience is that the height of the specific bands identified in brain tissue homogenates on Western blot is not identical to those in the CSF.

Testing antibody specificity in human samples can be challenging due to the lack of "pure" positive and negative controls (i.e., human samples lacking/overexpressing the target protein). Different types of reagents can be used to define specificity such as the recombinant full-protein, cell lysates, and/or animal tissue in which the target protein is overexpressed and/or downregulated (21). However, final conclusions for the specificity in human CSF or post-mortem tissue based only on reactivity observed in cells

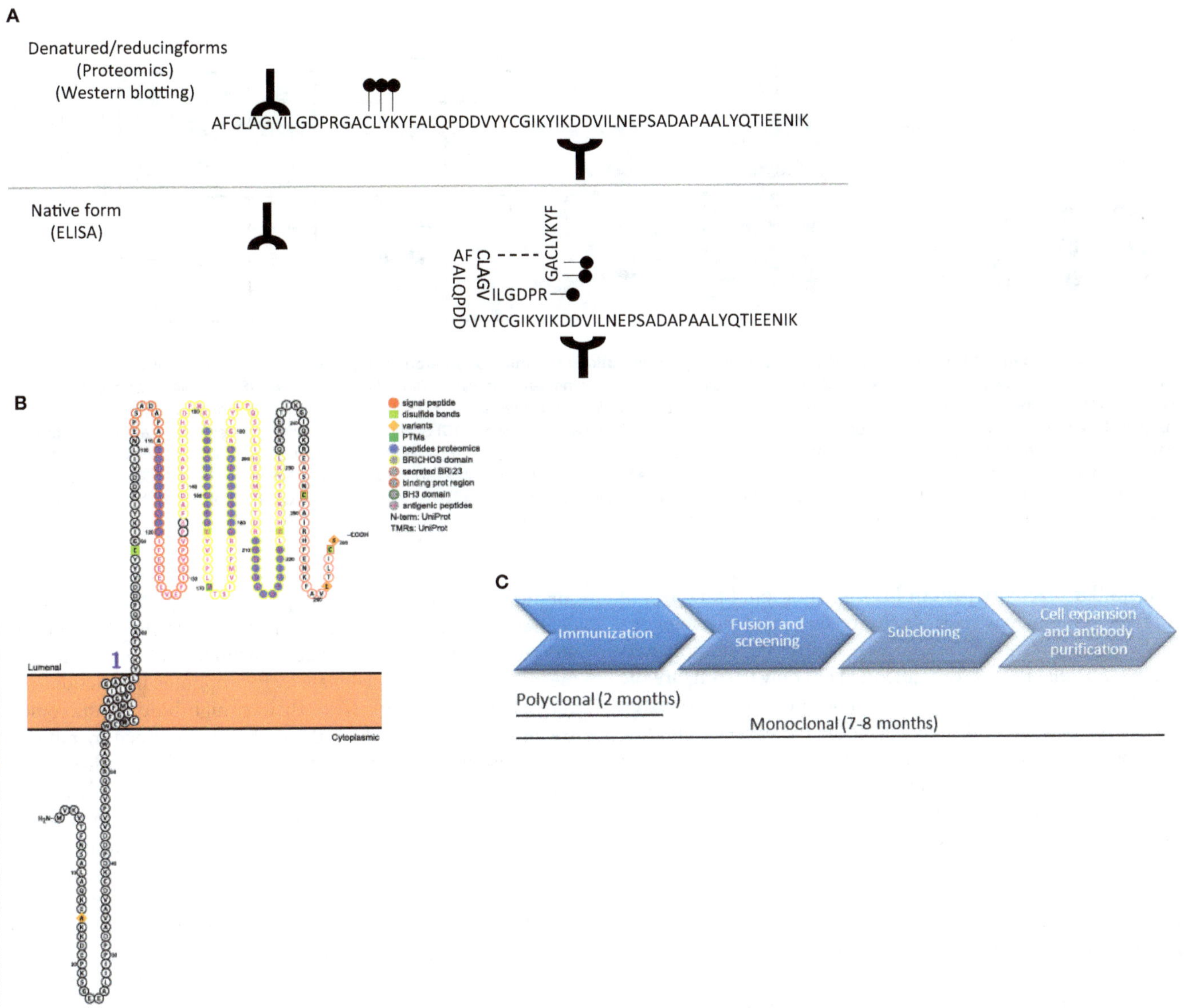

FIGURE 3 | Antibody design and production. **(A)** Schematic representation of a protein amino acid sequence in denatured/reducing conditions (upper) or in its native form (bottom). Green amino acids represent the peptides recognized by unbiased proteomics in the discovery phase. Antibodies (Y symbol), glycol groups (black dots), and disulfide bonds (dotted line) are also represented. Specific epitopes detected in the unbiased proteomics approach might be available in denatured conditions but might be masked in native conditions. **(B)** Graphical representation of a transmembrane protein using Protter (20), in which all protein characteristics are included. **(C)** Time-line differences in the production of polyclonal and monoclonal antibodies.

lysates or animal tissue must be drawn with due caution since this reactivity may not accurately represent the physiological form of the protein present in humans (21).

Antibody pre-adsorption with the antigenic peptide is also an easy and cost-effective alternative to test antibody specificity. If the signal obtained by Western blot using the antibody against the target matrix (e.g., CSF) is specific, it should be abrogated or remarkably reduced when the antibody is blocked with the antigenic peptide and be unaffected if similar but not identical peptides are used (34, 35). Unmodified reactivity after antibody pre-adsorption is non-specific and may derive from secondary antibody interactions or by contamination with other antibodies in the antibody solution (i.e., when the antibody has not been optimally affinity-purified). The reduced reactivity after antibody pre-adsorption does however not provide direct evidence of the specificity of the antibody, since the binding of the antibody to non-target proteins will be also inhibited. Thus, while persistent reactivity after pre-adsorption will indicate that the antibody is bad, reduced reactivity does not guarantee that the antibody is good (21, 36). Nonetheless, the binding to non-target proteins is unlikely to happen when antibodies have been produced against a unique sequence for the target protein. Further indirect evidence of antibody specificity comes from the comparison between the different antibodies, which should

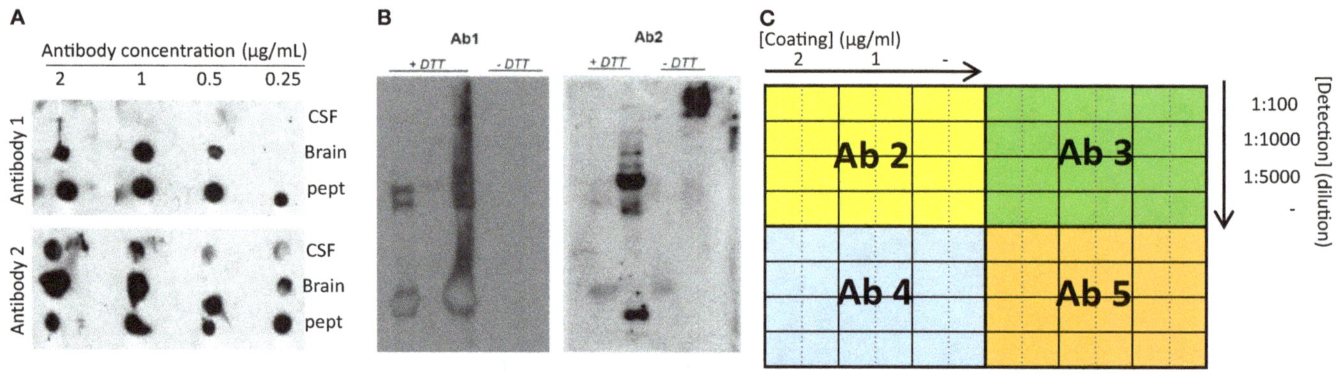

FIGURE 4 | Recommended experiments during antibody testing for an optimal selection of antibodies. **(A)** Example of a dot blot against CSF, human brain, or antigenic peptide using two antibodies recognizing two different epitopes of the same protein at different concentrations. **(B)** Two different samples analyzed by Western blot under reducing (+DTT) and non-reducing (−DTT) conditions and detected by two antibodies (Ab1 and Ab2) detecting two different epitopes of the same protein. Only Ab 2 can detect the protein of interest in CSF in native conditions. **(C)** Schematic representation exemplifying a checkerboard titration to test different antibody pairs for ELISA development. In this set-up, one antibody (Ab1) is used as capture antibody in three different concentrations (2 and 1 µg/mL and no capture antibody (−)). Four different antibodies are tested as detection antibodies (Ab 2–5) in four different dilutions (1:100, 1:1000, 1:5000, and no detection antibody (−)). A fixed concentration of the standard protein/peptide is used in every well (i.e., 0.5 µg/mL). The best combination will be the one giving the highest signal using the lowest amount of antibody (higher dilution) and with the lowest background (signal when no antibody is used).

give a similar reactivity pattern (35). In addition, homologs of the target protein may exist. If the recombinant homologous protein/fragments or the antibodies against the homologous protein are available, it is recommended not only to compare the reactivities between the antibodies but also to test whether the newly developed antibodies targeting the biomarker candidate can recognize homologous proteins. Those analyses will help to rule out possible cross-reactivity.

Direct evidence of the specificity could be obtained via isolation of the proteins recognized by the antibody through immunopurification (IP) followed by mass-spectrometry analysis. Those analyses can however be costly and time consuming since larger amounts of human CSF samples are usually needed to obtain a meaningful signal and to prepare the negative controls (IP without antibody and/or with an irrelevant antibody), and protein isolation from the antibody–protein complex may result difficult due to a strong binding.

Based on the resources available, a combination of the different approaches should be applied to determine the specificity of the different antibodies, as it was previously done for the monoclonal antibody that was subsequently used for a specific ELISA against $A\beta_{40}$ and not to other Aβ forms (37).

Recognition of Specific Physiological Protein Forms

For a successful ELISA development, it is important to know the different possible conformational states of the target protein (monomers, dimers, aggregates) in the corresponding matrix (i.e., CSF) and thus samples should be analyzed under different denaturing and reducing conditions (**Figure 4B**). In addition to Western blotting, it is recommended to analyze samples via direct ELISA, in order to further test which antibodies are able to recognize both the recombinant protein/peptide and CSF in native conditions. At this stage, the type of ELISA plate should also be defined. The most common ELISA plate is the flat-bottomed 96-well polystyrene microplate, which allows the adsorption of the antibodies to the well plate by hydrophobic interactions (low and medium binding). Nevertheless, high binding microplates are also available, in which the surface is modified by radiation to increase the binding strength between the antibodies and the plate (38).

Antibodies with proven specificity and ability to recognize the native protein in the human samples are the optimal ones for further immunoassay development. If no optimal antibodies are found, new antibodies detecting different epitopes should be produced. Usually, when good antibodies are produced, this phase will last approximately 3 months of one full-time equivalent, though it will also depend on the number of antibodies as well as the availability of all the reagents, samples, and expertise needed.

ELISA Development

Antibody Pair Selection

A prerequisite for a good sandwich ELISA is that the two different antibodies (capture and detection antibodies) optimally match. Thus, the best antibody pairs able to detect the target CSF biomarker are identified by screening every possible combination. In order to avoid false positive measurements due to, e.g., direct reactivity between the antibodies, the optimal concentration of capture and detection antibodies for each combination has to be established. This can be done performing a checkerboard titration using the recombinant protein fragments/peptides (or full protein if available) at one fixed concentration (i.e., 0.5 µg/mL) as a standard sample/calibrator (**Figure 4C**). As a starting point, a concentration up to 2 and 10 µg/mL for capture and detection antibodies, respectively, can be tested. During the subsequent steps, it is recommended to always include the standard calibrators and the pooled positive control CSF samples previously prepared (27).

Once the optimal antibody concentrations are established for each combination, both the standard sample and the CSF pools should be measured in serial dilutions to define which antibody pairs are able to detect the target CSF protein and the corresponding standard in a dose–response manner. Dose–response reactivity gives a good indication that the antibody pairs are detecting the corresponding protein. Sample dilution experiments will unravel the standard curve range as well as the optimal dilution factor of the CSF. If dose–response reactivity is not acquired, this may indicate that the reactivity observed is non-specific. The source of the non-specific signal should be identified, which may arise among other possibilities from the detection system used (i.e., secondary antibodies) or an inadequate blocking buffer (see below). If the source of the non-specific signal is not identified and mitigated, the corresponding antibody pairs should not be used for further assay development.

Once results are successful, i.e., at least one or two positive antibody pairs are present, production of monoclonal antibodies recognizing the same epitopes can be considered. It is expected that the produced monoclonal antibodies will behave similar to the corresponding polyclonal due to the limited epitopes that were used for immunization of the latter. Depending on the number of antibodies to be tested and whether non-specific signal is detected, this phase may last from 3 to 10 months approximately.

Assay Set-Up and Fine-Tuning

The different conditions and reagents used (i.e., incubation times, blocking buffers, assay diluent, secondary antibodies) can also play a critical role in the development of an ELISA (38). Blocking buffers are used to cover the unoccupied hydrophobic spaces of the ELISA plate wells once capture antibodies have been coated, reducing subsequent non-specific binding of the sample/reagents to the well. Different types of proteins are commonly used as a blocking agents, such as bovine serum albumin, non-fat dry milk, casein, normal serum, or fish gelatin, which can be diluted at different concentrations (ranging from 1 to 5%) in either phosphate- or tris-buffer saline (PBS or TBS). The different types of buffers and different protein concentrations should be tested since very low amount of blocking agent can lead to high background while excessive concentration may mask the binding epitope of the antibody. PBS can reduce signal of anti-phospho-epitope-specific antibodies, and in that case, TBS will be the first choice and should likewise be used for sample diluent. Non-ionic detergents can be added to the sample dilution buffer, such as Tween20 that disrupts low affinity protein–protein interactions and increases contact of the H_2O-component of the buffer to the surface. However, when background is high, it is recommended to add the protein used for blocking to the sample diluent, though at a lower concentration. This detergent buffer is also used during the washing steps between the different incubations of an ELISA procedure, but usually without added proteins. Selecting the optimal diluent helps to keep the background low, this will lead to an increase of sensitivity of the assay and can reduce matrix effects.

In addition to the buffer requirements, one should select the detection system used to create a quantitative signal. Enzymes (i.e., Horseradish Peroxidase, alkaline phosphatase) are commonly used, which are attached to either the detection antibody, to a secondary antibody or streptavidin when biotinylated detection antibodies are used. The enzyme reaction will produce a specific color once the corresponding chromogenic substrate or fluorochrome has been added (i.e., 3,5,3′,5′-tetramethylbenzidine, p-nitrophenyl phosphate). The amount of signal generated within the linear range of the assay is proportional to the activity of enzyme present and thus, to the concentration of the target protein.

Once the different buffers and reagents have been established, it is recommended to re-test the optimal concentration of the coating and detection antibodies, since the improvements achieved with the different conditions may allow one to reduce the antibody concentration. Taking into account that only optimal antibody pairs are tested in this phase, it may take a maximum of 3 months to establish the best conditions leading to the highest signal/noise ratio for each of the antibody pairs. At this stage, a small number of individual patient samples should be tested. If available, it is recommended to use the same samples that were used during the discovery phase in order to replicate the proteomics findings (qualification).

ELISA Validation

Initial ELISA Validation

Once an optimal assay has been developed or when it is commercially available, it is essential to test its analytical performance in the appropriate matrix (i.e., CSF) before assessing the clinical utility of the corresponding ELISA (28, 37, 39, 40). Several parameters need to be established such as precision, limits of detection, recovery, or parallelism among others. Validation of the assay will unravel whether the developed ELISA is accurate and robust in measuring the real levels of the candidate biomarker or if, on the contrary, the obtained values are influenced by other independent factors (i.e., pipetting errors, matrix effects, pre-analytical confounding factors). For example, the developed ELISA should have an optimal recovery, which is the ability of the assay to measure the specific candidate within the (complex) matrix (i.e., CSF) (41). During spike-recovery analysis, CSF samples with known concentration of the candidate biomarker are spiked with high, medium, low, and none amount of the calibrator. A bad recovery indicates that the different components of the matrix (i.e., CSF) affect the ability of the assay to measure the real concentration of the target molecule, which will affect the trueness of the results. Bad recoveries may be optimized by either using a different assay buffer mimicking better the matrix of interest or by further diluting the matrix of interest. ELISA validation will help to identify the different factors that compromise the reliability of the assay, which should be solved in order to draw accurate conclusions regarding the diagnostic performance of the biomarker candidate.

Previous guidelines have been published highlighting the parameters that should be stablished for the general validation of assays with different purposes (27, 41–45). This special issue in *Frontiers Neurology* contains a step-by-step and consensus standardized operating procedure (SOP) for a thorough ELISA validation for biomarkers for neurodegeneration (Andreasson et al.), developed by the members of the Joint Programming Neurodegenerative Disease (JPND) BIOMARKAPD (JPND-BIOMARKAPD), a consortium aiming to standardize the biomarker analysis for Alzheimer's and Parkinson's disease across Europe (46).

The fulfillment of the different parameters established by the JPND-BIOMARKAPD consortium as described by Andreasson and colleagues suggests that the assay is accurately measuring the candidate biomarker in CSF and thus a proof-of-concept analysis (verification) can be performed with a small cohort of individual samples (approximately 20 samples per clinical group). In case that some of the parameters are not fulfilled, it is recommended to re-analyze and test some of the incubation times, reagents, and concentrations established during assay development. Even if no changes in the concentration of the biomarker candidate are detected between the different clinical groups, it is worth to continue with a full-assay validation, since the assay might also be useful for other research purposes besides biomarker validation. However, full validation can only be performed on the final version of the assay. Noteworthy, when other matrices are used (i.e., post-mortem tissue, cell culture supernatants, cell lysates), an additional validation should always be performed to confirm the suitability of the assay for the corresponding matrix. The time frame for the completion of this phase typically lies between 2 and 8 months.

Full ELISA Validation

Once the new ELISA is fully developed, the novel assay should undergo an extensive validation for the targeted matrix in which other important parameters, including the reproducibility or the robustness of the assay, are tested as also indicated by Andreasson and colleagues in the current issue. The stability of the candidate biomarker under certain conditions should be also analyzed. Although the effect of pre-analytical variables have been likely minimized if the general guidelines for sample handling have been followed (31), some of the pre-analytical confounding factors should be specifically measured for the biomarker candidate to detect possible effects induced by different pre-analytical issues. Pre-analytical confounding factors include not only patient variables such as diurnal variation and fasting, but also processing factors such as the effect of freeze/thaw cycles and length of storage at different temperatures (28, 32, 47).

Since samples need to be prepared for pre-analytical variability testing (including storage over long time), this phase can take between 4 months and even a couple of years for long-term storage. Although the fulfillment of a complete ELISA validation ensures that the assay is suitable to measure the targeted molecule in the validated matrix, it is important to note that assay validation is a continuous process since reagents are continuously being renewed (i.e., quality control samples, standards, primary, and secondary antibodies). Thus, batch-to-batch variations should be always analyzed, tracked, and reported and, if needed, validation should be re-tested and an internal quality control program should be initiated. Nevertheless, since biomarker validation is a continuous process, current guidelines and workflows will have to be revised and updated regularly.

Clinical Assessment of the Biomarker

The different processes followed until this point allow to successfully develop and to analytically validate an assay that can specifically and accurately measure the novel discovered CSF biomarker candidate. In this latest stage, the assay can be used for clinical validation of the biomarker for the intended purpose (i.e., diagnosis, prognosis, treatment efficiency). A considerably larger number of samples must be analyzed compared to the discovery phase and thus a power analysis should be performed in order to define the optimal group size. Specificity and sensitivity of the corresponding biomarker should be calculated and the ability of the biomarker to discriminate between control and disease can be assessed using the receiver operating characteristic (ROC) curve and the area under the curve (AUC), alone and/or in combination with currently used CSF biomarker tests (i.e., $A\beta_{42}$, t-Tau, and p-Tau in AD) (48). According to international dementia biomarker criteria, a sensitivity and specificity of at least 85% is needed for a clinically useful biomarker (49). If a longitudinal study is performed, it might also be useful to assess the predictive value of the biomarkers that reflect the conversion from non-demented or mild cognitive impairment cases to the specific dementia with Cox proportional hazards models and Kaplan–Meier curves (50). When positive results are obtained, data should be independently replicated using larger cohorts, different populations and multi-center studies before its future possible implementation in routine analysis (51, 52).

Concluding Remarks and Perspectives for Future Assay Implementation in Routine Analysis

There is a great need to develop specific, sensitive, and practical tools to differentially diagnose AD and related dementias in its earliest possible phase. The gold standard format for biomarker analysis is ELISA, which usually needs to be developed when a novel biomarker candidate is identified. In order to facilitate the development of a novel ELISA and ease the validation of the potential candidate CSF biomarkers, here we suggest a straightforward workflow for ELISA development, which we divided into four different steps (**Figure 2**). In each step, different key issues need to be tested (**Table 1**). When a commercial ELISA is available, the corresponding assay should be validated for its use in the corresponding matrix (i.e., CSF) (**Figure 2**, step 3). In the last steps, a clinical assessment of the biomarker candidate should be performed using the validated ELISA.

Once the optimal assay has been fully developed and validated, and the diagnostic utility of the corresponding biomarker has been solidly established, it will be necessary to initiate the phase that will ultimately lead to the implementation of the diagnostic assay in routine diagnosis, i.e., to establish an *in vitro* diagnostic (IVD) test. Such tests are preferably developed on an automated platform (53, 54), which will strongly reduce variation between centers allowing the establishment of cut-off values. In order to implement in clinical practice, several governmental requirements need to be fulfilled, which can range from the reproducibility and stability of the analytical platform to proof of added diagnostic value of the discovered biomarker. The exact set of rules that need to be complied to implement an IVD test depends on the regulatory institution of each region, which is, for example, the 510(k) premarketing clearance oversight by the food and drug administration in United States (55) or the IVD Directive 98/97/EC established by the European Commission (56).

Developing a successful ELISA for the validation of novel protein biomarker candidates starts by taking the right decisions during early stages of the development, for which we believe the workflow described in this paper will be a very useful aid.

Acknowledgments

This work is part of the BIOMARKAPD project under the aegis of EU Joint Programme – Neurodegenerative Disease Research (JPND) – www.jpnd.eu, and the Memorabel program PRODIA, which are both supported through ZonMw (The Netherlands). We also acknowledge the support provided by the International Stichting Alzheimer Onderzoerk (ISAO), the association for frontotemporal degeneration (AFTD), and the Alzheimer's Drug Discovery Foundation (ADDF). We would like to also acknowledge all the members of Neurochemistry Laboratory of the Clinical Chemistry department at the VUmc (Amsterdam) for their expertise in assay development.

References

1. Alzheimer's Disease International. *World Alzheimer Report 2010. The Global Economic Impact of Dementia*. London: Alzheimer's disease International (2010).
2. Tapiola T, Alafuzoff I, Herukka S-K, Parkkinen L, Hartikainen P, Soininen H, et al. Cerebrospinal fluid {beta}-amyloid 42 and tau proteins as biomarkers of Alzheimer-type pathologic changes in the brain. *Arch Neurol* (2009) **66**:382–9. doi:10.1001/archneurol.2008.596
3. Blennow K, Hampel H, Weiner M, Zetterberg H. Cerebrospinal fluid and plasma biomarkers in Alzheimer disease. *Nat Rev Neurol* (2010) **6**:131–44. doi:10.1038/nrneurol.2010.4
4. Jack CR, Albert MS, Knopman DS, McKhann GM, Sperling RA, Carrillo MC, et al. Introduction to the recommendations from the National Institute on aging-Alzheimer's association workgroups on diagnostic guidelines for Alzheimer's disease. *Alzheimers Dement* (2011) **7**:257–62. doi:10.1016/j.jalz.2011.03.004
5. Ahmed RM, Paterson RW, Warren JD, Zetterberg H, O'Brien JT, Fox NC, et al. Biomarkers in dementia: clinical utility and new directions. *J Neurol Neurosurg Psychiatry* (2014) **85**:1426–34. doi:10.1136/jnnp-2014-307662
6. Craft GE, Chen A, Nairn AC. Recent advances in quantitative neuroproteomics. *Methods* (2013) **61**:186–218. doi:10.1016/j.ymeth.2013.04.008
7. Schutzer SE. Rapidly maturing field of proteomics: a gateway to studying diseases. *Proteomics* (2014) **14**:991–3. doi:10.1002/pmic.201400091
8. Frantzi M, Bhat A, Latosinska A. Clinical proteomic biomarkers: relevant issues on study design & technical considerations in biomarker development. *Clin Transl Med* (2014) **3**:7. doi:10.1186/2001-1326-3-7
9. Zhang J, Goodlett DR, Montine TJ. Proteomic biomarker discovery in cerebrospinal fluid for neurodegenerative diseases. *J Alzheimers Dis* (2005) **8**:377–86.
10. Kroksveen AC, Opsahl JA, Aye TT, Ulvik RJ, Berven FS. Proteomics of human cerebrospinal fluid: discovery and verification of biomarker candidates in neurodegenerative diseases using quantitative proteomics. *J Proteomics* (2011) **74**:371–88. doi:10.1016/j.jprot.2010.11.010
11. Rifai N, Gillette MA, Carr SA. Protein biomarker discovery and validation: the long and uncertain path to clinical utility. *Nat Biotechnol* (2006) **24**:971–83. doi:10.1038/nbt1235
12. Gao J, Garulacan L-A, Storm SM, Opiteck GJ, Dubaquie Y, Hefta SA, et al. Biomarker discovery in biological fluids. *Methods* (2005) **35**:291–302. doi:10.1016/j.ymeth.2004.08.020
13. Meng Z, Veenstra TD. Targeted mass spectrometry approaches for protein biomarker verification. *J Proteomics* (2011) **74**:2650–9. doi:10.1016/j.jprot.2011.04.011
14. Kroksveen AC, Aasebø E, Vethe H, Van Pesch V, Franciotta D, Teunissen CE, et al. Discovery and initial verification of differentially abundant proteins between multiple sclerosis patients and controls using iTRAQ and SID-SRM. *J Proteomics* (2013) **78**:312–25. doi:10.1016/j.jprot.2012.09.037
15. Cox KL, Devanarayan V, Kriauciunas A, Manetta J, Montrose C, Sittampalam S. Immunoassay methods. *Assay Guidance Manual*. Eli Lilly & Company and the National Center for Advancing Translational Sciences. Available from: http://www.ncbi.nlm.nih.gov/books/NBK92434/
16. Kelley M, DeSilva B. Key elements of bioanalytical method validation for macromolecules. *AAPS J* (2007) **9**:E156–63. doi:10.1208/aapsj0902017
17. Ramos-Vara JA. Technical aspects of immunohistochemistry. *Vet Pathol* (2005) **42**:405–26. doi:10.1354/vp.42-4-405
18. European Bioinformatics Institute (EMBL-EBI), SIB Swiss Institute of Bioinformatics, *Protein Information Resource (PIR). Universal Protein Resource (UniProt)*. Available from: http://www.uniprot.org/help/about
19. Bank RPD. *RCSB Protein Data Bank – RCSB PDB*. Available from: http://www.rcsb.org/pdb/home/home.do
20. Omasits U, Ahrens CH, Müller S, Wollscheid B. Protter: interactive protein feature visualization and integration with experimental proteomic data. *Bioinformatics* (2014) **30**:884–6. doi:10.1093/bioinformatics/btt607
21. Bordeaux J, Welsh AW, Agarwal S, Killiam E, Baquero MT, Hanna JA, et al. Antibody validation. *Biotechniques* (2010) **48**:197–209. doi:10.2144/000113382
22. Palomares LA, Estrada-Mondaca S, Ramírez OT. Production of recombinant proteins: challenges and solutions. *Methods Mol Biol* (2004) **267**:15–52. doi:10.1385/1-59259-774-2:015
23. Lipman NS, Jackson LR, Trudel LJ, Weis-Garcia F. Monoclonal versus polyclonal antibodies: distinguishing characteristics, applications, and information resources. *ILAR J* (2005) **46**:258–68. doi:10.1093/ilar.46.3.258
24. Leenaars M, Hendriksen CFM. Critical steps in the production of polyclonal and monoclonal antibodies: evaluation and recommendations. *ILAR J* (2005) **46**:269–79. doi:10.1093/ilar.46.3.269
25. Organization HP. *Human Antibody Initiative*. Available from: http://www.hupo.org/human-antibody-initiative/
26. Swedish Human Proteome Resource Program. *Protein Atlas*. Available from: http://www.proteinatlas.org/
27. Desilva B, Smith W, Weiner R, Kelley M, Smolec J, Lee B, et al. Recommendations for the bioanalytical method validation of ligand-binding assays to support pharmacokinetic assessments of macromolecules. *Pharm Res* (2003) **20**:1885–900. doi:10.1023/B:PHAM.0000003390.51761.3d
28. Koel-Simmelink MJA, Vennegoor A, Killestein J, Blankenstein MA, Norgren N, Korth C, et al. The impact of pre-analytical variables on the stability of neurofilament proteins in CSF, determined by a novel validated SinglePlex Luminex assay and ELISA. *J Immunol Methods* (2014) **402**:43–9. doi:10.1016/j.jim.2013.11.008
29. Bjerke M, Portelius E, Minthon L, Wallin A, Anckarsäter H, Anckarsäter R, et al. Confounding factors influencing amyloid Beta concentration in cerebrospinal fluid. *Int J Alzheimers Dis* (2010) **2010**:1–11. doi:10.4061/2010/986310
30. Teunissen CE, Verwey NA, Kester MI, van Uffelen K, Blankenstein MA. Standardization of assay procedures for analysis of the CSF biomarkers amyloid β((1-42)), tau, and phosphorylated tau in Alzheimer's disease: report of an international workshop. *Int J Alzheimers Dis* (2010) **2010**:635053. doi:10.4061/2010/635053
31. Teunissen CE, Tumani H, Engelborghs S, Mollenhauer B. Biobanking of CSF: international standardization to optimize biomarker development. *Clin Biochem* (2014) **47**:288–92. doi:10.1016/j.clinbiochem.2013.12.024

32. Del Campo M, Mollenhauer B, Bertolotto A, Engelborghs S, Hampel H, Simonsen AH, et al. Recommendations to standardize preanalytical confounding factors in Alzheimer's and Parkinson's disease cerebrospinal fluid biomarkers: an update. *Biomark Med* (2012) **6**:419–30. doi:10.2217/bmm.12.46
33. Reiber H, Peter JB. Cerebrospinal fluid analysis: disease-related data patterns and evaluation programs. *J Neurol Sci* (2001) **184**:101–22. doi:10.1016/S0022-510X(00)00501-3
34. Skliris G, Rowan B, Al-Dhaheri M, Williams C, Troup S, Begic S, et al. Immunohistochemical validation of multiple phospho-specific epitopes for estrogen receptor alpha (ERalpha) in tissue microarrays of ERalpha positive human breast carcinomas. *Breast Cancer Res Treat* (2009) **118**:443–53. doi:10.1016/j.biotechadv.2011.08.021.Secreted
35. Del Campo M, Hoozemans JJM, Dekkers L-L, Rozemuller AJ, Korth C, Müller-Schiffmann A, et al. BRI2-BRICHOS is increased in human amyloid plaques in early stages of Alzheimer's disease. *Neurobiol Aging* (2014) **35**:1596–604. doi:10.1016/j.neurobiolaging.2014.01.007
36. Holmseth S, Zhou Y, Follin-Arbelet VV, Lehre KP, Bergles DE, Danbolt NC. Specificity controls for immunocytochemistry: the antigen preadsorption test can lead to inaccurate assessment of antibody specificity. *J Histochem Cytochem* (2012) **60**:174–87. doi:10.1369/0022155411434828
37. Verwey NA, Veerhuis R, Twaalfhoven HAM, Wouters D, Hoozemans JJM, Bollen YJM, et al. Quantification of amyloid-beta 40 in cerebrospinal fluid. *J Immunol Methods* (2009) **348**:57–66. doi:10.1016/j.jim.2009.06.011
38. *Technical Guide for ELISA*. Available from: http://www.kpl.com/docs/techdocs/KPL%20ELISA%20Technical%20Guide.pdf
39. Petzold A, Altintas A, Andreoni L, Bartos A, Berthele A, Blankenstein MA, et al. Neurofilament ELISA validation. *J Immunol Methods* (2010) **352**:23–31. doi:10.1016/j.jim.2009.09.014
40. Smith BW, Strakova J, King JL, Erdman JW, O'Brien WD. Validated sandwich ELISA for the quantification of von Willebrand factor in rabbit plasma. *Biomark Insights* (2010) **2010**:119–27. doi:10.4137/BMI.S6051
41. Wharf C, Kingdom U. Guideline on bioanalytical method validation. *Eur Med Agency* (2012) **44**:1–23. Available from: http://www.ema.europa.eu/ema/index.jsp?curl=pages/includes/document/document_detail.jsp?webContentId=WC500109686&mid=WC0b01ac058009a3dc
42. Food and Drug Administration. *Guidance for Industry: Bioanalytical Method Validation*. US Dep Heal Hum Serv (2001). p. 4–10. Available from: http://www.labcompliance.de/documents/FDA/FDA-Others/Laboratory/f-507-bioanalytical-4252fnl.pdf
43. Valentin MA, Ma S, Zhao A, Legay F, Avrameas A. Validation of immunoassay for protein biomarkers: bioanalytical study plan implementation to support pre-clinical and clinical studies. *J Pharm Biomed Anal* (2011) **55**:869–77. doi:10.1016/j.jpba.2011.03.033
44. Lee JW, Devanarayan V, Barrett YC, Weiner R, Allinson J, Fountain S, et al. Fit-for-purpose method development and validation for successful biomarker measurement. *Pharm Res* (2006) **23**:312–28. doi:10.1007/s11095-005-9045-3
45. Lee JW, Hall M. Method validation of protein biomarkers in support of drug development or clinical diagnosis/prognosis. *J Chromatogr B Analyt Technol Biomed Life Sci* (2009) **877**:1259–71. doi:10.1016/j.jchromb.2008.11.022
46. BIOMARKAPD. *Biomarkers for Alzheimer's and Parkinson Disease*. Available from: http://www.neurodegenerationresearch.eu/initiatives/annual-calls-for-proposals/closed-calls/biomarkers-transnational-call/results-of-biomarker-call/biomarkapd/
47. Willemse EAJ, Teunissen CE. Importance of pre-analytical stability for CSF biomarker testing. *Cerebrospinal Fluid in Clinical Neurology*. p. 59–77. doi:10.1007/978-3-319-01225-4
48. Gnanapavan S, Hegen H, Khalil M, Hemmer B, Franciotta D, Hughes S, et al. Guidelines for uniform reporting of body fluid biomarker studies in neurologic disorders. *Neurology* (2014) **83**:1210–6. doi:10.1212/WNL.0000000000000809
49. The Ronald and Nancy Reagean Research Institute of the Alzheimer's Association and The National Institute on Aging Working Group 123. Consensus report of the working group on: "molecular and biochemical markers of Alzheimer's disease". *Neurobiol Aging* (1998) **19**:109–16.
50. Duits FH, Teunissen CE, Bouwman FH, Visser PJ, Mattsson N, Zetterberg H, et al. The cerebrospinal fluid "Alzheimer profile": easily said, but what does it mean? *Alzheimers Dement* (2014) **10**(6):713–23.e2. doi:10.1016/j.jalz.2013.12.023
51. Humpel C. Identifying and validating biomarkers for Alzheimer's disease. *Trends Biotechnol* (2011) **29**:26–32. doi:10.1016/j.tibtech.2010.09.007
52. Sackett D, Haynes R. The architecture of diagnostic research. *Br Med J* (2002) **324**:593–541. doi:10.1136/bmj.324.7336.539
53. Tighe PJ, Ryder RR, Todd I, Fairclough LC. ELISA in the multiplex era: potentials and pitfalls. *Proteomics Clin Appl* (2015) **9**(3–4):406–22. doi:10.1002/prca.201400130
54. Phillips KA, Van Bebber S, Issa AM. Diagnostics and biomarker development: priming the pipeline. *Nat Rev Drug Discov* (2006) **5**:463–9. doi:10.1038/nrd2033
55. Food and Drug Administration. *IVD Regulation*. Available from: http://www.fda.gov/MedicalDevices/DeviceRegulationandGuidance/IVDRegulatoryAssistance/ucm123682.htm#1
56. European Commission. *In Vitro Diagnostic Medical Devices. Directive 98/79/EC*. Available from: http://ec.europa.eu/growth/single-market/european-standards/harmonised-standards/iv-diagnostic-medical-devices/index_en.htm

18

Transmembrane amyloid-related proteins in CSF as potential biomarkers for Alzheimer's disease

Inmaculada Lopez-Font[1,2], *Inmaculada Cuchillo-Ibañez*[1,2], *Aitana Sogorb-Esteve*[1,2], *María-Salud García-Ayllón*[1,2,3] *and Javier Sáez-Valero*[1,2]*

[1] *Instituto de Neurociencias de Alicante, Universidad Miguel Hernández-CSIC, Sant Joan d'Alacant, Spain,* [2] *Centro de Investigación Biomédica en Red sobre Enfermedades Neurodegenerativas (CIBERNED), Sant Joan d'Alacant, Spain,* [3] *Unidad de Investigación, Fundación para el Fomento de la Investigación Sanitaria Biomédica de la Comunidad Valenciana (FISABIO), Hospital General Universitario de Elche, Elche, Spain*

Edited by:
Charlotte Elisabeth Teunissen,
VU University Medical Center
Amsterdam, Netherlands

Reviewed by:
Scott Ayton,
Florey Neuroscience Institute,
Australia
Henrik Zetterberg,
The Sahlgrenska Academy at the
University of Gothenburg, Sweden

Correspondence:
Javier Sáez-Valero,
Instituto de Neurociencias de Alicante,
Universidad Miguel Hernández-CSIC,
Av. Ramón y Cajal s/n, Sant Joan
d'Alacant E-03550, Spain
j.saez@umh.es

In the continuing search for new cerebrospinal fluid (CSF) biomarkers for Alzheimer's disease (AD), reasonable candidates are the secretase enzymes involved in the processing of the amyloid precursor protein (APP), as well as the large proteolytic cleavage fragments sAPPα and sAPPβ. The enzymatic activities of some of these secretases, such as BACE1 and TACE, have been investigated as potential AD biomarkers, and it has been assumed that these activities present in human CSF result from the soluble truncated forms of the membrane-bound enzymes. However, we and others recently identified soluble forms of BACE1 and APP in CSF containing the intracellular domains, as well as the multi-pass transmembrane presenilin-1 (PS1) and other subunits of γ-secretase. We also review recent findings that suggest that most of these soluble transmembrane proteins could display self-association properties based on hydrophobic and/or ionic interactions leading to the formation of heteromeric complexes. The oligomerization state of these potential new biomarkers needs to be taken into consideration for assessing their real potential as CSF biomarkers for AD by adequate molecular tools.

Keywords: Alzheimer's disease, cerebrospinal fluid, BACE1, soluble amyloid precursor protein, presenilin-1, TACE

Introduction

Alzheimer's disease (AD) is an age-related neurodegenerative disorder recognized as the most common cause of dementia among the elderly. The pathologic characteristics of AD are neurodegeneration and proteinaceous deposits, including extracellular plaques composed mostly of β-amyloid peptides (Aβ) and intracellular tangles of the microtubule-associated protein tau abnormally hyperphosphorylated (P-tau). Both pathological effectors, Aβ and P-tau, can be monitored in cerebrospinal fluid (CSF). In late-onset AD, concentrations of tau and P-tau in CSF are increased and probably reflect neuronal damage, but levels of Aβ peptides are decreased. These changes can be measured in CSF before the onset of any other symptoms, and, therefore, they can be used as a diagnostic marker for the disease [for a recent review, see Ref. (1)]. Although numerous laboratories have reported increased levels of P-tau and total tau (T-tau) in the CSF of AD patients, they are not specific, and also increase in other neuropathological disorders (2, 3). It is well recognized that Aβ peptides, and especially the Aβ42 species, are the most specific CSF biomarkers for AD.

According to the amyloid hypothesis, accumulation of Aβ in the brain, resulting from an imbalance between production and clearance, is the primary influence driving AD pathogenesis (4). The Aβ peptide is generated by processing a larger type I transmembrane spanning glycoprotein, the amyloid precursor protein (APP), through the successive action of proteolytic enzymes called secretases. Sequential processing of APP begins with either the action of α-secretase or β-secretase, followed by γ-secretase cleavage. When cleavage is carried out by β- and γ-secretase, the so-called amyloidogenic pathway, a 36–43 amino acid peptide is generated since γ-secretase acts on a domain with multiple potential cleavage sites (5). The Aβ40 peptide is the most common species, while the Aβ42 variant is the most amyloidogenic form of the peptide associated with AD progression. However, in the non-pathological condition, the majority of APP molecules are cleaved through the non-amyloidogenic pathway by the sequential action of α- and γ-secretases. α-Secretase cleaves APP within the Aβ domain, precluding the generation of the Aβ peptide [for a review, see Ref. (6)]. The existence in CSF of several shorter isoforms in addition to Aβ40 and Aβ42 has been explained by an alternative APP processing pathway involving concerted cleavages of APP by α- and β-secretase (7).

The predisposition for self-association of Aβ42 determines that while Aβ42 content is increased in the AD brain, its levels in CSF are decreased presumably due to its increasing deposition in brain tissue (2). In this context, with two dynamics playing out in opposite directions within the brain, increasing Aβ production and increasing deposition, the interpretation of CSF changes in Aβ levels in pre-symptomatic stages seems difficult. In fact, Jack et al. (8) proposed that Aβ-plaque biomarkers are dynamic early in the disease before the appearance of clinical symptoms, but have largely reached a plateau by the time clinical symptoms appear, determining that CSF Aβ does not change significantly over time in patients with AD. Moreover, in this context, it is difficult to anticipate, thus to evaluate, the outcomes expected from the CSF biochemical assessments of Aβ in AD subjects consequence of effective therapy with β- or γ-secretase inhibitors, potential disease-modifying therapeutics under development (9, 10).

In accordance with the mentioned challenges, there is a need to identify additional β-amyloid-related markers of AD. Reasonable candidates are proteins, such as secretases, involved in the pathological processing of APP, and the large proteolytic cleavage fragments sAPPα and sAPPβ. Since most of these secretases are transmembrane proteins, their assessments in CSF were not considered until recent years. The purpose of this article is to review recent evidence about the presence of secretase components in CSF and their potential as AD biomarkers. In addition, we summarize our recent findings about the presence of soluble full-length APP (sAPPf) in CSF and their oligomerization into heteromers. Our studies demonstrated that sAPP heteromers contribute to the estimation of sAPPα and sAPPβ levels, which needs to be taken into consideration for their assessment by ELISA. The suitability of applying adequate molecular tools for the assessment in CSF of hydrophobic proteins and soluble heteromeric aggregates is absolutely necessary to evaluate their potential as biomarkers.

Soluble Full-Length and Heteromers of sAPP in CSF

The processing of APP begins with the action of either α-secretase or β-secretase, initiating mandatory pathways. The initial shedding by α-secretase or β-secretase releases large soluble proteolytic cleavage fragments of APP, sAPPα and sAPPβ, respectively, both present in human CSF (11, 12). Since amyloidogenic processing of APP is expected to be altered in the Alzheimer brain, both large sAPP fragments have been postulated as potential new AD biomarkers, but no consistent changes in CSF sAPPα and sAPPβ levels have been identified to date [see review by Perneczky et al. (13)]. Interestingly, it has been suggested that full-length APP containing an intact cytoplasmic domain also exists as a soluble form (sAPPf) (14, 15). Recently, we confirmed that sAPPf is present in human CSF and demonstrated its contribution when estimating levels of large sAPP fragments (16). In consequence, the 6E10 antibody, a widely used anti-APP antibody that recognizes an epitope present in sAPPα and absent in sAPPβ, will detected not only sAPPα, but also sAPPf in CSF. Therefore, the use of 6E10 or similar antibodies in contraposition to pan-specific antibodies for the C-terminus of sAPPα should be considered as a contributing factor for contradictory findings between laboratories. Moreover, we have demonstrated that sAPPf co-exists in CSF with sAPPα and sAPPβ, and all forms are capable of assembling into heteromers [(16); see also **Figure 1A**]. The APP oligomerization status is particularly relevant, since most quantification of sAPPα and sAPPβ in CSF from AD subjects relies on ELISA determinations developed for monomeric species. Our data indicate that sAPP heteromers interfere with the measurement of sAPPα and sAPPβ in commercially available ELISA kits. Interestingly, an unexpected positive correlation has been consistently reported between both forms, indicating a similar shift for sAPPα and sAPPβ levels (17–20). Since the production of sAPPβ should be inversely proportional to that of sAPPα, this is an unexpected finding that we attributed, at least in part, to the existence of sAPPα/sAPPβ heteromers. In this context, early studies assessing sAPPα and sAPPβ levels by Western blot failed to demonstrate this positive correspondence (21). The assessment of sAPPα/sAPPβ levels is also of interest to monitor the biochemical effect of drugs targeting Aβ in clinical trials (22), particularly for β-/γ-secretase inhibitors since discouraging reports question this therapeutic strategy, even the amyloid cascade hypothesis (23). In this regard, β-secretase inhibition resulted in sAPPβ significant decrease, but also in increased concentration of sAPPα (24), suggesting that inhibition of β-secretase in humans resulted in a compensatory increase in non-amyloidogenic APP cleavage. The simultaneous determination of sAPPα and sAPPβ in CSF by protocols that prevents underestimation by heteromeric association is mandatory.

In conclusion, an optimal approach to quantify sAPPα and sAPPβ in CSF has been based on ELISA determinations, but the presence of heteromeric complexes of sAPP obligate adjusting protocols. Moreover, the characterization of a soluble transmembrane protein might be hindered by the difficulty in distinguishing it from the truncated species generated by cleavage of the transmembrane protein. The existence of different sAPP isoforms, generated from alternative exon splicing (26), adds complexity to the determination of sAPP as CSF biomarkers, but needs to be taken into consideration since large species of sAPP, which should correspond to APP751/770, appeared to increase AD CSF (16). Analysis of sAPPf splicing isoforms may be of particular interest

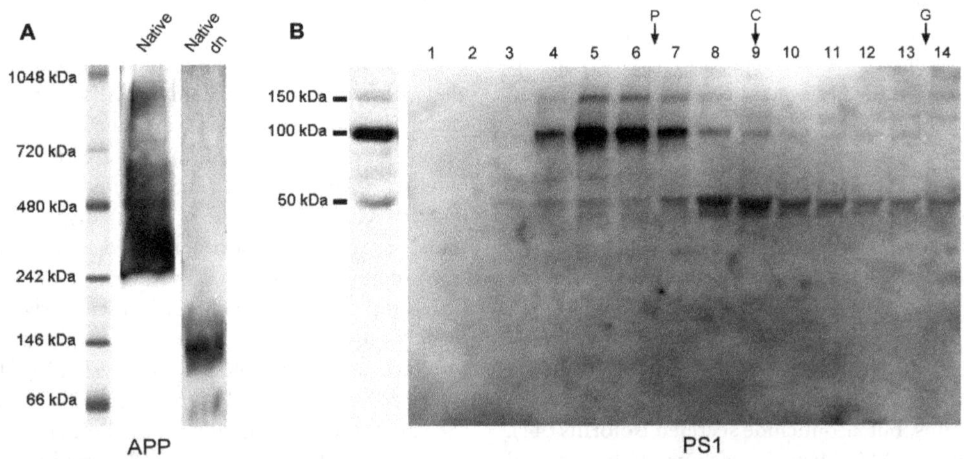

FIGURE 1 | sAPP and PS1 complexes in CSF. (A) APP complexes from CSF samples analyzed by blue native-PAGE and resolved with a C-terminal antibody (from Sigma), confirmed the presence of APP complexes. A CSF sample denatured by boiling at 95°C for 5 min under fully reducing conditions (Dn) was also analyzed by blue native-PAGE to warrant the migration of the monomeric sAPP band. A similar banding profile was obtained with sAPPα and sAPPβ specific antibodies (not shown). See Ref. (16) for further details. **(B)** CSF samples were fractionated in 5–20% sucrose density gradients (left panel: same CSF sample prior fractionation). The fractions (collected from the top) were immunoblotted for PS1 with an anti N-terminal antibody (from Calbiochem). Enzymes of known sedimentation coefficient, β-galactosidase (G, 16.0S; ~540 kDa), catalase (C, 11.4S; ~232 kDa), and alkaline phosphatase (P, 6.1S; ~140–160 kDa) were used as internal markers. Incubation of blots with antibodies for the different γ-secretase subunits confirmed that APH1 and PEN2, but not nicastrin, are present in CSF as complexes (see Ref. (25) to complete information). In all analyses performed on PS1, denaturation before electrophoresis was conducted at 50°C.

and needs to be more specifically addressed. More research is needed to design an appropriate strategy and assays for CSF sAPP. The validation of sAPP as a CSF biomarker may be of particular interest for assessing the effect of clinical trials based on β-secretase inhibition, where a decrease in newly generated sAPPβ is expected, but with an unclear effect on newly generated sAPPα (27).

β-Secretase and TACE/α-Secretase Activities in CSF

The major neuronal β-secretase has been identified as beta-site APP cleaving enzyme 1 [BACE1; (28)], though other proteases such as BACE2 and cathepsins might be involved as well (29, 30). Interestingly, both BACE1 protein and activity levels can be measured in CSF (31), but, to date, accurate determination of BACE1 remains a great challenge and there is no consensus as to whether its levels are consistently affected in CSF as dementia progresses (32). Most published results suggest that BACE1 activity increases in AD, preferentially in MCI cases with prodromal AD (31, 33, 34). However, such biochemical analysis often relies on APP fluorogenic substrates with modified APP β-cleavage sites, whose discrimination between BACE1 from other β-secretase enzymes like BACE2 and cathepsins is unclear [for a review, see Ref. (32)]. Currently, it is not known whether BACE1 activity reflects BACE1 protein content since it correlates poorly (33), and it is also unknown if the values measured are due to full-length BACE1 or a truncated form. Mature BACE1 holoprotein contains a single transmembrane domain and a short intracellular C-terminal (28). Membrane-bound BACE1 can be partly cleaved within its extracellular domain to generate soluble BACE1 for secretion (35, 36). Accordingly, it has been assumed that the BACE1 present in CSF is a truncated soluble form of the originally membrane-bound BACE1 missing the transmembrane and intracellular domains (37). Indeed, some studies failed to demonstrate the presence of BACE1 containing the C-terminal domain in human CSF and plasma (38, 39), but others detected immunoreactivity with BACE1 C-terminal antibodies (25, 31, 33), suggesting that full-length BACE1 exists in this fluid. The presence of full-length BACE1, together with its truncated form, has also been demonstrated in conditioned media from cultured neurons (40). The presence in CSF of an immature form of BACE1 protein, poorly active or inactive, has also been suggested (33). Future work will be required to elucidate if both the full-length and truncated BACE1 account for β-secretase in CSF.

Furthermore, similarly to APP, BACE1 occurred as a dimer in human brain tissue (41, 42). Therefore, we cannot discard the occurrence of BACE1 forming complexes in CSF, which needs to be taken into consideration, especially for the attempts to develop BACE1 ELISA assays (33, 43). In conclusion, extensive work remains to be accomplished to reinforce the interest of using CSF BACE1 levels and activity as AD biomarkers.

Regarding α-secretase, at least three members of the ADAM (a disintegrin and metalloproteinase) family, ADAM10, ADAM17 (TACE), and ADAM9 have been proposed as α-secretases (44), and other ADAM family members, such as ADAM8, has also demonstrated efficiency in cleavage of APP (45). Evidence indicates that ADAM10, but not ADAM9 or ADAM17, is the enzyme acting as a physiologically relevant constitutive α-secretase *in vivo* (46, 47). To our knowledge, the occurrence of ADAM-10/α-secretase activity in either CSF or plasma has not been reported to date, and ADAM10 has so far only been found in platelets (48) and other blood cells (49). However, elevated activity levels for ADAM17/TACE activity have been found in both CSF (50) and plasma (51, 52) from subjects with AD. TACE releases several transmembrane proteins into soluble forms, including APP, but also tumor necrosis factor α (TNFα) receptors (53). The synthetic peptide used for TACE enzymatic activity assays in CSF and plasma consists of a TACE-sensitive TNF sequence surrounding the TACE-specific cleaving site (50); thus, it constitutes a substrate favorable for TACE compared to ADAM10. α-Secretase accurately refers to the activity targeting APP and generating sAPPα; nonetheless, the general requirements for secretase cleavage are not strict and we cannot exclude the possibility that other enzymes, including ADAM10, may cleave peptides in human CSF and plasma. The presence in CSF of other ADAM family members, including ADAM10, deserves study.

Moreover, ADAM proteases, similarly to BACE1, are type I transmembrane proteins, but also include secreted isoforms (44). Indeed, ADAM10 and ADAM17 have been shown to be secreted outside the cells in exosomes (54). Thus, the occurrence of TACE activity in CSF and plasma has been attributed to soluble isoforms shedding from cell membranes after the cleavage of TNFα and the TNF receptors. Nonetheless, TACE protein has only been studied in plasma by Western blot using an anti-TACE polyclonal antibody (52), but not by the combination of N- and C-terminal antibodies allowing characterization of the full-length and truncated forms. Again, a parallel study of protein and enzyme activity is pending in order to define the most sensitive molecular tools necessary for using ADAM as CSF biomarkers.

Presenilin-1 and Other γ-Secretase Components are Present in CSF

γ-Secretase is an intramembrane protease complex composed of presenilin-1 (PS1), nicastrin, APH1 (anterior pharynx-defective 1), and PEN2 (presenilin enhancer 2) (55). Since most of the γ-secretase components contain several transmembrane domains, their presence in CSF was not assessed until recently. PS1 is a transmembrane aspartyl protease and the catalytic subunit of γ-secretase, and it is known to undergo endoproteolytic cleavage as part of its maturation, generating N- and C-terminal fragments (NTF and CTF) (56), with six- and three-transmembrane domains, respectively (57). APH1 also displays seven-transmembrane domains and PEN2 two transmembrane domains; only nicastrin contains a single transmembrane domain [for a review, see Ref. (58)]. Previously, the presence of soluble CTF–PS1 was reported in the media from cultured neurons (59). Recently, we demonstrated the presence of 100–150-kDa heteromeric complexes in CSF, composed of NTF and CTF PS1 [(25); see also **Figure 1B**]. The presence of the NTF and 20-kDa CTF fragments was only clearly detectable in *post-mortem* CSF, where artifacts are likely to appear. APH1 and PEN2, but not nicastrin, co-exist within these CSF–PS1 complexes. We were unable to detect γ-secretase activity in human CSF, and presumed that CSF–PS1 complexes may result from non-specific aggregation of these transmembrane proteins with large numbers of hydrophobic regions. PS1 aggregates have previously been described as temperature-sensitive (60); similarly, CSF–PS1 complexes are only detectable when denaturation before electrophoresis is conducted at 50°C (15 min). Thus, analysis performed with samples denatured at 98°C can underestimate and fail to detect PS1 complexes. Ultracentrifugation in sucrose density gradients confirmed the existence of stable complexes of 100–150-kDa, but also showed that large complexes, which sediment in regions closer to 200 and 250 kDa, are unstable during electrophoresis under denaturing conditions. Interestingly, when we assessed whether CSF–PS1 levels are altered in AD, ventricular *post-mortem* samples (disease at term) display higher levels of PS1 than those present in non-demented control cases, particularly the stable complexes resolved by sucrose density gradients. Lumbar CSF samples from probable AD cases (early stages of the disease) display only significant differences in the proportion of the PS1 stable complex, but not in total levels (25). The amount of PS1 stable complexes correlates with Aβ42. Our results suggest that the early and more significant phenomenon is the change in the dynamics of the assembly of PS1 complexes. The change in the proportion of stable complexes appears as a better marker for discriminating pathological samples than the estimation of total PS1 protein levels. Further characterization of CSF–PS1 complexes has yet to be conducted in order to define the appropriate methodological approach for evaluating their feasibility as a potential new AD biomarker, as well evaluation of its diagnostic performance in comparison with existing biomarkers such as Aβ.

Conclusion

Because CSF is in direct contact with the extracellular space of the central nervous system, biochemical changes in the brain could potentially be reflected in CSF. It is expected that potential AD biomarkers involved in AD pathogenesis will mirror AD progression. However, to date, no single biomarker has reached expectations. Several models of CSF secretion have been proposed (61–63), but the relationship with protein content and cellular origin of CSF protein composition remains unclear. Moreover, increasing evidence indicates the occurrence of soluble full-length membrane proteins in CSF. The mechanisms by which these membrane-bound proteins reached the CSF are unknown. Active secretion is unlikely, and it is still unclear if passive release from brain cells or neuronal death may be major contributing factors, as recently observed for BACE1 (43). Most of these forms could display self-association properties based on hydrophobic and/or ionic interactions, resulting in the formation of complexes. Indeed, proteins like presenilins, with large numbers of hydrophobic regions, may be highly unstable in CSF, and spontaneously form complexes. The occurrence of different types of protein complexes in CSF, forming heterogeneous components, should be considered to accurately determine their levels. In this sense, the presence in CSF of soluble oligomers, normally associated with protein-misfolding diseases, has been suggested for multiple sclerosis patients (64).

Our understanding of the potential roles for APP, BACE1, ADAM proteins, PS1, and other related proteins in CSF is lacking, but of interest in order to design adequate quantification strategies to assess their real potential as biomarkers for AD. Ultimately, it is anticipated that a combination of CSF biomarkers might serve for early diagnosis, but also for assessing disease progression and especially the efficiency of secretase inhibitors during the course of clinical trials. In this review, we presented evidence that most of the proteins related with APP processing are measurable in CSF. More investigation should focus on the possibility of monitoring soluble forms of APP and secretase components, and to evaluate the progress and feasibility of developing molecular tools for these potential new CSF biomarkers for AD.

Acknowledgments

This study was funded in part by the EU BIOMARKAPD-Joint Programming on Neurodegenerative Diseases (JPND) project. This project is supported through the Instituto de Salud Carlos III (ISCIII; grants PI11/03026 to JS-V), cofinanced by the Fondo Europeo de Desarrollo Regional (FEDER), and under the aegis of JPND, and through CIBERNED, ISC-III.

References

1. Blennow K, Dubois B, Fagan AM, Lewczuk P, de Leon MJ, Hampel H. Clinical utility of cerebrospinal fluid biomarkers in the diagnosis of early Alzheimer's disease. *Alzheimers Dement* (2015) **11**:58–69. doi:10.1016/j.jalz.2014.02.004
2. Blennow K, Hampel H, Weiner M, Zetterberg H. Cerebrospinal fluid and plasma biomarkers in Alzheimer disease. *Nat Rev Neurol* (2010) **6**:131–44. doi:10.1038/nrneurol.2010.4
3. Rosen C, Hansson O, Blennow K, Zetterberg H. Fluid biomarkers in Alzheimer's disease – current concepts. *Mol Neurodegener* (2013) **8**:20. doi:10.1186/1750-1326-8-20
4. Hardy J, Selkoe DJ. The amyloid hypothesis of Alzheimer's disease: progress and problems on the road to therapeutics. *Science* (2002) **297**:353–6. doi:10.1126/science.1072994
5. Steiner H, Fluhrer R, Haass C. Intramembrane proteolysis by gamma-secretase. *J Biol Chem* (2008) **283**:29627–31. doi:10.1074/jbc.R800010200
6. Thinakaran G, Koo EH. Amyloid precursor protein trafficking, processing, and function. *J Biol Chem* (2008) **283**:29615–9. doi:10.1074/jbc.R800019200
7. Portelius E, Price E, Brinkmalm G, Stiteler M, Olsson M, Persson R, et al. A novel pathway for amyloid precursor protein processing. *Neurobiol Aging* (2011) **32**:1090–8. doi:10.1016/j.neurobiolaging.2009.06.002
8. Jack CR Jr, Knopman DS, Jagust WJ, Shaw LM, Aisen PS, Weiner MW, et al. Hypothetical model of dynamic biomarkers of the Alzheimer's pathological cascade. *Lancet Neurol* (2010) **9**:119–28. doi:10.1016/S1474-4422(09)70299-6
9. Wolfe MS. γ-Secretase as a target for Alzheimer's disease. *Adv Pharmacol* (2012) **64**:127–53. doi:10.1016/B978-0-12-394816-8.00004-0
10. Yan R, Vassar R. Targeting the β secretase BACE1 for Alzheimer's disease therapy. *Lancet Neurol* (2014) **13**:319–29. doi:10.1016/S1474-4422(13)70276-X
11. Palmert MR, Podlisny MB, Witker DS, Oltersdorf T, Younkin LH, Selkoe DJ, et al. The beta-amyloid protein precursor of Alzheimer disease has soluble derivatives found in human brain and cerebrospinal fluid. *Proc Natl Acad Sci U S A* (1989) **86**:6338–42. doi:10.1073/pnas.86.16.6338
12. Ghiso J, Tagliavini F, Timmers WF, Frangione B. Alzheimer's disease amyloid precursor protein is present in senile plaques and cerebrospinal fluid: immunohistochemical and biochemical characterization. *Biochem Biophys Res Commun* (1989) **163**:430–7. doi:10.1016/0006-291X(89)92154-2
13. Perneczky R, Alexopoulos P, Kurz A. Soluble amyloid precursor proteins and secretases as Alzheimer's disease biomarkers. *Trends Mol Med* (2014) **20**:8–15. doi:10.1016/j.molmed.2013.10.001
14. Efthimiopoulos S, Vassilacopoulou D, Ripellino JA, Tezapsidis N, Robakis NK. Cholinergic agonists stimulate secretion of soluble full-length amyloid precursor protein in neuroendocrine cells. *Proc Natl Acad Sci U S A* (1996) **93**:8046–50. doi:10.1073/pnas.93.15.8046
15. Tezapsidis N, Li HC, Ripellino JA, Efthimiopoulos S, Vassilacopoulou D, Sambamurti K, et al. Release of nontransmembrane full-length Alzheimer's amyloid precursor protein from the lumenar surface of chromaffin granule membranes. *Biochemistry* (1998) **37**:1274–82. doi:10.1021/bi9714159
16. Cuchillo-Ibañez I, Lopez-Font I, Boix-Amorós A, Brinkmalm G, Blennow K, Molinuevo JL, et al. Heteromers of amyloid precursor protein in cerebrospinal fluid. *Mol Neurodegener* (2015) **10**:2. doi:10.1186/1750-1326-10-2
17. Lewczuk P, Kamrowski-Kruck H, Peters O, Heuser I, Jessen F, Popp J, et al. Soluble amyloid precursor proteins in the cerebrospinal fluid as novel potential biomarkers of Alzheimer's disease: a multicenter study. *Mol Psychiatry* (2010) **15**:138–45. doi:10.1038/mp.2008.84
18. Gabelle A, Roche S, Gény C, Bennys K, Labauge P, Tholance Y, et al. Correlations between soluble α/β forms of amyloid precursor protein and Aβ38, 40, and 42 in human cerebrospinal fluid. *Brain Res* (2010) **21**:175–83. doi:10.1016/j.brainres.2010.08.022
19. Mulugeta E, Londos E, Hansson O, Ballard C, Skogseth R, Minthon L, et al. Cerebrospinal fluid levels of sAPPα and sAPPβ in Lewy body and Alzheimer's disease: clinical and neurochemical correlates. *Int J Alzheimers Dis* (2011) **2011**:495025. doi:10.4061/2011/495025
20. Alexopoulos P, Tsolakidou A, Roselli F, Arnold A, Grimmer T, Westerteicher C, et al. Clinical and neurobiological correlates of soluble amyloid precursor proteins in the cerebrospinal fluid. *Alzheimers Dement* (2012) **8**:304–11. doi:10.1016/j.jalz.2011.04.009
21. Sennvik K, Fastbom J, Blomberg M, Wahlund LO, Winblad B, Benedikz E. Levels of alpha- and beta-secretase cleaved amyloid precursor protein in the cerebrospinal fluid of Alzheimer's disease patients. *Neurosci Lett* (2000) **278**:169–72. doi:10.1016/S0304-3940(99)00929-5
22. Blennow K. Biomarkers in Alzheimer's disease drug development. *Nat Med* (2010) **16**:1218–22. doi:10.1038/nm.2221
23. Karran E, Hardy J. Antiamyloid therapy for Alzheimer's disease – are we on the right road? *N Engl J Med* (2014) **370**:377–8. doi:10.1056/NEJMe1313943
24. May PC, Dean RA, Lowe SL, Martenyi F, Sheehan SM, Boggs LN, et al. Robust central reduction of amyloid-β in humans with an orally available, non-peptidic β-secretase inhibitor. *J Neurosci* (2011) **31**:16507–16. doi:10.1523/JNEUROSCI.3647-11.2011
25. García-Ayllón MS, Campanari ML, Brinkmalm G, Rábano A, Alom J, Saura CA, et al. CSF presenilin-1 complexes are increased in Alzheimer's disease. *Acta Neuropathol Commun* (2013) **1**:46. doi:10.1186/2051-5960-1-46
26. Tanaka S, Nakamura S, Ueda K, Kameyama M, Shiojiri S, Takahashi Y, et al. Three types of amyloid protein precursor mRNA in human brain: their differential expression in Alzheimer's disease. *Biochem Biophys Res Commun* (1988) **157**:472–9. doi:10.1016/S0006-291X(88)80273-0
27. Dobrowolska JA, Michener MS, Wu G, Patterson BW, Chott R, Ovod V, et al. CNS amyloid-β, soluble APP-α and -β kinetics during BACE inhibition. *J Neurosci* (2014) **34**:8336–46. doi:10.1523/JNEUROSCI.0540-14.2014
28. Vassar R, Kovacs DM, Yan R, Wong PC. The beta-secretase enzyme BACE in health and Alzheimer's disease: regulation, cell biology, function, and therapeutic potential. *J Neurosci* (2009) **29**:12787–94. doi:10.1523/JNEUROSCI.3657-09.2009
29. Dominguez D, Tournoy J, Hartmann D, Huth T, Cryns K, Deforce S, et al. Phenotypic and biochemical analyses of BACE1- and BACE2-deficient mice. *J Biol Chem* (2005) **280**:30797–806. doi:10.1074/jbc.M505249200
30. Haque A, Banik NL, Ray SK. New insights into the roles of endolysosomal cathepsins in the pathogenesis of Alzheimer's disease: cathepsin inhibitors as potential therapeutics. *CNS Neurol Disord Drug Targets* (2008) **7**:270–7. doi:10.2174/187152708784936653
31. Holsinger RM, McLean CA, Collins SJ, Masters CL, Evin G. Increased beta-secretase activity in cerebrospinal fluid of Alzheimer's disease subjects. *Ann Neurol* (2004) **55**:898–9. doi:10.1002/ana.20144
32. Decourt B, Sabbagh MN. BACE1 as a potential biomarker for Alzheimer's disease. *J Alzheimers Dis* (2011) **24**(Suppl 2):53–9. doi:10.3233/JAD-2011-110017
33. Zhong Z, Ewers M, Teipel S, Bürger K, Wallin A, Blennow K, et al. Levels of beta-secretase (BACE1) in cerebrospinal fluid as a predictor of risk in mild cognitive impairment. *Arch Gen Psychiatry* (2007) **64**:718–26. doi:10.1001/archpsyc.64.6.718
34. Zetterberg H, Andreasson U, Hansson O, Wu G, Sankaranarayanan S, Andersson ME, et al. Elevated cerebrospinal fluid BACE1 activity in incipient Alzheimer disease. *Arch Neurol* (2008) **65**:1102–7. doi:10.1001/archneur.65.8.1102

35. Benjannet S, Elagoz A, Wickham L, Mamarbachi M, Munzer JS, Basak A, et al. Post-translational processing of beta-secretase (beta-amyloid-converting enzyme) and its ectodomain shedding. The pro- and transmembrane/cytosolic domains affect its cellular activity and amyloid-beta production. *J Biol Chem* (2001) **276**:10879–87. doi:10.1074/jbc.M009899200
36. Hussain I, Hawkins J, Shikotra A, Riddell DR, Faller A, Dingwall C. Characterization of the ectodomain shedding of the beta-site amyloid precursor protein-cleaving enzyme 1 (BACE1). *J Biol Chem* (2003) **278**:36264–8. doi:10.1074/jbc.M304186200
37. Verheijen JH, Huisman LG, Neumann U, Paganetti P, Hack CE, Bouwman F. Detection of a soluble form of BACE-1 in human cerebrospinal fluid by a sensitive activity assay. *Clin Chem* (2006) **52**:1168–74. doi:10.1373/clinchem.2006.066720
38. Wu G, Sankaranarayanan S, Tugusheva K, Kahana J, Seabrook G, Shi XP, et al. Decrease in age-adjusted cerebrospinal fluid beta-secretase activity in Alzheimer's subjects. *Clin Biochem* (2008) **41**:986–96. doi:10.1016/j.clinbiochem.2008.04.022
39. Wu G, Sankaranarayanan S, Wong J, Tugusheva K, Michener MS, Shi X, et al. Characterization of plasma β-secretase (BACE1) activity and soluble amyloid precursor proteins as potential biomarkers for Alzheimer's disease. *J Neurosci Res* (2012) **90**:2247–58. doi:10.1002/jnr.23122
40. Murayama KS, Kametani F, Araki W. Extracellular release of BACE1 holoproteins from human neuronal cells. *Biochem Biophys Res Commun* (2005) **338**:800–7. doi:10.1016/j.bbrc.2005.10.015
41. Schmechel A, Strauss M, Schlicksupp A, Pipkorn R, Haass C, Bayer TA, et al. Human BACE forms dimers and colocalizes with APP. *J Biol Chem* (2004) **279**:39710–7. doi:10.1074/jbc.M402785200
42. Westmeyer GG, Willem M, Lichtenthaler SF, Lurman G, Multhaup G, Assfalg-Machleidt I, et al. Dimerization of beta-site beta-amyloid precursor protein-cleaving enzyme. *J Biol Chem* (2004) **279**:53205–12. doi:10.1074/jbc.M410378200
43. Barão S, Zhou L, Adamczuk K, Vanhoutvin T, van Leuven F, Demedts D, et al. BACE1 levels correlate with phospho-tau levels in human cerebrospinal fluid. *Curr Alzheimer Res* (2013) **10**:671–8. doi:10.2174/15672050113109990138
44. Vingtdeux V, Marambaud P. Identification and biology of α-secretase. *J Neurochem* (2012) **120**:34–45. doi:10.1111/j.1471-4159.2011.07477.x
45. Naus S, Reipschläger S, Wildeboer D, Lichtenthaler SF, Mitterreiter S, Guan Z, et al. Identification of candidate substrates for ectodomain shedding by the metalloprotease-disintegrin ADAM8. *Biol Chem* (2006) **387**:337–46. doi:10.1515/BC.2006.045
46. Jorissen E, Prox J, Bernreuther C, Weber S, Schwanbeck R, Serneels L, et al. The disintegrin/metalloproteinase ADAM10 is essential for the establishment of the brain cortex. *J Neurosci* (2010) **30**:4833–44. doi:10.1523/JNEUROSCI.5221-09.2010
47. Kuhn PH, Wang H, Dislich B, Colombo A, Zeitschel U, Ellwart JW, et al. ADAM10 is the physiologically relevant, constitutive alpha-secretase of the amyloid precursor protein in primary neurons. *EMBO J* (2010) **29**:3020–32. doi:10.1038/emboj.2010.167
48. Colciaghi F, Borroni B, Pastorino L, Marcello E, Zimmermann M, Cattabeni F, et al. α-Secretase ADAM10 as well as αAPPs is reduced in platelets and CSF of Alzheimer disease patients. *Mol Med* (2002) **8**:67–74.
49. Edwards DR, Handsley MM, Pennington CJ. The ADAM metalloproteinases. *Mol Aspects Med* (2008) **29**:258–89. doi:10.1016/j.mam.2008.08.001
50. Jiang H, Hampel H, Prvulovic D, Wallin A, Blennow K, Li R, et al. Elevated CSF levels of TACE activity and soluble TNF receptors in subjects with mild cognitive impairment and patients with Alzheimer's disease. *Mol Neurodegener* (2011) **6**:69. doi:10.1186/1750-1326-6-69
51. Bai L, Song N, Yu J, Tan L, Shen Y, Xie J, et al. Elevated plasma levels of soluble TNFRs and TACE activity in Alzheimer's disease patients of Northern Han Chinese descent. *Curr Alzheimer Res* (2013) **10**:57–62. doi:10.2174/1567205011310010008
52. Sun Q, Hampel H, Blennow K, Lista S, Levey A, Tang B, et al. Increased plasma TACE activity in subjects with mild cognitive impairment and patients with Alzheimer's disease. *J Alzheimers Dis* (2014) **41**:877–86. doi:10.3233/JAD-140177
53. Peschon JJ, Slack JL, Reddy P, Stocking KL, Sunnarborg SW, Lee DC, et al. An essential role for ectodomain shedding in mammalian development. *Science* (1998) **282**:1281–4. doi:10.1126/science.282.5392.1281
54. Stoeck A, Keller S, Riedle S, Sanderson MP, Runz S, Le Naour F, et al. A role for exosomes in the constitutive and stimulus-induced ectodomain cleavage of L1 and CD44. *Biochem J* (2006) **393**:609–18. doi:10.1042/BJ20051013
55. Kaether C, Haass C, Steiner H. Assembly, trafficking and function of gamma-secretase. *Neurodegener Dis* (2006) **3**:275–83. doi:10.1159/000095267
56. Thinakaran G, Borchelt DR, Lee MK, Slunt HH, Spitzer L, Kim G, et al. Endoproteolysis of presenilin 1 and accumulation of processed derivatives in vivo. *Neuron* (1996) **17**:181–90. doi:10.1016/S0896-6273(00)80291-3
57. Laudon H, Hansson EM, Melén K, Bergman A, Farmery MR, Winblad B, et al. A nine-transmembrane domain topology for presenilin 1. *J Biol Chem* (2005) **280**:35352–60. doi:10.1074/jbc.M507217200
58. Wakabayashi T, De Strooper B. Presenilins: members of the gamma-secretase quartets, but part-time soloists too. *Physiology (Bethesda)* (2008) **23**:194–204. doi:10.1152/physiol.00009.2008
59. Benussi L, Alberici A, Mayhaus M, Langer U, Ghidoni R, Mazzoli F, et al. Detection of the presenilin 1 COOH-terminal fragment in the extracellular compartment: a release enhanced by apoptosis. *Exp Cell Res* (2001) **269**:256–65. doi:10.1006/excr.2001.5329
60. De Strooper B, Beullens M, Contreras B, Levesque L, Craessaerts K, Cordell B, et al. Phosphorylation, subcellular localization, and membrane orientation of the Alzheimer's disease-associated presenilins. *J Biol Chem* (1997) **272**:3590–8. doi:10.1074/jbc.272.6.3590
61. Oresković D, Klarica M. The formation of cerebrospinal fluid: nearly a hundred years of interpretations and misinterpretations. *Brain Res Rev* (2010) **64**:241–62. doi:10.1016/j.brainresrev.2010.04.006
62. Damkier HH, Brown PD, Praetorius J. Cerebrospinal fluid secretion by the choroid plexus. *Physiol Rev* (2013) **93**:1847–92. doi:10.1152/physrev.00004.2013
63. Lehtinen MK, Bjornsson CS, Dymecki SM, Gilbertson RJ, Holtzman DM, Monuki ES. The choroid plexus and cerebrospinal fluid: emerging roles in development, disease, and therapy. *J Neurosci* (2013) **33**:17553–9. doi:10.1523/JNEUROSCI.3258-13.2013
64. David MA, Tayebi M. Detection of protein aggregates in brain and cerebrospinal fluid derived from multiple sclerosis patients. *Front Neurol* (2014) **5**:251. doi:10.3389/fneur.2014.00251

19

Antibody-free quantification of seven tau peptides in human CSF using targeted mass spectrometry

Pauline Bros[1,2†], *Jérôme Vialaret*[1†], *Nicolas Barthelemy*[1], *Vincent Delatour*[2], *Audrey Gabelle*[1,3], *Sylvain Lehmann*[1*] and *Christophe Hirtz*[1*]

[1] Laboratoire de Biochimie et de Protéomique Clinique - Institut de Médecine Régénérative et Biothérapies, Centre Hospitalier Universitaire de Montpellier, Montpellier, France, [2] Laboratoire National de Métrologie et d'Essais (LNE), Paris, France, [3] Centre Mémoire Ressources Recherche, Centre Hospitalier Universitaire de Montpellier, Hôpital Gui de Chauliac, Université Montpellier I, Montpellier, France

Edited by:
Raymond Scott Turner,
Georgetown University, USA

Reviewed by:
Michal Novak,
Slovak Academy of Sciences, Slovakia
Nicole Leclerc,
Université de Montréal, Canada

***Correspondence:**
Sylvain Lehmann and
Christophe Hirtz,
Laboratory of Biochemistry and Clinical Proteomics, Institute of Regenerative Medicine - Biotherapy, Centre Hospitalier Universitaire de Montpellier - Hôpital St. Eloi, 80, Av. A. Fliche, 34295 Montpellier Cedex 5, France
s-lehmann@chu-montpellier.fr;
c-hirtz@chu-montpellier.fr

† These authors have contributed equally to this work.

Tau protein concentration in cerebrospinal fluid (CSF) is currently used as a sensitive and specific biomarker for Alzheimer's disease. Its detection currently relies on ELISA but the perspective of using mass spectrometry (MS) to detect its different proteoforms represents an interesting alternative. This is however an analytical challenge because of its low concentration in the CSF, a biological fluid collected in small volume by lumbar puncture, and with a high structural heterogeneity. To overcome these issues, instead of using immunocapture as previously done, we rather relied on an original two steps pre-fractionation technique of CSF: perchloric acid (PCA) followed by micro solid phase extraction (μSPE). We could then measure seven tau trypsic peptides by Multiple Reaction Monitoring (MRM) on a triple quadrupole mass spectrometer. Quantification was performed using isotopically labeled ^{15}N- recombinant tau protein as internal standard and validated using CSF pools with low, medium, or high tau concentrations (HTCs). Repeatability, intermediate precision, linearity, limit of quantification (LOQ), and recovery were calculated for the different peptides. This new MRM assay, which allowed for the first time CSF tau protein quantification without immunocapture, has important potential application to follow tau metabolism in both diagnostic and therapeutic research.

Keywords: Alzheimer's disease, tau protein, human cerebrospinal fluid, LC-MS/MS, quantitative proteomic, triple quadrupole

Introduction

Alzheimer's disease (AD) is the most common form of dementia, a general term encompassing loss of memory and cognitive functions interfering therefore with activities of daily living. With 35 million of patients worldwide, AD represents 50–80% of cases of dementia and is reaching epidemic proportions in industrialized countries mainly because of the aging of the population.

Abbreviations: AD, Alzheimer Disease; CAV, Cell Accelerator Voltage; CE, Collision Energy; CSF, CerebroSpinal Fluid; ELISA, Enzyme Linked ImmunoAssay; FA, Formic Acid; HLB, Hydrophilic-Lipophilic-Balanced; LOQ, Limit of Quantification; MAPT, Microtubule-Associated Protein Tau; PCA, Perchloric Acid; TCA, Trifluoroacetic Acid; SPE, Solid Phase Extraction; MRM-MS, Multiple Reaction Monitoring Mass Spectrometry; PTM, Post Translational Modifications.

At neuro-pathological level, AD is characterized by the presence in the brain parenchyma of amyloid plaques and hyperphosphorylated tau (p-tau) proteins aggregated into neurofibrillary tangles (Gabelle et al., 2010). Tau protein is synthesized by a single microtubule-associated protein tau (MAPT) gene (chromosome 17q21) in humans (James et al., 2015) mainly expressed in neurons (Perrin et al., 2009). Tau protein is known to bind neuronal microtubules, promote their assembly, and stabilize them (Drechsel et al., 1992). The hyperphosphorylation occurring in case of AD caused its release from microtubules, destabilizing the axons, and triggering neuronal death (Sergeant et al., 2005). Quantification of tau in cerebrospinal fluid (CSF) is currently used as a sensitive and specific biomarker for AD diagnosis (Andreasen and Blennow, 2005). However, the full quantification of tau in CSF remained an analytical challenge. In fact, this protein has 6 different isoforms (ranging from 352 to 441 amino acids), and is subject to many different post-translational modifications like phosphorylation, glycosylation, and oxidation (Hernandez and Avila, 2007). Moreover, tau is present at very low concentration (Sjögren et al., 2001; Blennow and Vanmechelen, 2003) in CSF which is a highly complex matrix.

Currently, CSF tau quantification is performed in clinical daily routine by immunoassays (ELISA). If immunoassays are sensitive enough to detect low CSF tau concentrations, they present some boundaries: poor linearity, lack of specificity in regards to multiple tau proteoforms and no multiplexing. This is the reason why mass spectrometry (MS) is an interesting alternative in this context. In 2014, McAvoy et al. (2014) has published a quantitative LC-MS/MS method to measure tau in CSF with a sample preparation based on a immunoaffinity. Barthelemy et al. recently quantified 22 tau peptides by high resolution MS (Barthelemy, under review). Since this equipment is very rarely available in clinical laboratories, we used the same sample preparation protocol but quantification was performed on a triple quadrupole mass spectrometer. In this work, we describe the set-up of the first multiplex targeted MS quantification of tau in CSF without the need of immunocapture. The workflow includes a CSF protein precipitation and a solid phase extraction followed by a trypsic digestion. Seven tau proteotypic peptides located in different positions of the protein could be quantified by Selected Reaction Monitoring. This new method has important potential applications to follow tau metabolism in both diagnostic and therapeutic research.

Materials and Methods

Reagents

Perchloric acid (PCA), trifluoroacetic acid (TCA), and hydrogen peroxide (H_2O_2) were purchased from Sigma Aldrich (Saint Quentin Fallavier, France). Ammonium bicarbonate and trypsin were obtained from Fluka-Sigma Aldrich (Saint Quentin Fallavier, France) and Promega (Charbonnieres, France), respectively. Water, formic acid (FA), methanol (MeOH) were all ULC-MS grade and purchased from Biosolve (Dieuze, France). Normal Goat serum was obtained from Clinisciences (Nanterre, France). Protein LoBind tube 1.5 mL and Deepwell plate 96/500 μl Protein LoBind were purchased Eppendorf (Le Pecq, France). Oasis HLB μElution Plate 30 μm, was obtained from Waters (Guyancourt, France). Polypropylene vials and Zorbax 300 SB-C18 1 × 150 mm 3.5 μm were both purchased from Agilent Technologies (Santa Clara, CA, USA).

Human CSF Samples and ELISA CSF Tau Quantification

CSF samples were obtained from patients followed-up by the Montpellier neurological and Clinical Research Memory Centers (CMRR) for cognitive or behavioral disorders. They gave their informed consent for research and for the storage of their sample in an officially registered biological collection (#DC-2008-417) of the certified NFS 96-900 biobank of the CHRU of Montpellier (Ref: BB-0033-00031, www.biobanques.eu). CSF was collected in polypropylene tubes under standardized conditions, preferably between 9:00 a.m. and 1:00 p.m., to minimize the influence of diurnal variation. Each CSF sample was sent to the local laboratory within 4 h after collection and was centrifuged at 1000 g for 10 min at 4°C. CSF was aliquoted in polypropylene tubes of 1.5 mL and stored at −80°C until further analysis. Tau quantification was performed by ELISA InnoTest Tau from Fujirebio diagnostics following manufacturer's instructions.

Standards and Samples Preparation

Preparation of ^{14}N and ^{15}N recombinant tau protein (441) standards

^{14}N and ^{15}N recombinant tau protein (441) were obtained from Dr. Guy Lippens (UMR 8525, Lille Pasteur Institute, France). Lyophilized standards were resuspended at 1 mg/mL with ammonium bicarbonate 50 mmol/L. The solution was then aliquoted into 50 μL in LoBind tubes and stored at −80°C until use. Concentration of ^{14}N and ^{15}N tau primary calibrators was determined by amino acid analysis. Ten calibration standards were prepared gravimetrically using an analytical balance model Sartorius CPA224S-OCE (Sartorius Goettingen, Germany) by adding a fixed amount of ^{15}N tau to variable amounts of ^{14}N tau. Standards were diluted with 50 mmol/L ammonium bicarbonate and 1 mmol/L BSA and then further diluted in 0.5% goat serum so as to reach final concentration of 5 ng/mL for ^{15}N tau while that of ^{14}N tau ranged from 0.3 to 32.1 ng/mL.

Series of 8–10 human CSF samples with tau concentrations determined by ELISA were mixed to obtain 3 CSF pools with Low Tau Concentration (LTC), Medium Tau Concentration (MTC), and High Tau Concentration (HTC).

Precipitation, μSPE extraction and protein digestion

Sample extraction of tau peptides were performed according to Barthelemy et al. (Barthelemy, under review). Briefly, 450 μL of CSF or 0.5% serum samples were mixed with 50 μL of ^{15}N-tau-441 (50 ng/mL) in a LoBind tube. Protein precipitation was performed by adding 25 μL of 70% PCA. Samples were then vortexed, kept on ice for 15 min before centrifugation at 17,000 g at 4°C during 15 min to obtain a clear supernatant. Supernatants were acidified with 50 μL of 1% trifluoroacetic acid (TFA). SPE with a hydrophilic-lipophilic balance SPE 96-well plate was conditioned with 300 μL of MeOH and equilibrated with 500 μL of 0.1% TFA. Samples were loaded and washed with 500 µL of 0.1% TFA. For protein oxidation, 500 µL of 3% FA and 3% H_2O_2 solution in water was loaded on cartridge and kept 12 h at 4°C. Thereafter, cartridge was washed with 500 µL of 0.1%TFA. Oxidized tau proteins were eluted with 100 µL of 35% acetonitrile 0.1% TFA. Extracts were evaporated to dryness with a Speedvac instrument from LabConco (Kansas City, MO, USA) and resuspended with 40 µL of 1 ng/µL trypsin solution in 50 mM ammonium bicarbonate. The digestion was performed for 24 h at 37°C on a Thermomixer R from Eppendorf (Hambourg, Germany) and stopped with 5 µL of 10% FA and stored at −20°C prior to LC-MS/MS analysis (**Figure 1**).

LC-MS/MS

Liquid chromatography (LC) separation

LC separation was carried out on a 1290 LC system (Agilent technologies). Separation was performed with a reversed-phase Zorbax 300 SB-C18 column maintained at 60°C. The mobile phases consisted in (A) 0.1% FA in water and (B) 0.1% FA in MeOH. After an isocratic step of 2 min at 2% B, a linear gradient from 10 to 70% B was run over the next 13 min with a flow rate of 50 µL/min. The column was then washed for 1 min with 90% B and re-equilibrated during 5 min with 2% B. Eluent flow before 2 min and after 15 min was discarded with a divert valve to reduce contamination of the mass spectrometer.

MS/MS analysis

Mass spectrometric detection was performed using a 6490 triple quadrupole with an ESI source operating in positive mode and in dynamic MRM mode (Agilent technologies, Waldbronn, Germany). The control of the LC-MS/MS was done with MassHunter Software (Agilent technologies, Waldbronn, Germany). The ESI spray was set up according to the following settings: capillary tension 2500 V, gas flow 16 L/min with temperature of 140°C, sheath gas flow 7 L/min with temperature of 250°C, nebulizer 40 psi. Precursor ions were transferred inside the first quadrupole with high pressure ion funnel RF set to 150 V and low pressure in funnel RF set to 110 V. Collision energies (CE) and cell accelerator voltages (CA) were optimized for the peptide transitions of interest. The Skyline 2.6 version was used to conduct data treatment. All transitions per peptide were used as quantifiers and were automatically detected on specific retention time windows. LC-MS/MS were repeated 5 times for analytical validation.

Method Validation

The calibration curve was established by linear regression and its linearity was validated according to the criterion of a Pearson correlation $r^2 > 0.99$. The Limit of Quantification (LOQ) was defined as the concentration of the lowest calibration point with the relative standard deviation (RSD) of the area ratios ^{14}N tau peptide/^{15}N tau peptide was less than 20%. Absence of memory effects was tested by re-analyzing the calibrator point without adding any ^{14}N recombinant tau protein in the end of the analytical sequence.

The intermediate precision of the entire protocol was evaluated by preparing and measuring the 20 ng/mL calibration standard over 6 different days. LC-MS repeatability was tested on the 20 ng/mL calibration standard by injecting it 4 times in a row. RSD was calculated from the area ratios ^{14}N tau peptide/^{15}N tau peptide.

Recovery was evaluated by analyzing human CSF sample with LTC spiked to a final concentration of 6.6 ng/mL of ^{14}N tau. Recovery was calculated by applying the following equation: Recovery (%) = (Measured added concentration/Theoretical added concentration) × 100.

Results

Method Development, Linearity, and Recovery

Starting from 22 validated peptides of CSF tau protein obtained with high resolution MS in PRM mode (Barthelemy, under review), 7 peptides (GAAPPGQK, SGYSSPGSPGTPGSR, TPSLPTPPTREPK, TPSLPTPPTR, LQTPVPMPDLK, IGSTENLK, SPVVSGDTSPR) were validated using triple quadrupole in MRM mode (**Table 1**). One precursor ion and 2 products ion transitions were selected for the 22 peptides previously validated in PRM. We kept the most intense precursor ions (doubly charged) after optimization of the CE. Each transition was verified using Skyline Software. For the selection, three parameters were considered: signal intensities, presence of interferences and concentration in CSF pools (**Table 1**). The seven validated peptides (**Figure 2**) in human CSF had repeatable retention times with a mean RSD of 1.53% (**Table 2**).

Between successive LC-MS/MS analysis, no memory effect phenomenon was observed. The calibration linearity was assessed using 10 point calibration curves of ^{14}N tau standard spiked in normal goat serum 0.5%. MRM results showed linearity over 2–32.7 ng/mL concentration range (**Table 2**). Calibration curves were generated by linear regression analysis by plotting the peak area ratios (^{14}N tau/^{15}N tau) vs. concentration ratios for all measured peptides. The regression coefficients were calculated above 0.98 for the 7 considered peptides. Typical calibration curves are shown in **Figure 3**. The LOQs were determined over 0.3–2 ng/mL range depending on the peptide (**Table 2**). Calculated recovery rates were 121 ± 19% for the 7 tau peptides and using the 6.6 ng/mL calibration standard ($n = 3$). For the TPSLPTPPTR corresponding to the epitope of the ELISA capture antibody, a recovery of 107% was measured.

Precision Studies

Precision of the entire protocol (including both sample preparation and LC-MS/MS analysis) was evaluated using these samples. The RSD of the CSF pools processing was below 6% for the 7 targeted peptides. LC-MS/MS analysis was repeatable with RSD of less than 4% ($n = 4$).

Quantification of Tau Protein in CSF Pools

Tau concentrations measured in the 3 CSF pools (LTC, MTC, and HTC) displayed different results for the 7 peptides (**Table 2**). For the LTC, depending on the targeted peptide, MRM-calculated concentrations ranged from 0.3 to 6.6 ng/mL, for

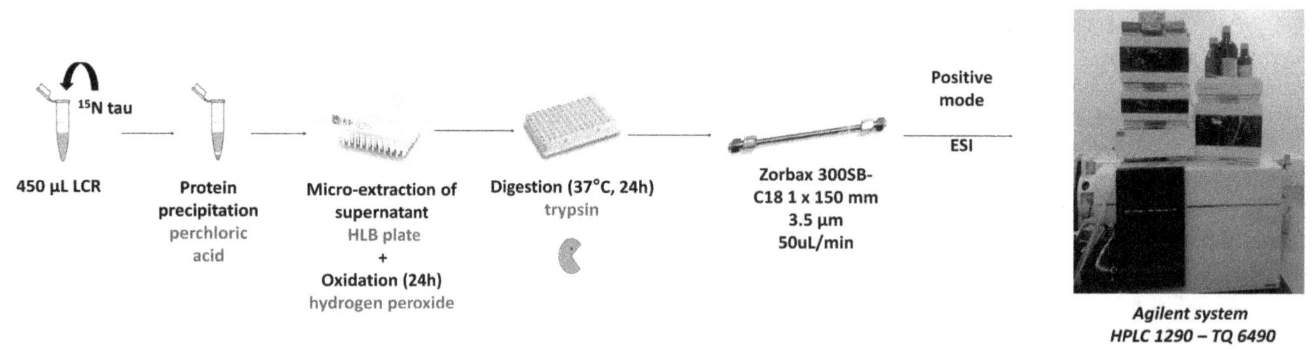

FIGURE 1 | Sample extraction: ^{15}N recombinant tau was spiked on CSF and proteins were then precipitated. Remaining proteins including tau in the supernatant were extracted on HLB cartridges. During extraction, an oxidation step was performed to oxidize methionine. Extracts were dried and then enzymatically digested by trypsin. Proteotypic peptides of tau protein were then quantified in the sample by LC-MS/MS.

TABLE 1 | Peptide selection: starting from 22 validated peptides of CSF tau protein obtained with high resolution mass spectrometry in PRM mode (Barthelemy, under review), the 7 quantifed peptides (GAAPPGQK, SGYSSPGSPGTPGSR, TPSLPTPPTREPK, TPSLPTPPTR, LQTPVPMPDLK, IGSTENLK, SPVVSGDTSPR) were selected by taking into account the three following parameters: signal intensities, presence of interferences, and concentration in CSF pools.

Peptide sequence	Peak intensity	Interfered	Increasing concentration in CSF pools	MRM validation
GAAPPGQK	**600**	**No**	**Yes**	**Yes**
TPPAPK	2200	No	No	No
TPPSSGEPPK	200	Yes	No	No
IGSTENLK	**100**	**No**	**Yes**	**Yes**
SPVVSGDTSPR	**100**	**No**	**Yes**	**Yes**
SGYSSPGSPGTPGSR	**300**	**No**	**Yes**	**Yes**
VQIINK	400	Yes	No	No
SRTPSLPTPPTREPK	0	Yes	No	No
IGSLDNITHVPGGGNK	0	Yes	No	No
ESPLQTPTEDGSEEPGSETSDAK	0	Yes	No	No
TPSLPTPPTREPK	**1200**	**No**	**Yes**	**Yes**
STPTAEDVTAPLVDEGAPGK	0	Yes	No	No
TPSLPTPPTR	**400**	**No**	**Yes**	**Yes**
QAAAQPHTEIPEGTTAEEAGIGDTPSLEDEAAGHVTQAR	0	Yes	No	No
HVPGGGSVQIVYKPVDLSK	0	Yes	No	No
TDHGAEIVYK	0	Yes	No	No
DQGGYTMHQDQEGDTDAGLK	0	Yes	No	No
LDLSNVQSK	0	Yes	No	No
QEFEVMEDHAGTYGLGDR	0	Yes	No	No
LQTAPVPMPDLK	**100**	**No**	**Yes**	**Yes**
HLSNVSSTGSIDM(diox)VDSPQLATLADEVSASLAK	0	Yes	No	No
KLDLSNVQSK	0	Yes	No	No

Bold and italics correspond to the 7 chosen tau peptides.
Underline characters (M) correspond to oxidized methionine.

the MTC from 1.6 to 12.5 ng/mL and for the HTC from 3.5 to 30.3 ng/mL. Calculated ratio between endogenous tau (^{14}N) and tau standard (^{15}N) are presented in **Figure 4**, showing the different concentrations obtained for each peptide in the three CSF pools. For the peptide TPSLPTPPTR corresponding to the epitope of the ELISA capture antibody, concentrations of 4.6 ng/mL for the LTC, 7.3 ng/mL for the MTC and 18.9 ng/mL for the HTC were obtained.

ELISA Quantitation and Correlation with MRM

Tau concentration determined in the LTC, MTC, and HTC pools using ELISA were 184 pg/mL, 399 pg/mL, and 1096 pg/mL, respectively. For the 7 peptides, concentrations obtained using MRM were highly correlated with those measured by ELISA (r^2 above 0.99) (see **Figure 5** for the TPSLPTPPTR peptide as an example). However, ELISA concentrations were 17–25 times lower than those measured by MRM.

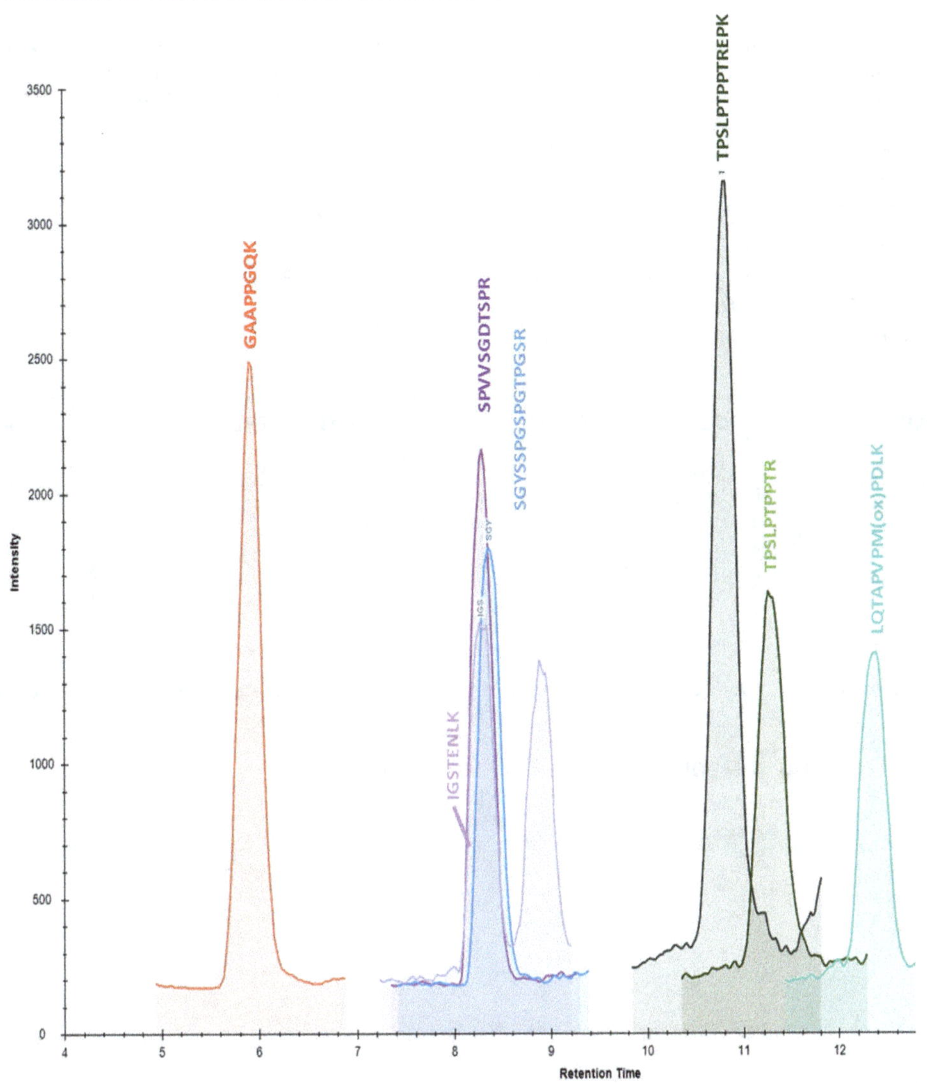

FIGURE 2 | Chromatogram of calibration standard at 32.1 ng/mL in 0.5% normal goat serum after sample preparation.

Discussion

In this work, we presented for the first time an MRM based multiplex assay for tau in the CSF that did not necessitate any immuno-capture. Thanks to an adaptation of the "protein standard for absolute quantification" (PSAQ) approach (Picard et al., 2012), to an original two step purification protocol, and to the latest generation of triple quadrupole MS analyzers, we realized the tour-de-force of quantifying in parallel 7 proteotypic peptides of the tau protein. Previous MS attempts to measure tau in the CSF of patients were in fact limited to a few peptides and/or rely on immuno-precipitation procedures that are potentially subject to cross-reactivity and difficulty to obtain reproducible results when using different batches of antibodies (Portelius et al., 2008; McAvoy et al., 2014). Our method was successfully applied to the analysis of CSF pools with different levels of tau protein. Based on previous data obtained using the same sample preparation workflow but using targeted high resolution mass spectrometry (PRM), we validated 7 peptides using our triple quadrupole (MRM) compared to the 22 beforehand validated by PRM on a high resolution mass spectrometer. If MRM can be considered to be less performing in terms of resolution, it has multiple advantages compared to PRM. Mainly, the method development is much easier, data amount generated are lighter and the data processing is highly facilitated thanks to the Skyline software. Additionally, our method can be much more easily be transferred in a clinical environment where most popular mass spectrometers are triple quadrupoles.

The MRM technology also provides several analytical advantages compared with standard ELISA methods (Lehmann et al., 2013). MRM is known to be highly selective and specific (Lehmann et al., 2013) allowing to determine the absolute concentration of the targeted protein, provided that appropriate calibration standards are available. The MRM

TABLE 2 | Method validation summary.

Peptide	Position in the tau protein sequence	Linear range (ng/mL)	LOQ (ng/mL)	Mean retention time (min)	Repeatability RSD (%)	Recovery at 6.6 ng/mL (%)	Measured tau concentration LTC (ng/mL)	Measured tau concentration MTC (ng/mL)	Measured tau concentration HTC (ng/mL)
GAAPPGQK	156 – 163	0.3 – 32.7	0.3	5.91	1.5	117	6.6	12.5	30.3
SGYSSPGSPGTPGSR	195 – 209	2.0 – 32.7	2.0	8.37	0.6	154	3.6	7.6	20.9
TPSLPTPPTREPK	212 – 224	2.0 – 32.7	2.0	10.80	1.2	109	3.2	8.1	15.7
TPSLPTPPTR*	212 – 223	1.0 – 32.7	1.0	11.31	1.6	107	4.6	7.3	18.9
LQTPVPMPDLK	243 – 254	0.5 – 32.7	0.5	12.32	3.1	98	1	2.5	17.3
IGSTENLK	260 – 267	1.0 – 32.7	1.0	8.28	3.2	137	2.1	4.9	9.5
SPVVSGDTSPR	396 – 406	0.5 – 32.7	0.5	8.28	1.3	130	0.3	1.6	3.5

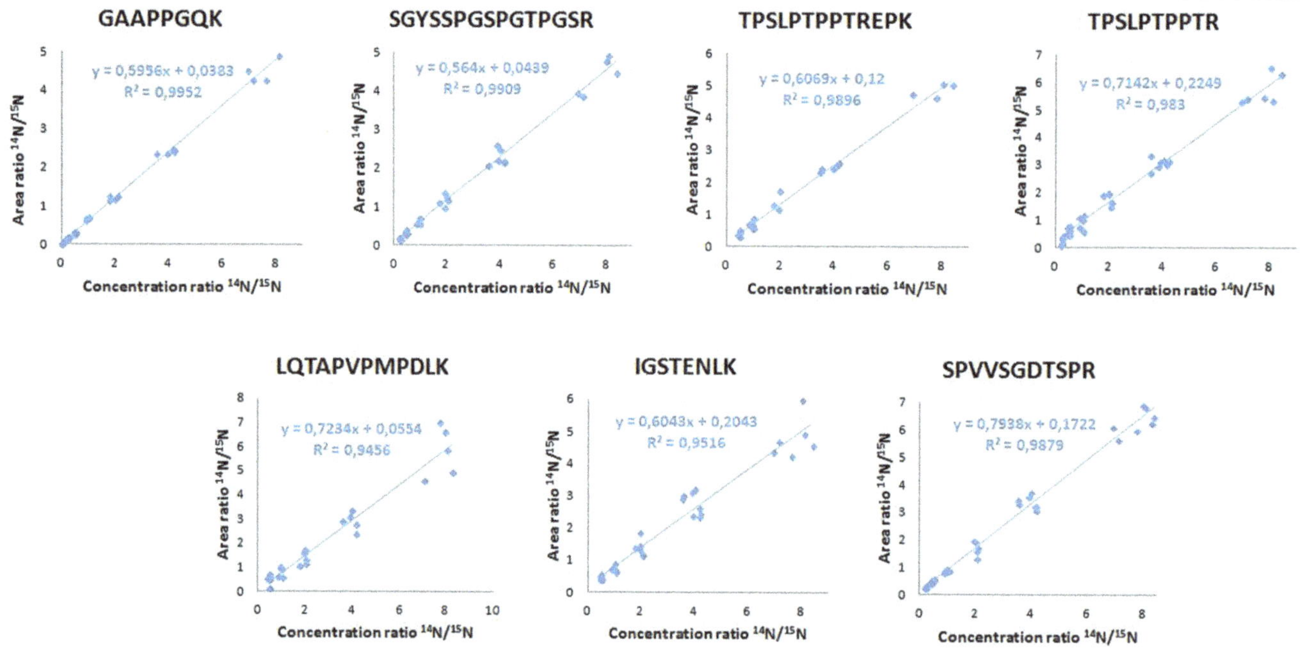

FIGURE 3 | Calibration curves of the 7 tau peptides.

absolute quantitation of the target protein takes benefit of the advantages of isotope dilution MS (Huillet et al., 2012). Adding a known amount of an isotopically labeled internal standard at the beginning of sample preparation protocol makes it possible to account for potential material non-recovery during sample preparation, which results in better accuracy and precision. MRM assay thus showed robust pre-analytical and analytical precision, matching current clinical needs.

Interestingly, the value obtained for the quantification of tau between the two approaches (MRM vs. ELISA) showed that the concentration measured with our MRM-MS assay with the TPSLPTPPTR peptide was around 17–25 times higher than that with the ELISA test. This result is in modest agreement with the work of McAvoy et al. (2014) who had found a correlation slope of 1.8 between MSD and their IA-MS method using the same peptide. The differences between the two LC-MS/MS approaches are probably due to the different sample preparation techniques (protein precipitation followed by SPE vs. immunoaffinity) and the different standards used to establish the calibration curves. The striking difference observed between LC-MS/MS and ELISA results raises the question of what method is the most accurate. However, a first evidence in favor of LC-MS/MS is that our results were in pretty good agreement with those published in McAvoy et al.: despite different sample preparation procedures and different calibration standards were used, the 2 studies shown that for Tau concentrations below 500 pg/mL, immunoassays are negatively biased against LC/MS. Another evidence that immunoassays underestimated tau concentration is that the concentration of our protein standard was 20 ng/mL when measured by amino acid analysis, 21.4 ng/mL by LC-MS/MS and around 2 ng/mL by ELISA (data not shown). However, we didn't check that the buffer in which standards were dissolved (ammonium bicarbonate 50 mM) is compatible with Innogenetics ELISA. It can't be ruled out that standards and even our 3 CSF pools were not commutable for ELISA tests, thereby introducing matrix effects that could explain

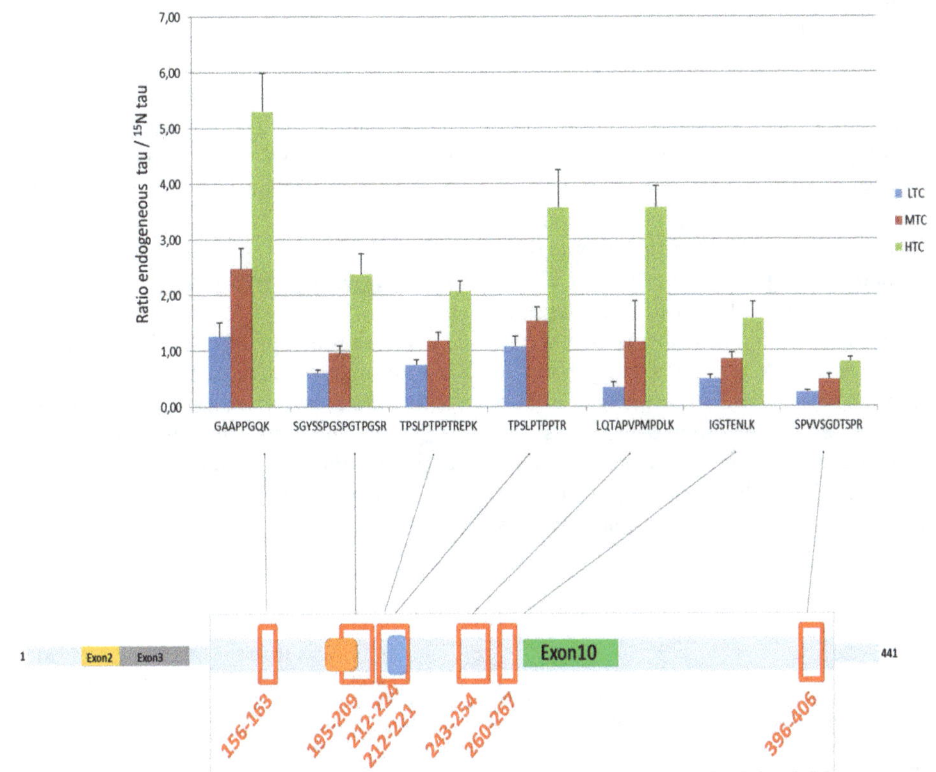

FIGURE 4 | Ratio endogenous tau/^{15}N tau in the three CSF pools (LTC, MTC, and HTC) for the 7 peptides. The scheme represents the localization of the 7 peptides on the tau protein.

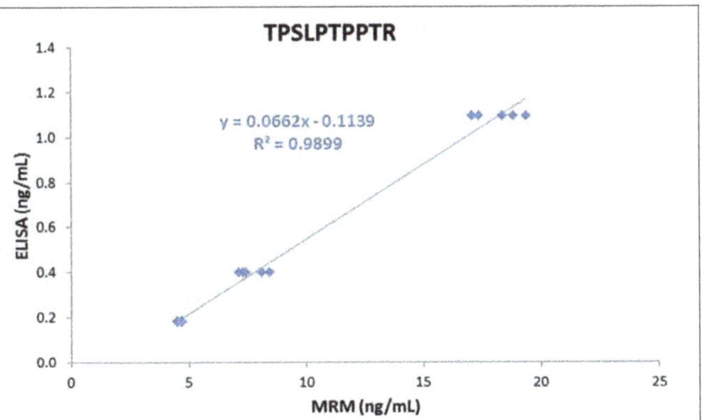

FIGURE 5 | Correlation between MRM and ELISA results.

the very large discrepancy between LC-MS/MS and ELISA results. In contrary, an argument in favor of ELISA is that there were important differences in the relative levels of the 7 measured tau peptides measured by LC-MS/MS, depending on their localization on the protein sequences; as illustrated in the **Figure 4**. This was observed with small variations in the different pools analyzed. This result can be explained by the strong structural heterogeneity of the tau protein. Indeed, it has many proteoforms (Smith and Kelleher, 2013): six isoforms (ranging from 352 to 441 amino acids), truncated forms and forms widely modified post-translationally by glycosylation, oxidation, and phosphorylation at more than 80 sites (Iqbal et al., 2010; Hanger et al., 2014). As phosphorylation and any other post-translational modification of tau peptides induce a mass shift that results in an underestimation of total tau concentration measured by LC-MS/MS, it could be suspected that LC-MS/MS results should have been even higher. This explains why total tau concentrations measured using different peptides were not in good agreement and suggests that total tau concentration can only be measured using peptides that are neither subject to any truncation nor post-translational modification. In this sense, the peptide GAAPPGQK appears to be the best candidate because it is short enough and it can't be phosphorylated. This hypothesis is supported by the fact that among the 7 considered peptides, total tau concentration was the highest when estimated with this peptide (see **Table 2**). Despite total tau concentrations estimated using all the 7 peptides are in insufficient agreement to support the use of peptides that can be phosphorylated, the results obtained with the 6 other peptides also show an excellent correlation between ELISA and LC-MS/MS, which suggest that they can have a clinical relevancy as independent biomarkers. However, to do the comparison with the 7 peptides, all phosphorylated forms should have been measured. The objective of measuring 7 peptides is not really to measure total tau concentration but rather to use the 7 peptides as independent biomarkers. As suggested in Höglund et al. (Höglund et al., 2015), having insights into tau structural characterization and providing the opportunity to simultaneously quantify several peptides whose concentration is directly proportional to that of given tau proteoforms will make it possible to discover potentially more predictive biomarkers of AD. A good example is P-Tau (181), that is known to be the most relevant and predictive proteoform of tau. This work thus illustrates the need but also the future perspectives associated with the quantification of a larger number of peptides. Especially, additional investigation using in particular MRM methods designed for phosphopeptides detection (e.g., prefractionation using titanium columns) will be needed to fully interpret our results and provide the analytical methods needed to determine which proteoforms of the tau protein are the most predictive of AD. Even if tau protein is considered as a major biomarker of AD, the protein is also increased when measured by ELISA in other tauopathies like Creutzfeldt–Jakob Disease or Fronto Temporal Dementia (Green et al., 1999; Wang et al., 2010). It will be interesting to use our new method to determine whether the multiplex quantification of the 7 tau peptides described in our study could help better differentiating pathologies with increased tau in the CSF. In any case, our MRM workflow realized without immunocapture in a clinical laboratory environment represents a major improvement to the state of the art and an interesting alternative and addition to classical ELISA. Further work on large clinical cohorts will be however needed to assess the clinical interest of this new approach.

Acknowledgments

This work was supported by the 2010 National PHRC "ProMara": Use of targeted quantitative proteomics and metabolic labeling with stable isotopes for the diagnosis and the investigation of neurological disorders and in particular Alzheimer Disease" and through the National French Alzheimer effort ("Plan Alzheimer"). The authors declare no potential conflicts of interest with respect to the authorship and/or publication of this article.

References

Andreasen, N., and Blennow, K. (2005). CSF biomarkers for mild cognitive impairment and early Alzheimer's disease. *Clin. Neurol. Neurosurg.* 107, 165–173. doi: 10.1016/j.clineuro.2004.10.011

Blennow, K., and Vanmechelen, E. (2003). CSF markers for pathogenic processes in Alzheimer's disease: diagnostic implications and use in clinical neurochemistry. *Brain Res. Bull.* 61, 235–242. doi: 10.1016/S0361-9230(03)00086-8

Drechsel, D. N., Hyman, A. A., Cobb, M. H., and Kirschner, M. W. (1992). Modulation of the dynamic instability of tubulin assembly by the microtubule-associated protein tau. *Mol. Biol. Cell* 3, 1141–1154. doi: 10.1091/mbc.3.10.1141

Gabelle, A., Roche, S., Geny, C., Bennys, K., Labauge, P., Tholance, Y., et al. (2010). Correlations between soluble alpha/beta forms of amyloid precursor protein and Abeta38, 40, and 42 in human cerebrospinal fluid. *Brain Res.* 1357, 175–183. doi: 10.1016/j.brainres.2010.08.022

Green, A. J., Harvey, R. J., Thompson, E. J., and Rossor, M. N. (1999). Increased tau in the cerebrospinal fluid of patients with frontotemporal dementia and Alzheimer's disease. *Neurosci. Lett.* 259, 133–135. doi: 10.1016/S0304-3940(98)00904-5

Hanger, D. P., Lau, D. H., Phillips, E. C., Bondulich, M. K., Guo, T., Woodward, B. W., et al. (2014). Intracellular and extracellular roles for tau in neurodegenerative disease. *J. Alzheimers. Dis.* 40(Suppl. 1), S37–S45. doi: 10.3233/JAD-132054

Hernandez, F., and Avila, J. (2007). Tauopathies. *Cell. Mol. Life Sci.* 64, 2219–2233. doi: 10.1007/s00018-007-7220-x

Höglund, K., Fourier, A., Perret-Liaudet, A., Zetterberg, H., Blennow, K., and Portelius, E. (2015). Alzheimer's disease - recent biomarker developments in relation to updated diagnostic criteria. *Clin. Chim. Acta.* doi: 10.1016/j.cca.2015.01.041. [Epub ahead of print].

Huillet, C., Adrait, A., Lebert, D., Picard, G., Trauchessec, M., Louwagie, M., et al. (2012). Accurate quantification of cardiovascular biomarkers in serum using Protein Standard Absolute Quantification (PSAQ) and selected reaction monitoring. *Mol. Cell. Proteomics* 11:M111.008235. doi: 10.1074/mcp.M111.008235

Iqbal, K., Liu, F., Gong, C. X., and Grundke-Iqbal, I. (2010). Tau in Alzheimer disease and related tauopathies. *Curr. Alzheimer Res.* 7, 656–664. doi: 10.2174/156720510793611592

James, O. G., Doraiswamy, P. M., and Borges-Neto, S. (2015). PET imaging of tau pathology in Alzheimer's disease and tauopathies. *Front. Neurol.* 6:38. doi: 10.3389/fneur.2015.00038

Lehmann, S., Hoofnagle, A., Hochstrasser, D., Brede, C., Glueckmann, M., Cocho, J. A., et al. (2013). Quantitative Clinical Chemistry Proteomics (qCCP) using mass spectrometry: general characteristics and application. *Clin. Chem. Lab. Med.* 51, 919–935. doi: 10.1515/cclm-2012-0723

McAvoy, T., Lassman, M. E., Spellman, D. S., Ke, Z., Howell, B. J., Wong, O., et al. (2014). Quantification of tau in cerebrospinal fluid by immunoaffinity enrichment and tandem mass spectrometry. *Clin. Chem.* 60, 683–689. doi: 10.1373/clinchem.2013.216515

Perrin, R. J., Fagan, A. M., and Holtzman, D. M. (2009). Multimodal techniques for diagnosis and prognosis of Alzheimer's disease. *Nature* 461, 916–922. doi: 10.1038/nature08538

Picard, G., Lebert, D., Louwagie, M., Adrait, A., Huillet, C., Vandenesch, F., et al. (2012). PSAQ standards for accurate MS-based quantification of proteins: from the concept to biomedical applications. *J. Mass Spectrom.* 47, 1353–1363. doi: 10.1002/jms.3106

Portelius, E., Hansson, S. F., Tran, A. J., Zetterberg, H., Grognet, P., Vanmechelen, E., et al. (2008). Characterization of tau in cerebrospinal fluid using mass spectrometry. *J. Proteome Res.* 7, 2114–2120. doi: 10.1021/pr7008669

Sergeant, N., Delacourte, A., and Buee, L. (2005). Tau protein as a differential biomarker of tauopathies. *Biochim. Biophys. Acta* 1739, 179–197. doi: 10.1016/j.bbadis.2004.06.020

Sjögren, M., Davidsson, P., Gottfries, J., Vanderstichele, H., Edman, A., Vanmechelen, E., et al. (2001). The cerebrospinal fluid levels of tau, growth-associated protein-43 and soluble amyloid precursor protein correlate in Alzheimer's disease, reflecting a common pathophysiological process. *Dement. Geriatr. Cogn. Disord.* 12, 257–264. doi: 10.1159/000051268

Smith, L. M., and Kelleher, N. L. (2013). Proteoform: a single term describing protein complexity. *Nat. Methods* 10, 186–187. doi: 10.1038/nmeth.2369

Wang, G. R., Gao, C., Shi, Q., Zhou, W., Chen, J. M., Dong, C. F., et al. (2010). Elevated levels of tau protein in cerebrospinal fluid of patients with probable Creutzfeldt-Jakob disease. *Am. J. Med. Sci.* 340, 291–295. doi: 10.1097/MAJ.0b013e3181e92a1f

20

Blood-based proteomic biomarkers of Alzheimer's disease pathology

Alison L. Baird, Sarah Westwood and Simon Lovestone*

Department of Psychiatry, University of Oxford, Oxford, UK

Edited by:
Charlotte Elisabeth Teunissen, VU University Medical Center Amsterdam, Netherlands

Reviewed by:
Jesus Avila, Centro de Biología Molecular Severo Ochoa, Spain
H. Bea Kuiperij, Radboud University Medical Center, Netherlands

***Correspondence:**
Alison L. Baird
alison.baird@psych.ox.ac.uk

The complexity of Alzheimer's disease (AD) and its long prodromal phase poses challenges for early diagnosis and yet allows for the possibility of the development of disease modifying treatments for secondary prevention. It is, therefore, of importance to develop biomarkers, in particular, in the preclinical or early phases that reflect the pathological characteristics of the disease and, moreover, could be of utility in triaging subjects for preventative therapeutic clinical trials. Much research has sought biomarkers for diagnostic purposes by comparing affected people to unaffected controls. However, given that AD pathology precedes disease onset, a pathology endophenotype design for biomarker discovery creates the opportunity for detection of much earlier markers of disease. Blood-based biomarkers potentially provide a minimally invasive option for this purpose and research in the field has adopted various "omics" approaches in order to achieve this. This review will, therefore, examine the current literature regarding blood-based proteomic biomarkers of AD and its associated pathology.

Keywords: Alzheimer's disease, biomarkers, blood, proteomics, dementia

INTRODUCTION

Dementia is now a huge public health priority, with 115.4 million people worldwide estimated to be living with dementia by 2050 (1). These numbers are not only alarming on an individual level, but they are also unsustainable for our economy. Dementia costs the global economy US$604 billion, and like prevalence rates this figure is also set to increase with an 85% rise in costs estimated by the year 2030 (2).

The most common form of dementia is Alzheimer's disease (AD), comprising approximately 50–70% of the elderly dementia population. AD is characterized by multiple cognitive deficits, which cause significant impairment to social or occupational functioning. The disease typically has a gradual onset followed by continuing cognitive decline, with a mean duration of approximately 8.5 years from the onset of clinical symptoms to the death of the patient (3).

Most clinical trials of potential therapeutic disease-modifying agents have involved individuals with clinically manifest dementia and have been relatively unsuccessful to date. Earlier stages of the disease are now being targeted, posing a challenge as it is difficult to detect individuals at this stage of AD; brain pathology is developing silently and cognitive symptoms if detectable are subtle. The underlying neuropathology characteristic of AD precedes symptom onset by many years, with the accumulation of amyloid-beta (Aβ) plaques believed to occur 15–20 years in advance of clinical manifestation of the disease (4), followed by the aggregation of abnormally phosphorylated tau in neurofibrillary tangles. A biological marker (biomarker) of these pathologic processes could serve as an indicator of disease presence, pathology, and progression. Moreover, they could have great utility

TABLE 1 | Search terms used for PubMed-based literature searches. Publications were filtered to include only studies in human species.

Search	Search terms
Plasma Aβ and Tau as biomarkers of AD	[alzheimer*(Title/Abstract) OR dementia(Title/Abstract) AND AD(Title/Abstract)] AND [blood(Title/Abstract) OR plasma(Title/Abstract) OR serum(Title/Abstract)] AND [proteomic*(Title/Abstract) OR proteome(Title/Abstract) OR protein(Title/Abstract) OR proteins(Title/Abstract)] AND [biomarker*(Title/Abstract) OR marker*(Title/Abstract)] AND [beta-amyloid(Title/Abstract) OR amyloid beta(Title/Abstract) OR abeta(Title/Abstract) OR tau(Title/Abstract)]
Plasma biomarkers of AD (case–control studies)	[alzheimer*(Title/Abstract) OR dementia(Title/Abstract) AND AD(Title/Abstract)] AND [blood(Title/Abstract) OR plasma(Title/Abstract) OR serum(Title/Abstract)] AND [proteomic*(Title/Abstract) OR proteome(Title/Abstract) OR protein(Title/Abstract) OR proteins(Title/Abstract)] AND [biomarker*(Title/Abstract) OR marker*(Title/Abstract)] AND [diagnos*(Title/Abstract) OR prognos*(Title/Abstract) OR progression(Title/Abstract)]
Plasma biomarkers of brain atrophy	[alzheimer*(Title/Abstract) OR dementia(Title/Abstract) AND AD(Title/Abstract)] AND [blood(Title/Abstract) OR plasma(Title/Abstract) OR serum(Title/Abstract)] AND [proteomic*(Title/Abstract) OR proteome(Title/Abstract) OR protein(Title/Abstract) OR proteins(Title/Abstract)] AND [biomarker*(Title/Abstract) OR marker*(Title/Abstract)] AND [atrophy(Title/Abstract) OR brain volume(Title/Abstract) OR sMRI(Title/Abstract) OR structural magnetic resonance imaging(Title/Abstract) OR structural MRI(Title/Abstract)]
Plasma biomarkers of cognitive decline	[alzheimer*(Title/Abstract) OR dementia(Title/Abstract) AND AD(Title/Abstract)] AND [blood(Title/Abstract) OR plasma(Title/Abstract) OR serum(Title/Abstract)] AND [proteomic*(Title/Abstract) OR proteome(Title/Abstract) OR protein(Title/Abstract) OR proteins(Title/Abstract)] AND [biomarker*(Title/Abstract) OR marker*(Title/Abstract)] AND [cognitive decline(Title/Abstract) OR cognition(Title/Abstract) OR MMSE(Title/Abstract) OR ADAS(Title/Abstract) OR CDR(Title/Abstract)]
Plasma biomarkers of PET amyloid	[alzheimer*(Title/Abstract) OR dementia(Title/Abstract) AND AD(Title/Abstract)] AND [blood(Title/Abstract) OR plasma(Title/Abstract) OR serum(Title/Abstract)] AND [proteomic*(Title/Abstract) OR proteome(Title/Abstract) OR protein(Title/Abstract) OR proteins(Title/Abstract)] AND [biomarker*(Title/Abstract) OR marker*(Title/Abstract)] AND [pib(Title/Abstract) OR Pittsburgh compound b(Title/Abstract) OR florbetapir(Title/Abstract) OR flutemetamol(Title/Abstract) OR florbetaben(Title/Abstract) OR amyloid PET(Title/Abstract) OR brain amyloid(Title/Abstract)]

in drug development and clinical trials, in particular for use in patient stratification and cohort enrichment.

In this review, we will discuss various studies that have utilized proteomic-based approaches to discover blood-based biomarkers for early and ideally preclinical detection of AD pathological processes and their use in clinical trials. We performed literature searches on PubMed[1] using the search terms detailed in **Table 1**. The literature included for review was supplemented with other known applicable papers that were not identified in the searches.

BIOMARKERS FOR AD

Today, the biomarkers used most extensively in clinical trials for dementia and to some extent in clinical practice are structural magnetic resonance imaging (MRI), molecular imaging of amyloid deposition using positron emission tomography (PET), imaging of metabolism using fluoro-deoxy-D-glucose (FDG)-PET, and cerebrospinal fluid (CSF) measures of Aβ and tau. However, structural changes measured using MRI are most likely relatively late events in the disease course and PET imaging is relatively expensive and limited in availability. Moreover, structural MRI and FDG-PET are not direct measures of the core pathological hallmarks of AD (Aβ and tau) and may, therefore, be relatively non-specific for AD in some cases (5) (**Figure 1**).

The most well-characterized and validated tissue fluid molecular-based biomarker for AD is the decrease in Aβ and increase in tau and phospho-tau (pTau) observed in the CSF of people with AD, with a number of studies documenting discrimination of AD patients from healthy controls with good sensitivity and specificity, as reviewed by others (6). However, the clinical utility of this biomarker is limited by the relatively invasive nature of obtaining CSF (lumbar puncture), particularly from elderly individuals. This may limit its use in longitudinal studies or for clinical progression monitoring, for which repeated CSF measures would be required. Also, attention needs to be paid to standardization of measurement of these biomarkers, given that large inter-laboratory variation in the concentrations measured of these biomarkers are observed (7).

In a revised model of the temporal relationship between key biomarkers of AD pathology, Jack et al. (8) suggested that changes in CSF $A\beta_{1-42}$ are the earliest detectable biomarker of AD pathology, followed by the PET detection of changes in brain amyloid, changes in CSF tau levels, and finally MRI-based detection of hippocampal atrophy and FDG-PET measures of brain glucose metabolism, all of which occur prior to the emergence of clinical symptoms of the disease (8). This hypothesis is corroborated by the recent findings of a non-linear association between CSF $A\beta_{1-42}$ and florbetapir F-18 PET imaging of brain amyloid load at the extreme ends of the clinical scale, while strongest association is seen at the mid-range of clinically measured disease severity (9). These findings would suggest that the two measures could reflect different aspects of AD Aβ pathology, with PET ligands having poor affinity for diffuse plaques, which develop early. At this stage, the plaques retain Aβ and, hence, CSF measures of Aβ may be more sensitive than PET earlier on in the disease (9). It is, therefore, of importance to consider the sensitivity of these biomarkers in relation to the staging of disease when designing biomarker studies.

BLOOD-BASED BIOMARKERS

The minimally invasive and potentially inexpensive nature of tests using blood-based proteomic biomarkers make these approaches

[1] http://www.ncbi.nlm.nih.gov/pubmed

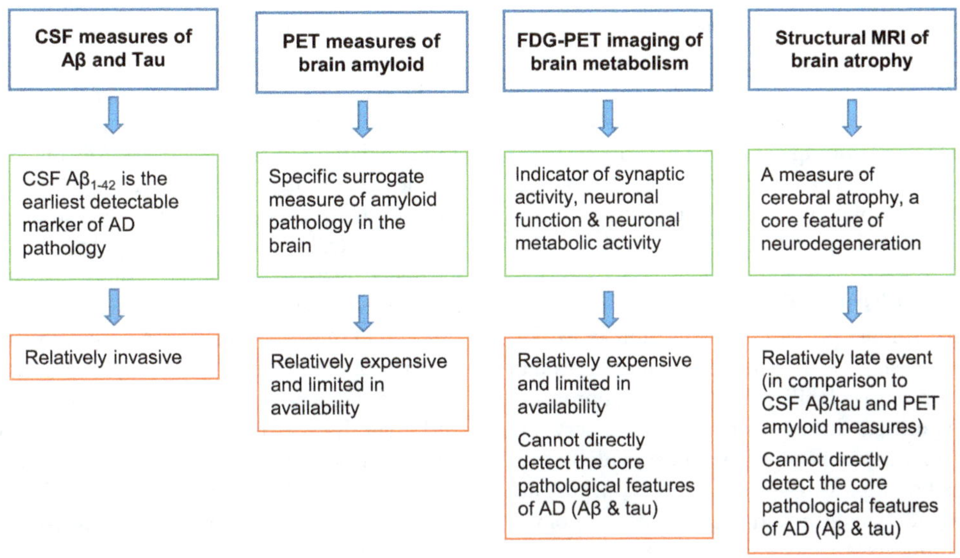

FIGURE 1 | Advantages (green boxes) and disadvantages (red boxes) of the biomarkers that are currently most widely used in clinical trials.

practical to implement, allowing for repeated sampling in large cohorts, and, therefore, might have significant advantages over other biomarker modalities. However, the use of blood as a matrix for measurement of biomarkers has the inherent disadvantage of its complex composition and subsequently poses technical difficulties for biomarker detection.

The most challenging of many obstacles to developing blood-based biomarkers is the massive dynamic range of proteins in blood, spanning up to 12 orders of magnitude (10). Furthermore, changes within the blood are often very small and reflect a wide range of both peripheral and central processes and, therefore, pinpointing AD-specific changes can be challenging. Separated by the blood–brain barrier the relationship between analytes found in the blood and changes in the brain is still uncertain. However, with aging and in AD, the blood–brain barrier is disrupted resulting in increased permeability, and this is thought to be a relatively early event in the aging brain, worsening with increased cognitive impairment (11). Blood–brain barrier disruption should only strengthen the relationship between blood and brain, and as an early event this would support the possibility of detecting protein-based markers related to AD at the early stages of disease. Nevertheless, concentrations of most known potential biomarkers are considerably lower in the blood than reported in CSF. For example, Aβ peptide concentration is 100-fold lower in blood than in CSF (12). Additionally, highly abundant plasma proteins such as albumin and IgG may mask the presence of less abundant proteins that may serve as potential biomarkers.

TECHNIQUES FOR BLOOD-BASED BIOMARKER DISCOVERY

The complexity of blood as a source of biomarkers is reflected in the limitations of various proteomic techniques that have been employed to investigate blood-based biomarkers for AD. In the following section, we will provide a brief overview of some of the tools available for proteomic biomarker discovery in blood, including mass spectrometry (MS), immunocapture, and aptamer-based techniques. Each of these approaches has their advantages and disadvantages and to date studies have combined a number of these approaches in the discovery pipeline for identifying protein biomarkers related to AD.

Mass Spectrometry-Based Assays

For discovery-level proteomics, a key attribute required of the technique used is the ability to measure multiple targets simultaneously in a multiplexing manner. MS-based approaches have been widely used in this way and possess the inherent advantage of there being no requirement for prior knowledge of the proteins being identified, hence, allowing for unbiased hypothesis-free biomarker discovery. Moreover, to facilitate multiplexing capabilities of MS-based protein quantification, approaches for labeling peptides or intact proteins have been developed, for example, the use of isobaric tags (13). This allows for the pooling of labeled samples for subsequent MS analysis, hence, increasing throughput. However, disadvantages of labeling may include increased complexity in sample preparation compared to label-free approaches. Furthermore, quantitative information can only be provided for peptides that contain the labeled amino acid, limiting the quantitative coverage of the sample to the labeled peptides alone.

However, the huge abundance of a select few proteins in plasma and serum limits the detection of lower molecular weight proteins by MS. In plasma and serum, albumin and the immunoglubulins (IgG, IgA, IgM, and IgD) represent 75% of the total protein weight, and 99% of these samples are constituted by only 22 different protein species (14). Fractionation of the sample is one of the approaches that can be taken to reduce this sample complexity (15). Immunoaffinity-based depletion of the most abundant proteins is another approach that can be used to improve the detection of lower molecular weight proteins and the use of several different immunoaffinity depletion reagents have been documented (16–18). However, a disadvantage of depletion is the potential removal of lower molecular weight proteins, in addition to the high molecular weight targets for depletion. This is mainly an issue due to the binding nature of the protein targets for depletion, such as albumin, and, therefore, by removal of albumin, inadvertently albumin-bound lower molecular weight proteins may also be removed.

Immunocapture-Based Assays

The gold standard for soluble protein quantification is ELISA. However, with the increasing need to measure multiple protein targets, with limited sample availability, multiplexing approaches for targeted and hypothesis-driven biomarker discovery are now increasingly being used. Two of the most widely used immunocapture-based multiplexing systems for this purpose are mesoscale discovery (MSD) and the Luminex xMAP technology.

Both MSD and Luminex xMAP technologies are similar to the "sandwich" ELISA in priniciple. However, in an MSD assay, the capture antibodies are coated on specific spot regions at the base of the wells of a microtiter plate. Capture antibodies for different targets can be coated on each of the different spots, thus, allowing for multiple protein targets to be captured simultaneously in a single sample. Electrochemiluminescence (SULFO-TAG) labels are then bound to the detection antibodies and upon electrical stimulation the SULFO-TAG labels emit light, which is used to quantify the amount of target protein present. Luminex xMAP assays, in contrast, use microsphere-based technology, which involves coating of the capture antibody to microspheres "beads" in suspension, and fluorescently labeled detection antibodies for detection and quantification. In this way, multiple beads may be coated with multiple capture antibodies for multiplexing protein measurements in a single sample. Whichever approach to multiplexed affinity capture is used, the method is dependent on the quality, binding characteristics, and batch stability of the primary (and indeed secondary) antibodies used.

Given the targeted nature of immunocapture-based assays, these approaches are not necessarily suitable for unbiased hypothesis-free approaches for biomarker discovery. Furthermore, protein quantification by immunocapture methods will be epitope specific, and the quantitative values obtained will relate to the region of the protein recognized by the antibodies used within the assay. This is an important property to note when using immunocapture-based methods for replication of findings that may have been discovered on a different methodological platform, such as MS. Where failure to technically replicate data between platforms is observed, it could be due to differences in the region of the protein being recognized by the different assays. Platform and assay differences in protein quantification are, therefore, important points to consider when designing the pipeline for biomarker discovery and development.

Aptamer-Based Assays

Aptamer-based approaches also provide another approach for relative quantification of multiple proteins in a multiplexing manner. Aptamers are single-stranded oligonucleotides, which recognize and bind target proteins with high affinity and specificity. Using this technology, the protein signal is effectively transformed to a nucleotide signal for subsequent microarray-based quantification of the relative fluorescence levels. An example of this approach is the panel that Somalogic has developed, which measures over 1300 analytes in a single sample[2]. Advantages of this technology are clearly the large and unrivaled number of protein targets that can be quantified simultaneously in a single sample, making this platform ideal for extensive proteomic analysis in samples of limited availability. However, proteins quantified in this way are limited to those for which aptamers have been designed just as immunoaffinity approaches are limited by antibody availability.

Each of the proteomic techniques described here have inherent advantages and disadvantages for both hypothesis-generating and hypothesis-driven biomarker discovery. Furthermore, as described earlier, platform and assay differences may impact upon the ability to technically replicate findings at the discovery level, and should, therefore, be considered carefully when designing biomarker studies.

BLOOD-BASED MEASURES OF Aβ AND TAU

In the CSF, $A\beta_{42}$ (along with tau and pTau) shows good sensitivity and specificity for classifying AD patients from healthy controls (19). Given the success in developing CSF markers of Aβ and tau as biomarkers it is unsurprising, therefore, that parallel approaches have been attempted in blood.

Amyloid Beta

Amyloid-beta fragments are produced by β and γ-secretase metabolism of the protein APP. β-secretase cleavage of APP produces sAPPβ and a 99 amino acid membrane bound fragment, which upon subsequent γ-secretase cleavage produces various Aβ species (20). Of these Aβ species, $A\beta_{40}$ is the most abundant, while the highly hydrophobic and insoluble $A\beta_{42}$ is the principal component of amyloid plaques in the AD brain (21), although deposition of insoluble $A\beta_{40}$ in plaques of the AD brain has also been observed (22).

To date, $A\beta_{42}$ and $A\beta_{40}$ are the predominant species that have been investigated in blood, however, as reviewed extensively by others (23, 24), the results of these studies have been somewhat contradictory. To illustrate this, a reduction in plasma levels of $A\beta_{42}$ in mild cognitive impairment (MCI) and AD subjects compared to healthy controls has been shown (25), while no difference between AD and cognitively healthy controls in serum $A\beta_{42}$ has also been reported by others (26).

In terms of disease progression, the results are equally contradictory. An association of decreased plasma $A\beta_{42}$ with more rapid cognitive decline in AD (27), progression from healthy to MCI (28), and conversion from MCI to AD (29) has been shown. Yet an opposite trend has also been reported, including increased $A\beta_{42}$ with conversion from cognitively healthy to MCI (30) and elevated baseline plasma $A\beta_{42}$ in participants who converted to

[2]www.somalogic.com

AD versus participants who remained cognitively healthy over a 5-year period (31). Moreover, Mayeux et al. showed that the increase in plasma $A\beta_{42}$ was followed by a decrease in individuals with the onset of AD (31), a pattern that has been mirrored in healthy elderly participants, who demonstrated higher baseline plasma $A\beta_{42}$ followed by greater reductions in plasma $A\beta_{42}$ with cognitive decline (32).

The results of blood $A\beta_{40}$ as an AD biomarker have also been conflicting and are perhaps not as promising as that of $A\beta_{42}$. For example, both increased serum $A\beta_{40}$ (26, 33) and decreased plasma $A\beta_{40}$ (34) have been shown in AD versus healthy controls. Reduced levels of plasma $A\beta_{40}$ have also been associated with more rapid cognitive decline in AD (27), while no change in plasma $A\beta_{40}$ between cognitively stable MCI and MCI to AD converters (29) or association with risk of developing dementia (35) have been observed.

Given the differing results of plasma $A\beta_{42}$ and $A\beta_{40}$ in relation to AD, it is not surprising that studies examining the potential of $A\beta_{42}/A\beta_{40}$ in blood as an AD marker have also been conflicting in their results. A number of studies have documented reduced plasma $A\beta_{42}/A\beta_{40}$ in association with AD-related parameters, including in MCI and AD subjects compared to healthy controls (25, 28), with progression from MCI to AD compared to cognitively stable MCI (29) and with risk of developing MCI and AD (36). However, increased plasma $A\beta_{42}/A\beta_{40}$ has also been related to increased risk of developing AD (37).

Very recently, however, a much larger, prospective, community-based study examined the levels of plasma $A\beta_{42}$ and $A\beta_{40}$ in over 2000 dementia-free individuals, and followed these individuals for dementia/AD over an 8-year period (35). In this study, Chouraki et al., found that lower levels of plasma $A\beta_{42}$ were associated with an increased risk of developing dementia, which given the size of the study may be one of the most promising plasma Aβ results to date.

The conflicting findings of different Aβ studies may perhaps suggest that the utility of plasma Aβ as a marker is quite disease-stage specific, as postulated by Blasko et al. Their findings of a relationship of plasma Aβ with conversion from cognitively healthy to MCI, but not later in the disease course when participants convert from MCI to AD, would indicate that plasma Aβ may be more successful as a marker of pathology at the preclinical stages of disease. This theory would also be in line with why plasma $A\beta_{42}$ appears to perform as a marker of risk for developing dementia over an 8-year period, as documented by Chouraki et al.

Relationship Between Plasma and CSF Aβ

Given that CSF Aβ is normally cleared in blood (38), it could be hypothesized that a reduction in plasma $A\beta_{42}$ would be observed following the decrease observed in CSF $A\beta_{42}$ in late-onset AD (39). However, a number of studies have actually reported that CSF and plasma levels of $A\beta_{42}$ and $A\beta_{40}$ do not correlate well (40–42). There are several theories that could be proposed to explain this. First, the relationship between CSF and plasma levels of Aβ may only exist at specific stages of the disease, relating to the degree of aggregation of brain amyloid in plaques. Second, it is thought that plasma Aβ may have a causal role in the development of microvascular dysfunction (43) and given the considerable incidence of cerebrovascular pathology in the AD brain (44), it has been proposed that this heterogeneity in pathology could also impact upon the levels of Aβ measured in blood.

Plasma Aβ and Neuropathology

The relationship between plasma Aβ and brain pathology is also not yet resolved. Levels of $A\beta_{40}$ and $A\beta_{42}$ 1 year prior to post-mortem brain tissue collection were not associated with frontal and temporal necortex $A\beta_{40}$ and $A\beta_{42}$ burden at post mortem (45). However, using PET measures of brain amyloid burden does suggest a relationship between plasma Aβ and brain amyloid load, with an association between reduced plasma $A\beta_{42}/A\beta_{40}$ and increased brain amyloid load being shown (28, 46, 47). Moreover, the ratio of the plasma proteins APP669-711 (cleavage product of the amyloid precursor protein) and $A\beta_{42}$ was increased in individuals of high amyloid burden subjects and demonstrated good sensitivity and specificity (93 and 96% respectively) for discrimination of amyloid negative and positive subjects (48).

These findings indicate a potential relationship between plasma Aβ species and the neuropathology of AD, however, given the contradictory results of plasma Aβ as a marker of AD diagnosis and clinical progression, it is clear that further work is required in order to consolidate the findings. As mentioned earlier, potential theories for the variability in the blood Aβ study results have been suggested and include disease-heterogeneity effects upon Aβ levels, and a disease-stage-specific nature of Aβ as a marker, with perhaps Aβ acting as an effective marker of preclinical rather than established disease. While these are valid theories that likely are having an impact, they are not able to explain the full extent of variability between the different Aβ study findings.

Important additional issues that likely contribute to the variability observed between studies are the technical challenges encountered with measuring Aβ. First, Abdullah et al. reported high intra-subject differences in plasma Aβ measures, as assessed by ELISA in two to three separate blood samples retrieved within a 4-week period from each individual (26). This variation in part may be related to the performance of the Aβ assays, with perhaps variation in the measurements being introduced due to lack of sensitivity of these assays. However, it is worth noting that plasma Aβ exhibits a circadian rhythm in its levels (49) and, therefore, in order to use Aβ as a reliable marker, standardization in time of sampling will be required.

Second, it should be noted that many of the studies documented here have assessed plasma Aβ by immunocapture-based approaches, including commercially available and in-house optimized ELISAs (25–27, 29–31, 33, 36, 37, 42, 45, 46), luminex xMAP assays (25, 28, 35, 41, 42), and immunomagnetic reduction (IMR) assays (47). While ELISAs are the gold standard for protein quantification, it is possible that inter-study variation in the results could be introduced by the use of different assays, which use antibodies that recognize different epitopes of Aβ. In this situation, standardization in the assay used across studies so that blood Aβ measures were epitope specific would be advisable.

Another factor to be considered is the technical difficulties of measuring Aβ, which is present at low concentrations in blood and will readily bind other circulating proteins, such as albumin, lipoproteins, and complement factors (50). One way to help overcome this issue might, therefore, be to develop an assay that can measure both free and cell/protein-bound Aβ. This is an approach that has been used to develop the AB test, which quantifies $A\beta_{40}$ and $A\beta_{42}$ peptides that are free in plasma and bound to other proteins in plasma and blood cells[3]. The AB test shows promise for measuring Aβ in an AD-based cohort (51). Chiu and colleagues also report quantification of plasma Aβ by another highly sensitive immunoassay, developed using a technology known as superconducting quantum interference device (SQUID) IMR assay. This technology is based on measuring the magnetic signals produced from nanoparticles, bound to the target molecule of interest and is able to detect plasma Aβ levels as low as 1 pg/ml for $A\beta_{40}$ and 10 pg/ml for $A\beta_{42}$. This is lower than that of standard $A\beta_{42}$ ELISAs, of which the lower limit of detection is generally around 50 pg/ml (52). Furthermore, the SQUID-IMR technology involves the use of iron-nanoparticles and it has been suggested that the iron-chelating effect may inhibit Aβ oligomerization, hence, reducing the issue of non-quantifiable Aβ oligomers (52). While the results of these new assays for Aβ are promising, validation of these assays in further larger and independent cohort studies is required.

Tau

To date the investigation of plasma tau-based measures and their utility as biomarkers for AD have also been limited, primarily due to tau being an axonal protein and, therefore, of low abundance in blood. Efforts have, therefore, been made to develop more sensitive assays for detection and reliable quantification.

First, Henriksen et al. have reported measurement of specific tau fragments using an ELISA method. These assays quantified specific tau fragments in serum [ADAM10-generated fragment (Tau-A) and caspase-3-generated fragment (Tau-C)] (53, 54). Using this method, measures of serum Tau-A, Tau-C, and the Tau-A/Tau-C ratio were shown to be associated with cognitive change in AD, although no association of the serum tau fragments with CSF tau and pTau were observed (54). A second approach that has been reported for measuring tau utilizes a digital array-based technology (55). This approach involves the isolation and detection of single enzyme molecules using femtolitre-sized reaction chambers, known as single-molecule arrays (SiMOA). This method facilitates the detection of the target at low concentrations by ensuring that the fluorophores are confined to small volumes and, hence, the concentration of fluorescently labeled target is high (56). Using this assay, elevated levels of plasma tau in AD in comparison to controls and MCI were shown, although a considerable overlap in the range of plasma tau across the diagnostic groups was also found (55). Moreover, no correlation between plasma and CSF tau levels were observed (55). Lastly, Chiu and colleagues reported quantification of plasma Tau by SQUID-IMR (as described earlier for detection of plasma Aβ) and showed an increase in plasma tau in MCI and AD, along with an association of plasma tau with clinical measures of cognition and regional brain volume (57). This is all early but promising work, and moving forward, as with blood Aβ measures, further replication of these findings in larger independent cohorts will be crucial for ascertaining the robustness of blood-based tau as an AD-related biomarker.

[3] www.araclon.com

DISCOVERY OF BLOOD-BASED BIOMARKERS OF AD USING A CASE–CONTROL STUDY DESIGN

Since the blood–brain barrier damage that occurs in AD would facilitate movement of proteins between brain and blood (58), research has also focused upon the detection of other blood-based proteins, in addition to Aβ and tau, which may serve as markers for AD. Using both untargeted and candidate-based proteomic approaches and a case–control study design, a substantial number of proteins related to a diagnosis of AD or MCI have been identified (33, 59–95).

However, a panel of proteins rather than single protein candidates may have greater sensitivity and specificity as a biomarker and may collectively better describe and characterize the disease and its pathology. A number of studies, including from our group, have, therefore, taken an approach of analyzing multivariate signatures for prediction of AD and/or MCI status, and have identified and evaluated different proteins that collectively demonstrate sensitivity and specificity for classifying AD and/or MCI to varying degrees (96–118).

Alzheimer's disease biomarker studies premised upon a case–control study design have been extensively reviewed by others (119, 120) and as would be expected, many of the candidates identified in these studies can be related to aspects of the disease pathology, for example, having roles in inflammatory and amyloidogenic processes.

These studies comparing established disease to non-disease or prediction of rate of progression in established disease are promising but of more value would be marker sets that detected preclinical or prodromal disease. One design enabling such discovery is the prediction of conversion from MCI by using historical samples from research cohort participants with MCI comparing those who subsequently converted to dementia in a given time-frame to those who did not. One of the first such studies identified an 18 plasma protein signature that not only classified AD from control subjects with 90% accuracy but was also able to predict MCI patients who would convert to AD within 5 years (97). However, replication of the 18 protein biomarker panel in subsequent studies has so far been unsuccessful (103, 121, 122). Yang et al. also demonstrated prediction of MCI conversion to AD with 79% accuracy using a 60 protein biomarker set (123), while we identified a panel of 10 proteins that were shown to strongly associate with both the degree of disease severity and to predict MCI progression to AD with 87% accuracy (124). More recently, Apostolova et al. reported prediction of MCI progression to AD with 73% accuracy by plasma IL-6R combined with clinical measures and *APOE* genotype (125).

Although a number of plasma protein signatures of AD diagnosis, disease severity, and progression have been identified in discovery-based studies, a key concern for the field has been the lack of reproducibility of these results. As yet there has been no single blood-based proteomic signature that can successfully distinguish between AD and MCI and cognitively healthy elderly in a reproducible manner. The reason for such non-reproducibility is unknown. It might be the inherent heterogeneity of the disease and the differences, therefore, between cohort studies. It might also be technical variability, including assay variation and sample collection and curation variation, or it might be that the findings are in fact artifactual and there is no consistent proteomic signature to be found in blood. However, another reason for the failure to replicate might be the intrinsic limitation of case–control studies in a condition with such a long prodrome.

First, it is important to consider the heterogeneity of dementia and the extensive comorbidity and differential environmental exposure in the elderly. As well as multiple dementia conditions being hard to distinguish from each other, the AD group itself can be clinically heterogeneous as can MCI. Moreover, comorbid conditions are common in AD, and might not only alter the blood proteome directly but the associated polypharmacy prevalent in the elderly could also have an impact.

Second, case–control-based studies have inherent limitations when the target of discovery is in prodromal, or, worse, preclinical disease. In the context of AD research, the goal of biomarker discovery is primarily to detect individuals harboring early pathological change but without manifest dementia, as these individuals might be the most likely to respond to disease modifying agents. And yet in case–control studies such individuals will be included in studies not in the "case" group but in the "control" group. Clearly, this study design is at best non-optimal and at worse, destined for failure.

The recent failure of phase III clinical trials of antibody therapies targeting amyloid pathology, in part probably due to the absence of brain amyloid pathology in a considerable proportion of the participants (126, 127), highlights the important role biomarkers predictive of core AD neuropathology could play in recruitment to clinical trials. However, the inevitable screen failures using such approaches would be costly and increase the time to recruitment. Therefore, the development of a minimally invasive blood-based biomarker of AD pathology could have real utility as a first pass or triage marker, to identify potential participants more likely to harbor pathology and to reduce screen failure and, hence, facilitate trials conduct.

DISCOVERY OF BLOOD-BASED BIOMARKERS OF AD PATHOLOGY USING AN ENDOPHENOTYPE APPROACH

Endophenotype-based approaches for blood-based biomarker discovery have begun to be implemented and have utilized various AD-related measures to identify blood-based biomarkers reflective of disease activity and pathology, including at the preclinical stages. These studies have included endophenotypes defined by measures such as brain atrophy (structural MRI), rate of cognitive decline, and brain amyloid β burden (Pittsburgh B (PiB) PET brain imaging), with change in PiB PET amyloid burden being the earliest event of these in the disease course. These studies have identified a number of different potential proteomic biomarkers (**Tables 2** and **3**).

Blood-Based Biomarkers of Brain Atrophy and Rate of Cognitive Decline

We began by focusing on endophenotype approaches using mostly the AddNeuroMed, a European multicentre study (143) and the neuroimaging substudy of the Baltimore Longitudinal Study for Aging (BLSA) (144). Two key pathology endophenotypes were employed; structural neuroimaging of atrophy as a proxy measure of *in vivo* pathology and rate of clinical progression (**Table 2**), which was calculated based on retrospective and prospective measures of cognitive decline.

In 2010, we published a study that utilized a 2DGE-MS/MS-based approach to discover plasma protein markers of both of these outcome variables in AD (128). This work identified seven proteins (complement C3, γ-fibrinogen, serum albumin, complement factor-I, clusterin, α-1-microglobulin, and serum amyloid-P) that were able to explain 34% of the variance in hippocampal volume in MCI and AD, and five proteins (complement component C4a, complement C8, clusterin, ApoA1, and transthyretin) that were able to discriminate fast from slow progressing AD groups. These proteins were then selected for replication studies, including in an independent AD/MCI/control-based cohort, using an orthogonal immunoassay-based approach. In this study, we replicated the association of complement C3, complement factor-I, γ-fibrinogen and α-1-microglobulin with brain atrophy, and along with complement C3a, these five proteins were able to explain 35% of whole brain volume in AD (129). In a separate study, we also replicated the association of transthyretin with an increased rate of cognitive decline in AD (136).

However, the most promising candidate marker identified in this discovery study was the protein clusterin, which associated with both hippocampal atrophy and clinical progression (128). We also showed in this same study but in an independent (AD/MCI/control) cohort, an association of clusterin with cognitive measures and with brain atrophy, specifically in the entorhinal cortex and with PiB PET measures of fibrillary amyloid burden in the entorhinal cortex of a non-demented elderly cohort (128). While very recently increased plasma clusterin levels have been associated with increased risk of conversion to AD and rate of cognitive decline in an independent study (145). These findings indicate that changes in plasma clusterin may be an early event in the disease course, which occurs with amyloid deposition but prior (or without) onset of clinical symptoms. Moreover, in this same study, we demonstrated colocalization of clusterin with Aβ in plaques in the brains of a transgenic mouse model of AD (TASTPM) (128), thus, adding further support to the theory that clusterin may be implicated in amyloid formation and clearance (146).

Adding weight to our hypothesis that changes in plasma clusterin were an early event, increased levels of plasma clusterin in association with slower rates of brain atrophy in MCI were demonstrated (131). However, to the contrary, Song et al. demonstrated an association of increased plasma clusterin with reduced white matter volume in MCI/cognitively healthy elderly over a 2-year period (130). These findings are somewhat contradictory, and could be explained in part by the evidence for clusterin having both neuroprotective and pro-amyloidegenic properties,

TABLE 2 | Summary of the significant findings of studies examining plasma protein markers of brain atrophy and rate of cognitive decline.

Proteins	Outcome variables (subjects)	Analytical platform	Study
Endophenotype: structural MRI measures of brain atrophy			
C3, FGG, albumin, CFI, clusterin, A1M and SAP	Hippocampal atrophy (AD and MCI)	2DGE LC-MS/MS	(128)
C3, C3a, CFI, FGG, and A1M	Whole brain volume (AD)	ELISA and western blots	(129)
ApoB/ApoA1[a], ApoC3[b], ApoE[b], and Clusterin[b,c]	Hippocampal volume[a], gray matter volume[b], and white matter volume[c] (MCI and non-demented elderly)	Luminex xMAP (Myriad RBM)	(130)
Clusterin	Rate of brain atrophy (multiple brain regions in MCI)	ELISA	(131)
IL-1ra[d] IL-6[d], IL-10[d], IL-13[e], and TNF-α[f]	Ventricular volume[d], entorhinal cortex volume[e], and whole brain volume[f] (AD)	Luminex xMAP	(132)
MIP1α, IGFBP2, CgA, and cortisol	SPARE-AD measures of brain atrophy (AD, MCI, and non-demented elderly)	Luminex xMAP (Myriad RBM)	(133)
RANTES[g], NSE[g,h], TTR[g,h], clusterin[g], A1AT[h], ApoC3[h], ApoA1[h], ApoE[h], BDNF[h] and $A\beta_{40}$[h]	Atrophy in multiple brain regions (MCI[g] and AD[h])	Luminex xMAP	(124)
PPY, fetuin B, PSA-ACT, and ChkT	Entorhinal cortex and hippocampal volume (AD, MCI, and non-demented elderly)	SOMAscan	(134)
ApoE	Hippocampal volume (MCI, non demented elderly)	Luminex xMAP (Myriad RBM)	(135)
Endophenotype: rate of cognitive decline			
C4a, C8, clusterin, ApoA1, and TTR	Rate of cognitive decline (AD)	2DGE LC-MS/MS	(128)
ApoA1, ApoA2, ApoH, and ApoB/ApoA1 ratio	Risk of cognitive decline (non-demented elderly)	Luminex xMAP (Myriad RBM	(130)
TTR	Rate of cognitive decline (AD)	ELISA	(136)
IL-4, IL-10, G-CSF, IL-2, IFN-γ, and PDGF	Rate of cognitive decline (AD)	Luminex xMAP	(132)
NCAM, sRAGE, and ICAM	Rate of cognitive decline (AD)	Luminex xMAP	(124)
Clusterin and NAP2	Rate of cognitive decline (AD)	SOMAscan	(134)

C3, complement C3; FGG, γ-fibrinogen; CF1, complement factor-I; A1M, α-1-microglobulin; SAP, serum amyloid-P; C3a, complement C3a; ApoB, apolipoprotein B; ApoA1, apolipoprotein A1; ApoC3, apolipoprotein C3; ApoE, apolipoprotein E; ApoC4, apolipoprotein C4; IL-1ra, interleukin 1 receptor antagonist; IL-6, interleukin-6; IL-10, interleukin-10; IL-13, interleukin-13; TNF-α, tumor necrosis factor alpha; MIP1α, macrophage inhibitory protein 1α; IGFBP2, insulin-like growth factor binding protein 2; CgA, chromogranin A; RANTES, regulated on activation normal T cell expressed and secreted; NSE, neuron-specific enolase; TTR, transthyretin; A1AT, alpha 1 antitrypsin; BDNF, brain derived neurotrophic factor; $A\beta_{40}$, amyloid beta 1-40; PPY, pancreatic polypeptide; PSA-ACT, prostate-specific antigen complexed to α1-antichymotrypsin; Chk2, serine/threonine-protein kinase Chk2; C4a, complement component C4a; C8, complement C8; ApoA2, apolipoprotein A-2; ApoH, apolipoprotein-H; IL-4, interleukin-4; G-CSF, granulocyte-colony-stimulating factor; IL-2, interleukin-2; IFN-γ, interferon-gamma; PDGF, platelet-derived growth factor; NCAM, neural cell adhesion molecule; sRAGE, soluble receptor for advanced glycation end products; ICAM, intercellular adhesion molecule; NAP2, nucleosome assembly protein 2.

TABLE 3 | Summary of the significant findings of studies examining plasma protein markers of PET amyloid.

Protein(s)	Outcome variable (subjects)	Analytical platform	Study
Clusterin	PiB PET amyloid (non-demented elderly)	ELISA	(128)
ApoE, C3, albumin, plasminogen, haptoglobin and IgG C chain region	PiB PET amyloid (non-demented elderly)	2DGE LC-MS/MS	(137)
C-peptide, fibrinogen, A1AT, PPY, C3, vitronectin, cortisol, AXL receptor kinase, IL-3, IL-13, MMP9, ApoE, and IgE (this panel of proteins combined with covariates predicts amyloid positive subjects with 92 and 55% sensitivity and specificity, respectively)	PiB PET amyloid (AD, MCI, and non-demented elderly)	Luminex xMAP (Myriad RBM)	(138)
Aβ1–42, CXCL-13, IL-17, IgM-1, PPY, and VCAM-1 (this panel of proteins with age, *APOE* genotype, and CDR sum of boxes predicts NAB with 79 and 76% sensitivity and specificity, respectively)	PiB PET amyloid (AD, MCI, and non-demented elderly)	Luminex xMAP (Myriad RBM)	(139)
A2M, CFHR1, and FGG. (FGG in combination with age predicts NAB with 59 and 78% sensitivity and specificity, respectively)	PiB PET amyloid (AD, MCI, and non-demented elderly)	TMT LC-MS/MS	(140)
IL-6R, ApoE, and clusterin (in combination with clinical measures: trails B, AVLT, MMSE, education, *APOE* genotype and mean hippocampal volume predicts NAB with 79 and 83% sensitivity and specificity)	CSF Aβ and PiB PET amyloid (MCI)	Luminex xMAP (Myriad RBM)	(125)
BDNF	PiB PET amyloid (AD, MCI and non-demented elderly)	Luminex xMAP (Myriad RBM)	(141)
PPY and IgM*	PiB PET amyloid (AD, MCI, and non-demented elderly, *non-demented elderly only)	SOMAscan	(142)

ApoE, apolipoprotein E; C3, complement C3; A1AT, alpha 1 antitrypsin; PPY, pancreatic polypeptide; IL-3, interleukin-3; IL-13, interleukin-13; MMP9, matrix metalloproteinase-9 total; ApoE, apolipoprotein E; IgE, immunoglobulin E; CKCL-13, chemokine ligand 13; IL-17, interleukin-17; IgM-1, immunoglobulin M; VCAM-1, vascular cell adhesion protein; A2M, alpha 2 macroglobulin; CFHR1, CFH-related protein 1; FGG, fibrinogen gamma chain; NAB, neocortical amyloid burden.
**non demented elderly only.*

dependent on its concentration relative to Aβ. Clusterin is implicated in Aβ aggregation and clearance (146–151) and at high concentrations, clusterin binds Aβ, thus, preventing its aggregation. Yet when Aβ levels are high, clusterin instead is incorporated with amyloid in insoluble aggregates (148). Furthermore, clusterin possesses neurotoxic properties, as demonstrated by its involvement in non-canonical wnt signaling (the wnt–PCP–JNK pathway), which mediates Aβ toxicity (152). It could, therefore, be postulated that clusterin is playing different roles in these studies that demonstrate opposing relationships of plasma clusterin with brain atrophy. Nonetheless, these studies add further evidence for the role of clusterin in AD pathology. It is also worth noting that evidence for clusterin being implicated in AD pathology has also been provided on the genetic level, with an association of the variant rs11136000 in the clusterin gene with AD risk (153, 154), increased rates of cognitive decline at the pre-symptomatic stages of the disease (155) and brain volume and structure (volumetric expansion and lateral ventricle surface morphology) in AD, MCI, and elderly control subjects (156).

To date, clusterin is likely to be the most promising potential biomarker of AD-related phenotypes that we have identified in our studies, as supported by an association on the proteomic level with both clinical and neuroimaging measures of AD pathology, on the genetic level with AD risk and on a mechanistic level with amyloid function and processing.

Following the identification of clusterin using a dual endophenotype-based approach founded upon both brain atrophy and cognitive decline measures, we sought to extend this approach further to find biomarkers of these endophenotypes using different proteomic methods, which may be more sensitive for detection of alternative groups of proteins. One such study was reported by Sattlecker et al. who utilized the SOMAscan technology for plasma protein biomarker discovery in a cohort of AD, MCI, and controls. The strongest findings of this study included an association of clusterin with cognitive decline, replicating the findings of Thambisetty et al. (128), along with an association of fetuin B and pancreatic polypeptide with brain atrophy, and an association of pancreatic polypeptide and PSA-ACT with a diagnosis of AD (134).

In addition to hypothesis generating discovery approaches, targeted hypothesis-driven approaches have also been successful in identifying potential biomarkers of brain atrophy and cognitive decline. For example, the apolipoprotein family is widely implicated in neurodegeneration (157, 158) and in a targeted study, Song et al. showed a negative correlation of plasma clusterin and ApoE with gray matter volume and an association of ApoA1, ApoA2, ApoH, and the ApoB/ApoA1 ratio with risk of cognitive decline in cognitively normal individuals (130). As these proteins are associated with pathology-related outcomes at the preclinical stage of disease, this would suggest that the apolipoproteins may be markers in an early phase of the disease pathogenesis. More recently, Teng et al. also showed an association of plasma ApoE levels with hippocampal volume in a cohort of AD, MCI, and control included in the Alzheimer's disease neuroimaging initiative (ADNI) cohort (135).

We have also taken a targeted approach to examine the biomarker potential of inflammatory proteins (132), given the evidence for an inflammatory component in AD pathology (159, 160). We observed five proteins that were associated with brain atrophy measures (IL-1ra, IL-6, IL-10, TNF-α, and IL-13) and six proteins that were associated with rate of cognitive decline in AD (IL-4, IL-10, G-CSF, IL-2, IFN-γ, and PDGF) (132). Of note was the association of IL-10 with both brain atrophy and rate of cognitive decline, adding further confidence to the finding of its association with AD-related endophenotypes (132). Toledo et al. also published findings of inflammatory proteins (macrophage inflammatory protein 1 alpha, chromogranin A) along with proteins implicated in the stress response (cortisol) and insulin response (insulin-like growth factor binding protein 2) as markers of brain atrophy (133).

Following the identification of various plasma proteins related to AD and proxy measures of disease activity (neuroimaging measured of brain atrophy and clinical measures of cognitive decline), we next sought to validate the most promising and disease-relevant protein markers. To do this, we used multiplex bead assays to measure candidate proteins in a larger ($N > 1000$) cohort of AD/MCI/control participants (124). Interestingly, we found that different sets of proteins were associated with brain atrophy in MCI compared to AD, indicating that these markers are disease-phase specific, and the strongest associations with brain atrophy were observed for clusterin in the MCI group and ApoE in the AD group (124). Furthermore, we identified three proteins NCAM, sRAGE, and ICAM as being associated with rate of cognitive decline and we, therefore, hypothesized that these markers may be predictive of conversion from MCI to AD. When we tested this, we found that there were a panel of 10 proteins (transthyretin, clusterin, cystatin C, A1AcidG, ICAM1, complement component C4, PEDF, A1AT, RANTES, and ApoC3) along with *APOE* genotype, which were able to predict MCI conversion to AD with 87% accuracy, 85% sensitivity, and 88% specificity, as described earlier (124).

Blood-Based Biomarkers of Brain Amyloid Burden

Blood-based biomarkers of neocortical Aβ (extracellular β-amyloid) burden (NAB) as measured by PET brain imaging have also been sought (**Table 3**). These studies have used the Australian Imaging, Biomarker and Lifestyle Flagship Study of Ageing (AIBL) (161), the ADNI[4], and the BLSA (144) for the purpose of finding plasma proteomic markers of brain amyloid burden.

The first study we carried out used the BLSA study to discover plasma proteins that were associated with NAB in non-demented elderly individuals (137). Using a 2DGE-MS/MS-based approach, this study identified six proteins (ApoE, Complement C3, Albumin, Plasminogen, Haptoglobin and IgG C chain region) that discriminated "high" from "low" PiB PET brain amyloid burden subjects in discovery-based studies, and a further association of ApoE with amyloid burden in the medial temporal lobe in an independent validation study (137).

[4]www.adni-info.org

Following this, we carried out a separate study to examine the association of plasma proteins with NAB in AD, MCI, and control subjects included in the ADNI[5] (138). Plasma proteins were measured by the Myriad Rules-Based Medicine (RBM) panel using commercially available multiplexed luminex assays. This work identified 13 plasma proteins (c-peptide, fibrinogen, A1AT, pancreatic polypeptide, complement C3, vitronectin, cortisol, AXL receptor kinase, IL-3, IL-13, matrix metalloproteinase-9 total, ApoE, and IgE), which in combination with covariates were able to discriminate PiB-positive from PiB-negative individuals with 92 and 55% sensitivity and specificity, respectively (138).

Shortly after this, Burnham et al. published a study that again utilized the RBM panel for identifying plasma proteins predictive of NAB in an AD, MCI, and control-based population; however, this study utilized the AIBL study for discovery, followed by validation of potential biomarkers of NAB in the ADNI (139). In summary, Burnham et al. identified six plasma proteins ($A\beta_{42}$, chemokine ligand 13, IL-17, IgM-1, pancreatic polypeptide and VCAM-1) that contributed to a biomarker signature that was able to predict NAB with 79 and 76% sensitivity and specificity in the ADNI-based validation cohort (139).

More recently, a study carried out in an ADNI-based MCI cohort revealed that plasma IL-6 receptor, clusterin, and ApoE levels coupled with a number of clinical and demographic measures, *APOE* genotype and mean hippocampal volume, achieved 79 and 83% sensitivity and specificity for prediction of NAB (125). Hwang et al. also reported an association of reduced plasma BDNF levels with increased regional measures of NAB in an ADNI cohort (141).

We also recently reported the results of an LC-MS/MS-based approach for the discovery of plasma protein biomarkers of NAB in AD, MCI, and healthy controls enrolled in the AIBL study (140). Using this approach, a number of plasma proteins were shown to be significantly associated with NAB, including A2M, CFH-related protein 1, and γ-fibrinogen. Moreover, the association of γ-fibrinogen in combination with age was found to predict NAB with 59 and 78% sensitivity and specificity, respectively (140).

Although the exact protein biomarker panels identified by these studies for prediction of NAB differs between the studies, it is of note that there are some commonalities in the proteins included in these biomarker panels, including ApoE (125, 137, 138), complement C3 (137, 138), and pancreatic polypeptide (138, 139). A recent study, therefore, sought to replicate these findings in an independent cohort of AD, MCI, and control subjects in the AIBL study (142). This work replicated an association of two proteins with NAB; pancreatic polypeptide across the cohort of AD, MCI, and cognitively healthy elderly, and IgM in the cognitively healthy elderly group, while the association of the other protein candidates with NAB was not replicated (142). This lack of replication between studies is disappointing; however, it is quite possible that this could be in part due to technical platform differences, as the discovery studies used both MS (137, 140) and immunocapture-based approaches (125, 138, 139, 141), while replication was sought using the SOMAscan platform (142). As mentioned earlier, platform and assay differences may provide differing quantitative proteomic results, given that there are key differences in the nature of the protein being measured by these techniques. MS approaches measure denatured protein in a peptide-specific manner, while immunocapture-based assays use antibodies for epitope-specific native protein measures. The SOMAscan platform also measures native protein, but by binding of an aptamer to a tertiary structure-specific epitope. Therefore, differences in the region and confirmation of the protein target being measured by these different techniques may result in varying quantitative results.

These various studies utilizing an AD pathology endophenotype-based approach for biomarker discovery show promise in identifying biomarkers reflective of core AD pathology and disease activity. However, it is important to note that there are some issues surrounding the approach of predicating blood-based biomarker discovery on PET amyloid measures. First, PiB PET detects insoluble fibrillary but not insoluble oligomeric Aβ, which are known to possess neurotoxic and synaptotoxic properties (162). Therefore, blood-based biomarkers of PiB PET amyloid may not be the most relevant markers of brain amyloid pathology. Second, it is possible that the relationship of plasma proteins with PiB PET amyloid measures could be specific to the technical aspects of the PET imaging technique used. For example, variability in the amyloid measure could be introduced by the use of alternative radiotracers or alternative methods of PET data analysis.

Therefore, in order to assess the reproducibility and robustness of plasma proteins biomarkers of amyloid (as indicated by PiB PET), it will be essential to perform replication and validation studies examining their association with brain amyloid burden (1) in larger independent cohorts, (2) using orthogonal technical platforms for biomarker quantification, and (3) using alternative measures indicative of amyloid (for example, alternative PET amyloid radiotracers and CSF Aβ).

Other Potential Endophenotype Approaches

While endophenotype-based designs founded upon rates of cognitive decline, brain atrophy, and brain amyloid burden show promise, there are further measures of AD and other aspects of core AD neuropathology that warrant investigation as potential endophenotypes for biomarker discovery. FDG-PET measures cerebral metabolic glucose utilization rate and serves as an indicator of synaptic activity, neuronal function, and neuronal metabolic activity (163). FDG-PET has been reported to have an average diagnostic accuracy of 93% (96% sensitivity and 90% specificity) for differentiating AD from cognitively healthy elderly subjects (164), and can discriminate between different dementia-types with around 94% accuracy (165). Using FDG-PET as an endophenotype of pathology for blood-based biomarker discovery could, therefore, aid in the development of biomarkers relating to synaptic and neuronal function, and the prodromal stage of disease, given that hypometabolism is known to occur in amnestic MCI (165, 166). Moreover, glucose metabolism

[5] adni.loni.ucla.edu

is thought to be more closely associated with certain memory, language, and visuospatial clinical variants of AD than measures of Aβ deposition and so plasma protein biomarkers of FDG-PET cerebral glucose metabolism could be of utility in detecting these clinical aspects of the disease (167).

With the development of tau imaging comes the opportunity to investigate blood-based biomarkers related specifically to brain tau pathology, which could obviously be of potential utility beyond AD and for tauopathies such as fronto-temporal dementia. The development of tau imaging has been challenging due to the deposition of tau protein being intracellular, which impacts upon radiotracer binding and image contrast (168). However, current research to develop various tau brain imaging tracers is underway, including the tracers 18F-THK523, [F-18]-T807, and [F-18]-T808 (169–171). PET imaging of tau could, therefore, provide another endophenotype parameter for the design of studies that seek to uncover peripheral proteomic biomarkers relating specifically to tau pathology in the brain.

Moreover, other types of biomarkers detectable in the blood show promise as potential markers of AD, including, for example, metabolomic (172–175) and transcriptomic-based markers (176, 177). Further research to examine how these markers may be related to pathology endophenotypes and the potential of combining these markers as a multimodal signature of AD pathology will be important.

CONCLUSION

Much research has sought blood-based proteomic biomarkers that may have diagnostic utility in discriminating AD cases from control, with limited success in identifying a reproducible signature of diagnostic or trials utility.

An alternative approach, which we have increasingly employed is using surrogates for disease activity – endophenotypes – such as cerebral atrophy imaging or molecular markers of amyloid pathology and rate of decline. Such an approach yields different but overlapping panels of markers. It is, therefore, possible that such markers predicated on pathological processes might be more reproducible and ultimately of more utility in diagnostic, prognostic, predictive, and other utilities especially in the context of clinical trials.

However, it seems intrinsically unlikely to us that a blood-based biomarker would replace relatively specific and reliable markers such as molecular markers in CSF or PET imaging markers that are more proximal to the disease state. Rather, we predict that blood-based biomarkers might be less specific but possibly more sensitive and certainly more readily conducted repeatedly in the context of large-scale, community-based studies and where repeated measures to track change is required. This then raises the prospect of what might be termed the biomarker funnel, a series of tests and investigations starting with the minimally invasive, highly sensitive, poorly specific marker set leading toward a technologically demanding or invasive test that is highly specific. This would be a blood test triage or selection process for CSF or PET tests in effect. Such a funnel is commonplace in medicine – fasting glucose before a glucose tolerance test, mammography before biopsy are examples, but there are many others. A biomarker funnel with blood-based markers as an early step toward a pathological diagnosis in life would be a very substantial step forward and maybe an essential step before clinical trials can be both effective and achievable.

AUTHOR CONTRIBUTIONS

AB, SW, and SL all contributed to the design of the review and interpretation of the studies included within it. AB, SW, and SL all contributed to the drafting and revision of the content and provided final approval of this version to be published.

ACKNOWLEDGMENTS

Research in the authors' laboratories is supported by Alzheimer's Research UK, Alzheimer's Society, MRC, NIHR, Parkinson's UK, Wellcome trust, and the EU.

REFERENCES

1. Prince M, Bryce R, Albanese E, Wimo A, Ribeiro W, Ferri CP. The global prevalence of dementia: a systematic review and metaanalysis. *Alzheimers Dement* (2013) **9**:63–75.e2. doi:10.1016/j.jalz.2012.11.007
2. Wimo A, Prince M. *World Alzheimer Report 2010: The Global Economic Impact of Dementia*. London : Alzheimer's Disease International (2010).
3. Francis PT, Palmer AM, Snape M, Wilcock GK. The cholinergic hypothesis of Alzheimer's disease: a review of progress. *J Neurol Neurosurg Psychiatry* (1999) **66**:137–47. doi:10.1136/jnnp.66.2.137
4. Villemagne VL, Pike KE, Chetelat G, Ellis KA, Mulligan RS, Bourgeat P, et al. Longitudinal assessment of Abeta and cognition in aging and Alzheimer disease. *Ann Neurol* (2011) **69**:181–92. doi:10.1002/ana.22248
5. Johnson KA, Fox NC, Sperling RA, Klunk WE. Brain imaging in Alzheimer disease. *Cold Spring Harb Perspect Med* (2012) **2**:a006213. doi:10.1101/cshperspect.a006213
6. Kang JH, Korecka M, Toledo JB, Trojanowski JQ, Shaw LM. Clinical utility and analytical challenges in measurement of cerebrospinal fluid amyloid-beta(1-42) and tau proteins as Alzheimer disease biomarkers. *Clin Chem* (2013) **59**:903–16. doi:10.1373/clinchem.2013.202937
7. Teunissen CE, Verwey NA, Kester MI, Van Uffelen K, Blankenstein MA. Standardization of assay procedures for analysis of the CSF biomarkers amyloid beta((1-42)), tau, and phosphorylated tau in Alzheimer's disease: report of an international workshop. *Int J Alzheimers Dis* (2010) **35**:271–8. doi:10.4061/2010/635053
8. Jack CR Jr, Knopman DS, Jagust WJ, Petersen RC, Weiner MW, Aisen PS, et al. Tracking pathophysiological processes in Alzheimer's disease: an updated hypothetical model of dynamic biomarkers. *Lancet Neurol* (2013) **12**:207–16. doi:10.1016/S1474-4422(12)70291-0
9. Toledo JB, Bjerke M, Da X, Landau SM, Foster NL, Jagust W, et al. Nonlinear association between cerebrospinal fluid and florbetapir F-18 beta-amyloid measures across the spectrum of Alzheimer disease. *JAMA Neurol* (2015) **72**:571–81. doi:10.1001/jamaneurol.2014.4829
10. Anderson NL, Anderson NG. The human plasma proteome. *Mol Cell Proteomics* (2002) **1**:845–67. doi:10.1074/mcp.R200007-MCP200
11. Montagne A, Barnes SR, Sweeney MD, Halliday MR, Sagare AP, Zhao Z, et al. Blood-brain barrier breakdown in the aging human hippocampus. *Neuron* (2015) **85**:296–302. doi:10.1016/j.neuron.2014.12.032
12. Lewczuk P, Esselmann H, Bibl M, Paul S, Svitek J, Miertschischk J, et al. Electrophoretic separation of amyloid beta peptides in plasma. *Electrophoresis* (2004) **25**:3336–43. doi:10.1002/elps.200406068
13. Westbrook JA, Noirel J, Brown JE, Wright PC, Evans CA. Quantitation with chemical tagging reagents in biomarker studies. *Proteomics Clin Appl* (2015) **9**:295–300. doi:10.1002/prca.201400120

14. Tirumalai RS, Chan KC, Prieto DA, Issaq HJ, Conrads TP, Veenstra TD. Characterization of the low molecular weight human serum proteome. *Mol Cell Proteomics* (2003) **2**:1096–103. doi:10.1074/mcp.M300031-MCP200
15. Mostovenko EH, Rattke C, Deelder J, Van Veelen PA, Palmblad M. Comparison of peptide and protein fractionation methods in proteomics. *EuPA Open Proteom* (2013) **1**:30–7. doi:10.1016/j.euprot.2013.09.001
16. Liao Q, Zhao L, Chen X, Deng Y, Ding Y. Serum proteome analysis for profiling protein markers associated with carcinogenesis and lymph node metastasis in nasopharyngeal carcinoma. *Clin Exp Metastasis* (2008) **25**:465–76. doi:10.1007/s10585-008-9152-8
17. Kaur P, Reis MD, Couchman GR, Forjuoh SN, Greene JF, Asea A. Serpine 1 links obesity and diabetes: a pilot study. *J Proteomics Bioinform* (2010) **3**:191–9. doi:10.4172/jpb.1000139
18. Tang HY, Beer LA, Barnhart KT, Speicher DW. Rapid verification of candidate serological biomarkers using gel-based, label-free multiple reaction monitoring. *J Proteome Res* (2011) **10**:4005–17. doi:10.1021/pr2002098
19. Mulder C, Verwey NA, van der Flier WM, Bouwman FH, Kok A, van Elk EJ, et al. Amyloid-beta(1-42), total tau, and phosphorylated tau as cerebrospinal fluid biomarkers for the diagnosis of Alzheimer disease. *Clin Chem* (2010) **56**:248–53. doi:10.1373/clinchem.2009.130518
20. Murphy MP, LeVine H. Alzheimer's disease and the amyloid-beta peptide. *J Alzheimers Dis* (2010) **19**:311–23. doi:10.3233/JAD-2010-1221
21. Masters CL, Simms G, Weinman NA, Multhaup G, McDonald BL, Beyreuther K. Amyloid plaque core protein in Alzheimer disease and Down syndrome. *Proc Natl Acad Sci U S A* (1985) **82**:4245–9. doi:10.1073/pnas.82.12.4245
22. Wang J, Dickson DW, Trojanowski JQ, Lee VM. The levels of soluble versus insoluble brain Abeta distinguish Alzheimer's disease from normal and pathologic aging. *Exp Neurol* (1999) **158**:328–37. doi:10.1006/exnr.1999.7085
23. Song F, Poljak A, Valenzuela M, Mayeux R, Smythe GA, Sachdev PS. Meta-analysis of plasma amyloid-beta levels in Alzheimer's disease. *J Alzheimers Dis* (2011) **26**:365–75. doi:10.3233/JAD-2011-101977
24. Koyama A, Okereke OI, Yang T, Blacker D, Selkoe DJ, Grodstein F. Plasma amyloid-beta as a predictor of dementia and cognitive decline: a systematic review and meta-analysis. *Arch Neurol* (2012) **69**:824–31. doi:10.1001/archneurol.2011.1841
25. Lui JK, Laws SM, Li QX, Villemagne VL, Ames D, Brown B, et al. Plasma amyloid-beta as a biomarker in Alzheimer's disease: the AIBL study of aging. *J Alzheimers Dis* (2010) **20**:1233–42. doi:10.3233/JAD-2010-090249
26. Abdullah L, Paris D, Luis C, Quadros A, Parrish J, Valdes L, et al. The influence of diagnosis, intra- and inter-person variability on serum and plasma Abeta levels. *Neurosci Lett* (2007) **428**:53–8. doi:10.1016/j.neulet.2007.09.058
27. Locascio JJ, Fukumoto H, Yap L, Bottiglieri T, Growdon JH, Hyman BT, et al. Plasma amyloid beta-protein and C-reactive protein in relation to the rate of progression of Alzheimer disease. *Arch Neurol* (2008) **65**:776–85. doi:10.1001/archneur.65.6.776
28. Rembach A, Faux NG, Watt AD, Pertile KK, Rumble RL, Trounson BO, et al. Changes in plasma amyloid beta in a longitudinal study of aging and Alzheimer's disease. *Alzheimers Dement* (2014) **10**:53–61. doi:10.1016/j.jalz.2012.12.006
29. Fei M, Jianghua W, Rujuan M, Wei Z, Qian W. The relationship of plasma Abeta levels to dementia in aging individuals with mild cognitive impairment. *J Neurol Sci* (2011) **305**:92–6. doi:10.1016/j.jns.2011.03.005
30. Blasko I, Jellinger K, Kemmler G, Krampla W, Jungwirth S, Wichart I, et al. Conversion from cognitive health to mild cognitive impairment and Alzheimer's disease: prediction by plasma amyloid beta 42, medial temporal lobe atrophy and homocysteine. *Neurobiol Aging* (2008) **29**:1–11. doi:10.1016/j.neurobiolaging.2006.09.002
31. Mayeux R, Honig LS, Tang MX, Manly J, Stern Y, Schupf N, et al. Plasma A[beta]40 and A[beta]42 and Alzheimer's disease: relation to age, mortality, and risk. *Neurology* (2003) **61**:1185–90. doi:10.1212/01.WNL.0000091890.32140.8F
32. Pomara N, Willoughby LM, Sidtis JJ, Mehta PD. Selective reductions in plasma Abeta 1-42 in healthy elderly subjects during longitudinal follow-up: a preliminary report. *Am J Geriatr Psychiatry* (2005) **13**:914–7. doi:10.1097/00019442-200510000-00012
33. Wang T, Xiao S, Liu Y, Lin Z, Su N, Li X, et al. The efficacy of plasma biomarkers in early diagnosis of Alzheimer's disease. *Int J Geriatr Psychiatry* (2014) **29**:713–9. doi:10.1002/gps.4053
34. Buerger K, Frisoni G, Uspenskaya O, Ewers M, Zetterberg H, Geroldi C, et al. Validation of Alzheimer's disease CSF and plasma biological markers: the multicentre reliability study of the pilot European Alzheimer's disease neuroimaging initiative (E-ADNI). *Exp Gerontol* (2009) **44**:579–85. doi:10.1016/j.exger.2009.06.003
35. Chouraki V, Beiser A, Younkin L, Preis SR, Weinstein G, Hansson O, et al. Plasma amyloid-beta and risk of Alzheimer's disease in the Framingham Heart Study. *Alzheimers Dement* (2015) **11**:249–57. doi:10.1016/j.jalz.2014.07.001
36. Graff-Radford NR, Crook JE, Lucas J, Boeve BF, Knopman DS, Ivnik RJ, et al. Association of low plasma Abeta42/Abeta40 ratios with increased imminent risk for mild cognitive impairment and Alzheimer disease. *Arch Neurol* (2007) **64**:354–62. doi:10.1001/archneur.64.3.354
37. van Oijen M, Hofman A, Soares HD, Koudstaal PJ, Breteler MM. Plasma Abeta(1-40) and Abeta(1-42) and the risk of dementia: a prospective case-cohort study. *Lancet Neurol* (2006) **5**:655–60. doi:10.1016/S1474-4422(06)70501-4
38. Ghersi-Egea JF, Gorevic PD, Ghiso J, Frangione B, Patlak CS, Fenstermacher JD. Fate of cerebrospinal fluid-borne amyloid beta-peptide: rapid clearance into blood and appreciable accumulation by cerebral arteries. *J Neurochem* (1996) **67**:880–3. doi:10.1046/j.1471-4159.1996.67020880.x
39. Motter R, Vigo-Pelfrey C, Kholodenko D, Barbour R, Johnson-Wood K, Galasko D, et al. Reduction of beta-amyloid peptide42 in the cerebrospinal fluid of patients with Alzheimer's disease. *Ann Neurol* (1995) **38**:643–8. doi:10.1002/ana.410380413
40. Mehta PD, Pirttila T, Patrick BA, Barshatzky M, Mehta SP. Amyloid beta protein 1-40 and 1-42 levels in matched cerebrospinal fluid and plasma from patients with Alzheimer disease. *Neurosci Lett* (2001) **304**:102–6. doi:10.1016/S0304-3940(01)01754-2
41. Le Bastard N, Aerts L, Leurs J, Blomme W, De Deyn PP, Engelborghs S. No correlation between time-linked plasma and CSF Abeta levels. *Neurochem Int* (2009) **55**:820–5. doi:10.1016/j.neuint.2009.08.006
42. Bateman RJ, Xiong C, Benzinger TL, Fagan AM, Goate A, Fox NC, et al. Clinical and biomarker changes in dominantly inherited Alzheimer's disease. *N Engl J Med* (2012) **367**:795–804. doi:10.1056/NEJMoa1202753
43. Thomas T, Thomas G, McLendon C, Sutton T, Mullan M. Beta-amyloid-mediated vasoactivity and vascular endothelial damage. *Nature* (1996) **380**:168–71. doi:10.1038/380168a0
44. Petrovitch H, Ross GW, Steinhorn SC, Abbott RD, Markesbery W, Davis D, et al. AD lesions and infarcts in demented and non-demented Japanese-American men. *Ann Neurol* (2005) **57**:98–103. doi:10.1002/ana.20318
45. Freeman SH, Raju S, Hyman BT, Frosch MP, Irizarry MC. Plasma Abeta levels do not reflect brain Abeta levels. *J Neuropathol Exp Neurol* (2007) **66**:264–71. doi:10.1097/NEN.0b013e31803d3ae4
46. Devanand DP, Schupf N, Stern Y, Parsey R, Pelton GH, Mehta P, et al. Plasma Abeta and PET PiB binding are inversely related in mild cognitive impairment. *Neurology* (2011) **77**:125–31. doi:10.1212/WNL.0b013e318224afb7
47. Tzen KY, Yang SY, Chen TF, Cheng TW, Horng HE, Wen HP, et al. Plasma Abeta but not tau is related to brain PiB retention in early Alzheimer's disease. *ACS Chem Neurosci* (2014) **5**:830–6. doi:10.1021/cn500101j
48. Kaneko N, Nakamura A, Washimi Y, Kato T, Sakurai T, Arahata Y, et al. Novel plasma biomarker surrogating cerebral amyloid deposition. *Proc Jpn Acad Ser B Phys Biol Sci* (2014) **90**:353–64. doi:10.2183/pjab.90.353
49. Huang Y, Potter R, Sigurdson W, Kasten T, Connors R, Morris JC, et al. Beta-amyloid dynamics in human plasma. *Arch Neurol* (2012) **69**:1591–7. doi:10.1001/archneurol.2012.18107
50. Kuo YM, Emmerling MR, Lampert HC, Hempelman SR, Kokjohn TA, Woods AS, et al. High levels of circulating Abeta42 are sequestered by plasma proteins in Alzheimer's disease. *Biochem Biophys Res Commun* (1999) **257**:787–91. doi:10.1006/bbrc.1999.0552
51. Sotolongo-Grau O, Pesini P, Valero S, Lafuente A, Buendia M, Perez-Grijalba V, et al. Association between cell-bound blood amyloid-beta(1-40) levels and hippocampus volume. *Alzheimers Res Ther* (2014) **6**:56. doi:10.1186/s13195-014-0056-3
52. Chiu MJ, Yang SY, Chen TF, Chieh JJ, Huang TZ, Yip PK, et al. New assay for old markers-plasma beta amyloid of mild cognitive impairment and Alzheimer's disease. *Curr Alzheimer Res* (2012) **9**:1142–8. doi:10.2174/156720512804142967
53. Henriksen K, Wang Y, Sorensen MG, Barascuk N, Suhy J, Pedersen JT, et al. An enzyme-generated fragment of tau measured in serum shows an inverse

correlation to cognitive function. *PLoS One* (2013) **8**:e64990. doi:10.1371/journal.pone.0064990

54. Henriksen K, Byrjalsen I, Christiansen C, Karsdal MA. Relationship between serum levels of tau fragments and clinical progression of Alzheimer's disease. *J Alzheimers Dis* (2015) **43**:1331–41. doi:10.3233/JAD-140984
55. Zetterberg H, Wilson D, Andreasson U, Minthon L, Blennow K, Randall J, et al. Plasma tau levels in Alzheimer's disease. *Alzheimers Res Ther* (2013) **5**:9. doi:10.1186/alzrt163
56. Rissin DM, Kan CW, Campbell TG, Howes SC, Fournier DR, Song L, et al. Single-molecule enzyme-linked immunosorbent assay detects serum proteins at subfemtomolar concentrations. *Nat Biotechnol* (2010) **28**:595–9. doi:10.1038/nbt.1641
57. Chiu MJ, Chen YF, Chen TF, Yang SY, Yang FP, Tseng TW, et al. Plasma tau as a window to the brain-negative associations with brain volume and memory function in mild cognitive impairment and early Alzheimer's disease. *Hum Brain Mapp* (2014) **35**:3132–42. doi:10.1002/hbm.22390
58. Zipser BD, Johanson CE, Gonzalez L, Berzin TM, Tavares R, Hulette CM, et al. Microvascular injury and blood-brain barrier leakage in Alzheimer's disease. *Neurobiol Aging* (2007) **28**:977–86. doi:10.1016/j.neurobiolaging.2006.05.016
59. Bush AI, Whyte S, Thomas LD, Williamson TG, Van Tiggelen CJ, Currie J, et al. An abnormality of plasma amyloid protein precursor in Alzheimer's disease. *Ann Neurol* (1992) **32**:57–65. doi:10.1002/ana.410320110
60. Kennard ML, Feldman H, Yamada T, Jefferies WA. Serum levels of the iron binding protein p97 are elevated in Alzheimer's disease. *Nat Med* (1996) **2**:1230–5. doi:10.1038/nm1196-1230
61. Lombardi VR, Cacabelos R. 19/20 kDa low molecular weight serum protein pattern: a novel potential biochemical prognostic marker for different types of dementia. *Neurosci Lett* (1999) **260**:61–4. doi:10.1016/S0304-3940(98)00960-4
62. Diamandis EP, Yousef GM, Petraki C, Soosaipillai AR. Human kallikrein 6 as a biomarker of Alzheimer's disease. *Clin Biochem* (2000) **33**:663–7. doi:10.1016/S0009-9120(00)00185-5
63. Kalman J, Marki-Zay J, Juhasz A, Santha A, Dux L, Janka Z. Serum and cerebrospinal fluid cystatin C levels in vascular and Alzheimer's dementia. *Acta Neurol Scand* (2000) **101**:279–82. doi:10.1034/j.1600-0404.2000.09011.x
64. Ueno I, Sakai T, Yamaoka M, Yoshida R, Tsugita A. Analysis of blood plasma proteins in patients with Alzheimer's disease by two-dimensional electrophoresis, sequence homology and immunodetection. *Electrophoresis* (2000) **21**:1832–45. doi:10.1002/(SICI)1522-2683(20000501)21:9<1832::AID-ELPS1832>3.0.CO;2-7
65. Licastro F, Pedrini S, Davis LJ, Caputo L, Tagliabue J, Savorani G, et al. Alpha-1-antichymotrypsin and oxidative stress in the peripheral blood from patients with probable Alzheimer disease: a short-term longitudinal study. *Alzheimer Dis Assoc Disord* (2001) **15**:51–5. doi:10.1097/00002093-200101000-00007
66. Schmidt R, Schmidt H, Curb JD, Masaki K, White LR, Launer LJ. Early inflammation and dementia: a 25-year follow-up of the Honolulu-Asia Aging Study. *Ann Neurol* (2002) **52**:168–74. doi:10.1002/ana.10265
67. Mocali A, Cedrola S, Della Malva N, Bontempelli M, Mitidieri VA, Bavazzano A, et al. Increased plasma levels of soluble CD40, together with the decrease of TGF beta 1, as possible differential markers of Alzheimer disease. *Exp Gerontol* (2004) **39**:1555–61. doi:10.1016/j.exger.2004.07.007
68. Zhang R, Barker L, Pinchev D, Marshall J, Rasamoelisolo M, Smith C, et al. Mining biomarkers in human sera using proteomic tools. *Proteomics* (2004) **4**:244–56. doi:10.1002/pmic.200300495
69. van Oijen M, Witteman JC, Hofman A, Koudstaal PJ, Breteler MM. Fibrinogen is associated with an increased risk of Alzheimer disease and vascular dementia. *Stroke* (2005) **36**:2637–41. doi:10.1161/01.STR.0000189721.31432.26
70. Liu HC, Hu CJ, Chang JG, Sung SM, Lee LS, Yuan RY, et al. Proteomic identification of lower apolipoprotein A-I in Alzheimer's disease. *Dement Geriatr Cogn Disord* (2006) **21**:155–61. doi:10.1159/000090676
71. Guerreiro RJ, Santana I, Bras JM, Santiago B, Paiva A, Oliveira C. Peripheral inflammatory cytokines as biomarkers in Alzheimer's disease and mild cognitive impairment. *Neurodegener Dis* (2007) **4**:406–12. doi:10.1159/000107700
72. Liao PC, Yu L, Kuo CC, Lin C, Kuo YM. Proteomics analysis of plasma for potential biomarkers in the diagnosis of Alzheimer's disease. *Proteomics Clin Appl* (2007) **1**:506–12. doi:10.1002/prca.200600684
73. Ozturk C, Ozge A, Yalin OO, Yilmaz IA, Delialioglu N, Yildiz C, et al. The diagnostic role of serum inflammatory and soluble proteins on dementia subtypes: correlation with cognitive and functional decline. *Behav Neurol* (2007) **18**:207–15. doi:10.1155/2007/432190
74. Guntert A, Campbell J, Saleem M, O'brien DP, Thompson AJ, Byers HL, et al. Plasma gelsolin is decreased and correlates with rate of decline in Alzheimer's disease. *J Alzheimers Dis* (2010) **21**:585–96. doi:10.3233/JAD-2010-100279
75. Laske C, Stransky E, Hoffmann N, Maetzler W, Straten G, Eschweiler GW, et al. Macrophage colony-stimulating factor (M-CSF) in plasma and CSF of patients with mild cognitive impairment and Alzheimer's disease. *Curr Alzheimer Res* (2010) **7**:409–14. doi:10.2174/156720510791383813
76. Mueller C, Zhou W, Vanmeter A, Heiby M, Magaki S, Ross MM, et al. The heme degradation pathway is a promising serum biomarker source for the early detection of Alzheimer's disease. *J Alzheimers Dis* (2010) **19**:1081–91. doi:10.3233/JAD-2010-1303
77. Han SH, Jung ES, Sohn JH, Hong HJ, Hong HS, Kim JW, et al. Human serum transthyretin levels correlate inversely with Alzheimer's disease. *J Alzheimers Dis* (2011) **25**:77–84. doi:10.3233/JAD-2011-102145
78. Ijsselstijn L, Dekker LJ, Stingl C, van der Weiden MM, Hofman A, Kros JM, et al. Serum levels of pregnancy zone protein are elevated in presymptomatic Alzheimer's disease. *J Proteome Res* (2011) **10**:4902–10. doi:10.1021/pr200270z
79. Teunissen CE, Veerhuis R, De Vente J, Verhey FR, Vreeling F, Van Boxtel MP, et al. Brain-specific fatty acid-binding protein is elevated in serum of patients with dementia-related diseases. *Eur J Neurol* (2011) **18**:865–71. doi:10.1111/j.1468-1331.2010.03273.x
80. Henkel AW, Muller K, Lewczuk P, Muller T, Marcus K, Kornhuber J, et al. Multidimensional plasma protein separation technique for identification of potential Alzheimer's disease plasma biomarkers: a pilot study. *J Neural Transm* (2012) **119**:779–88. doi:10.1007/s00702-012-0781-3
81. Wu G, Sankaranarayanan S, Wong J, Tugusheva K, Michener MS, Shi X, et al. Characterization of plasma beta-secretase (BACE1) activity and soluble amyloid precursor proteins as potential biomarkers for Alzheimer's disease. *J Neurosci Res* (2012) **90**:2247–58. doi:10.1002/jnr.23122
82. Yang MH, Yang YH, Lu CY, Jong SB, Chen LJ, Lin YF, et al. Activity-dependent neuroprotector homeobox protein: a candidate protein identified in serum as diagnostic biomarker for Alzheimer's disease. *J Proteomics* (2012) **75**:3617–29. doi:10.1016/j.jprot.2012.04.017
83. Androsova LV, Mikhailova NM, Zozulia SA, Dupin AM, Rassadina GA, Lavrent'eva NV, et al. Inflammatory markers in Alzheimer's disease and vascular dementia. *Zh Nevrol Psikhiatr Im S S Korsakova* (2013) **113**:49–53.
84. Gaiottino J, Norgren N, Dobson R, Topping J, Nissim A, Malaspina A, et al. Increased neurofilament light chain blood levels in neurodegenerative neurological diseases. *PLoS One* (2013) **8**:e75091. doi:10.1371/journal.pone.0075091
85. Gezen-Ak D, Dursun E, Hanagasi H, Bilgic B, Lohman E, Araz OS, et al. BDNF, TNFalpha, HSP90, CFH, and IL-10 serum levels in patients with early or late onset Alzheimer's disease or mild cognitive impairment. *J Alzheimers Dis* (2013) **37**:185–95. doi:10.3233/JAD-130497
86. Johansson P, Aberg D, Johansson JO, Mattsson N, Hansson O, Ahren B, et al. Serum but not cerebrospinal fluid levels of insulin-like growth factor-I (IGF-I) and IGF-binding protein-3 (IGFBP-3) are increased in Alzheimer's disease. *Psychoneuroendocrinology* (2013) **38**:1729–37. doi:10.1016/j.psyneuen.2013.02.006
87. Perneczky R, Guo LH, Kagerbauer SM, Werle L, Kurz A, Martin J, et al. Soluble amyloid precursor protein beta as blood-based biomarker of Alzheimer's disease. *Transl Psychiatry* (2013) **3**:e227. doi:10.1038/tp.2013.11
88. Sun L, Tan MS, Hu N, Yu JT, Tan L. Exploring the value of plasma BIN1 as a potential biomarker for Alzheimer's disease. *J Alzheimers Dis* (2013) **37**:291–5. doi:10.3233/JAD-130392
89. Shih YH, Tsai KJ, Lee CW, Shiesh SC, Chen WT, Pai MC, et al. Apolipoprotein C-III is an amyloid-beta-binding protein and an early marker for Alzheimer's disease. *J Alzheimers Dis* (2014) **41**:855–65. doi:10.3233/JAD-140111
90. Hertze J, Nagga K, Minthon L, Hansson O. Changes in cerebrospinal fluid and blood plasma levels of IGF-II and its binding proteins in Alzheimer's disease: an observational study. *BMC Neurol* (2014) **14**:64. doi:10.1186/1471-2377-14-64
91. Song F, Poljak A, Kochan NA, Raftery M, Brodaty H, Smythe GA, et al. Plasma protein profiling of mild cognitive impairment and Alzheimer's

disease using iTRAQ quantitative proteomics. *Proteome Sci* (2014) **12**:5. doi:10.1186/1477-5956-12-5

92. Baranowska-Bik A, Bik W, Styczynska M, Chodakowska-Zebrowska M, Barcikowska M, Wolinska-Witort E, et al. Plasma leptin levels and free leptin index in women with Alzheimer's disease. *Neuropeptides* (2015) **52**:73–8. doi:10.1016/j.npep.2015.05.006
93. Hare DJ, Doecke JD, Faux NG, Rembach A, Volitakis I, Fowler CJ, et al. Decreased plasma iron in Alzheimer's disease is due to transferrin desaturation. *ACS Chem Neurosci* (2015) **6**:398–402. doi:10.1021/cn5003557
94. Muenchhoff J, Poljak A, Song F, Raftery M, Brodaty H, Duncan M, et al. Plasma protein profiling of mild cognitive impairment and Alzheimer's disease across two independent cohorts. *J Alzheimers Dis* (2015) **43**:1355–73. doi:10.3233/JAD-141266
95. Qin W, Jia X, Wang F, Zuo X, Wu L, Zhou A, et al. Elevated plasma angiogenesis factors in Alzheimer's disease. *J Alzheimers Dis* (2015) **45**:245–52. doi:10.3233/JAD-142409
96. Hye A, Lynham S, Thambisetty M, Causevic M, Campbell J, Byers HL, et al. Proteome-based plasma biomarkers for Alzheimer's disease. *Brain* (2006) **129**:3042–50. doi:10.1093/brain/awl279
97. Ray S, Britschgi M, Herbert C, Takeda-Uchimura Y, Boxer A, Blennow K, et al. Classification and prediction of clinical Alzheimer's diagnosis based on plasma signaling proteins. *Nat Med* (2007) **13**:1359–62. doi:10.1038/nm1653
98. Ait-Ghezala G, Abdullah L, Volmar CH, Paris D, Luis CA, Quadros A, et al. Diagnostic utility of APOE, soluble CD40, CD40L, and Abeta1-40 levels in plasma in Alzheimer's disease. *Cytokine* (2008) **44**:283–7. doi:10.1016/j.cyto.2008.08.013
99. Cutler P, Akuffo EL, Bodnar WM, Briggs DM, Davis JB, Debouck CM, et al. Proteomic identification and early validation of complement 1 inhibitor and pigment epithelium-derived factor: two novel biomarkers of Alzheimer's disease in human plasma. *Proteomics Clin Appl* (2008) **2**:467–77. doi:10.1002/prca.200780101
100. Gomez Ravetti M, Moscato P. Identification of a 5-protein biomarker molecular signature for predicting Alzheimer's disease. *PLoS One* (2008) **3**:e3111. doi:10.1371/journal.pone.0003111
101. O'Bryant SE, Xiao G, Barber R, Reisch J, Doody R, Fairchild T, et al. A serum protein-based algorithm for the detection of Alzheimer disease. *Arch Neurol* (2010) **67**:1077–81. doi:10.1001/archneurol.2010.215
102. Laske C, Leyhe T, Stransky E, Hoffmann N, Fallgatter AJ, Dietzsch J. Identification of a blood-based biomarker panel for classification of Alzheimer's disease. *Int J Neuropsychopharmacol* (2011) **14**:1147–55. doi:10.1017/S1461145711000459
103. Marksteiner J, Kemmler G, Weiss EM, Knaus G, Ullrich C, Mechtcheriakov S, et al. Five out of 16 plasma signaling proteins are enhanced in plasma of patients with mild cognitive impairment and Alzheimer's disease. *Neurobiol Aging* (2011) **32**:539–40. doi:10.1016/j.neurobiolaging.2009.03.011
104. O'Bryant SE, Xiao G, Barber R, Huebinger R, Wilhelmsen K, Edwards M, et al. A blood-based screening tool for Alzheimer's disease that spans serum and plasma: findings from TARC and ADNI. *PLoS One* (2011) **6**:e28092. doi:10.1371/journal.pone.0028092
105. O'Bryant SE, Xiao G, Barber R, Reisch J, Hall J, Cullum CM, et al. A blood-based algorithm for the detection of Alzheimer's disease. *Dement Geriatr Cogn Disord* (2011) **32**:55–62. doi:10.1159/000330750
106. Doecke JD, Laws SM, Faux NG, Wilson W, Burnham SC, Lam CP, et al. Blood-based protein biomarkers for diagnosis of Alzheimer disease. *Arch Neurol* (2012) **69**:1318–25. doi:10.1001/archneurol.2012.1282
107. Hu WT, Holtzman DM, Fagan AM, Shaw LM, Perrin R, Arnold SE, et al. Plasma multianalyte profiling in mild cognitive impairment and Alzheimer disease. *Neurology* (2012) **79**:897–905. doi:10.1212/WNL.0b013e318266fa70
108. Soares HD, Potter WZ, Pickering E, Kuhn M, Immermann FW, Shera DM, et al. Plasma biomarkers associated with the apolipoprotein E genotype and Alzheimer disease. *Arch Neurol* (2012) **69**:1310–7. doi:10.1001/archneurol.2012.1070
109. Guo LH, Alexopoulos P, Wagenpfeil S, Kurz A, Perneczky R. Plasma proteomics for the identification of Alzheimer disease. *Alzheimer Dis Assoc Disord* (2013) **27**:337–42. doi:10.1097/WAD.0b013e31827b60d2
110. Liang F, Jia J, Wang S, Qin W, Liu G. Decreased plasma levels of soluble low density lipoprotein receptor-related protein-1 (sLRP) and the soluble form of the receptor for advanced glycation end products (sRAGE) in the clinical diagnosis of Alzheimer's disease. *J Clin Neurosci* (2013) **20**:357–61. doi:10.1016/j.jocn.2012.06.005
111. Llano DA, Devanarayan V, Simon AJ. Evaluation of plasma proteomic data for Alzheimer disease state classification and for the prediction of progression from mild cognitive impairment to Alzheimer disease. *Alzheimer Dis Assoc Disord* (2013) **27**:233–43. doi:10.1097/WAD.0b013e31826d597a
112. Zhang J, Jia J, Qin W, Wang S. Combination of plasma tumor necrosis factor receptors signaling proteins, beta-amyloid and apolipoprotein E for the detection of Alzheimer's disease. *Neurosci Lett* (2013) **541**:99–104. doi:10.1016/j.neulet.2013.03.007
113. Marksteiner J, Imarhiagbe D, Defrancesco M, Deisenhammer EA, Kemmler G, Humpel C. Analysis of 27 vascular-related proteins reveals that NT-proBNP is a potential biomarker for Alzheimer's disease and mild cognitive impairment: a pilot-study. *Exp Gerontol* (2014) **50**:114–21. doi:10.1016/j.exger.2013.12.001
114. Agarwal S, Ghanty P, Pal NR. Identification of a small set of plasma signalling proteins using neural network for prediction of Alzheimer's disease. *Bioinformatics* (2015) **31**:2505–13. doi:10.1093/bioinformatics/btv173
115. Delaby C, Gabelle A, Blum D, Schraen-Maschke S, Moulinier A, Boulanghien J, et al. Central nervous system and peripheral inflammatory processes in Alzheimer's disease: biomarker profiling approach. *Front Neurol* (2015) **6**:181. doi:10.3389/fneur.2015.00181
116. Peng M, Jia J, Qin W. Plasma gelsolin and matrix metalloproteinase 3 as potential biomarkers for Alzheimer disease. *Neurosci Lett* (2015) **595**:116–21. doi:10.1016/j.neulet.2015.04.014
117. Uchida K, Shan L, Suzuki H, Tabuse Y, Nishimura Y, Hirokawa Y, et al. Amyloid-β sequester proteins as blood-based biomarkers of cognitive decline. *Alzheimers Dement* (2015) **1**:270–80. doi:10.1016/j.dadm.2015.04.003
118. Zhao X, Lejnine S, Spond J, Zhang C, Ramaraj TC, Holder DJ, et al. A candidate plasma protein classifier to identify Alzheimer's disease. *J Alzheimers Dis* (2015) **43**:549–63. doi:10.3233/JAD-141149
119. Zurbig P, Jahn H. Use of proteomic methods in the analysis of human body fluids in Alzheimer research. *Electrophoresis* (2012) **33**:3617–30. doi:10.1002/elps.201200360
120. Lista S, Faltraco F, Prvulovic D, Hampel H. Blood and plasma-based proteomic biomarker research in Alzheimer's disease. *Prog Neurobiol* (2013) **10**(1–102):1–17. doi:10.1016/j.pneurobio.2012.06.007
121. Soares HD, Chen Y, Sabbagh M, Roher A, Schrijvers E, Breteler M. Identifying early markers of Alzheimer's disease using quantitative multiplex proteomic immunoassay panels. *Ann N Y Acad Sci* (2009) **1180**:56–67. doi:10.1111/j.1749-6632.2009.05066.x
122. Bjorkqvist M, Ohlsson M, Minthon L, Hansson O. Evaluation of a previously suggested plasma biomarker panel to identify Alzheimer's disease. *PLoS One* (2012) **7**:e29868. doi:10.1371/journal.pone.0029868
123. Yang H, Lyutvinskiy Y, Herukka SK, Soininen H, Rutishauser D, Zubarev RA. Prognostic polypeptide blood plasma biomarkers of Alzheimer's disease progression. *J Alzheimers Dis* (2014) **40**:659–66. doi:10.3233/JAD-132102
124. Hye A, Riddoch-Contreras J, Baird AL, Ashton NJ, Bazenet C, Leung R, et al. Plasma proteins predict conversion to dementia from prodromal disease. *Alzheimers Dement* (2014) **10**:799–807. doi:10.1016/j.jalz.2014.05.1749
125. Apostolova LG, Hwang KS, Avila D, Elashoff D, Kohannim O, Teng E, et al. Brain amyloidosis ascertainment from cognitive, imaging, and peripheral blood protein measures. *Neurology* (2015) **84**:729–37. doi:10.1212/WNL.0000000000001231
126. Doody RS, Thomas RG, Farlow M, Iwatsubo T, Vellas B, Joffe S, et al. Phase 3 trials of solanezumab for mild-to-moderate Alzheimer's disease. *N Engl J Med* (2014) **370**:311–21. doi:10.1056/NEJMoa1312889
127. Salloway S, Sperling R, Fox NC, Blennow K, Klunk W, Raskind M, et al. Two phase 3 trials of bapineuzumab in mild-to-moderate Alzheimer's disease. *N Engl J Med* (2014) **370**:322–33. doi:10.1056/NEJMoa1304839
128. Thambisetty M, Simmons A, Velayudhan L, Hye A, Campbell J, Zhang Y, et al. Association of plasma clusterin concentration with severity, pathology, and progression in Alzheimer disease. *Arch Gen Psychiatry* (2010) **67**:739–48. doi:10.1001/archgenpsychiatry.2010.78
129. Thambisetty M, Simmons A, Hye A, Campbell J, Westman E, Zhang Y, et al. Plasma biomarkers of brain atrophy in Alzheimer's disease. *PLoS One* (2011) **6**:e28527. doi:10.1371/journal.pone.0028527

130. Song F, Poljak A, Crawford J, Kochan NA, Wen W, Cameron B, et al. Plasma apolipoprotein levels are associated with cognitive status and decline in a community cohort of older individuals. *PLoS One* (2012) **7**:e34078. doi:10.1371/journal.pone.0034078
131. Thambisetty M, An Y, Kinsey A, Koka D, Saleem M, Guntert A, et al. Plasma clusterin concentration is associated with longitudinal brain atrophy in mild cognitive impairment. *Neuroimage* (2012) **59**:212–7. doi:10.1016/j.neuroimage.2011.07.056
132. Leung R, Proitsi P, Simmons A, Lunnon K, Guntert A, Kronenberg D, et al. Inflammatory proteins in plasma are associated with severity of Alzheimer's disease. *PLoS One* (2013) **8**:e64971. doi:10.1371/journal.pone.0064971
133. Toledo JB, Da X, Bhatt P, Wolk DA, Arnold SE, Shaw LM, et al. Relationship between plasma analytes and SPARE-AD defined brain atrophy patterns in ADNI. *PLoS One* (2013) **8**:e55531. doi:10.1371/journal.pone.0055531
134. Sattlecker M, Kiddle SJ, Newhouse S, Proitsi P, Nelson S, Williams S, et al. Alzheimer's disease biomarker discovery using SOMAscan multiplexed protein technology. *Alzheimers Dement* (2014) **10**:724–34. doi:10.1016/j.jalz.2013.09.016
135. Teng E, Chow N, Hwang KS, Thompson PM, Gylys KH, Cole GM, et al. Low plasma ApoE levels are associated with smaller hippocampal size in the Alzheimer's disease neuroimaging initiative cohort. *Dement Geriatr Cogn Disord* (2015) **39**:154–66. doi:10.1159/000368982
136. Velayudhan L, Killick R, Hye A, Kinsey A, Guntert A, Lynham S, et al. Plasma transthyretin as a candidate marker for Alzheimer's disease. *J Alzheimers Dis* (2012) **28**:369–75. doi:10.3233/JAD-2011-110611
137. Thambisetty M, Tripaldi R, Riddoch-Contreras J, Hye A, An Y, Campbell J, et al. Proteome-based plasma markers of brain amyloid-beta deposition in non-demented older individuals. *J Alzheimers Dis* (2010) **22**:1099–109. doi:10.3233/JAD-2010-101350
138. Kiddle SJ, Thambisetty M, Simmons A, Riddoch-Contreras J, Hye A, Westman E, et al. Plasma based markers of [11C] PiB-PET brain amyloid burden. *PLoS One* (2012) **7**:e44260. doi:10.1371/journal.pone.0044260
139. Burnham SC, Faux NG, Wilson W, Laws SM, Ames D, Bedo J, et al. A blood-based predictor for neocortical Abeta burden in Alzheimer's disease: results from the AIBL study. *Mol Psychiatry* (2014) **19**:519–26. doi:10.1038/mp.2013.40
140. Ashton NJ, Kiddle SJ, Graf J, Ward M, Baird AL, Hye A, et al. Blood protein predictors of brain amyloid for enrichment in clinical trials? *Alzheimers Dement (Amst)* (2015) **1**:48–60. doi:10.1016/j.dadm.2014.11.005
141. Hwang KS, Lazaris AS, Eastman JA, Teng E, Thompson PM, Gylys KH, et al. Plasma BDNF levels associate with Pittsburgh compound B binding in the brain. *Alzheimers Dement (Amst)* (2015) **1**:187–93. doi:10.1016/j.dadm.2015.01.005
142. Voyle N, Baker D, Burnham SC, Covin A, Zhang Z, Sangurdekar DP, et al. Blood protein markers of neocortical amyloid-beta burden: a candidate study using SOMAscan technology. *J Alzheimers Dis* (2015) **46**:947–61. doi:10.3233/JAD-150020
143. Lovestone S, Francis P, Kloszewska I, Mecocci P, Simmons A, Soininen H, et al. AddNeuroMed – the European collaboration for the discovery of novel biomarkers for Alzheimer's disease. *Ann N Y Acad Sci* (2009) **1180**:36–46. doi:10.1111/j.1749-6632.2009.05064.x
144. Resnick SM, Goldszal AF, Davatzikos C, Golski S, Kraut MA, Metter EJ, et al. One-year age changes in MRI brain volumes in older adults. *Cereb Cortex* (2000) **10**:464–72. doi:10.1093/cercor/10.5.464
145. Jongbloed W, Van Dijk KD, Mulder SD, van de Berg WD, Blankenstein MA, van der Flier W, et al. Clusterin levels in plasma predict cognitive decline and progression to Alzheimer's disease. *J Alzheimers Dis* (2015) **46**:1103–10. doi:10.3233/JAD-150036
146. Wilson MR, Yerbury JJ, Poon S. Potential roles of abundant extracellular chaperones in the control of amyloid formation and toxicity. *Mol Biosyst* (2008) **4**:42–52. doi:10.1039/B712728F
147. DeMattos RB, Cirrito JR, Parsadanian M, May PC, O'dell MA, Taylor JW, et al. ApoE and clusterin cooperatively suppress Abeta levels and deposition: evidence that ApoE regulates extracellular Abeta metabolism in vivo. *Neuron* (2004) **41**:193–202. doi:10.1016/S0896-6273(03)00850-X
148. Yerbury JJ, Poon S, Meehan S, Thompson B, Kumita JR, Dobson CM, et al. The extracellular chaperone clusterin influences amyloid formation and toxicity by interacting with prefibrillar structures. *FASEB J* (2007) **21**:2312–22. doi:10.1096/fj.06-7986com
149. Nuutinen T, Suuronen T, Kauppinen A, Salminen A. Clusterin: a forgotten player in Alzheimer's disease. *Brain Res Rev* (2009) **61**:89–104. doi:10.1016/j.brainresrev.2009.05.007
150. Yu JT, Tan L. The role of clusterin in Alzheimer's disease: pathways, pathogenesis, and therapy. *Mol Neurobiol* (2012) **45**:314–26. doi:10.1007/s12035-012-8237-1
151. Li X, Ma Y, Wei X, Li Y, Wu H, Zhuang J, et al. Clusterin in Alzheimer's disease: a player in the biological behavior of amyloid-beta. *Neurosci Bull* (2014) **30**:162–8. doi:10.1007/s12264-013-1391-2
152. Killick R, Ribe EM, Al-Shawi R, Malik B, Hooper C, Fernandes C, et al. Clusterin regulates beta-amyloid toxicity via Dickkopf-1-driven induction of the wnt-PCP-JNK pathway. *Mol Psychiatry* (2014) **19**:88–98. doi:10.1038/mp.2012.163
153. Harold D, Abraham R, Hollingworth P, Sims R, Gerrish A, Hamshere ML, et al. Genome-wide association study identifies variants at CLU and PICALM associated with Alzheimer's disease. *Nat Genet* (2009) **41**:1088–93. doi:10.1038/ng1009-1156d
154. Lambert JC, Heath S, Even G, Campion D, Sleegers K, Hiltunen M, et al. Genome-wide association study identifies variants at CLU and CR1 associated with Alzheimer's disease. *Nat Genet* (2009) **41**:1094–9. doi:10.1038/ng.439
155. Thambisetty M, Beason-Held LL, An Y, Kraut M, Nalls M, Hernandez DG, et al. Alzheimer risk variant CLU and brain function during aging. *Biol Psychiatry* (2013) **73**:399–405. doi:10.1016/j.biopsych.2012.05.026
156. Roussotte FF, Gutman BA, Madsen SK, Colby JB, Thompson PM; Alzheimer's Disease Neuroimaging Initiative. Combined effects of Alzheimer risk variants in the CLU and ApoE genes on ventricular expansion patterns in the elderly. *J Neurosci* (2014) **34**:6537–45. doi:10.1523/JNEUROSCI.5236-13.2014
157. Lewis TL, Cao D, Lu H, Mans RA, Su YR, Jungbauer L, et al. Overexpression of human apolipoprotein A-I preserves cognitive function and attenuates neuroinflammation and cerebral amyloid angiopathy in a mouse model of Alzheimer disease. *J Biol Chem* (2010) **285**:36958–68. doi:10.1074/jbc.M110.127829
158. Lopez MF, Krastins B, Ning M. The role of apolipoprotein E in neurodegeneration and cardiovascular disease. *Expert Rev Proteomics* (2014) **11**:371–81. doi:10.1586/14789450.2014.901892
159. Akiyama H, Barger S, Barnum S, Bradt B, Bauer J, Cole GM, et al. Inflammation and Alzheimer's disease. *Neurobiol Aging* (2000) **21**:383–421. doi:10.1016/S0197-4580(00)00124-X
160. Mrak RE, Griffin WS. Potential inflammatory biomarkers in Alzheimer's disease. *J Alzheimers Dis* (2005) **8**:369–75.
161. Ellis KA, Bush AI, Darby D, De Fazio D, Foster J, Hudson P, et al. The Australian imaging, biomarkers and lifestyle (AIBL) study of aging: methodology and baseline characteristics of 1112 individuals recruited for a longitudinal study of Alzheimer's disease. *Int Psychogeriatr* (2009) **21**:672–87. doi:10.1017/S1041610209009405
162. Walsh DM, Selkoe DJ. A beta oligomers – a decade of discovery. *J Neurochem* (2007) **101**:1172–84. doi:10.1111/j.1471-4159.2006.04426.x
163. Sokoloff L. Relationships among local functional activity, energy metabolism, and blood flow in the central nervous system. *Fed Proc* (1981) **40**:2311–6.
164. Bohnen NI, Djang DS, Herholz K, Anzai Y, Minoshima S. Effectiveness and safety of 18F-FDG PET in the evaluation of dementia: a review of the recent literature. *J Nucl Med* (2012) **53**:59–71. doi:10.2967/jnumed.111.096578
165. Mosconi L, Tsui WH, Herholz K, Pupi A, Drzezga A, Lucignani G, et al. Multicenter standardized 18F-FDG PET diagnosis of mild cognitive impairment, Alzheimer's disease, and other dementias. *J Nucl Med* (2008) **49**:390–8. doi:10.2967/jnumed.107.045385
166. Morbelli S, Piccardo A, Villavecchia G, Dessi B, Brugnolo A, Piccini A, et al. Mapping brain morphological and functional conversion patterns in amnestic MCI: a voxel-based MRI and FDG-PET study. *Eur J Nucl Med Mol Imaging* (2010) **37**:36–45. doi:10.1007/s00259-009-1218-6
167. Laforce R Jr, Tosun D, Ghosh P, Lehmann M, Madison CM, Weiner MW, et al. Parallel ICA of FDG-PET and PiB-PET in three conditions with underlying Alzheimer's pathology. *Neuroimage Clin* (2014) **4**:508–16. doi:10.1016/j.nicl.2014.03.005

168. Shokouhi S, Claassen D, Riddle W. Imaging brain metabolism and pathology in Alzheimer's disease with positron emission tomography. *J Alzheimers Dis Parkinsonism* (2014) **4**:143. doi:10.4172/2161-0460.1000143
169. Fodero-Tavoletti MT, Okamura N, Furumoto S, Mulligan RS, Connor AR, McLean CA, et al. 18F-THK523: a novel in vivo tau imaging ligand for Alzheimer's disease. *Brain* (2011) **134**:1089–100. doi:10.1093/brain/awr038
170. Chien DT, Bahri S, Szardenings AK, Walsh JC, Mu F, Su MY, et al. Early clinical PET imaging results with the novel PHF-tau radioligand [F-18]-T807. *J Alzheimers Dis* (2013) **34**:457–68. doi:10.3233/JAD-122059
171. Chien DT, Szardenings AK, Bahri S, Walsh JC, Mu F, Xia C, et al. Early clinical PET imaging results with the novel PHF-tau radioligand [F18]-T808. *J Alzheimers Dis* (2014) **38**:171–84. doi:10.3233/JAD-130098
172. Han X, Rozen S, Boyle SH, Hellegers C, Cheng H, Burke JR, et al. Metabolomics in early Alzheimer's disease: identification of altered plasma sphingolipidome using shotgun lipidomics. *PLoS One* (2011) **6**:e21643. doi:10.1371/journal.pone.0021643
173. Gonzalez-Dominguez R, Garcia A, Garcia-Barrera T, Barbas C, Gomez-Ariza JL. Metabolomic profiling of serum in the progression of Alzheimer's disease by capillary electrophoresis-mass spectrometry. *Electrophoresis* (2014) **35**:3321–30. doi:10.1002/elps.201400196
174. Mapstone M, Cheema AK, Fiandaca MS, Zhong X, Mhyre TR, Macarthur LH, et al. Plasma phospholipids identify antecedent memory impairment in older adults. *Nat Med* (2014) **20**:415–8. doi:10.1038/nm.3466
175. Whiley L, Sen A, Heaton J, Proitsi P, Garcia-Gomez D, Leung R, et al. Evidence of altered phosphatidylcholine metabolism in Alzheimer's disease. *Neurobiol Aging* (2014) **35**:271–8. doi:10.1016/j.neurobiolaging.2013.08.001
176. Desire L, Blondiaux E, Carriere J, Haddad R, Sol O, Fehlbaum-Beurdeley P, et al. Blood transcriptomic biomarkers of Alzheimer's disease patients treated with EHT 0202. *J Alzheimers Dis* (2013) **34**:469–83. doi:10.3233/JAD-121501
177. Lunnon K, Sattlecker M, Furney SJ, Coppola G, Simmons A, Proitsi P, et al. A blood gene expression marker of early Alzheimer's disease. *J Alzheimers Dis* (2013) **33**:737–53. doi:10.3233/JAD-2012-121363

Expanding the repertoire of biomarkers for Alzheimer's disease: targeted and non-targeted approaches

*Douglas Galasko**

Department of Neurosciences, Shiley-Marcos Alzheimer's Disease Research Center, University of California, San Diego, La Jolla, CA, USA

Edited by:
Charlotte Elisabeth Teunissen, VU University Medical Center Amsterdam, Netherlands

Reviewed by:
Davide Chiasserini, University of Perugia, Italy
Hugo Marcel Vanderstichele, ADx NeuroSciences, Belgium
Claire Bridel, VU University Medical Center Amsterdam, Netherlands

***Correspondence:**
Douglas Galasko
dgalasko@ucsd.edu

The first biofluid markers developed for Alzheimer's disease (AD) used targeted approaches for discovery. These initial biomarkers were directed at key protein constituents of the hallmark brain lesions in AD. Biomarkers for plaques targeted the amyloid beta protein (Aβ) and for tangles, the microtubule-associated protein tau. Cerebrospinal fluid levels of Aβ and tau have excellent diagnostic utility and can be used to monitor aspects of therapeutic development. Recent research has extended our current concepts of AD, which now include a slow buildup of pathology during a long pre-symptomatic period, a complex cascade of pathological pathways in the brain that may accelerate once symptoms develop, the potential of aggregated proteins to spread across brain pathways, and interactions with vascular and other age-associated brain pathologies. There are many potential roles for biomarkers within this landscape. A more diverse set of biomarkers would provide a better picture of the staging and state of pathological events in the brain across the stages of AD. The aim of this review is to focus on methods of biomarker discovery that may help to expand the currently accepted biomarkers. Opportunities and approaches for targeted and non-targeted (or –omic) biomarker discovery are highlighted, with examples from recent studies. How biomarker discoveries can be developed and integrated to become useful tools in diagnostic and therapeutic efforts is discussed.

Keywords: Alzheimer's disease, biomarker, biofluid, amyloid, tau, synapse, proteomics

INTRODUCTION

Biomarkers have many potential uses in Alzheimer's disease (AD), related neurodegenerative disorders and brain aging. Initial efforts to develop diagnostic biomarkers for AD were focused on the hallmark pathological lesions of senile plaques and neurofibrillary tangles. Amyloid beta-protein (Aβ), an integral component of plaques, and the microtubule-associated protein tau, the major protein found in tangles, were detected in cerebrospinal fluid (CSF). Sensitive enzyme-linked immunosorbent assays (ELISAs) were developed to selectively detect pathogenic forms of Aβ (Aβ42) and tau, with the later advent of assays for phosphorylated forms of tau (P-tau) (1–3). Different phosphor-epitopes of tau have been identified in CSF and are increased in AD, including tau phosphorylated at threonine181 (the form most commonly measured), serine 199, and serine

231 (4). Increased levels of P-tau are more specific for AD than other dementias and may add value in differential diagnosis (4, 5). The profile of decreased Aβ42 and increased total tau and P-tau in CSF has high diagnostic value for AD (6) and has been a mainstay of AD biomarker research. Changes in CSF biomarkers are apparent in early symptomatic stages of AD, such as mild cognitive impairment (MCI) (7), and also occur pre-symptomatically (8). In these settings, the core biomarkers can provide prognostic information, for example, which patients with MCI may progress to AD dementia (7, 9–11). Also, studies have shown that patients with MCI or AD with higher baseline levels of CSF tau or P-tau (12, 13), and more recently higher baseline levels of the postsynaptic protein neurogranin (14) may show more rapid progression. This indicates the value of CSF biomarkers for predicting progression, e.g., for prognosis in preclinical stages of AD. Many forms of A-beta exist in CSF, and profiling N-terminal truncated forms was shown to increase prognostic value in MCI in one study (15).

Several themes that have emerged from AD research highlight the increased need for biomarkers, and also set the stage for how they may be used. First, AD is now viewed as a chronic and slowly progressive disorder, with a long buildup of pathology that precedes symptoms by a decade or longer (16). Also, among people with late-onset AD, autopsy studies highlight the frequent co-occurrence of other brain pathologies, such as vascular changes (macro-infarcts, lacunes and micro-infarcts, amyloid angiopathy, arteriosclerosis, and microbleeds) and other protein aggregates (e.g., alpha-Synuclein and TDP43) (17, 18). These may contribute to dementia and can be difficult to detect during life. In patients with atypical presentations, such as younger onset of dementia, the clinical picture may not be clear, and biomarkers can provide pointers to underlying pathology. Finally, treatment interventions for AD are shifting to earlier intervention, including stages of prodromal AD, where symptoms are mild, and most recently to prevention studies, where cognition falls within normal limits. Biomarkers have valuable roles to play in this pre-symptomatic stage to provide measures that may guide therapeutics. By measuring several biomarkers in CSF through individual or multiplex assays, it may be possible to index a number of biochemical processes in the brain that are informative about AD and related neurodegenerative disorders simultaneously. This enhances the value of CSF sampling. This review will summarize the potential roles for biomarkers and how approaches to biomarker discovery can help to build a pipeline that will address these needs and inform risk assessment, diagnosis, and treatment (**Figure 1**).

SOURCES OF FLUID BIOMARKERS

The most obvious source of biomarkers relevant to the brain is CSF, which bathes the brain and spinal cord. CSF biomarkers reflect overall brain biochemistry, and processes such as neuronal damage, synapse loss, and inflammation may result in detectable biomarker changes in CSF if they are extensive enough. CSF is sampled through the lumbar space and may have different concentrations of analytes compared to the ventricular CSF. Typically, analytes are more concentrated in lumbar CSF, as noted for Aβ40, Aβ42, and tau (19). The question of concentration gradients within the lumbar CSF arises for many analytes and needs to be studied – this is not a major problem for Tau, P-tau, and Aβ42. Blood derivatives, such as plasma and serum, are easier to access than CSF, but typically reflect the body as a whole. If a brain-specific protein crosses into the blood, it may be subject to dilution, the action of proteases, and clearance by the liver and kidney, rendering it difficult to detect. As a further complication, systemic features of AD, such as weight loss or lower physical activity may result in subtle changes in blood biomarker levels.

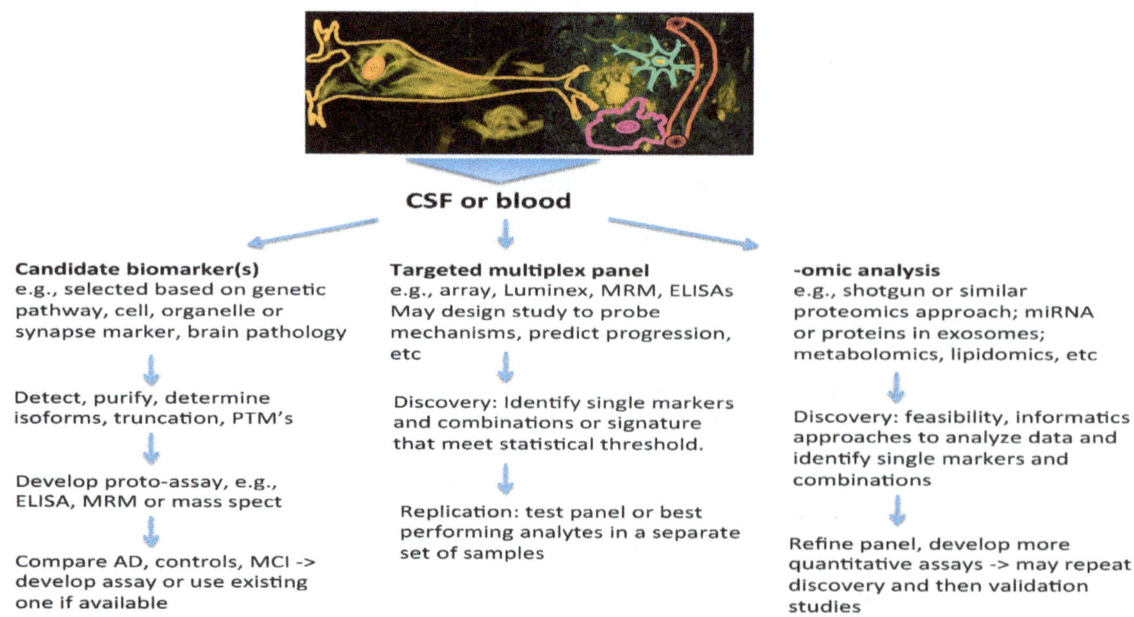

FIGURE 1 | Biomarker discovery for Alzheimer's disease – approaches.

These are many of the reasons why it has been extremely difficult to identify a blood biomarker that directly reflects the state of neurodegeneration (20, 21).

There are other questions or areas where blood biomarkers may have utility. Some plasma or serum analytes may relate to traits that predispose to neurodegeneration, for example, biomarkers that may be influenced by susceptibility genes. If age or environmental risk factors related to dementia have systemic effects, then these may be evident through the analysis of blood biomarkers. Blood biomarkers are particularly helpful as measures of drug levels and can provide peripheral indices of target engagement. Blood cells, e.g., lymphocytes or leukocytes, may be used to derive immune signatures or measures of RNA expression that may be indices of susceptibility for AD. Plasma and blood biomarkers are influenced by genetic factors and a wide spectrum of environmental factors, for example, diet, systemic illness, and physical activity. A recent paper studied over 300 plasma analytes longitudinally in twins, and identified variability that could be attributed to all of these factors. These findings suggest that a search for peripheral markers for AD may be extremely complicated, because in addition to these variables, aging is yet another factor that may impact on levels of peripheral markers. Plasma levels of Aβ, including ratios between different forms of Aβ (such as the ratio of Aβ42/Aβ40) have been inconsistent across studies, are only weakly correlated with CSF levels of Aβ or with markers of amyloid brain imaging, and although they may have some predictive value for the development of AD, this is relatively low [reviewed in Ref. (22)]. Peripheral issue may be a source of pathological proteins if there are systemic features of a neurodegenerative disease. This has been identified in Parkinson's disease (PD), where nerve endings can be stained for abnormal forms of alpha-synuclein in skin and salivary gland biopsy (23).

Regardless of whether a biomarker is measured in blood, CSF, or in biopsy material, data that shed light on how the biomarker is produced, released, cleared, and metabolized should be sought. To understand the biomarker comprehensively, it may require data from cell, model organism, and animal studies, as well as human biofluids and postmortem tissue. A recent development is the ability to study kinetics of CSF and plasma analytes by administering stable isotopes intravenously or orally to human subjects (24, 25). Examining the relationships between different types of biomarkers can also inform about pathogenetic processes, for example, by correlating biofluid biomarker changes with neuroimaging markers. This also allows modeling of when the biomarker becomes abnormal and how it changes during the early course of AD (26).

EXPANDED ROLES FOR BIOMARKERS IN AD

There are many potential roles of biomarkers for AD and neurodegenerative disorders (**Table 1**). New biomarker discovery efforts need to take into consideration the current landscape of AD diagnosis and treatment efforts. The clinical diagnosis of typical AD by experts is often highly accurate; therefore, diagnostic biomarkers should be sensitive enough to help in early diagnosis, e.g., at stages of MCI or prodromal AD (27, 28). Because the sensitivity of CSF Aβ42, tau, and P-tau to discriminate prodromal AD from cognitively normal individuals is high, it may be challenging for additional biomarkers to improve on this. The differential diagnosis of unusual or atypical cases is a situation where biomarkers may clearly augment clinical judgment. Evaluating whether non-AD pathology may be present is an important question, particularly in elderly individuals with cognitive problems, and additional biomarkers could be helpful if they inform about processes, such as alpha-Synuclein, TDP-43, or vascular brain pathology. Mixed pathology is often present in the brains of elderly individuals with dementia, and a biomarker panel that allowed clear prediction of the types of underlying pathology would be useful.

Therapeutic efforts for AD are shifting to earlier intervention, including studies of secondary prevention, and even primary prevention in people with genetic predisposition. Potential uses of CSF biomarkers in clinical trials for AD and PD were recently reviewed in detail (46). Neuropathology and clinical research have shown that there are preclinical stages of AD during which amyloid and tau pathology accumulates, before the onset of memory decline (47). This provides an opportunity to start treatment interventions with the goal of delaying the onset of AD. Changes in biomarkers may provide a clearer early readout from prevention studies than changes in cognitive measures. Biomarkers are critical to identifying the presence of amyloid or tau brain pathology in this situation. For studies of early intervention, screening biomarkers, e.g., blood tests, that can improve the likelihood of detecting pathological brain changes through a more definitive test, such as molecular brain imaging and lumbar puncture, would be a great asset.

Biomarkers may help to improve the understanding of risk factors and mechanisms of disease. One would expect that causative or susceptibility genetic factors should be easy to link to biomarkers in biofluids. This has only been demonstrated in a few instances. For example, in AD, the APOE e4 allele has not yet been associated with a unique biomarker profile but modulates levels of the ApoE protein (48, 49). Inflammation plays a role in AD and other neurodegenerative disorders, and genetic variants related to the TREM2 gene increase the risk of AD and other dementias (50). In CSF, levels of a secreted soluble form of TREM were recently found to be decreased in AD (51). Other inflammatory biomarkers, such as secreted cytokines and chemokines, are unchanged or slightly increased in CSF in AD (52, 53). CSF biomarkers have been used as endophenotypes to discover genetic variants related to their levels, for example, CSF tau in AD (39), and CSF biomarkers related to inflammation (54). Genetic forms of non-AD dementia have provided clues for novel biomarkers. For example, inherited forms of frontotemporal dementia (FTD) due to mutations in the progranulin gene result in haplo-insufficiency with decreased production of granulin. Correspondingly, levels of granulin in plasma and CSF are markedly (and diagnostically) decreased (55). Burgeoning research on AD pathology has identified abnormalities in many biological processes, and it is likely that many pathogenic steps and events are occurring in a cascade (56). It may be feasible to develop biomarkers that can help to track many of these events,

TABLE 1 | Roles for fluid biomarkers in Alzheimer's disease.

Roles in diagnosis, staging, and prognosis	Examples of biofluid markers	Comments	Reference
Screening or diagnosis with a blood test	Plasma Aβ42/Aβ40	Weak predictive value Not diagnostic	Toledo et al. (22)
	Multi-analyte test panels, e.g., phospholipids Multi-analyte protein screening (e.g., Somascan)	Initial good discrimination, needs replication	Mapstone et al. (29), Sattlecker et al. (30)
	Plasma t-Tau	Slight increase in AD; much overlap	Zetterberg et al. (31)
	Auto-antibody profile; peptoids	Needs replication	Reddy et al. (32), Nagele et al. (33)
Diagnosis of AD vs. control	CSF Aβ42, t-Tau, P-Tau	Validated extensively	Skillbäck et al. (5)
Diagnosis of AD pathology at prodromal or MCI stage	CSF Aβ42, t-Tau, P-Tau	Validated extensively	Mattsson et al. (7)
Differential diagnosis	CSF Aβ42, t-Tau, P-Tau	Validated extensively	Skillbäck et al. (5)
Predict progression, e.g., from control to AD, MCI to AD, and rate of progression in AD	High levels of CSF t-Tau, P-Tau Ratios e.g., Aβ42/t-Tau Low CSF Aβ42	Validated extensively Aβ42 alone does not predict AD progression rate	Shaw et al. (10)
	N-terminal truncated CSF Aβ42	MCI progression	Vanderstichele et al. (15)
	Neurogranin	MCI progression	Kvartsberg et al. (14)
	YKL40	MCI progression, control progression when combined with Aβ42	Craig-Schapiro et al. (34)
	Visinin-like protein-1	MCI progression; control progression especially when combined with Aβ42	Tarawneh et al. (35)
Diagnosis of non-AD disorders	Few specific markers, but ratios and patterns help, e.g., very high tau in CJD; ratio of P-tau/T-tau in FTLD-tau; high neurofilament-L levels in vascular cognitive impairment, PSP and FTLD		Skillbäck et al. (36), Hu et al. (37)
	α-Synuclein	Decreased in Parkinson's but sensitivity is not diagnostically useful	Parnetti et al. (38)
Understand genetic and other risk factors	CSF t-Tau, P-tau, Aβ42 ApoE protein, clusterin, inflammatory cytokines TREM-2	Genes or SNPs associated with AD genetic risk may relate to levels of CSF biomarkers	Cruchaga et al. (39)
Markers of pathobiology Synaptic damage Neuronal damage Axonal tracts Inflammation	Neurogranin, SNAP-25 Visinin-like-protein-1; t-Tau NFL Cytokines, chemokines, c3, YKL-40	Many other potential pathways and processes may be reflected in CSF	
Blood–brain barrier integrity and small vessel CNS ischemia	CSF: serum albumin ratio, IgG index, MMP 2, 3, and 9; NFL	Altered in vascular cognitive impairment	Rosenberg et al. (40)
Roles in therapeutics	**Examples**	**Comments**	**Reference**
Preclinical drug development	Aβ42, t-Tau, P-Tau sAPPα and sAPPβ Oligomeric forms of Aβ and Tau	Can be used to evaluate compounds in cell and animal models	Liu et al. (41), Jeppsson et al. (42)
Target engagement in pharmacodynamic studies	Aβ40 and 42 in CSF and plasma for gamma-secretase inhibitors sAPPα, sAPPβ, and Aβ for BACE inhibitors	Has helped with dose finding	Fleisher et al. (43)
Detailed studies of synthesis and clearance	SILK studies for Aβ metabolism	Used to characterize detailed pharmacodynamics of anti-Aβ therapeutics	Bateman et al. (24)
Patient selection or stratification	CSF Aβ42, t-Tau, P-tau	Enroll patients with AD signature	Coric et al. (44)
Identify toxicity	Increases in CSF biomarkers of neuronal damage or of inflammation		Van Gool et al. (45)
Provide biological support for treatment effect	Changes in CSF Aβ-related biomarkers indicating target engagement and of t-Tau, P-Tau, or synaptic markers such as neurogranin in a direction indicating reduction of neurodegeneration	Changes in a group of markers could support anti-amyloid therapeutics	

This table is not intended as a comprehensive listing, but shows representative biomarkers that can aid in diagnostic or therapeutic efforts. The biomarkers in this table are discussed in the text. The majority of markers are proteins discovered through candidate approaches, but there is room for an expanded suite of markers using diverse discovery approaches to improve our understanding of AD.

t-Tau, total tau levels; α-Syn, alpha-Synuclein; sAPP, secreted amyloid protein precursor; NFL, neurofilament light; TREM2, triggering receptor expressed on myeloid cells 2; MBP, myelin basic protein; MMP, matrix metalloprotease; BACE, beta-site APP cleaving enzyme 1; SILK, stable isotope kinetic labeling; CJD, Creutzfeld–Jacob disease; PSP, progressive supranuclear palsy; FTLD, fronto-temporal lobar degeneration.

for example, microglial activation, inflammation, synaptic damage, and dysfunction (discussed later). This approach, together with neuroimaging methods, offers an opportunity to build a more complete picture of neurodegeneration in living patients at different stages of disease.

There are many potential therapeutic applications of biomarkers in AD. These typically have involved targeted biomarkers. During preclinical development, screening for gamma-secretase inhibitors and modulators and BACE inhibitors in cell and animal models have obtained their readout by using assays for the same secreted forms of Aβ that are used in AD diagnosis (57–59). These assays can be further applied to animal models and in human studies to identify target engagement and pharmacodynamic effects. A more detailed application is through CSF catheter placement to sample CSF during 24–36 h. This has been extended using stable isotope labeling kinetics (SILK) to estimate the fractional production and clearance rates of Aβ from CSF (24). In clinical trials, CSF biomarkers may be used to select patients or to stratify treatment. For example, in trials that aim to enroll patients with MCI due to AD, requiring a baseline CSF biomarker profile can increase confidence that the study population has symptoms due to AD rather than other causes. Target engagement may be demonstrated for certain types of amyloid-related interventions, in particular, secretase inhibitors. For example, gamma-secretase inhibitors that were studied in human clinical trials (43) and Beta-secretase inhibitors (60) showed robust effects in decreasing secreted forms of APP as well as Aβ in early phase studies, and the gamma-secretase inhibitor semagacestat showed plasma biomarker evidence of target activation in a phase 3 trial (61). Mass spectrometry (MS) characterization has identified a specific Aβ peptide signature after BACE inhibitor treatment (60). However, it is more challenging to show target engagement by antibodies directed against Aβ, because these bind Aβ and alter its levels in CSF and plasma. As novel drug targets are identified, efforts to identify companion biomarkers that help to identify immediate and downstream effects of drug action should be pursued.

Changes in levels of tau and P-tau in CSF have been examined as prototypic AD biomarkers of neurodegeneration or neuronal damage, with the hypothesis that neuroprotective or disease-modifying drug effects may result in a decrease of these markers. It is likely that profiling biomarkers more broadly could be more informative. For example, biomarkers that index aspects of pre- and postsynaptic change, microglial activation, and astrocytic responses combined with neuroimaging could provide greater insights into the dynamics and interactions of neurons and glial cells in response to interventions. In efforts to make a claim to support drug efficacy, biofluid biomarkers are expected to play a supporting rather than a primary role. For example, if one of the effects of a drug treatment is to slow neurodegeneration enough to produce a meaningful cognitive readout, biomarker changes could be used to identify which disease-related pathways have been affected. To better understand events during neurodegeneration or disease progression, further exploration using non-targeted –omic approaches is worth pursuing. A complicated situation arises if biomarker changes are present in the absence of an appropriate clinical readout; this could indicate that the drug hit its target and influenced biomarkers but this is ineffective clinically, or that the changes in the biomarker are ambiguous. For example, CSF P-tau levels have been shown to decrease significantly in patients who received bapineuzumab, with a trend for total tau to decrease, but this did not correlate with clinical efficacy (62).

APPROACHES TO DISCOVER BIOMARKERS IN BIOFLUIDS

Protein and peptide biomarkers in biofluids have formed the mainstay of clinical diagnostic tests in AD and other neurodegenerative disorders. As discussed above, despite over two decades of research, we have identified only a small number of fluid biomarkers for AD. The currently available biomarkers of CSF Aβ, tau, and P-tau have problems with measurement and standardization issues (63) that have hindered their routine and widespread use. The development of quality standards, a MS assay, and second-generation assays for these analytes are likely to improve this situation. As yet there are no established biomarkers for other neurodegenerative disorders and for vascular cognitive impairment. In view of the complexity of AD, the coexistence of mixed pathology in late-onset dementia, and the increasing emphasis for early diagnosis of AD and other neurodegenerative disorders, the search for additional biomarkers is highly warranted. One challenge is that CSF and plasma both contain proteins whose concentration spans several orders of magnitude, and almost all other proteins are overshadowed in concentration by albumin. Methods to identify novel biomarkers, in particular, proteomics, have improved, allowing post-translational modifications to be sought, and low abundance proteins (members of the "deep proteome") to be detected. Two main strategies for biomarker discovery have emerged, namely, targeted or candidate biomarker discovery, and multiplex or –omic approaches.

Targeted Approaches to Identify and Develop Protein and Peptide Biomarkers

The search for targeted or candidate biomarkers for AD met with significant early successes. Based on the expectation that abnormal forms of Aβ and tau could be found in CSF, methods to detect forms of these proteins in CSF and plasma were developed. Many important and complex steps have been involved in understanding and translating these hallmark AD biomarkers. To start, assays that selectively detected the longer and more aggregation-prone form of Aβ, Aβ42, were required. Total levels of Aβ in CSF were unchanged in AD, and the paradox that levels of Aβ42 were selectively decreased in CSF in AD (1) has been "explained" by aggregation of this peptide within the brain, leaving less to diffuse into the CSF. CSF levels of Aβ42 were later found to correlate inversely with the extent of fibrillar brain amyloid deposition as measured by amyloid PET imaging (64, 65). Although increased levels of CSF tau were present in AD relative to controls, why this occurred was not clear – CSF tau is not a marker of tangle formation, but is increased in situations of significant neuronal damage, for example, after acute stroke (66) or in Creutzfeld–Jacob disease (36). Assays for specifically P-tau also showed increases in AD, and CSF P-tau had higher specificity for AD than did increases of total tau. Only a few studies have tried to identify the forms of tau that are released into CSF. These were found to be N-terminal fragments of tau, with little if any of the full-length protein present (67, 68). The mechanisms of the release of tau into CSF remain unclear. Although converging data across many laboratories and studies have confirmed the profile of decreased Aβ42 and increased total and P-tau in CSF, cutoffs vary across laboratories (63, 69). Extensive quality control efforts have helped to decrease the variability. There are new efforts under way to develop fully automated assays for these key analytes, which will dramatically improve standardization.

Selecting a candidate biomarker has several advantages. Defined biochemical pathways and pathological mechanisms can help to relate the candidate to AD or to another neurodegenerative disorder, which may help to "make sense" of findings regarding the biomarker. Tools for detecting candidate biomarkers may be available, and sensitive detection methods can be developed. As a recent example, tau is released into CSF after neuronal injury. Increased levels of tau can be detected in plasma using ultrasensitive assay methods and were found to be transiently increased in boxers after bouts (70). Post-translational modifications of candidate biomarkers may also be sought and may provide markers related to mechanisms of disease. For example, phosphorylation is important in regulatory and signaling pathways and has been implicated in altering the solubility and promoting aggregation of proteins. P-tau (4) and alpha-synuclein (71) are detectable in CSF and may provide insights into processes relevant to AD and PD, respectively.

Although CSF Aβ42 and tau reflect certain steps of pathology in the brain, much attention has focused on small oligomeric aggregates of these proteins. Evidence suggests that oligomeric forms of Aβ may be the culprits responsible for toxicity (72–74) and also suggests that oligomers and aggregates of tau are species that contribute to neurodegeneration and correlate with cognitive loss in postmortem studies (75, 76). Also, aggregated or oligomeric forms of Aβ and tau may contribute to propagation of pathology (77). Despite the development of sensitive assays that can detect extremely low levels of Aβ oligomers, these have not been consistently or reliably identified in CSF in relation to AD (78, 79).

Several further examples of recent candidate biomarker discovery highlight the continued value of candidate approaches. A candidate approach led to the identification of the neuronal calcium sensor protein visinin-like protein-1 in CSF, and levels were found to be increased in AD relative to controls and predicted progression from non-demented to mild dementia (35) Similarly, a candidate approach was recently used to identify the dendritic protein neurogranin, which is involved in long-term potentiation and calcium regulation, and is decreased and mislocalized in brain tissue in AD. After initial characterization in CSF by HPLC and MS methods an ELISA was developed. Levels of neurogranin were reported to be increased in CSF in AD, even at the stage of MCI (80), and predicted progression from prodromal AD to dementia, as well as rate of progression of MRI change in AD (14). As a second example, genetic studies have implicated variation in the gene that encodes TREM2 as a risk factor in some patients with late-onset AD and later for other neurodegenerative disorders [reviewed in Ref. (81)]. Studies into the biology of cells derived from people homozygous for TREM2 mutations revealed impaired secretion of a cleaved fragment of TREM2. Decreased levels of this fragment were detected using an ELISA in CSF samples from patients with AD (51). Another example is the measurement of levels of granulin to identify people with mutations in the progranulin gene that predisposes to FTD. Progranulin mutations result in haplo-insufficiency and therefore people who carry mutations have a marked decrease in levels of secreted granulin in plasma and CSF (82).

One further example of an important application of CSF biomarkers relates to blood–brain barrier (BBB) integrity. An increased CSF:serum ratio of albumin is an established index used for many years as an indicator of loss of BBB integrity, and together with the IgG index and measurement of myelin basic protein levels, has been used as a diagnostic aid in multiple sclerosis. More recently, other markers of BBB integrity have emerged, particularly in relation to vascular cognitive impairment, and analysis of matrix metalloproteases and neurofilament-light levels have been proposed to supplement the albumin ratio and increase the diagnostic utility for subcortical small vessel disease (40).

A broader targeted approach to discovery is to multiplex known assays in combination [e.g., Luminex panels of assays of secreted proteins; multiple reagent monitoring (MRM) methods to examine selected panels of analytes with spiked in calibrator peptides for quantitation]. Several studies in AD have used arrays or multiplex ELISA-type assays for known secreted proteins to identify biomarkers in plasma and CSF (83, 84). Findings have been inconsistent, and different panels of plasma biomarkers have emerged from different studies, depending on analytical as well as biostatistical methods. Some of the analytes measured in these panels of secreted proteins in CSF showed correlations with cognitive test scores (85), or neuroimaging changes (86) although a validated panel of markers capable of tracking progression in AD has not yet emerged. Data from these studies were used to examine genetic variation associated with CSF levels of 59 proteins, and there were associations for proteins involved in inflammatory signaling (54). There are no validated CSF biomarkers for most non-AD dementias, although patterns of biomarkers, such as CSF P-tau181/total tau ratio, may be helpful in discriminating tauopathies from TDP43-associated FTLD disorders (37).

Targeted biomarker approaches have some disadvantages. Their detection and analysis need specific reagents, e.g., antibodies with high affinity, and antibodies against different regions are typically required to enable quantitative assays to be established and post-translational modifications to be analyzed. Finally, carrying out serial studies of candidate biomarkers and running individual assays to obtain multi-analyte data can be time consuming.

Highly Sensitive Assays

Many analytes detectable in plasma or CSF occur at low levels. This can pose a challenge to routine methods of analysis, such as ELISA. Recent technological refinements have resulted in ultrasensitive assay methods, capable of quantitation over low picomolar or femtomolar levels of analytes (87). For example, immuno-PCR, in which an oligonucleotide is conjugated to a detector antibody in a sandwich format, then amplified, has been developed and refined to allowed multiplex assays (88). Another refinement, single molecule arrays (SIMOA), which divides samples into microwells and allows higher detection of signal to background, has been used to identify changes in plasma Aβ in patients who had experienced cardiac arrest (89) and increases in serum or plasma levels of tau in professional athletes after concussion (90), in combat-related traumatic brain injury (TBI) (91), and in patients with major brain trauma (92). Plasma levels of tau are slightly increased in AD compared to controls but are not diagnostically useful (31).The general theme that measuring multiple analytes may paint a more detailed and clearer picture applies to the setting of TBI: recent studies have shown that biomarkers of neuronal, axonal, and astroglial injury appear acutely after the injury, and that axonal markers such as neurofilament protein persist longer in plasma and CSF than markers such as tau (93).

Non-Targeted Approaches to Protein and Peptide Biomarker Discovery

Non-targeted approaches to biomarker discovery typically involve multiplex and –omic methods, which range from analyzing 10 to 100 analytes to performing large-scale unbiased proteomic or metabolomic screens. These approaches have the advantages of providing coverage of a wide range of potential biomarkers, and of identifying novel markers and mechanisms that may not have been obvious from pathogenic mechanisms or pathology. Also, analyses of interactions between markers, and of how markers relate to biological pathways, can be undertaken. There are several challenges to conducting, analyzing and interpreting large-scale –omic studies. For single analyte assays, a great deal of effort typically goes into development, standardization, and quantitation. By contrast, the analytes in large-scale –omic or similar methods may not be accurately quantified across their dynamic range. Both plasma and CSF have a few dominant proteins, in particular albumin, which are orders of magnitude higher in concentration than the vast majority of proteins and peptides. Methods to deplete the most dominant proteins are often used in –omic studies, but these preparation steps may alter the proteome. It is encouraging that test–retest proteomic analyses after immunodepletion of major proteins in CSF from subjects who underwent repeated lumbar punctures about 1 week apart provided evidence for a reasonably stable proteome (94). Detecting truncated forms of proteins or post-translational modifications may be more difficult in –omic studies using biofluids. Study design and data analysis need to be carefully considered to take proteomic studies from the stage of description or annotation to searching for group differences and the complex series of downstream steps that may lead to identification of candidate peptides and potential markers (95, 96). It is easy to identify false positive biomarker hits when hundreds of potential markers are analyzed and multiple comparisons are made, therefore separate cohorts for discovery and validation are essential. When interpreting findings, it is important to consider what factors may have contributed to the significant group of analytes. For example, vascular disease often coexists with AD, and vascular risk factors may be over-represented in AD patients compared to controls. Especially for proteomic studies of plasma, it is important to take factors such as hypertension, diabetes, weight loss, and decreased physical activity into account during data analyses. As an example of the promise of proteomic studies, recent promising results were reported in a large-scale effort to identify potential biomarkers related to aging through proteomic analysis of plasma, and strategies used in this project are summarized in Ref. (96).

Many non-targeted large-scale proteomic studies of CSF have been conducted in AD. It is interesting to note that Aβ42 and tau have not been detected as AD biomarkers in proteomic analyses of CSF. Early methods of separation, such as 2-dimensional gel electrophoresis (2DGE), resulted in detection and annotation of members of the CSF proteome, but few consistent markers specific for AD appeared. An extension of 2DGE called DIGE uses different fluorescent labels for biosamples from different groups of subjects (e.g., controls and those with disease) and allows for subtle differences to be identified. This has resulted in the discovery of a few novel biomarkers for AD, notably YKL40, a molecule secreted by astrocytes whose levels are increased in CSF in AD (34). MS methods remain the workhorse of proteomics and have been refined and improved in recent years. Analyses of CSF have continued to expand the catalog of proteins detectable in CSF, and a recent study identified and annotated over 2,500 proteins, each identified by at least 2 unique peptides [Ref. (97); database available at http://129.177.231.63/csf-pr/].

Technical improvements in MS have greatly improved the reproducibility of sample runs. Isobaric labeling of peptides, followed by a MS pipeline, can be used to compare samples from different groups of subjects. An approach that resembles the methods used in DIGE yielded several candidate peptide biomarkers for AD (98). Other approaches have allowed targeted quantitative analysis of selected peptides, as well as multiplexing (99, 100). By spiking in samples with heavily labeled known peptides as calibrators, a series of analytes may be analyzed quantitatively, termed MRM or selective reaction monitoring (SRM). For example, an exploratory proteomic study using CSF from patients with familial AD and controls yielded a set of novel candidate biomarkers (101), but these have not been replicated. Another study examined a panel of 39 candidate CSF biomarkers using MRM, and identified 4 that changed over 12 months with progression of AD (102). Recent studies of PD have explored whether a panel of analytes monitored using MRM may have value in diagnosis or relate to cognitive impairment (103). A pipeline for incorporating SRM methods into novel proteomic biomarker discovery has been proposed and its feasibility was demonstrated in a mouse cancer model (104). The sensitivity of MRM is much higher than that of untargeted proteomics, but it still is easier to quantify more abundant proteins, and antibody methods for highly sensitive assays have advantages for lower abundance analytes. Another analytical approach, immunoprecipitation followed by MS, allows differently processed forms of the same protein to be measured in biofluid samples. This targeted approach of MS has been used for the analysis of different forms of Aβ peptides with a variety of different N- and C-terminal amino acids and has provided signatures of the effects of BACE inhibitors on APP processing (60).

Novel approaches to multiplex detection, such as the use of aptamer-based assays or antibody arrays, have allowed the profiling of hundreds to over one thousand analytes simultaneously from small starting volumes of biofluid sample, although the data generated are not truly quantitative (105). Aptamer approaches to screen for plasma biomarkers for AD are under way and have shown some initial promise. For example, in one study, a panel of 13 proteins predicted AD with an area under the ROC curve of 0.7 (30). Other studies that used this technology have found differences between patients with MCI and AD compared to controls, but the specific analytes that were most highly predictive have differed across studies (106, 107). Aptamer technology has also been applied to identify members of the plasma proteome that are changed with aging. In an aging twin study that was followed by replication in several other cohorts, 13 plasma proteins were identified that showed robust changes with aging, some of which are growth factors (108). About 26% of the variability of the markers measured in twins could be explained by a heritable component. Understanding more about the biology of analytes that are detected by aptamer-based tests, and conducting replication studies will be helpful to advance this novel approach to protein biomarker identification.

Non-Protein and "Unconventional" Biomarkers

Antibodies directed against novel antigens have been sought in serum or plasma as diagnostic markers for AD. Results have not always been consistent, and biomarkers have not yet been established using this method. One approach is to look for antibodies against pathogenic proteins, such as different forms of Aβ, e.g., by screening plasma or serum using micro-arrays. In recent examples, studies that screened for novel conformational forms of pathogenic proteins or unknown antigens that may be diagnostically altered in AD, PD, or other disorders have used auto-antibody and peptoid approaches [e.g., Ref. (32, 33, 109)]. Although initial hits emerged from these studies have not been replicated and the approaches have not yet matured into readily usable assays.

Metabolomic approaches measure small molecules that are substrates or products of metabolic processes. Two analytical methods are typically used, namely MS, which can identify large numbers of metabolites but has slow throughput, and magnetic resonance spectroscopy (MRS), which has higher throughput but lower sensitivity. Several recent small-scale studies have been able to distinguish patterns in CSF samples from AD patients and controls (110, 111). These studies will require extension and replication. Methods to standardize acquisition of metabolomics data are needed in order for these to be able to be readily used by reference laboratories. Increased statistical rigor and the need for extensive replication strongly need to be applied to metabolomic studies (112). Lipidomic analyses have also been applied to AD, with inconsistent findings. One recent study identified a panel of lipid-related biomarkers in plasma that predicted conversion to AD (29). Although clinical assessment, sample handling, and biomarker analysis were carefully standardized in this study, the number of subjects who progressed from normal cognition to impairment was small. This panel of biomarkers has not yet been replicated. Another lipidomic study identified changes in long chain cholesteryl esters in plasma that discriminated patients with AD and controls, but lacked replication cohorts (113). Careful study design with large enough numbers and replication cohorts are essential to make progress in this area. Also, robust assay platforms will need to be developed that will allow a set of lipidomic assays to be routinely run as a mature assay.

Exosomes are a subset of microvesicles and are released from cells under physiological and pathological conditions and circulate in body fluids. Exosomes are smaller than microparticles, and are usually defined as <100 nM in diameter. This small size poses a challenge to current methods of detection using flow cytometry. Exosomes arise from intracellular microvesicular bodies, whereas microparticles originate from the plasma membranes of cells or from apoptotic bodies. Exosomes may be implicated in neurodegenerative disorders in altered intercellular communication, for example, by transporting microRNA (miRNA), or by contributing to the spread of misfolded proteins (114). Methods to isolate exosomes have not been well standardized, and commercial kits yield mixed populations of exosomes and other particles. Extracellular vesicles, including exosomes, are found in CSF and their proteome has been characterized (115, 116). To date, there are no clear diagnostic markers that distinguish AD based on CSF exosomes, but much work is ongoing. Recent reports have isolated and analyzed exosomes in plasma, after using an immunopurification step to isolate a subset that have surface markers suggesting their neuronal origin, such as L1 cellular adhesion molecule (L1CAM) (117, 118). Subsequent protein analyses using ELISA identified differences in levels of AD protein biomarkers of Aβ42 and tau (118) between AD and controls. These are promising initial findings, but much further work is needed to replicate and extend the findings. For example, it is unclear how exosomes might traffic from the CNS to the bloodstream, and therefore whether these truly reflect neuronal pathophysiology. Also, the multiple steps necessary to isolate exosomes and then assay their contents poses challenges to assay standardization.

MicroRNAs are small RNA species that control gene expression by binding to sets of target mRNAs and may play roles in intracellular communication. They can be isolated from exosomes or directly from biofluids. There are technical problems in quantifying levels of miRNAs, and the development of methods and standards are still in their early stages. Studies in AD have identified profiles of miRNAs in CSF that may distinguish patients from controls but have been inconsistent across studies (119–121). Levels of miRNA levels are affected by the presence of cells, so that careful standardization will be necessary for studies using CSF (121). Studies of miRNA are reviewed in more detail in this collection of reviews (122).

Peripheral cells, such as mononuclear cells and lymphocytes, as well as platelets have been the subjects of many types of biomarker studies in AD. The nature of these studies and the types of biomarkers that have been sought are too diverse to be easily summarized here. Although an enormous number of markers and biological processes can be interrogated using cells, to date, no consistent biomarker profiles have emerged that were subsequently widely replicated.

VALIDATING AND UNDERSTANDING BIOMARKERS

The initial validation of biomarkers requires the development of quantitative, sensitive, and reliable assays, and identifying pre-analytical and analytical factors that may influence the levels that are measured (123). As examples of pre-analytical factors, for Aβ, polypropylene collection tubes are required, whereas for alpha-synuclein, measuring the extent of contamination by hemoglobin is important (124). Effects of storage, freeze–thaw cycles, and sample handling need to be carefully determined. Assay performance metrics, the type of analytical platform to be used, preparation and use of analytical standards and biological replicates also need to be standardized. Appropriately scaled clinical studies aimed at determining cutoff points, sensitivity, and specificity need to be conducted. Depending on the proposed use of the biomarker, longitudinal studies and postmortem confirmation of pathological features of brain pathology may add credence to claims for sensitivity and specificity. Meta-analyses or pooled analyses of multi-center data can provide information about effects of age and APOE genotype on CSF biomarkers (65). Assays typically progress through different stages of qualification. Much effort has gone into comparisons of A-beta and tau assays, including round robin efforts, which also were recently applied to MS assays for A-beta (125), and international quality control efforts. Next-generation assays for A-beta42, tau, and P-tau may help to decrease variability and to develop rigorous and standardized cutoff points that are readily applicable across laboratories. Understanding the phenomena that the biomarkers are measuring goes beyond these validation steps that have been outlined, and it is a critical step in determining the use of biomarkers, particularly regarding therapeutic studies. As a sobering observation, although increased CSF levels of tau and P-tau are routinely detected in AD, the mechanisms whereby these biomarkers are released into the CSF are not well understood.

There are many opportunities to study genetics in relation to biomarkers, some of which have been discussed earlier. Large-scale studies of patients with inherited forms of early onset AD are helping to expand the map and timeline of biomarkers (126). Because age is the strongest risk factor for sporadic AD, it is important to continue to study how biomarkers and related brain processes change during aging. As an example, studies of Aβ metabolism using SILK have shown that there are marked changes in parameters related to production and clearance of Aβ from the CSF in association with aging (127).

TOWARD AN EXPANDED SUITE OF BIOMARKERS

Biomarkers in biofluids have provided several important insights into AD, and currently have a role both in diagnosis and in the development of therapy. An attainable future goal is to improve and standardize current assays for Aβ, tau, and P-tau to permit routine and widespread clinical use. Progress will continue to be made in the development of assays to allow early and pre-symptomatic detection of AD to facilitate therapeutic studies (128). An ambitious goal will be to identify biomarkers that predict who is at risk for beginning to developing amyloid deposition in the brain before these deposits arise. In the area of diagnostics, the development of multi-analyte panels that are able to provide indices of non-AD degenerative disorders and important biological processes will remain an important area of research. As an illustrative example, a recent study of a nine analyte panel of CSF biomarkers had good differential diagnostic ability to distinguish between atypical movement disorders, PD and AD (129).

For clinical trials, a suite of biomarkers to evaluate amyloid processing exists, but markers related to oligomers remain elusive. Biomarkers that inform about target engagement for other therapeutic areas, for example, tau therapeutics, require further development. Prognostic, predictive, and companion biomarkers have not yet been identified and can be sought in the context of longitudinal studies. Relationships between biofluid markers, brain imaging, and cognitive testing will help to refine the roadmap of progression along the way to dementia in AD, especially during preclinical and prodromal stages. The potential for plasma biomarkers to provide screening, diagnostic, or prognostic tools merits continued study, but the design and validation of a plasma biomarker may be more complex than for a CSF biomarker.

The growth of research and development of new technologies gives hope that we may be able to develop a more comprehensive suite of biomarkers to build a detailed picture of the brain, that may integrate markers related to different cell types, important cellular structures such as synapses, biological processes such as transport, lipid metabolism, and exosome release, and effects of damage, oxidative stress, and inflammation. Progress in these areas holds the promise of greatly extending the reach of biofluid biomarkers for AD and related disorders.

REFERENCES

1. Motter R, Vigo-Pelfrey C, Kholodenko D, Barbour R, Johnson-Wood K, Galasko D, et al. Reduction of beta-amyloid peptide42 in the cerebrospinal fluid of patients with Alzheimer's disease. *Ann Neurol* (1995) **38**:643–8. doi:10.1002/ana.410380413
2. Vandermeeren M, Mercken M, Vanmechelen E, Six J, van de Voorde A, Martin JJ, et al. Detection of tau proteins in normal and Alzheimer's disease cerebrospinal fluid with a sensitive sandwich enzyme-linked immunosorbent assay. *J Neurochem* (1993) **61**:1828–34. doi:10.1111/j.1471-4159.1993.tb09823.x
3. Andreasen N, Sjögren M, Blennow K. CSF markers for Alzheimer's disease: total tau, phospho-tau and Abeta42. *World J Biol Psychiatry* (2003) **4**:147–55. doi:10.1080/15622970310029912
4. Hampel H, Buerger K, Zinkowski R, Teipel SJ, Goernitz A, Andreasen N, et al. Measurement of phosphorylated tau epitopes in the differential diagnosis of Alzheimer disease: a comparative cerebrospinal fluid study. *Arch Gen Psychiatry* (2004) **61**:95–102. doi:10.1001/archpsyc.61.1.95
5. Skillbäck T, Farahmand BY, Rosén C, Mattsson N, Nägga K, Kilander L, et al. Cerebrospinal fluid tau and amyloid-β1-42 in patients with dementia. *Brain* (2015) **138**(Pt 9):2716–31. doi:10.1093/brain/awv181
6. Olsson B, Zetterberg H, Hampel H, Blennow K. Biomarker-based dissection of neurodegenerative diseases. *Prog Neurobiol* (2011) **95**:520–34. doi:10.1016/j.pneurobio.2011.04.006
7. Mattsson N, Zetterberg H, Hansson O, Andreasen N, Parnetti L, Jonsson M, et al. CSF biomarkers and incipient Alzheimer's disease in patients with mild cognitive impairment. *JAMA* (2009) **302**:385–93. doi:10.1001/jama.2009.1064
8. Vos SJ, Xiong C, Visser PJ, Jasielec MS, Hassenstab J, Grant EA, et al. Preclinical Alzheimer's disease and its outcome: a longitudinal cohort study. *Lancet Neurol* (2013) **12**:957–65. doi:10.1016/S1474-4422(13)70194-7
9. Hansson O, Zetterberg H, Buchhave P, Londos E, Blennow K, Minthon L. Association between CSF biomarkers and incipient Alzheimer's disease in patients with mild cognitive impairment: a follow-up study. *Lancet Neurol* (2006) **5**:228–34. doi:10.1016/S1474-4422(06)70355-6
10. Shaw LM, Vanderstichele H, Knapik-Czajka M, Clark CM, Aisen PS, Petersen RC, et al. Cerebrospinal fluid biomarker signature in Alzheimer's disease neuroimaging initiative subjects. *Ann Neurol* (2009) **65**:403–13. doi:10.1002/ana.21610
11. Buchhave P, Minthon L, Zetterberg H, Wallin AK, Blennow K, Hansson O. Cerebrospinal fluid levels of β-amyloid 1-42, but not of tau, are fully changed already 5 to 10 years before the onset of Alzheimer dementia. *Arch Gen Psychiatry* (2012) **69**:98–106. doi:10.1001/archgenpsychiatry.2011.155
12. Kester MI, van der Vlies AE, Blankenstein MA, Pijnenburg YA, van Elk EJ, Scheltens P, et al. CSF biomarkers predict rate of cognitive decline in Alzheimer disease. *Neurology* (2009) **73**:1353–8. doi:10.1212/WNL.0b013e3181bd8271
13. Degerman Gunnarsson M, Lannfelt L, Ingelsson M, Basun H, Kilander L. High tau levels in cerebrospinal fluid predict rapid decline and increased dementia mortality in Alzheimer's disease. *Dement Geriatr Cogn Disord* (2015) **37**:196–206. doi:10.1159/000355556
14. Kvartsberg H, Duits FH, Ingelsson M, Andreasen N, Öhrfelt A, Andersson K. Cerebrospinal fluid levels of the synaptic protein neurogranin correlates with cognitive decline in prodromal Alzheimer's disease. *Alzheimers Dement* (2015) **2015**(11):1180–90. doi:10.1016/j.jalz.2014.10.009
15. Vanderstichele H, De Meyer G, Andreasen N, Kostanjevecki V, Wallin A, Olsson A, et al. Amino-truncated beta-amyloid42 peptides in cerebrospinal fluid and prediction of progression of mild cognitive impairment. *Clin Chem* (2005) **51**:1650–60. doi:10.1373/clinchem.2005.051201
16. Braak H, Braak E. Frequency of stages of Alzheimer-related lesions in different age categories. *Neurobiol Aging* (1997) **18**:351–7. doi:10.1016/S0197-4580(97)00056-0
17. Schneider JA, Arvanitakis Z, Bang W, Bennett DA. Mixed brain pathologies account for most dementia cases in community-dwelling older persons. *Neurology* (2007) **69**:2197–204. doi:10.1212/01.wnl.0000271090.28148.24
18. Rahimi J, Kovacs GG. Prevalence of mixed pathologies in the aging brain. *Alzheimers Res Ther* (2014) **6**:82. doi:10.1186/s13195-014-0082-1
19. Brandner S, Thaler C, Lelental N, Buchfelder M, Kleindienst A, Maler JM, et al. Ventricular and lumbar cerebrospinal fluid concentrations of Alzheimer's disease biomarkers in patients with normal pressure hydrocephalus and posttraumatic hydrocephalus. *J Alzheimers Dis* (2014) **41**:1057–62. doi:10.3233/JAD-132708
20. Galasko D, Golde TE. Biomarkers for Alzheimer's disease in plasma, serum and blood – conceptual and practical problems. *Alzheimers Res Ther* (2013) **5**:10. doi:10.1186/alzrt164
21. Hu WT, Holtzman DM, Fagan AM, Shaw LM, Perrin R, Arnold SE, et al. Plasma multianalyte profiling in mild cognitive impairment and Alzheimer disease. *Neurology* (2011) **79**:897–905. doi:10.1212/WNL.0b013e318266fa70
22. Toledo JB, Shaw LM, Trojanowski JQ. Plasma amyloid beta measurements – a desired but elusive biomarker. *Alzheimers Res Ther* (2013) **5**:8. doi:10.1186/alzrt162
23. Beach TG, Adler CH, Sue LI, Vedders L, Lue L, White III CL, et al. Multi-organ distribution of phosphorylated alpha-synuclein histopathology in subjects with Lewy body disorders. *Acta Neuropathol* (2010) **119**:689–702. doi:10.1007/s00401-010-0664-3
24. Bateman RJ, Munsell LY, Morris JC, Swarm R, Yarasheki KE, Holtzman DM. Human amyloid-beta synthesis and clearance rates as measured in cerebrospinal fluid in vivo. *Nat Med* (2006) **12**:856–61. doi:10.1038/nm1438
25. Fanara P, Wong PY, Husted KH, Liu S, Liu VM, Kohlstaedt LA, et al. Cerebrospinal fluid-based kinetic biomarkers of axonal transport in monitoring neurodegeneration. *J Clin Invest* (2012) **122**:3159–69. doi:10.1172/JCI64575
26. Sutphen CL, Jasielec MS, Shah AR, Macy EM, Xiong C, Vlassenko AG, et al. Longitudinal cerebrospinal fluid biomarker changes in preclinical Alzheimer disease during middle age. *JAMA Neurol* (2015) **72**(9):1029–42. doi:10.1001/jamaneurol.2015.1285
27. Dubois B, Feldman HH, Jacova C, Hampel H, Molinuevo JL, Blennow K, et al. Advancing research diagnostic criteria for Alzheimer's disease: the IWG-2 criteria. *Lancet Neurol* (2014) **13**:614–29. doi:10.1016/S1474-4422(14)70090-0
28. Sperling RA, Aisen PS, Beckett LA, Bennett DA, Craft S, Fagan AM, et al. Toward defining the preclinical stages of Alzheimer's disease: recommendations from the National Institute on Aging – Alzheimer's Association workgroups on diagnostic guidelines for Alzheimer's disease. *Alzheimers Dement* (2011) **7**:280–92. doi:10.1016/j.jalz.2011.03.003
29. Mapstone M, Cheema AK, Fiandaca MS, Zhong X, Mhyre TR, MacArthur LH, et al. Plasma phospholipids identify antecedent memory impairment in older adults. *Nat Med* (2014) **20**:415–8. doi:10.1038/nm.3466
30. Sattlecker M, Kiddle SJ, Newhouse S, Proitsi P, Nelson S, Williams S, et al. Alzheimer's disease biomarker discovery using SOMAscan multiplexed protein technology. *Alzheimers Dement* (2014) **10**(6):724–34. doi:10.1016/j.jalz.2013.09.016
31. Zetterberg H, Wilson D, Andreasson U, Minthon L, Blennow K, Randall J. Plasma tau levels in Alzheimer's disease. *Alzheimers Res Ther* (2013) **5**(2):9. doi:10.1186/alzrt163
32. Reddy MM, Wilson R, Wilson J, Connell S, Gocke A, Hynan L, et al. Identification of candidate IgG biomarkers for Alzheimer's disease via combinatorial library screening. *Cell* (2011) **144**:132–42. doi:10.1016/j.cell.2010.11.054
33. Nagele E, Han M, Demarshall C, Belinka B, Nagele R. Diagnosis of Alzheimer's disease based on disease-specific autoantibody profiles in human sera. *PLoS One* (2011) **6**:e23112. doi:10.1371/journal.pone.0023112
34. Craig-Schapiro R, Perrin RJ, Roe CM, Xiong C, Carter D, Cairns NJ, et al. YKL-40: a novel prognostic fluid biomarker for preclinical Alzheimer's disease. *Biol Psychiatry* (2010) **68**:903–12. doi:10.1016/j.biopsych.2010.08.025
35. Tarawneh R, D'Angelo G, Macy E, Xiong C, Carter D, Cairns NJ. Visinin-like protein-1: diagnostic and prognostic biomarker in Alzheimer disease. *Ann Neurol* (2011) **70**:274–85. doi:10.1002/ana.22448
36. Skillbäck T, Rosén C, Asztely F, Mattsson N, Blennow K, Zetterberg H. Diagnostic performance of cerebrospinal fluid total tau and phosphorylated tau in Creutzfeldt-Jakob disease: results from the Swedish mortality registry. *JAMA Neurol* (2014) **71**:476–83. doi:10.1001/jamaneurol.2013.6455
37. Hu WT, Watts K, Grossman M, Glass J, Lah JJ, Hales C, et al. Reduced CSF p-Tau181 to Tau ratio is a biomarker for FTLD-TDP. *Neurology* (2013) **81**(22):1945–52. doi:10.1212/01.wnl.0000436625.63650.27
38. Parnetti L, Castrioto A, Chiasserini D, Persichetti E, Tambasco N, El-Agnaf O. Cerebrospinal fluid biomarkers in Parkinson disease. *Nat Rev Neurol* (2013) **9**(3):131–40. doi:10.1038/nrneurol.2013.10

39. Cruchaga C, Kauwe JS, Harari O, Jin SC, Cai Y, Karch CM. GWAS of cerebrospinal fluid tau levels identifies risk variants for Alzheimer's disease. *Neuron* (2013) **78**:256–68. doi:10.1016/j.neuron.2013.02.026
40. Rosenberg GA, Wallin A, Wardlaw JM, Markus HS, Montaner J, Wolfson L, et al. Consensus statement for diagnosis of subcortical small vessel disease. *J Cereb Blood Flow Metab* (2015). doi:10.1038/jcbfm.2015.172
41. Liu Q, Waltz S, Woodruff G, Ouyang J, Israel MA, Herrera C. Effect of potent γ-secretase modulator in human neurons derived from multiple presenilin 1-induced pluripotent stem cell mutant carriers. *JAMA Neurol* (2014) **71**:1481–9. doi:10.1001/jamaneurol.2014.2482
42. Jeppsson F, Eketjäll S, Janson J, Karlström S, Gustavsson S, Olsson LL, et al. Discovery of AZD3839, a potent and selective BACE1 inhibitor clinical candidate for the treatment of Alzheimer disease. *J Biol Chem* (2012) **287**:41245–57. doi:10.1074/jbc.M112.409110
43. Fleisher AS, Raman R, Siemers ER, Becerra L, Clark CM, Dean RA, et al. Phase 2 safety trial targeting amyloid beta production with a gamma-secretase inhibitor in Alzheimer disease. *Arch Neurol* (2008) **65**:1031–8. doi:10.1001/archneur.65.8.1031
44. Coric V, Salloway S, van Dyck CH, Dubois B, Andreasen N, Brody M, et al. Targeting prodromal Alzheimer disease with avagacestat: a randomized clinical trial. *JAMA Neurol* (2015) **72**(11):1324–33. doi:10.1001/jamaneurol.2015.0607
45. Van Gool SW, Van Kerschaver E, Brock P, Pottel H, Hulstaert F. Disease- and treatment-related elevation of the neurodegenerative marker tau in children with hematological malignancies. *Leukemia* (2000) **14**:2076–84. doi:10.1038/sj.leu.2401934
46. Lleó A, Cavedo E, Parnetti L, Vanderstichele H, Herukka SK, Andreasen N. Cerebrospinal fluid biomarkers in trials for Alzheimer and Parkinson diseases. *Nat Rev Neurol* (2015) **11**:41–55. doi:10.1038/nrneurol.2014.232
47. Jack CR, Knopman DS, Jagust WJ, Petersen RC, Weiner MW, Aisen PS, et al. Tracking pathophysiological processes in Alzheimer's disease: an updated hypothetical model of dynamic biomarkers. *Lancet Neurol* (2013) **12**:207–16. doi:10.1016/S1474-4422(12)70291-0
48. Cruchaga C, Kauwe JSK, Nowotny P, Bales K, Pickering ES, Mayo K, et al. Cerebrospinal fluid APOE levels: an endophenotype for genetic studies of Alzheimer's disease. *Hum Mol Genet* (2012) **21**:4558–71. doi:10.1093/hmg/dds296
49. Toledo JB, Da X, Weiner MW, Wolk DA, Xie SX, Arnold SE. CSF ApoE levels associate with cognitive decline and MRI changes. *Acta Neuropathol* (2014) **1127**:621–32. doi:10.1007/s00401-013-1236-0
50. Jonsson T, Stefansson H, Steinberg S, Jonsdottir I, Jonsson PV, Snaedal J, et al. Variant of TREM2 associated with the risk of Alzheimer's disease. *N Engl J Med* (2013) **368**:107–16. doi:10.1056/NEJMoa1211103
51. Kleinberger G, Yamanishi Y, Suárez-Calvet M, Czirr E, Lohmann E, Cuyvers E, et al. TREM2 mutations implicated in neurodegeneration impair cell surface transport and phagocytosis. *Sci Transl Med* (2014) **6**(243):243ra86. doi:10.1126/scitranslmed.3009093
52. Galasko D, Montine TJ. Biomarkers of oxidative damage and inflammation in Alzheimer's disease. *Biomark Med* (2010) **4**:27–36. doi:10.2217/bmm.09.89
53. Brosseron F, Krauthausen M, Kummer M, Heneka MT. Body fluid cytokine levels in mild cognitive impairment and Alzheimer's disease: a comparative overview. *Mol Neurobiol* (2014) **50**:534–44. doi:10.1007/s12035-014-8657-1
54. Kauwe JS, Bailey MH, Ridge PG, Perry R, Wadsworth ME, Hoyt KL, et al. Genome-wide association study of CSF levels of 59 Alzheimer's disease candidate proteins: significant associations with proteins involved in amyloid processing and inflammation. *PLoS Genet* (2014) **10**(10):e1004758. doi:10.1371/journal.pgen.1004758
55. Finch N, Baker M, Crook R, Swanson K, Kuntz K, Surtees R, et al. Plasma progranulin levels predict progranulin mutation status in frontotemporal dementia patients and asymptomatic family members. *Brain* (2009) **132**:583–91. doi:10.1093/brain/awn352
56. Hardy J. The amyloid hypothesis for Alzheimer's disease: a critical reappraisal. *J Neurochem* (2009) **110**:1129–34. doi:10.1111/j.1471-4159.2009.06181.x
57. Lanz TA, Hosley JD, Adams WJ, Merchant KM. Studies of Abeta pharmacodynamics in the brain, cerebrospinal fluid, and plasma in young (plaque-free) Tg2576 mice using the gamma-secretase inhibitor N2-[(2S)-2-(3,5-difluorophenyl)-2-hydroxyethanoyl]-N1-[(7S)-5-methyl-6-oxo-6,7-dihydro-5H-dibenzo[b,d]azepin-7-yl]-L-alaninamide (*LY-411575*). *J Pharmacol Exp Ther* (2004) **309**:49–55.
58. Eketjall S, Janson J, Jeppson F, Svanhangen A, Kolmodin K, Gustavsson S. AZ-4217: a high potency BACE inhibitor displaying acute central efficacy in different in vivo models and reduced amyloid deposition in tg2576 mice. *J Neurosci* (2013) **33**:10075–84. doi:10.1523/JNEUROSCI.1165-13.2013
59. Wagner SL, Zhang C, Cheng S, Nguyen P, Zhang X, Rynearson KD, et al. Soluble γ-secretase modulators selectively inhibit the production of the 42-amino acid amyloid β peptide variant and augment the production of multiple carboxy-truncated amyloid β species. *Biochemistry* (2014) **53**:702–13. doi:10.1021/bi401537v
60. Portelius E, Dean RA, Andreasson U, Mattsson N, Westerlund A, Olsson M, et al. β-site amyloid precursor protein-cleaving enzyme 1(BACE1) inhibitor treatment induces Aβ5-X peptides through alternative amyloid precursor protein cleavage. *Alzheimers Res Ther* (2014) **6**(5–8):75. doi:10.1186/s13195-014-0075-0
61. Doody RS, Raman R, Sperling RA, Seimers E, Sethuraman G, Mohs R, et al. Peripheral and central effects of γ-secretase inhibition by semagacestat in Alzheimer's disease. *Alzheimers Res Ther* (2015) **7**(1):36. doi:10.1186/s13195-015-0121-6
62. Blennow K, Zetterberg H, Rinne JO, Salloway S, Wei J, Black R. Effect of immunotherapy with bapineuzumab on cerebrospinal fluid biomarker levels in patients with mild to moderate Alzheimer disease. *Arch Neurol* (2012) **69**:1002–10. doi:10.1001/archneurol.2012.90
63. Mattsson N, Andreasson U, Persson S, Carrillo MC, Collins S, Chalbot S, et al. CSF biomarker variability in the Alzheimer's association quality control program. *Alzheimers Dement* (2013) **9**:251–61. doi:10.1016/j.jalz.2013.01.010
64. Mattsson N, Insel PS, Landau S, Jagust W, Donohue M, Shaw LM, et al. Diagnostic accuracy of CSF A-beta42 and Florbetapir PET for Alzheimer's disease. *Ann Clin Transl Med* (2014) **1**:534–43. doi:10.1002/acn3.81
65. Toledo JB, Bjerke M, Da X, Landau SM, Foster NL, Jagust W, et al. Nonlinear association between cerebrospinal fluid and florbetapir F-18 β-amyloid measures across the spectrum of Alzheimer disease. *JAMA Neurol* (2015) **72**:571–81. doi:10.1001/jamaneurol.2014.4829
66. Hesse C, Rosengren L, Andreasen N, Davidsson P, Vanderstichele H, Vanmechelen E, et al. Transient increase in total tau but not phospho-tau in human cerebrospinal fluid after acute stroke. *Neurosci Lett* (2001) **297**:187–90. doi:10.1016/S0304-3940(00)01697-9
67. Johnson GVW, Seubert P, Cox TM, Motter R, Brown JP, Galasko D. The tau protein in human cerebrospinal fluid in Alzheimer's disease consists of proteolytically derived fragments. *J Neurochem* (1997) **43**(0–433):1997.
68. Meredith JE Jr, Sankaranarayanan S, Guss V, Lanzetti AJ, Berisha F, Neely RJ, et al. Characterization of novel CSF Tau and ptau biomarkers for Alzheimer's disease. *PLoS One* (2013) **8**(10):e76523. doi:10.1371/journal.pone.0076523
69. Vos SJ, Visser PJ, Verhey F, Aalten P, Knol D, Ramakers I, et al. Variability of CSF Alzheimer's disease biomarkers: implications for clinical practice. *PLoS One* (2014) **9**:e100784. doi:10.1371/journal.pone.0100784
70. Neselius S, Zetterberg H, Blennow K, Randall J, Wilson D, Marcusson J, et al. Olympic boxing is associated with elevated levels of the neuronal protein tau in plasma. *Brain Inj* (2013) **27**:425–33. doi:10.3109/02699052.2012.750752
71. Wang Y, Shi M, Chung KA, Zabetian CP, Leverenz JB, Berg D, et al. Phosphorylated α-synuclein in Parkinson's disease. *Sci Transl Med* (2012) **4**:121ra20. doi:10.1126/scitranslmed.3002566
72. Walsh DM, Klyubin I, Shankar GM, Townsend M, Fadeeva JV, Betts V, et al. The role of cell-derived oligomers of Abeta in Alzheimer's disease and avenues for therapeutic intervention. *Biochem Soc Trans* (2005) **33**:1087–90. doi:10.1042/BST20051087
73. Benilova I, Karran E, De Strooper B. The toxic Aβ oligomer and Alzheimer's disease: an emperor in need of clothes. *Nat Neurosci* (2012) **15**:349–57. doi:10.1038/nn.3028
74. Klein WL. Synaptotoxic amyloid-β oligomers: a molecular basis for the cause, diagnosis, and treatment of Alzheimer's disease? *J Alzheimers Dis* (2013) **33**(Suppl 1):S49–S65. doi:10.3233/JAD-2012-129039
75. Spires-Jones TL, Hyman BT. The intersection of amyloid beta and tau at synapses in Alzheimer's disease. *Neuron* (2014) **82**:756–71. doi:10.1016/j.neuron.2014.05.004
76. Musiek ES, Holtzman DM. Three dimensions of the amyloid hypothesis: time, space and 'wingmen'. *Nat Neurosci* (2015) **18**:800–6. doi:10.1038/nn.4018

77. Jucker M, Walker LC. Self-propagation of pathogenic protein aggregates in neurodegenerative diseases. *Nature* (2013) **501**(7465):45–51. doi:10.1038/nature12481
78. Esparza TJ, Zhao H, Cirrito JR, Cairns NJ, Bateman RJ, Holtzman DM, et al. Amyloid-β oligomerization in Alzheimer dementia versus high-pathology controls. *Ann Neurol* (2013) **73**:104–19. doi:10.1002/ana.23748
79. Yang T, O'Malley TT, Kanmert D, Jerecic J, Zieske LR, Zetterberg H, et al. A highly sensitive novel immunoassay specifically detects low levels of soluble Aβ oligomers in human cerebrospinal fluid. *Alzheimers Res Ther* (2015) **7**(1):14. doi:10.1186/s13195-015-0100-y
80. De Vos A, Jacobs D, Struyfs H, Fransen E, Andersson K, Portelius E, et al. C-terminal neurogranin is increased in cerebrospinal fluid but unchanged in plasma in Alzheimer's disease. *Alzheimers Dement* (2015). doi:10.1016/j.jalz.2015.05.012
81. Karch CM, Goate AM. Alzheimer's disease risk genes and mechanisms of disease pathogenesis. *Biol Psychiatry* (2015) **77**:43–51. doi:10.1016/j.biopsych.2014.05.006
82. Ghidoni R, Benussi L, Glionna M, Franzoni M, Binetti G. Low plasma progranulin levels predict progranulin mutations in frontotemporal lobar degeneration. *Neurology* (2008) **71**:1235–9. doi:10.1212/01.wnl.0000325058.10218.fc
83. Britschgi M, Rufibach K, Huang SL, Clark CM, Kaye JA, Li G. Modeling of pathological traits in Alzheimer's disease based on systemic extracellular signaling proteome. *Mol Cell Proteomics* (2011) **10**:M111.008862. doi:10.1074/mcp.M111.008862
84. Hu WT, Holtzman DM, Fagan AM, Shaw LM, Perrin R, Arnold SE, et al. *Neurology* (2012) **79**(9): 897–905.
85. Hu WT, Chen-Plotkin A, Arnold SE, Grossman M, Clark CM, Shaw LM, et al. Biomarker discovery for Alzheimer's disease, frontotemporal lobar degeneration, and Parkinson's disease. *Acta Neuropathol* (2010) **120**:385–99. doi:10.1007/s00401-010-0723-9
86. Paterson RW, Bartlett JW, Blennow K, Fox NC; Alzheimer's Disease Neuroimaging Initiative, Shaw LM, et al. Cerebrospinal fluid markers including trefoil factor three are associated with neurodegeneration in amyloid positive individuals. *Transl Psychiatry* (2014) **4**:e419. doi:10.1038/tp.2014.58
87. Fischer SK, Joyce A, Spengler M, Yang TY, Zhuang Y, Fjording MS, et al. Emerging technologies to increase ligand binding assay sensitivity. *AAPS J* (2015) **17**(1):93–101. doi:10.1208/s12248-014-9682-8
88. Niemeyer CM, Adler M, Wacker R. Detecting antigens by quantitative immuno-PCR. *Nat Protoc* (2007) **2**(8):1918–30. doi:10.1038/nprot.2007.267
89. Zetterberg H, Mörtberg E, Song L, Chang L, Provuncher GK, Patel PP, et al. Hypoxia due to cardiac arrest induces a time-dependent increase in serum amyloid β levels in humans. *PLoS One* (2011) **6**(12):e28263. doi:10.1371/journal.pone.0028263
90. Shahim P, Tegner Y, Wilson DH, Randall J, Skillbäck T, Pazooki D, et al. Blood biomarkers for brain injury in concussed professional ice hockey players. *JAMA Neurol* (2014) **71**:684–92. doi:10.1001/jamaneurol.2014.367
91. Olivera A, Lejbman N, Jeromin A, French LM, Kim HS, Cashion A, et al. Peripheral total tau in military personnel who sustain traumatic brain injuries during deployment. *JAMA Neurol* (2015) **72**:1109–16. doi:10.1001/jamaneurol.2015.1383
92. Liliang PC, Liang CL, Weng HC, Lu K, Wang KW, Chen HJ, et al. Tau proteins in serum predict outcome after severe traumatic brain injury. *J Surg Res* (2010) **160**:302–7. doi:10.1016/j.jss.2008.12.022
93. Zetterberg H, Blennow K. Fluid markers of traumatic brain injury. *Mol Cell Neurosci* (2015) **66**(Pt B):99–102. doi:10.1016/j.mcn.2015.02.003
94. Schutzer SE, Liu T, Natelson BH, Angel TE, Schepmoes AA, Purvine SO, et al. Establishing the proteome of normal human cerebrospinal fluid. *PLoS One* (2010) **5**(6):e10980. doi:10.1371/journal.pone.0010980
95. McGuire JN, Overgaard J, Pociot F. Mass spectrometry is only one piece of the puzzle in clinical proteomics. *Brief Funct Genomic Proteomic* (2008) **7**:74–83. doi:10.1093/bfgp/eln005
96. Griffiths HR, Augustyniak EM, Bennett SJ, Debacq-Chainiaux F, Dunston CR, Kristensen P, et al. Novel ageing-biomarker discovery using data-intensive technologies. *Mech Ageing Dev* (2015) **151**:114–21. doi:10.1016/j.mad.2015.05.010
97. Zhang Y, Guo Z, Zou L, Yang Y, Zhang L, Ji N, et al. A comprehensive map and functional annotation of the normal human cerebrospinal fluid proteome. *J Proteomics* (2015) **119**:90–9. doi:10.1016/j.jprot.2015.01.017
98. Hölttä M, Minthon L, Hansson O, Holmén-Larsson J, Pike I, Ward M. An integrated workflow for multiplex CSF proteomics and peptidomics-identification of candidate cerebrospinal fluid biomarkers of Alzheimer's disease. *J Proteome Res* (2015) **14**(2):654–63. doi:10.1021/pr501076j
99. Sajic T, Liu Y, Aebersold R. Using data-independent, high-resolution mass spectrometry in protein biomarker research: perspectives and clinical applications. *Proteomics Clin Appl* (2015) **9**:307–21. doi:10.1002/prca.201400117
100. Chahrour O, Cobice D, Malone J. Stable isotope labelling methods in mass spectrometry-based quantitative proteomics. *J Pharm Biomed Anal* (2015) **113**:2–20. doi:10.1016/j.jpba.2015.04.013
101. Ringman JM, Schulman H, Becker C, Jones T, Bai Y, Immermann F, et al. Proteomic changes in cerebrospinal fluid of presymptomatic and affected persons carrying familial Alzheimer disease mutations. *Arch Neurol* (2012) **6**:96–104. doi:10.1001/archneurol.2011.642
102. Wildsmith KR, Schauer SP, Smith AM, Arnott D, Zhu Y. Identification of longitudinally dynamic biomarkers in Alzheimer's disease cerebrospinal fluid by targeted proteomics. *Mol Neurodegener* (2014) **9**:22. doi:10.1186/1750-1326-9-22
103. Lehnert S, Jesse S, Rist W, Steinacker P, Soininen H, Herukka SK, et al. iTRAQ and multiple reaction monitoring as proteomic tools for biomarker search in cerebrospinal fluid of patients with Parkinson disease dementia. *Exp Neurol* (2012) **234**:499–504. doi:10.1016/j.expneurol.2012.01.024
104. Whiteaker JR, Lin C, Kennedy J, Hou L, Trute M, Sokal I, et al. A targeted proteomics-based pipeline for validation of biomarkers in plasma. *Nat Biotechnol* (2011) **29**:629–34. doi:10.1038/nbt.1900
105. Brody EN, Gold L, Lawn RM, Walker JJ, Zichi D. High-content affinity-based proteomics: unlocking protein biomarker discovery. *Expert Rev Mol Diagn* (2010) **10**:1013–22. doi:10.1586/erm.10.89
106. Hye A, Riddoch-Contreras J, Baird AL, Ashton NJ, Bazenet C, Leung R, et al. Plasma proteins predict conversion to dementia from prodromal disease. *Alzheimers Dement* (2014) **10**:799–807. doi:10.1016/j.jalz.2014.05.1749
107. Zhao X, Lejnine S, Spond J, Zhang C, Ramaraj TC, Holder DJ, et al. A candidate plasma protein classifier to identify Alzheimer's disease. *J Alzheimers Dis* (2015) **43**:549–63. doi:10.3233/JAD-141149
108. Menni C, Kiddle SJ, Mangino M, Viñuela A, Psatha M. Circulating proteomic signatures of chronological age. *J Gerontol A Biol Sci Med Sci* (2015) **70**:809–16. doi:10.1093/gerona/glu121
109. Tian H, Davidowitz E, Lopez P, He P, Schulz P, Moe J, et al. Isolation and characterization of antibody fragments selective for toxic oligomeric tau. *Neurobiol Aging* (2015) **36**:1342–55. doi:10.1016/j.neurobiolaging.2014.12.002
110. Trushina E, Dutta T, Persson X-MT, Mielke MM, Petersen RC. Identification of altered metabolic pathways in CSF and plasma in mild cognitive impairment and Alzheimer's disease using metabolomics. *PLoS One* (2013) **8**:e63644. doi:10.1371/journal.pone.0063644
111. Kaddurah-Daouk R, Zhu H, Sharma S, Bogdanov M, Rozen SG, Matson W, et al. Alterations in metabolic pathways and networks in Alzheimer's disease. *Transl Psychiatry* (2013) **3**:e244. doi:10.1038/tp.2013.18
112. Xia J, Broadhurst DI, Wilson M, Wishart DS. Translational biomarker discovery in clinical metabolomics: an introductory tutorial. *Metabolomics* (2013) **9**:280–99. doi:10.1007/s11306-012-0482-9
113. Proitsi P, Kim M, Whiley L, Pritchard M, Leung R. Plasma lipidomics analysis finds long chain cholesteryl esters to be associated with Alzheimer's disease. *Transl Psychiatry* (2015) **5**:e494. doi:10.1038/tp.2014.127
114. Schneider A, Simons M. Exosomes: vesicular carriers for intercellular communication in neurodegenerative disorders. *Cell Tissue Res* (2013) **352**:33–47. doi:10.1007/s00441-012-1428-2
115. Street JM, Barran PE, Mackay CL, Weidt S, Balmforth C, Walsh TS, et al. Identification and proteomic profiling of exosomes in human cerebrospinal fluid. *J Transl Med* (2012) **10**:5. doi:10.1186/1479-5876-10-5
116. Chiasserini D, van Weering JR, Piersma SR, Pham TV, Malekzadeh A, Teunissen CE, et al. Proteomic analysis of cerebrospinal fluid extracellular vesicles: a comprehensive dataset. *J Proteomics* (2014) **106**:191–204. doi:10.1016/j.jprot.2014.04.028
117. Shi M, Liu C, Cook TJ, Bullock KM, Zhao Y, Ginghina C, et al. Plasma exosomal α-synuclein is likely CNS-derived and increased in Parkinson's disease. *Acta Neuropathol* (2014) **128**(5):639–50. doi:10.1007/s00401-014-1314-y
118. Fiandaca MS, Kapogiannis D, Mapstone M, Boxer A, Eitan E, Schwartz JB, et al. Identification of preclinical Alzheimer's disease by a profile of pathogenic proteins in neurally derived blood exosomes: a case-control study. *Alzheimers Dement* (2015) **11**:600–7. doi:10.1016/j.jalz.2014.06.008

119. Cogswell JP, Ward J, Taylor IA, Waters M, Shi Y. Identification of miRNA changes in Alzheimer's disease brain and CSF yields putative biomarkers and insights into disease pathways. *J Alzheimers Dis* (2008) **14**:27–41.
120. Sala Frigerio C, Lau P, Salta E, Tournoy J, Bossers K, Vandenberghe R, et al. Reduced expression of hsa-miR-27a-3p in CSF of patients with Alzheimer disease. *Neurology* (2013) **81**:2103–6. doi:10.1212/01.wnl.0000437306.37850.22
121. Müller M, Jäkel L, Bruinsma IB, Claassen JA, Kuiperij HB, Verbeek MM. microRNA-29a is a candidate biomarker for Alzheimer's disease in cell-free cerebrospinal fluid. *Mol Neurobiol* (2015). doi:10.1007/s12035-015-9156-8
122. Zhao Y, Bhattacharjee S, Dua P, Alexandrov PN, Lukiw WJ. microRNA-based biomarkers and the diagnosis of Alzheimer's disease. *Front Neurol* (2015) **6**:162. doi:10.3389/fneur.2015.00162
123. Vanderstichele H, Bibl M, Engelborghs S, Le Bastard N, Lewczuk P, Molinuevo JL, et al. Standardization of preanalytical aspects of cerebrospinal fluid biomarker testing for Alzheimer's disease diagnosis: a consensus paper from the Alzheimer's biomarkers standardization initiative. *Alzheimers Dement* (2012) **8**:65–73. doi:10.1016/j.jalz.2011.07.004
124. del Campo M, Mollenhauer B, Bertolotto A, Engelborghs S, Hampel H, Simonsen AH, et al. Recommendations to standardize preanalytical confounding factors in Alzheimer's and Parkinson's disease cerebrospinal fluid biomarkers: an update. *Biomark Med* (2012) **6**:419–30. doi:10.2217/bmm.12.46
125. Pannee J, Gobom J, Shaw LM, Korecka M, Chambers EE, Lame M, et al. Round robin test on quantification of amyloid-β 1-42 in cerebrospinal fluid by mass spectrometry. *Alzheimers Dement* (2015). doi:10.1016/j.jalz.2015.06.1890
126. Bateman RJ, Xiong C, Benzinger TL, Fagan AM, Goate A, Fox NC. Clinical and biomarker changes in dominantly inherited Alzheimer's disease. *N Engl J Med* (2012) **367**:795–804. doi:10.1056/NEJMoa1202753
127. Patterson BW, Elbert DL, Mawuenyega KG, Kasten T, Ovod V, Ma S, et al. Age and amyloid effects on human central nervous system amyloid-beta kinetics. *Ann Neurol* (2015) **78**(3):439–53. doi:10.1002/ana.24454
128. Toledo JB, Zetterberg H, van Harten AC, Glodzik L, Martinez-Lage P, Bocchio-Chiavetto L, et al. Alzheimer's disease cerebrospinal fluid biomarker in cognitively normal subjects. *Brain* (2015) **138**(Pt 9):2701–15. doi:10.1093/brain/awv199
129. Magdalinou NK, Paterson RW, Schott JM, Fox NC, Mummery C, Blennow K, et al. A panel of nine cerebrospinal fluid biomarkers may identify patients with atypical parkinsonian syndromes. *J Neurol Neurosurg Psychiatry* (2015) **86**(11):1240–7. doi:10.1136/jnnp-2014-309562

22

Plasma 24-metabolite panel predicts preclinical transition to clinical stages of Alzheimer's disease

*Massimo S. Fiandaca[1,2], Xiaogang Zhong[3], Amrita K. Cheema[4], Michael H. Orquiza[5], Swathi Chidambaram[6], Ming T. Tan[3], Carole Roan Gresenz[7], Kevin T. FitzGerald[8], Mike A. Nalls[9], Andrew B. Singleton[9], Mark Mapstone[1] and Howard J. Federoff[1]**

[1] Department of Neurology, University of California Irvine, Irvine, CA, USA, [2] Department of Neurological Surgery, University of California Irvine, Irvine, CA, USA, [3] Department of Bioinformatics, Biostatistics and Biomathematics, Georgetown University Medical Center, Washington, DC, USA, [4] Departments of Oncology and Biochemistry, Georgetown University Medical Center, Washington, DC, USA, [5] Department of Neuroscience, Georgetown University Medical Center, Washington, DC, USA, [6] School of Medicine, Georgetown University Medical Center, Washington, DC, USA, [7] Department of Economics, Sociology and Statistics, RAND Corporation, Arlington, VA, USA, [8] Pellegrino Center for Clinical Bioethics, Georgetown University Medical Center, Washington, DC, USA, [9] Laboratory of Neurogenetics, National Institute on Aging, National Institutes of Health, Bethesda, MD, USA

Edited by:
Charlotte Elisabeth Teunissen, VU University Medical Center Amsterdam, Netherlands

Reviewed by:
Anja Hviid Simonsen, Copenhagen University Hospital, Denmark; Rigshospitalet, Denmark
Sarah Westwood, University of Oxford, UK

***Correspondence:**
Howard J. Federoff
federoff@uci.edu

We recently documented plasma lipid dysregulation in preclinical late-onset Alzheimer's disease (LOAD). A 10 plasma lipid panel, predicted phenoconversion and provided 90% sensitivity and 85% specificity in differentiating an at-risk group from those that would remain cognitively intact. Despite these encouraging results, low positive predictive values limit the clinical usefulness of this panel as a screening tool in subjects aged 70–80 years or younger. In this report, we re-examine our metabolomic data, analyzing baseline plasma specimens from our group of phenoconverters ($n = 28$) and a matched set of cognitively normal subjects ($n = 73$), and discover and internally validate a panel of 24 plasma metabolites. The new panel provides a classifier with receiver operating characteristic area under the curve for the discovery and internal validation cohort of 1.0 and 0.995 (95% confidence intervals of 1.0–1.0, and 0.981–1.0), respectively. Twenty-two of the 24 metabolites were significantly dysregulated lipids. While positive and negative predictive values were improved compared to our 10-lipid panel, low positive predictive values provide a reality check on the utility of such biomarkers in this age group (or younger). Through inclusion of additional significantly dysregulated analyte species, our new biomarker panel provides greater accuracy in our cohort but remains limited by predictive power. Unfortunately, the novel metabolite panel alone may not provide improvement in counseling and management of at-risk individuals but may further improve selection of subjects for LOAD secondary prevention trials. We expect that external validation will remain challenging due to our stringent study design, especially compared with more diverse subject cohorts. We do anticipate, however, external validation of reduced plasma lipid species as a predictor of phenoconversion to either prodromal or manifest LOAD.

Keywords: Alzheimer's disease, biomarkers, economics, ethics, lipids, metabolomics, risk assessment

INTRODUCTION

A major push in neurology and neurological research related to late-onset Alzheimer's disease (LOAD) in the last 5 years has been to better define the preclinical pathological stages that herald the development of clinically overt disease (1). As it relates to this paper, when we use the term AD, we mean LOAD, the most common clinical form of the disease and featuring a combination of genetic and epigenetic etiologies. In this context, we define preclinical LOAD as the separate stages of pathobiologic development that immediately precede prodromal amnestic mild cognitive impairment (aMCI) and manifest LOAD. We define, therefore, aMCI and LOAD to comprise the clinical stages of AD. Since treatments initiated during the preclinical stages may be more effective due to a more receptive brain substrate, the discovery and validation of biomarkers that define such a preclinical period has gained significant momentum (1). Our current investigative efforts focus on defining a more accurate and predictive set of plasma-based metabolomic biomarkers compared to those from our previous study (2). While the majority of LOAD biomarker studies to date have been carried out via case–control comparisons, our investigations arise from data developed from a 5-year longitudinal observation study. Longitudinal studies allow direct assessment of pathobiology during times of transition, while case–control studies primarily infer these transition events by comparing health to disease. Cerebrospinal fluid (CSF), neuroimaging, and a variety of other blood-based biomarkers have also been proposed via case–control analyses (3) but have not gained favor due to their associated risk, cost, and/or lack of requisite sensitivity and specificity values. There are few longitudinal investigations in the literature that define which neurocognitively intact subjects will progress to either prodromal or manifest LOAD. Our recent plasma lipid biomarker study (2) provided receiver operating characteristic area under the curve (ROC AUC) values of 0.96 and 0.92 with 95% confidence interval of 0.93–0.99 and 0.87–0.98, respectively, in the discovery and internal validation cohorts analyzed. The calculated positive predictive value (PPV), but not the negative predictive value (NPV), estimates remained low due to the low prevalence in this age group, arguing against the use of such a panel as a screening tool in a similarly aged, asymptomatic population. While sensitivity and specificity reflect on accuracy provided by a test, predictive values address the meaning of test results given a particular context (i.e., age-dependent prevalence) (4). The discovery and internal validation metabolomic analyses that were originally advanced, however, provided support to the lipid irregularities previously associated with LOAD (5), and our 5-year longitudinal study design allowed identification of biomarkers that predict the pending phenoconversion to the clinical stages of LOAD. Herein, we describe the discovery and internal validation of an expanded panel of plasma metabolites, from the same baseline asymptomatic subjects previously reported (2). The expanded metabolite panel provides increased sensitivity and specificity and improved predictive values within our cohort. In addition, the specific analytes in the panel further strengthen the links between dysregulated brain and plasma lipid species during the preclinical stages of LOAD. Our expanded biomarker panel, therefore, provides significant potential benefits, as well as burdens that must be considered by individuals and society at large. Such a biomarker panel for preclinical LOAD must initially play a role in selecting subjects for secondary prevention trials and, possibly, monitoring their therapeutic success or failure. Eventually, however, it will be critical that biomarker panels of disease stimulate the development of new or repurposed therapeutics. A diagnostic test without an associated viable treatment option is always limited. Eventually, a highly accurate panel such as proposed might be applicable in a general clinical practice, identifying older adults with a high risk of phenoconversion to the clinical stages of LOAD, and allowing initiation of treatment that could modify the course of disease.

MATERIALS AND METHODS

Participants

The study design for this investigation is structured in a manner similar to that used in our original study (2) but features discovery and internal validation sets that include only subjects who maintain a cognitively normal status [normal control (NC)] and those who phenoconvert from cognitive normality at baseline ($\text{Converter}_{\text{pre}}$) to either aMCI or AD by either year 3 or year 5 of the Rochester/Orange County Aging Study (**Figure 1**). As part of a 5-year observational study, we enrolled a total of 525 community-dwelling participants from two distinct geographic regions, aged 70 and older, and who were otherwise healthy. Health records and medications were fully documented, and subjects were excluded only if major neurologic or oncologic illness was present. All study participants provided informed consent for study inclusion and use of their neurocognitive results and peripheral blood specimens for analyses. Institutional review boards (IRBs) at each institution approved the protocols and informed consent documents. As opposed to including the incident aMCI/AD group, as described in our original investigation (2), the primary inclusion and comparison for this analysis was limited to those subjects who remained cognitively normal throughout the study and those who phenoconverted to aMCI or AD during the 5-year study. Subjects were continuously enrolled in the study over 5 years. In a planned midpoint analysis, we selected those who remained cognitively normal or phenoconverted from baseline to year 3 for the discovery cohort and those who were subsequently enrolled or who subsequently phenoconverted during year 3 to 5 for the internal validation cohort. As shown in **Table 1**, the 71 discovery subjects include 53 NC and 18 $\text{Converter}_{\text{pre}}$ individuals. The discovery cohort $\text{Converter}_{\text{pre}}$ subjects consisted of 2 individuals who phenoconverted to AD and 16 who transitioned to aMCI. Of this group, three of those converting to aMCI carried an *APOE* ϵ4 allele. The 30 internal validation subjects featured 20 NC and 10 $\text{Converter}_{\text{pre}}$ individuals. Internal validation cohort phenoconverters consisted of five individuals who developed AD and five meeting criteria for aMCI. In the internal validation cohort, two of the AD converters carried an *APOE* ϵ4 allele. The discovery and internal validation cohorts did not share any common subjects. **Figure 1** further depicts how the $\text{Converter}_{\text{pre}}$ subjects were selected (number that phenoconverted by year 3 and the remaining that

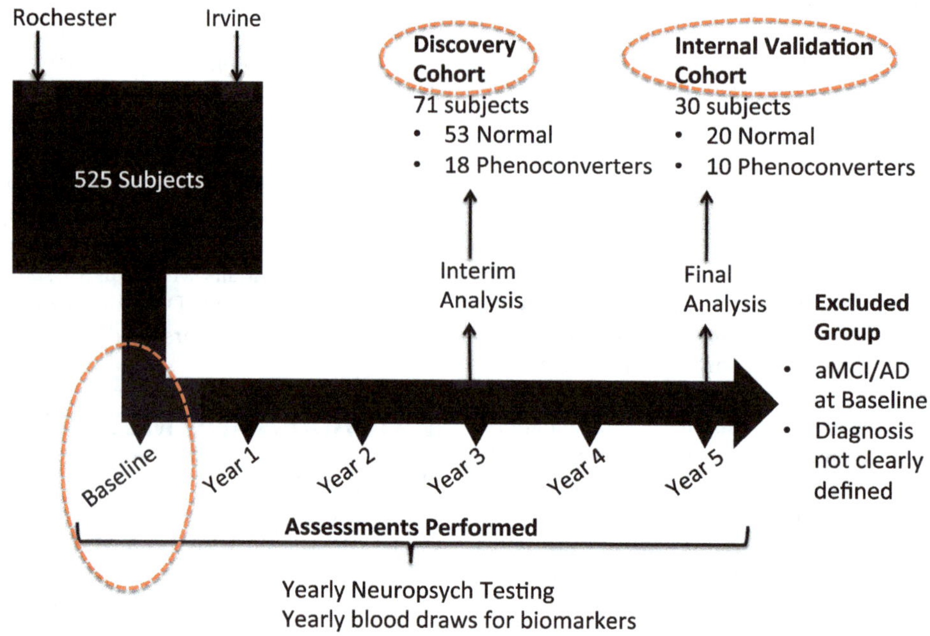

FIGURE 1 | Schematic representation of overall study design and specific analyses reported in this paper. Clinical subjects for the 5-year observational study were selected for participation at the University of Rochester and the University of California Irvine. An interim analysis was performed at year 3 of the study, comparing 53 subjects who maintained normal cognition since baseline study entry, to a group of 18 subjects who were cognitively normal at baseline but had phenoconverted to either aMCI or AD by year 3. This group made up our discovery cohort from which initial biomarker discovery was performed. With complete neuropsychological assessments available by study termination, an additional group of 10 subjects were noted to have phenoconverted during year 4 and year 5. This latter group was combined with a group of 20 matched subjects who maintained normal cognition throughout the study, and together were designated as the internal validation group (or cohort). All subjects included in this analysis (Discovery and Internal Validation cohorts) had only their baseline blood specimens assessed for metabolomic biomarker comparisons (dashed red circles).

TABLE 1 | Discovery and internal validation cohort demographic details.

Clinical groups	n (M/F)	Mean age years [SD]	Mean education years [SD]	% *APOE* ϵ4
Normal control (NC)				
Discovery	53 (18/35)	81.6 [3.6]	15.7 [2.3]	24.6
Internal validation	20 (9/11)	81.4 [3.3]	15.1 [2.5]	20
$\text{Converter}_{\text{pre}}$				
Discovery	18 (8/10)	80.7 [2.3]	15.3 [3.1]	16.7
Internal validation	10 (4/6)	79.3 [5.5]	14.5 [1.8]	20
Total discovery	71 (26/45)	81.8 [3.0]	15.5 [2.7]	20.7
Total internal validation	30 (13/17)	80.9 [4.4]	14.8 [2.2]	20.0

n, number of subjects; F, female subjects; M, male subjects; SD, standard deviation; % APOE ϵ4, percent having at least a single APOE ϵ4 allele.
Gender, age, education, and APOE ϵ4 status were not significantly different (Chi-square $p > 0.05$) between discovery and internal validation groups.

phenoconverted by year 5) and matched to NC subjects, for this manuscript as well as our previous lipidomic study. The number of subjects in our discovery ($n = 71$) and internal validation ($n = 30$) groups (or cohorts), therefore, approaches the accepted biostatistical standards (6) for discovery and validation groupings of 2/3 and 1/3, respectively. This study focused solely on biomarker comparisons between subject groups categorized as fulfilling the cognitively normal state ($\text{Converter}_{\text{pre}}$ vs. NC) at baseline. Excluded from this and our previous analysis (2) were a significant number of the total longitudinal study participants who could not be categorized based on the strict neurocognitive grouping parameters. We believe that rigorous clinical classification is necessary to increase signal in the biological samples for new metabolomic discovery. In any study with clinical characterization such as ours, we can clearly identify the cases (aMCI or LOAD), but not all remaining subjects should be considered NCs. Thus, in our work, we specifically define criteria for NCs and those who do not meet either definition (case or control) are not included in the specific study analysis. Subject data from the excluded individuals are undergoing separate analyses, not specifically related to the diagnosis of LOAD. The goal of this analysis, therefore, was to develop a biomarker model that would more accurately predict whether phenoconversion would or would not occur in cognitively normal subjects of our aging cohort within 5 years from study entry. Herein, we compare those cognitively normal ($\text{Converter}_{\text{pre}}$ or preclinical LOAD, $n = 28$) individuals, who developed memory impairment, with or without functional impairment, within 5 years of study entry, to those subjects who remained cognitively normal (NC, $n = 73$) over the same 5-year study period (**Table 1**) (total study group analyzed, $n = 101$). Of the 28 subjects who phenoconverted, 21 developed aMCI, and 7 developed AD within the 5-year study. We reiterate that the 101 subjects in this analysis are a subset of those reported in our previous publication (that also included those with incident aMCI/AD) (2).

Our discovery and internal validation groups of cognitively normal individuals at baseline assessment (including both NC and Converter$_{pre}$) were matched for age, gender, and education and featured similar *APOE* allele status (**Table 1**). Our internal validation group consisted of approximately one-third of all subjects included in our analysis and was composed of phenoconverters from years 3 to 5 and their matched set of control subjects. All study participants underwent phlebotomy between 8:00 a.m. and 10:00 a.m., on a yearly basis, while fasting and withholding their morning medications, and as close as possible to the same day each year of study participation. Blood specimens were initially placed on ice, and the blood components were separated within 24 h, yielding multiple plasma aliquots that were frozen immediately thereafter at −80°C until undergoing metabolomic analyses. Smaller plasma aliquots allowed a single freeze-thaw cycle prior to metabolomic processing for all specimens. All metabolomic data used for this analysis had been previously made available online (2), and untargeted discovery and targeted internal validation data had been obtained from baseline plasma specimens for all reported study participants. Glycerophospholipids were the most significantly dysregulated class of metabolites in our original untargeted discovery data. Discovery group data for this investigation resulted from 71 baseline subject specimens who underwent a targeted multiple reaction monitoring-stable isotope dilution-mass spectrometry (MRM-SID-MS) analysis using the Biocrates Absolute-IDQ P180 Kit (Biocrates Life Sciences, Innsbruck, Austria), which evaluates five classes of metabolites, including acylcarnitines (ACs), amino acids, hexoses, phospho- and sphingo-lipids, and biogenic amines, in an effort to reduce bias toward a particular class of metabolites. A subsequent internal validation study was completed on an additional 30 baseline subject specimens that underwent similar metabolomic analyses (**Figure 1**). These data were preprocessed, as previously described (2), prior to statistical consideration.

Statistical Analysis

Statistical treatment of the data in this study was according to the same overall methods as described in our previous publication (2). The abundance measurements for metabolites (with a specific mass/charge ratio, m/z) in both positive and negative modes were expressed as intensity units that were initially normalized using log transformation and quantile normalization (**Figure 2**). For the 71 subjects in the discovery cohort, we calculated the level of differential expression for each metabolite using a t-test, comparing NC and Converter$_{pre}$, constrained by p-value <0.05. Among these differentially expressed metabolites, we performed the feature selection using a regularized learning technique, which uses the least absolute shrinkage and selection operator (LASSO) penalty (7, 8). We first obtained the regularization path over a grid of values for the tuning parameter lambda (λ) through 10-fold cross-validation. The optimal value for λ obtained by the cross-validation procedure was used to fit the model. All the features with nonzero coefficients were deemed as biomarker candidates. This technique is known to reduce overfitting and variance in classification.

The classification performance of the selected metabolites was assessed using the ROC curve AUC. To maintain rigor of independent validation, the simple logistic model from the discovery set was fixed. The statistical team was blinded to the sample group identities of the internal validation cohort, which consisted of different NCs and Converter$_{pre}$ subjects than those used in the discovery cohort. Any separation in values between NC and Converter$_{pre}$ subjects for the final panel was evaluated using a robust method, the hidden logistic regression model with the maximum estimated likelihood (MEL) estimator (9). A combined classifier, based on the final biomarker panel for 101 subjects, within the discovery and internal validation groups, was developed to determine differences between NC and Converter$_{pre}$ groups. The resulting combined classifier allowed the development of a plasma metabolite index (PMI), which provides a single predictive value of risk of phenoconversion in cognitively normal subjects observed over the 5-year interval. The PMI is obtained by mapping the log odds in a regularized logistic regression model on a 0–100 scale.

Positive and negative predictive value calculations used in this paper feature the direct measures of sensitivity and specificity defined from the ROC curves (10, 11) as well as the clinical prevalence from the literature (12), based on the disease in the specific population tested (13). Accuracy measures, which combine sensitivity and specificity for our biomarkers, were calculated for the 10-lipid and new metabolite panels. Accuracy values are calculated for potential cutoff probabilities of being diagnosed Converter$_{pre}$ based on the ROC curve.

RESULTS

The clinical groups (see **Table 1**) were not significantly different ($p \geq 0.05$) from each other based on gender, age, education, and *APOE* ϵ4 allele carrier percentages. *APOE* allele status was not a significant covariate, as previously reported (2). The ROC AUC with and without inclusion of *APOE* ϵ4 allele status in the classifier was not significantly different ($p \geq 0.05$). Cognitive and phenoconversion details for the cohorts associated with this study are provided in **Table 2**. The memory Z-scores clearly decline from baseline to the post conversion (Converter$_{post}$) state. Mean time to phenoconversion for all converters was 2.1 years. The discovery group had a mean time to phenoconversion of 1.5 years, while the internal validation group's mean time to phenoconversion was 3.1 years. The mean time to phenoconversion was significantly longer for the internal validation group compared to the discovery group (Mann–Whitney U Z-score = −3.21, p = 0.0013).

A total of 174 significant ($p < 0.05$) differentially expressed metabolites were defined in the discovery cohort. Of this group, 24 metabolites [13 glycerophosphatidylcholines (PCs), 9 ACs, 1 amino acid, and 1 biogenic amine] (**Table 3**) fulfilled the specific selection criteria established for the new biomarker panel. Three of the 24 metabolites, all belonging to the AC group (see bottom 3 entities in **Table 3**; **Figure 3**), had significantly increased levels, while quantities of the remaining metabolites were all significantly reduced in Converter$_{pre}$ subjects compared to NC, for both discovery and internal validation groups (**Table 3**; **Figure 3**). Seven of the 24 metabolites were featured in our previously reported panel of 10 plasma lipids (2) (see top 7 in **Table 3**; **Figure 3**), and include a single AC (C3, proprionyl-L-carnitine), a single lysophosphatidylcholine (lysoPC a C18:2),

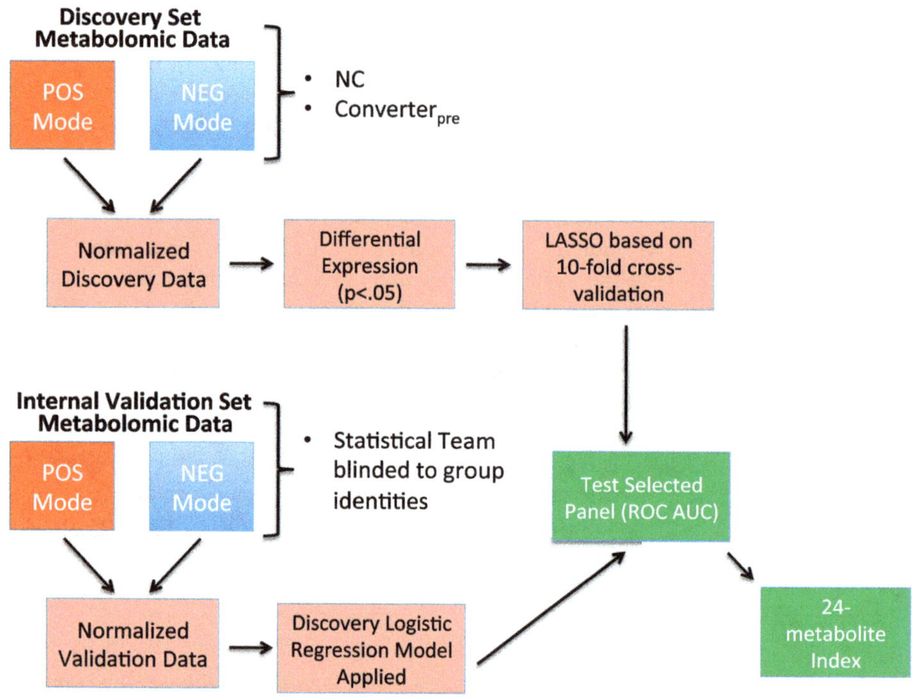

FIGURE 2 | Flow chart showing steps in biomarker model development. Discovery cohort information was obtained from baseline specimen metabolomic data from subjects who remained cognitively normal (NC) throughout the study and baseline specimens from those that phenoconverted ($Converter_{pre}$) during the study's first 3 years. Discovery metabolomic data from positive and negative modes underwent normalization, followed by selection of significantly altered metabolites ($p < 0.05$), which were then annotated. The significant, annotated biomarker panel was then defined via a regularized learning method that features the LASSO restriction. The discovery biomarker panel selected is then tested using the receiver operating characteristic area under the curve (ROC AUC) method. With the statistical team blinded to group identities, the Internal Validation cohort data were similarly normalized and annotated. Internal Validation data were subjected to the results of the discovery logistic regression classifier and tested using the ROC AUC method. Combined data from the discovery and internal validation sets were used to develop a 24-metabolite index.

TABLE 2 | Cognitive *Z*-scores and conversion diagnosis.

	Cognitive *Z*-scores					Conversion Dx (aMCI/ AD)	Years to phenoconversion [SEM]
	Z_{att} [SEM]	Z_{exe} [SEM]	Z_{lan} [SEM]	Z_{mem} [SEM]	Z_{vis} [SEM]		
Normal control (NC)							
Discovery	−0.17 [0.1]	−0.06 [0.1]	0.03 [0.1]	0.08 [0.1]	0.06 [0.1]	n.a.	n.a.
Internal validation	0.03 [0.1]	0.06 [0.2]	0.06 [0.1]	−0.05 [0.1]	0.27 [0.2]	n.a.	n.a.
$Converter_{pre}$							
Discovery	−0.35 [0.2]	−0.54 [0.2]	−0.58 [0.3]	−0.81 [0.1]	−0.48 [0.3]	n.a.	n.a.
Internal validation	−0.42 [0.2]	−0.42 [0.4]	−0.03 [0.4]	−0.02 [0.1]	0.35 [0.3]	n.a.	n.a.
$Converter_{post}$							
Discovery	−0.33 [0.2]	−0.60 [0.2]	−0.88 [0.3]	−1.7 [0.1]	−0.39 [0.3]	(16/2)	1.5 [0.5]
Internal validation	−0.31 [0.2]	−1.0 [0.4]	−0.75 [0.4]	−1.7 [0.1]	0.06 [0.3]	(5/5)	3.1* [1.2]

Z_{att}, attention composite Z score; Z_{exe}, executive composite Z score; Z_{lan}, language composite Z score; Z_{mem}, memory composite Z score; Z_{vis}, visuoperceptual composite Z score. Conversion Dx represents the number of individuals who phenoconverted to the specific diagnosis: n.a., not applicable; aMCI, amnestic mild cognitive impairment; AD, Alzheimer's disease. Note the prominent decline in Z_{mem} for the Converter subjects from $Converter_{pre}$ to $Converter_{post}$ consistent with phenoconversion to memory impairment. Also, note decline in other cognitive domains consistent with the diagnosis of AD in some subjects, which requires impairment in memory plus one other cognitive domain.

**Mean time to phenoconversion was significantly longer for the internal validation converter group compared to the discovery converter group (Mann–Whitney U Z-score = −3.21, $p < 0.01$); SEM, standard error of the mean.*

and 5 PCs, with either ester (a) or ether (e) linkages (PC aa 36:6; PC aa 38:0; PC aa 38:6; PC aa 40:1; and PC ae 40:6). Nine novel ACs in the current panel include valeryl-L-carnitine (C5), hydroxyvaleryl-L-carnitine/methylmalonyl-L-carnitine (C5-OH/C3-DC-M), non-ayl-L-carnitine (C9), decenoyl-L-carnitine (C10:1), decadienyl-L-carnitine (C10:2)dodecenoyl-L-carnitine (C12:1), hexadecadienyl-L-carnitine (C16:2), and hydroxyoctadecenoyl-L-carnitine (C18:1-OH). This new panel

TABLE 3 | Components of the 24 metabolite biosignature for determining risk of phenoconversion from normal cognition to aMCI or AD.

Metabolite name	Discovery cohort			Internal validation cohort	
	p-value	Log ratio (mean)	Log ratio (median)	Log ratio (mean)	Log ratio (median)
PC ae C40:6	0.0380	−0.3039	−0.0809	−0.2980	−0.2445
PC aa C40:1	0.0414	−0.2040	−0.0779	−1.1414	−0.1909
PC aa C38:6	0.0365	−0.3372	−0.2081	−0.9792	−0.1445
PC aa C38:0	0.0391	−0.2510	−0.0533	−0.5129	−0.1469
PC aa C36:6	0.0446	−0.3695	−0.1270	−0.2383	−0.1472
lysoPC a C18:2	0.0299	−0.3326	−0.0409	−0.3801	−0.1235
C3	0.0031	−0.4574	−0.2728	−1.2751	−0.3337
PC ae C36:4	0.0428	−0.3994	−0.0769	−0.6625	−0.2740
C10:2	0.0403	−0.4042	−0.1914	−0.1913	−0.2948
C9	0.0070	−0.4044	−0.2231	−0.8499	−0.2433
PC ae C42:1	0.0073	−0.4980	−0.3428	−1.3565	−0.3138
PC aa C38:3	0.0432	−0.4141	−0.1500	−0.8084	−0.2387
C5	0.0013	−0.2769	−0.1959	−0.6762	−0.2451
ADMA	0.0163	−0.2962	−0.1144	−1.0761	−1.5794
Asn	0.0441	−0.1788	−0.0891	−0.8982	−0.1933
PC aa C34:4	0.0346	−0.4353	−0.1906	−0.1430	−0.0835
C18:1-OH	0.0182	−0.2676	−0.3349	−1.2507	−0.2383
PC ae C34:0	0.0148	−0.4064	−0.2323	−1.2721	−0.4404
C5-OH (C3-DC-M)	0.0003	−0.4214	−0.3204	−2.1235	−2.0212
PC aa C40:5	0.0298	−0.4349	−0.1534	−0.5866	−0.4183
PC aa C32:0	0.0150	−0.4014	−0.1843	−1.4605	−0.6273
C16:2	0.0108	0.2767	0.0789	0.5001	0.0419
C12:1	0.0001	0.5075	0.3435	0.8748	0.2055
C10:1	0.0026	0.3642	0.2172	0.6121	0.0184

In the metabolites listed, C_ species (e.g., C3) denote acylcarnitines (ACs). Phosphocholine (PC) metabolites display combined numbers of carbon atoms for their two acyl groups (sn_1 and sn_2 positions) (e.g., C38), whereas the combined number of double bonds (unsaturation) is displayed after the colon (e.g., C38:6). Acyl group linkages to choline backbone for PCs feature ester (a) or ether (e) linkage (e.g., PC ae C36:4). Asn, asparagine. ADMA, asymmetric dimethylarginine. LysoPC, lysophosphatidylcholine species, with only one acyl group, typically in the sn_1 position. The discovery cohort provided significant differentially expressed metabolites between $Converter_{pre}$ and NC. The column of p values indicates the significant differences for mean analyte values between the clinical groups for the discovery cohort. Log ratios represent the difference of the log-transformed values (mean or median) for $Converter_{pre}$ and NC subjects. Negative log values indicate that levels (mean or median) of the analyte in $Converter_{pre}$ < NC, while positive log values indicate that levels (mean or median) in $Converter_{pre}$ > NC. NC, normal control subjects.

also features asparagine (Asn), an amino acid, and asymmetric dimethylarginine (ADMA), a biogenic amine. All 7 novel PCs in this panel contain pairs of long chain fatty acids (FAs) (13–21 carbons), as did those in our previous report (2). The new PCs include PC aa C32:0, PC aa C34:0, PC aa C34:4, PC ae C36:4, PC aa C38:3, PC aa C40:5, and PC ae C42:1.

Receiver operating characteristic analyses (**Figures 4A,B**) of the plasma 24-metabolite panel yielded AUC measures of 1.00 and 0.995, for the discovery and internal validation groups, respectively. As a test on the accuracy of the 24-metabolite panel, a support vector machine (SVM) classifier was also developed on the discovery set and provided a similar ROC AUC (0.98) measure. Such precision allows the development of a plasma 24 metabolite index (P24MI) (**Figure 4C**) based on a regularized logistic regression model using the combined discovered and validated 24 metabolite values. The P24MI provides 100% confidence that subjects in our study with scores of ≥49 will phenoconvert to either aMCI or AD over the next 5 years.

Comparisons of our 10-lipid panel and expanded 24-metabolite panel are presented in **Table 4**, which define the comprehensive improvement provided by the expanded panel. Importantly, the presented PPV and NPV in **Table 4** are derived using a conservative calculation method (10), and they feature similar published prevalence estimates of LOAD for female and male subjects aged 71–79 years: 2.33% for females, and 2.30% for males (12). Gender differences in LOAD prevalence grow significantly in subsequent decades, much higher in women, and is most likely due to their longer life expectancy (14).

DISCUSSION

We present an expanded plasma metabolite panel that attempts to maximize sensitivity, specificity, PPV, NPV, and accuracy in predicting risk of phenoconversion in a clinically asymptomatic cohort of seniors participating in a 5-year observational study. We included predictive assessments in the presentation of this 24-metabolite panel and in the retrospective analysis of our published 10-lipid panel (2) (see **Table 4**). It is important to note that our original lipidomic panel, while demonstrating the feasibility of risk identification using blood-based biomarkers for the preclinical stages of LOAD, was specifically defined to achieve approximately 90% sensitivity and specificity of classification utilizing the smallest number of analytes. These particular selection criteria were meant to provide interpretive simplicity and ease of implementation on a path toward a putative diagnostic assay. Since then, other investigators (15–17) have reported similar

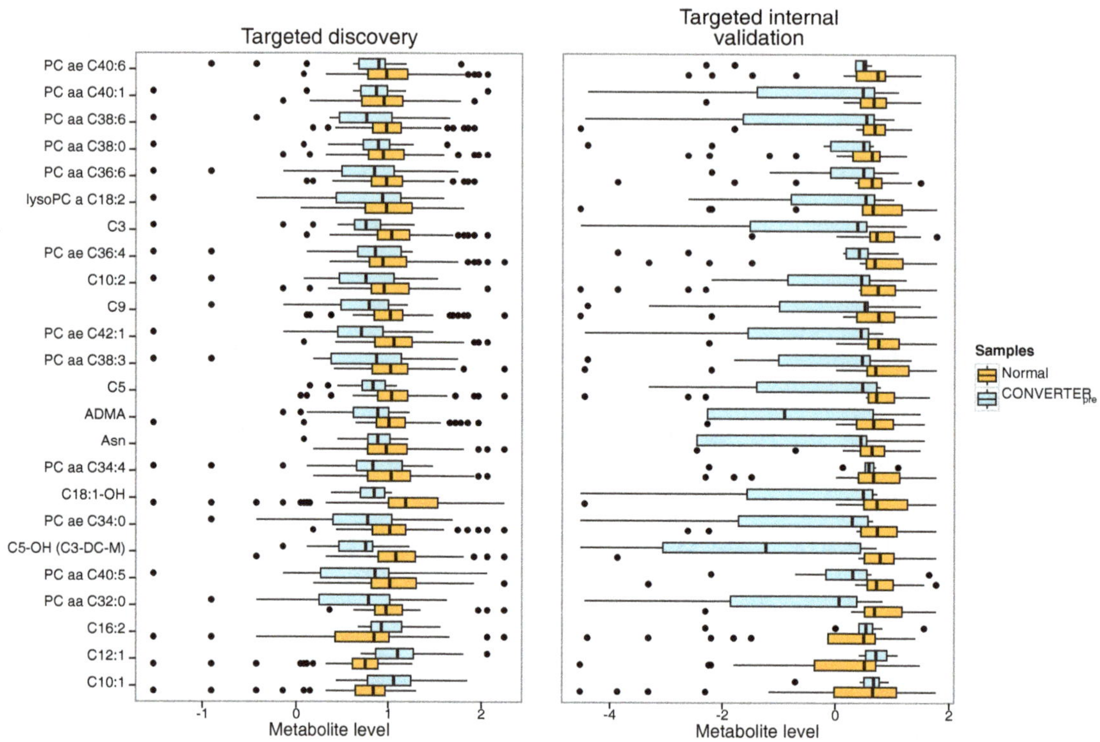

FIGURE 3 | Horizontal box and whisker plots of plasma 24 metabolite panel results for clinical groups in discovery and internal validation cohorts. Comparative ranges of plasma metabolite levels for the targeted discovery and internal validation studies are displayed, allowing appraisal of metabolite results in the cognitively intact normal (orange) versus Converter$_{pre}$ (light blue) groups. The box defines the interquartile range (IQR) with the vertical black line within the box representing the median value. The whiskers define the upper and lower 25% limits of the data, while the dots represent outliers (≥1.5 IQR lengths from the ends of the box). The normal group featured 53 subjects in the discovery and 20 in the internal validation cohorts, while the Converter$_{pre}$ group included 18 and 10 subjects, for discovery and internal validation cohorts, respectively. Individual analytes are listed on the left vertical axis, while normalized metabolite levels are shown on the horizontal axis. All the Converter$_{pre}$ analyte results are reduced in comparison to NC levels, except for three acylcarnitine species (bottom of figure), C16:2, C12:1, and C10:1, which are elevated. Note the higher variability of the internal validation set compared to the discovery set, due to less than half of the number of subjects in the former compared to the latter.

groups of phospholipids depleted in the blood of Alzheimer's disease (AD) patients, while a recent nutritional intervention study provided an alternative validation of our initial lipidomic findings (18). Since the ultimate utility of a clinical diagnostic test will depend, at least in part, on a combination of safety, predictive accuracy, and cost, especially if used as a screening tool in asymptomatic subjects, we now provide a new metabolomic panel that maximizes predictive accuracy in the examined age group while maintaining safety and relatively low cost.

Despite the significant differences in time to phenoconversion between our discovery and internal validation groups (**Table 2**), we are encouraged that our metabolomic profile developed under a time to phenoconversion of 1.5 years also appears accurate up to 3 years prior to phenoconversion. We believe that analysis of serial specimens from our participants would provide extremely valuable information regarding analyte changes over time. Such analyses are yet to be finalized due to the associated expenses. However, we believe that insights on whether expansion of our metabolomic biomarker panel could be useful in raising predictive accuracy of phenoconversion risk would be independent of these serial analyses. While test sensitivity and specificity was improved, PPV and NPV, especially PPV remained limited by the low prevalence used for our age range (12). Importantly, our 24-metabolite panel provides an improved risk assessment regarding which subjects will develop aMCI or AD, and more importantly, which subjects will not.

The revised selection criteria for our 24-metabolite panel accounts for the inclusion of seven significantly dysregulated plasma lipid species from our original report (2), and 15 additional abnormal plasma lipids, a single amino acid, and a single biogenic amine. The 3 lipids included in our original 10-lipid panel but excluded from the current 24-metabolite panel were likely not considered due to more significant metabolites and the LASSO exclusion to avoid co-linearity. We assert that this novel plasma metabolite panel provides concordant, significantly altered analytes based on the specific selection criteria and statistical stringency used. These plasma biosignatures of phenoconversion risk primarily feature dysregulated lipid species, with the majority being reduced in plasma compared to normal. The significant reduction in both PC and AC species in peripheral blood supports the hypothesis put forth by our group (2) and others (5, 15, 18–20) that abnormalities in lipid networks may not only represent biomarkers for, but may be integral to the development of specific neurodegenerative

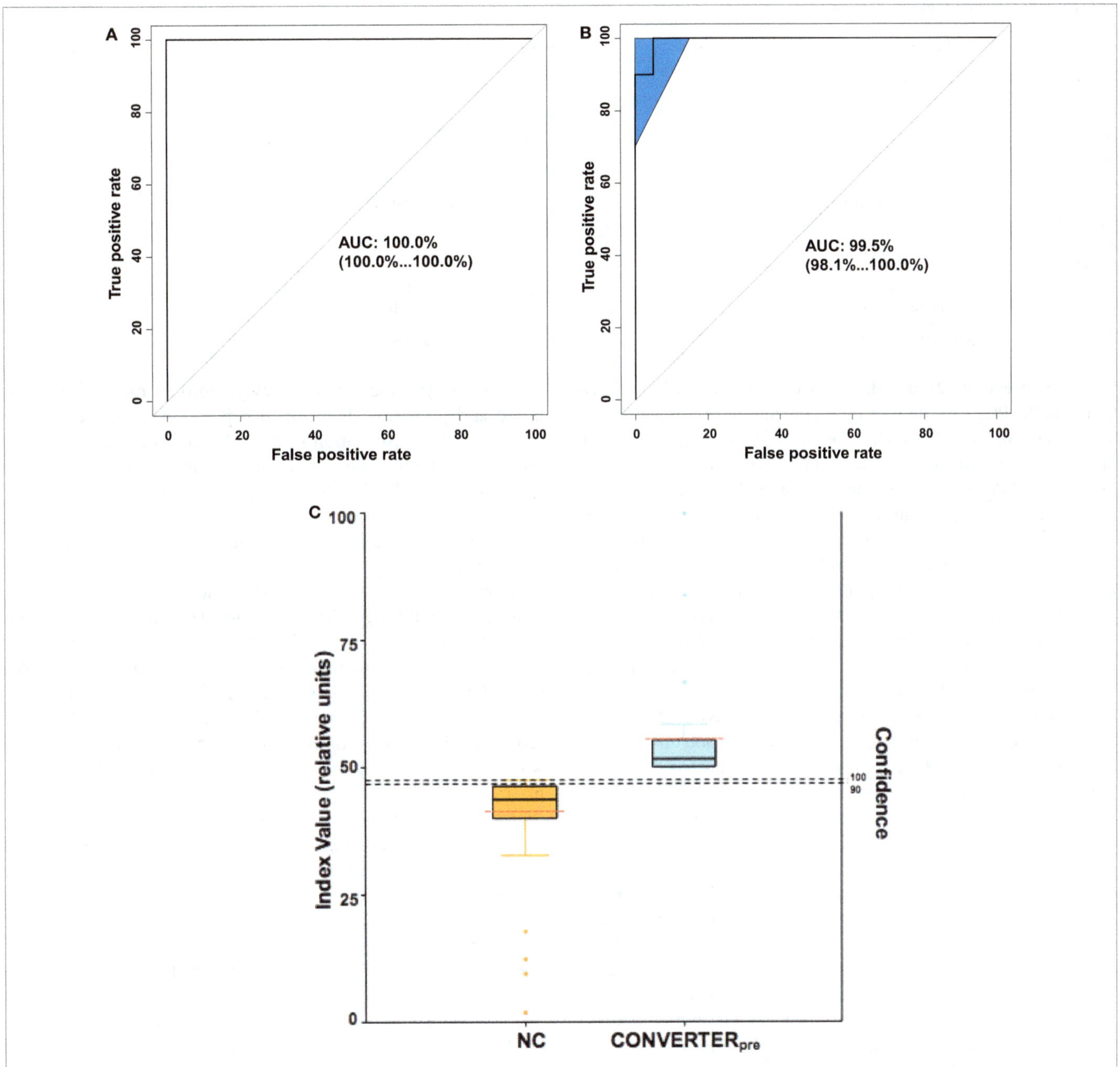

FIGURE 4 | Analytic representations to discriminate Converter$_{pre}$ from normal control (NC) subjects. **(A,B)** provide receiver operating characteristic (ROC) curves, whereas **(C)** depicts the calculated plasma 24 metabolite index (P24MI). **(A)** ROC area under the curve (AUC) for the Discovery cohort was equal to 1.00 with 95% confidence interval (in parentheses) ranging from 1.00 to 1.00. **(B)** ROC AUC for the internal validation cohort was 0.995, with 95% confidence interval (shaded area on plot) ranging from 0.981 to 1.00. **(C)** The P24MI results are depicted in vertical boxplots based on the logistic regression model that distinguishes between Converter$_{pre}$ and NC groups. Solid black horizontal lines represent the mean value, while the dashed red horizontal lines represent the median value. Orange and light blue dots represent outliers (≥1.5 IQR lengths from the ends of the box). The higher index values (left vertical axis) are associated with an increased risk of phenoconversion to aMCI or AD, as seen in our Converter$_{pre}$ subjects, with confidence (right vertical axis) of predicting phenoconversion transitioning from 90 to 100% at an relative index value of 48. Based on the calculated P24MI in our current dataset, a relative index value ≥49 represents a Converter$_{pre}$ individual and a risk of phenoconversion of 100% within the 5-year study range. Note the relatively low variability of the P24MI for both the NC group and the Converter$_{pre}$ group, with no overlap.

pathologies, including LOAD. Similarities in the dysregulated lipid networks within brains from human LOAD and transgenic mouse models of early-onset AD (EOAD) suggest disruptions in the levels of certain bioactive lipids, including glycerophospholipids, ceramides, and sphingomyelins, highlighting the utility of lipidomics for investigating these conditions (21). Future assessments may elucidate shared as well as distinct etiologic mechanisms in both EOAD and LOAD and dictate particular therapeutic options to target the differences in their pathobiologic networks.

TABLE 4 | Biomarker panel comparisons.

Biomarker panel		Sensitivity	Specificity	ROC AUC	PPV/NPV (%)	Accuracy (%)
Gender	Cohort					
10 lipid (2)		0.9	0.85			85
Male					12.4/99.7	
Female					12.5/99.7	
	Discovery			0.96		
	Internal validation			0.92		
24 metabolite		1.00	0.95			95
Male					32.0/100	
Female					32.3/100	
	Discovery			1.00		
	Internal validation			0.995		

ROC AUC, receiver operating characteristic area under the curve; PPV, positive predictive value; NPV, negative predictive value.

In our previous (2) as well as our current plasma biomarker panel, all the PCs are notably reduced during the preclinical stages of LOAD. Similar PC reductions have been documented in AD brains (22) and attributed to pathologic activation of phospholipase A_2 (PLA_2) (22, 23). Using current analytic methods, dysregulated lipid metabolism has been confirmed, with reductions in specific PCs noted in brain (24), plasma (5), and serum (25) of AD subjects compared to controls. With PLA_2 activity known to form lyso PCs, lack of significant central elevations in this phospholipid byproduct may relate to their rapid re-acylation to form PCs for repair (or attempted repair) of membranes (26) or to generation of downstream metabolites. The mechanistic link between reduction of brain lipid in association with LOAD, and in peripheral blood, has yet to be fully elucidated. Interestingly, the PCs in our 24-metabolite panel all feature polyunsaturated fatty acids (PUFAs) (**Table 3**), as has been reported by others (25, 27). While the brain has the capacity to generate all the lipid species it requires for normal function, along with most saturated and monounsaturated FAs (28, 29), specific substrates required to maintain brain lipid homeostasis, especially sources of energy and certain PUFAs, are delivered to the brain via the bloodstream. In normal brain metabolic processing, phospholipid components are efficiently recycled and have relatively long central half-lives (28). Essential PUFAs such as docosahaxaenoic acid (DHA; 22:6 n-3) and arachidonic acid (AA; 20:4 n-6) provide structural functionality as phospholipid components in bilayer membranes. Once released, either directly or through byproducts, they are known to participate in signal transduction processes that have positive and negative consequences within cells (30). Under conditions where brain membrane lipids undergo catabolism (e.g., oxidative stress, or neuroinflammation), the downstream intermediates often are not recycled to the membrane and thereby increase the demand for lipid precursors from the bloodstream (**Figure 5**). Such precursors exist in plasma as unesterified FAs ($\leq$22 carbons) bound to albumin, or as esterified FA species (>22 carbons) within phospholipids preferentially transported within circulating lipoproteins (30). Esterified FAs can be converted to unesterified forms via lipases within the lipoproteins or circulating within the blood (31–33). Flux of unesterified FAs into the brain, across the blood–brain barrier (BBB), is rapid and occurs via simple diffusion and possibly via facilitated transport (30). All unesterified FAs entering the brain are immediately esterified by acetyl-CoA-synthase (34–37), preventing their diffusion back to blood and preparing them for incorporation into lipid biosynthetic pathways. Activation of phospholipases (e.g., PLA_2) with increased oxidative stress is implicated in diminishing PUFAs from membrane lipids (16). We have observed elevated levels of oxidative lipid metabolites in our at-risk preclinical subjects, that do not reach statistical significance, but reach significant elevation in plasma from symptomatic LOAD subjects compared to controls [unpublished data][1]. Hartmann and colleagues (18) provided an indirect test to this hypothesis of depleted substrates (**Figure 5A**), in their investigation of a medically regulated nutritional supplement (Souvenaid®) in a randomized, placebo-controlled, double-blind clinical trial in subjects having mild dementia, attempting to stimulate *de novo* PC synthesis via the Kennedy pathway (38). They report significant elevations in five specific blood-derived PCs with the supplemental agents, including members of our original plasma 10-lipid panel. Restoration of blood lipids with dietary supplements has been proposed as beneficial in both preclinical and mild AD by stabilizing synaptic membrane function (39), and network connectivity (40). In another recent publication (41), the authors propose that redox reactive autoantibodies are produced in CSF and blood as a result of exposure to oxidizing agents (in prodromal or manifest AD). Moreover, they proposed utilizing the autoantibody levels as disease biomarkers to differentiate control subjects from those with MCI or AD. From our perspective, such phospholipid autoantibodies are poised to preferentially bind to specific plasma phospholipids, with resultant clearance of the conjugates from blood plasma, making brain lipid substrates less available for entry into the brain. Recent data indicate a role for ACs beyond β-oxidation (42), including neuroprotection by increasing antioxidant activity, modulating membrane composition, assisting with lipid biosynthesis, participating in gene regulation, enhancing cholinergic neurotransmission, and improving mitochondrial function. Altered AC levels in those destined to phenoconvert to AD, therefore, may parallel central alterations in neuroprotection and/or bioenergetic capacity.

Finally, the reduced abundance of asparagine (asp) and asymmetric dimethylarginine (ADMA), in $Converter_{pre}$ compared to NC, provide insights into orthogonal dysregulated networks in the

[1]Cheema AK, Personal communication (2015)

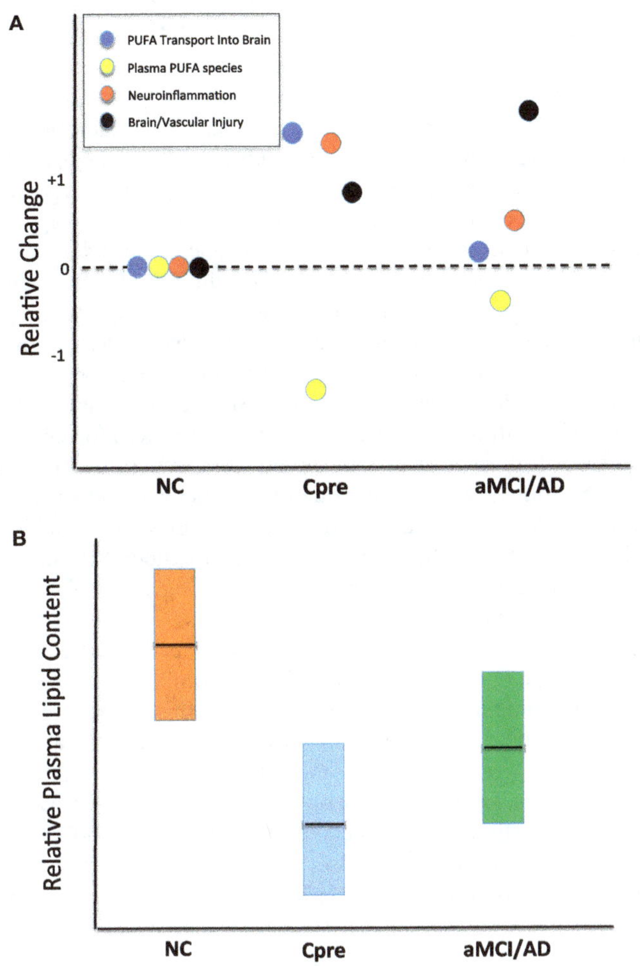

FIGURE 5 | Schematic representations of potential alterations within brain and peripheral blood responsible for reduced plasma phospholipid levels. **(A)** Qualitative dot plot of differential changes occurring in cognitively normal control (NC), cognitively normal Converter$_{pre}$ (C$_{pre}$) subjects, and those with amnestic mild cognitive impairment or Alzheimer's disease (aMCI/AD). Note that all four processes (represented within boxed legend) are at the zero relative level in the NC subjects. The C$_{pre}$ subjects could show significant polyunsaturated fatty acid (PUFA) transport into brain to replenish lost substrate as a result of neuroinflammation or other brain injury. The increase in PUFA flux into the brain is an attempt to compensate for ongoing injury and results in a marked reduction in the plasma levels of molecules carrying those lipid species. Dark horizontal line within boxes represents proposed mean. **(B)** Qualitative plasma phospholipid biomarker results, previously quantified (2), which may be better interpreted via the theory proposed in **(A)**. Dark horizontal line within boxes represents proposed mean. The full explanation for this metabolic phenomenon in the C$_{pre}$ subjects remains to be elucidated.

preclinical stages of LOAD. CSF and plasma asparagine levels are known to be reduced in AD subjects compared to controls (43). Depletion of asparagine from the CNS has been associated with reversible altered mental status in children and adults, including short-term memory impairment in the elderly (44). Asparagine's primary role is within proteins (45), affording a common site for N-glycosylation and providing unique structural characteristics at the ends of α-helices and within β-sheets (46). The brain, compared to peripheral organs, is particularly dependent on intrinsic production of asparagine due to limited transport across the BBB (47). ADMA is produced from a post-translational modification of polypeptides by specific methyltransferases, with subsequent release into plasma following cellular protein turnover (48). Elevated ADMA levels in blood have been consistently associated with cardiovascular disease (CVD) risk factors, such as hypertension or hypercholesterolemia (48, 49). Within blood and other tissues, ADMA is considered the primary inhibitor of nitric oxide synthase (NOS), and thereby, a regulator of nitric oxide (NO) production. Brain-specific NOS (nNOS or NOS1) (50), and consequently NO production, is regulated by the relative concentrations of substrate, arginine, versus ADMA (48). Although increased NO concentrations have been associated with neuronal cell death, NO has been implicated in important synaptic actions, including learning and memory (51). While ADMA levels in CSF and blood of AD patients have not provided consistent findings (52), we have not found previous reports of ADMA plasma levels in preclinical AD subjects. The reduced ADMA levels in our preclinical AD (Converter$_{pre}$) subjects, and thereby the implied elevation of NO vasodilator activity compared to matched controls, may indicate a compensatory process, possibly triggered by the presence of oxidative stress that increases NO production in the early stages of AD (53). Additional investigations are required to further elucidate these associations.

The potential for a highly accurate early screening test for AD raises important questions about the value of such testing, especially given that AD is a condition for which no cure exists and treatment options are extremely limited. In other contexts, the potential disutility associated with receiving bad health news (54, 55) and with discrimination based on test results, particularly in an employment or insurance context, has been recognized (56). On the other hand, information from early screening may produce utility by reducing uncertainty about the future and allowing individuals to optimize key economic decisions related to consumption, retirement, and future planning (57, 58). In addition, because significant limitations and rapid declines in financial capacity are a hallmark of patients with early stage AD (59–62), earlier diagnosis may also yield value in the form of averted financial losses. Individuals with AD that is too early to diagnose may be susceptible to financial exploitation and may have trouble managing day-to-day household financial responsibilities such as paying bills on time. Accurate LOAD testing may help families better recognize and respond to those financial decision-making deficits – such as by changing the financial head of household or instituting other checks and balances (58) – before major financial problems occur. The scale and scope of negative financial outcomes associated with AD in the prediagnosis period may be substantial but as yet remain unquantified. Finally, the advent of a predictive LOAD diagnostic is likely to advance researchers' ability to develop and test novel AD therapeutics. Responding to the projected future financial burden imposed by LOAD, and the potential sources of value from predictive testing, many states have prioritized early detection in their future preparations for AD (63).

As highlighted in the most recent report of the Presidential Commission for the Study of Bioethical Issues (64), ethical reflection and review need to be integrated into the research process from the planning phase to produce treatments and therapies that best meet the patient's values and goals. Procedures should be implemented to ensure patient and public participation in the design of ethical research protocols, development of diagnostics and treatments, and a delivery process for predictive AD diagnostics. To achieve these goals, accurate and transparent public communication is needed, along with an emphasis on pre- and post-test counseling, as underscored in recent guidelines for AD testing (65).

We acknowledge the residual limitations provided by the relatively small, homogenous cohort of subjects used in this investigation, which is a subset of our previously reported study participants (2). We believe that there are advantages to a longitudinal study design that cannot be replicated in larger cross-sectional or case–control studies, however, especially for defining and directly investigating the preclinical state. Despite the added cost and time required, longitudinal observational studies allow the direct determination of the included preclinical period and to time the transition to clinical disease quite accurately. It is through analyses of preclinical biospecimens directly determined through such observations that specific, temporally related disease mechanisms can be accurately determined. As a result of longitudinal clinical and limited correlative biomarker determinations, we have helped define potential preclinical dysregulated plasma lipids and other metabolites within our study group. Similar preclinical mechanisms can only be inferred using methods that compare health to disease. We remain committed to a full analysis of all of our longitudinal specimens obtained from our Rochester/Orange County Aging Study subjects. In the meantime, however, an external validation study is underway in which we are evaluating plasma specimens from a larger, more ethnically diverse, and slightly younger subject cohort to discern the applicability of our current metabolomic biomarker panels beyond our strictly defined cohort (2). External validation of our findings remains a critical component that currently limits the impact and utility of our results.

We also acknowledge the possibility of overfitting of the classifier model to our limited set of subjects in this investigation, despite our attempt to minimize such effects with the statistical methods used. We present the current findings as a starting point, therefore, for the external validation studies that are currently underway. Optimal external validation of our biomarker panels will require plasma samples that are obtained in similar subjects, under comparable rigorous collection and processing procedures. In our case, specific details to be followed would include morning blood collections in a limited time window, following an overnight fast and withholding morning medications, and minimizing plasma freeze-thaw cycles prior to metabolomic analysis. It seems unlikely that currently available specimens from external cohorts will meet such strict criteria, but application of our biomarker panels to such disparate specimens will instruct us regarding what similarities, if any, may exist related to preclinical disease biosignatures despite different demographics and sample collection/processing methods.

The alteration in specific analyte species during the preclinical stages of LOAD from our studies is consistent with results from other groups (25, 27, 38) and provides evidence for unique metabolomic dysregulation, especially related to plasma lipids, during the preclinical and clinical LOAD stages. While the theoretical basis for the significant preclinical lipid reductions within plasma during preclinical LOAD remains unconfirmed, there are several mechanistic reasons for their occurrence that can be readily tested. We encourage other investigators to advance our understanding of such postulates through independent validation studies. The dysregulated analyte species found in our study subjects appear to suggest at least several altered metabolic networks, distinct from amyloid and tau, during the preclinical LOAD stages, which if supported by additional investigations, may encourage development of new potentially disease-modifying interventions. The current shift toward diagnostics that help define preclinical LOAD (i.e., biomarkers from blood, CSF, and neuroimaging) is expected to stimulate a new class of secondary prevention clinical trials that feature novel or repurposed therapeutics. Enrichment of asymptomatic at-risk individuals for participation in such trials would depend on using accurate, safe, and inexpensive subject selection methods. The optimal biomarker method(s) could also allow serial monitoring of specific pathobiologic networks that could herald therapeutic failure (or success). Such biomarker approaches may not only allow improved patient safety but also mitigate overall study costs. Novel capabilities provided by preclinical biomarkers, we believe, will help stimulate resurgence in therapeutic development for LOAD by the biopharmaceutical industry. We remain encouraged that through a heightened awareness of all stakeholders in our society regarding the possible utility of preclinical biomarkers, through education and dialog, we may be better positioned to cope with and eventually overcome the devastating effects of LOAD on the world's population.

AUTHORS CONTRIBUTION

MF, AC, MM, and HF conceived this investigation. MM was primarily responsible for coordinating the recruitment of patient samples and clinical data collection. AC was primarily responsible for the metabolomic analyses. XZ, MT, and MN provided statistical analyses of the metabolomic data and classifier development. MF, XZ, AC, MT, MN, AS, MM, and HF participated in data interpretation. MF, XZ, and MM produced all tables and figures. MF, SZ, AC, MO, SC, and MM performed the literature search. CG provided neuro-economics perspectives. KF provided the neuro-ethics perspectives. All the authors participated in writing the manuscript and editing for content. Final manuscript preparation and edits were performed by MF and HF.

ACKNOWLEDGMENTS

We thank R. Padilla, I. Conteh, J. McCann, and D. Phelps for processing and storage of the biorepository specimens in preparation for metabolomic analyses, and R. Singh and P. Kaur for technical assistance in developing the metabolomics data. We thank Eileen Johnson, RN, for collecting blood samples associated with this study.

REFERENCES

1. Sperling RA, Aisen PS, Beckett LA, Bennett DA, Craft S, Fagan AM, et al. Toward defining the preclinical stages of Alzheimer's disease: recommendations from the National Institute on Aging-Alzheimer's Association workgroups on diagnostic guidelines for Alzheimer's disease. *Alzheimers Dement* (2011) **7**:280–92. doi:10.1016/j.jalz.2011.03.003
2. Mapstone M, Cheema AK, Fiandaca MS, Zhong X, Mhyre TR, Macarthur LH, et al. Plasma phospholipids identify antecedent memory impairment in older adults. *Nat Med* (2014) **20**:415–8. doi:10.1038/nm.3466
3. Fiandaca MS, Mapstone M, Cheema AK, Federoff HJ. The critical need for defining preclinical biomarkers in Alzheimer's disease. *Alzheimers Dement* (2014) **10**:S195–211. doi:10.1016/j.jalz.2014.04.015
4. Zweig MH, Campbell G. Receiver-operating characteristic (ROC) plots: a fundamental evaluation tool in clinical medicine. *Clin Chem* (1993) **39**:561–77.
5. Whiley L, Sen A, Heaton J, Proitsi P, Garcia-Gomez D, Leung R, et al. Evidence of altered phosphatidylcholine metabolism in Alzheimer's disease. *Neurobiol Aging* (2014) **35**:271–8. doi:10.1016/j.neurobiolaging.2013.08.001
6. Guyon I. *A Scaling Law for the Validation Set Training Set Ratio*. Homdel, NJ: AT&T Bell Laboratories (1996).
7. Tibshirani R. Regression shrinkage and selection via the lasso. *J R Stat Soc B* (1996) **58**:267–88.
8. Hastie T, Tibshirani R, Friedman J. *The Elements of Statistical Learning; Data Mining, Inference, and Prediction*. New York, NY: Springer-Verlag (2008).
9. Rousseeuw PJ, Christmann A. Robustness against separation and outliers in logistic regression. *Comput Stat Data Anal* (2003) **43**:315–32. doi:10.1016/S0167-9473(02)00304-3
10. Youden WJ. Index for rating diagnostic tests. *Cancer* (1950) **3**:32–5. doi:10.1002/1097-0142(1950)3:1<32::AID-CNCR2820030106>3.0.CO;2-3
11. Vermont J, Bosson JL, Francois P, Robert C, Rueff A, Demongeot J. Strategies for graphical threshold determination. *Comput Methods Programs Biomed* (1991) **35**:141–50. doi:10.1016/0169-2607(91)90072-2
12. Plassman BL, Langa KM, Fisher GG, Heeringa SG, Weir DR, Ofstedal MB, et al. Prevalence of dementia in the United States: the aging, demographics, and memory study. *Neuroepidemiology* (2007) **29**:125–32. doi:10.1159/000109998
13. Steinberg DM, Fine J, Chappell R. Sample size for positive and negative predictive value in diagnostic research using case-control designs. *Biostatistics* (2009) **10**:94–105. doi:10.1093/biostatistics/kxn018
14. Alzheimer's A. 2014 Alzheimer's disease facts and figures. *Alzheimers Dement* (2014) **10**:e47–92. doi:10.1016/j.jalz.2014.02.001
15. Chatterjee P, Lim WLF, Gupta VB, Sorhabi HR, Taddei K, Brown B, et al. Altered plasma phospholipid composition in autosomal dominant Alzheimer's disease: a DIAN study. *Alzheimers Dement* (2014) **10**:260. doi:10.1016/j.jalz.2014.04.412
16. Gonzalez-Dominguez R, Garcia-Barrera T, Gomez-Ariza JL. Using direct infusion mass spectrometry for serum metabolomics in Alzheimer's disease. *Anal Bioanal Chem* (2014) **406**:7137–48. doi:10.1007/s00216-014-8102-3
17. Proitsi P, Kim M, Whiley L, Pritchard M, Leung R, Soininen H, et al. Plasma lipidomics analysis finds long chain cholesteryl esters to be associated with Alzheimer's disease. *Transl Psychiatry* (2015) **5**:e494. doi:10.1038/tp.2014.127
18. Hartmann T, Van Wijk N, Wurtman RJ, Olde Rikkert MG, Sijben JW, Soininen H, et al. A nutritional approach to ameliorate altered phospholipid metabolism in Alzheimer's disease. *J Alzheimers Dis* (2014) **41**:715–7. doi:10.3233/JAD-141137
19. Martin V, Fabelo N, Santpere G, Puig B, Marin R, Ferrer I, et al. Lipid alterations in lipid rafts from Alzheimer's disease human brain cortex. *J Alzheimers Dis* (2010) **19**:489–502. doi:10.3233/JAD-2010-1242
20. Hadaczek P, Wu G, Sharma N, Ciesielska A, Bankiewicz K, Davidow AL, et al. GDNF signaling implemented by GM1 ganglioside; failure in Parkinson's disease and GM1-deficient murine model. *Exp Neurol* (2015) **263**:177–89. doi:10.1016/j.expneurol.2014.10.010
21. Chan RB, Oliveira TG, Cortes EP, Honig LS, Duff KE, Small SA, et al. Comparative lipidomic analysis of mouse and human brain with Alzheimer disease. *J Biol Chem* (2012) **287**:2678–88. doi:10.1074/jbc.M111.274142
22. Nitsch RM, Blusztajn JK, Pittas AG, Slack BE, Growdon JH, Wurtman RJ. Evidence for a membrane defect in Alzheimer disease brain. *Proc Natl Acad Sci U S A* (1992) **89**:1671–5. doi:10.1073/pnas.89.5.1671
23. Klein J. Membrane breakdown in acute and chronic neurodegeneration: focus on choline-containing phospholipids. *J Neural Transm* (2000) **107**:1027–63. doi:10.1007/s007020070051
24. Grimm MO, Grosgen S, Riemenschneider M, Tanila H, Grimm HS, Hartmann T. From brain to food: analysis of phosphatidylcholins, lyso-phosphatidylcholins and phosphatidylcholin-plasmalogens derivates in Alzheimer's disease human post mortem brains and mice model via mass spectrometry. *J Chromatogr A* (2011) **1218**:7713–22. doi:10.1016/j.chroma.2011.07.073
25. Gonzalez-Dominguez R, Garcia-Barrera T, Gomez-Ariza JL. Metabolomic study of lipids in serum for biomarker discovery in Alzheimer's disease using direct infusion mass spectrometry. *J Pharm Biomed Anal* (2014) **98**:321–6. doi:10.1016/j.jpba.2014.05.023
26. Farooqui AA, Horrocks LA, Farooqui T. Glycerophospholipids in brain: their metabolism, incorporation into membranes, functions, and involvement in neurological disorders. *Chem Phys Lipids* (2000) **106**:1–29. doi:10.1016/S0009-3084(00)00128-6
27. Conquer JA, Tierney MC, Zecevic J, Bettger WJ, Fisher RH. Fatty acid analysis of blood plasma of patients with Alzheimer's disease, other types of dementia, and cognitive impairment. *Lipids* (2000) **35**:1305–12. doi:10.1007/s11745-000-0646-3
28. Edmond J. Essential polyunsaturated fatty acids and the barrier to the brain: the components of a model for transport. *J Mol Neurosci* (2001) **16**:181–93; discussion 215–121.
29. Bazinet RP, Laye S. Polyunsaturated fatty acids and their metabolites in brain function and disease. *Nat Rev Neurosci* (2014) **15**:771–85. doi:10.1038/nrn3820
30. Rapoport SI. In vivo fatty acid incorporation into brain phosholipids in relation to plasma availability, signal transduction and membrane remodeling. *J Mol Neurosci* (2001) **16**:243–61; discussion 279–284.
31. Brecher P, Kuan HT. Lipoprotein lipase and acid lipase activity in rabbit brain microvessels. *J Lipid Res* (1979) **20**:464–71.
32. Purdon D, Arai T, Rapoport S. No evidence for direct incorporation of esterified palmitic acid from plasma into brain lipids of awake adult rat. *J Lipid Res* (1997) **38**:526–30.
33. Spector AA. Plasma free fatty acid and lipoproteins as sources of polyunsaturated fatty acid for the brain. *J Mol Neurosci* (2001) **16**:159–65; discussion 215–121.
34. Sugiura T, Kudo N, Ojima T, Mabuchi-Itoh K, Yamashita A, Waku K. Coenzyme A-dependent cleavage of membrane phospholipids in several rat tissues: ATP-independent acyl-CoA synthesis and the generation of lysophospholipids. *Biochim Biophys Acta* (1995) **1255**:167–76. doi:10.1016/0005-2760(94)00237-S
35. Deutsch J, Rapoport SI, Purdon AD. Relation between free fatty acid and acyl-CoA concentrations in rat brain following decapitation. *Neurochem Res* (1997) **22**:759–65. doi:10.1023/A:1022030306359
36. Rabin O, Deutsch J, Grange E, Pettigrew KD, Chang MC, Rapoport SI, et al. Changes in cerebral acyl-CoA concentrations following ischemia-reperfusion in awake gerbils. *J Neurochem* (1997) **68**:2111–8. doi:10.1046/j.1471-4159.1997.68052111.x
37. Rapoport SI, Chang MCJ, Spector AA. Delivery and turnover of plasma-derived essential PUFAs in mammalian brain. *J Lipid Res* (2001) **42**:678–85.
38. Kennedy EP, Weiss SB. The function of cytidine coenzymes in the biosynthesis of phospholipides. *J Biol Chem* (1956) **222**:193–214.
39. van Wijk N, Broersen LM, De Wilde MC, Hageman RJ, Groenendijk M, Sijben JW, et al. Targeting synaptic dysfunction in Alzheimer's disease by administering a specific nutrient combination. *J Alzheimers Dis* (2014) **38**:459–79. doi:10.3233/JAD-130998
40. de Waal H, Stam CJ, Lansbergen MM, Wieggers RL, Kamphuis PJ, Scheltens P, et al. The effect of souvenaid on functional brain network organisation in patients with mild Alzheimer's disease: a randomised controlled study. *PLoS One* (2014) **9**:e86558. doi:10.1371/journal.pone.0086558
41. McIntyre JA, Ramsey CJ, Gitter BD, Saykin AJ, Wagenknecht DR, Hyslop PA, et al. Antiphospholipid autoantibodies as blood biomarkers for detection of early stage Alzheimer's disease. *Autoimmunity* (2015) **48**(5):344–51. doi:10.3109/08916934.2015.1008464
42. Jones LL, Mcdonald DA, Borum PR. Acylcarnitines: role in brain. *Prog Lipid Res* (2010) **49**:61–75. doi:10.1016/j.plipres.2009.08.004
43. Jimenez-Jimenez FJ, Molina JA, Gomez P, Vargas C, De Bustos F, Benito-Leon J, et al. Neurotransmitter amino acids in cerebrospinal fluid of patients

with Alzheimer's disease. *J Neural Transm* (1998) **105**:269–77. doi:10.1007/s007020050073
44. Holland J, Fasanello S, Onuma T. Psychiatric symptoms associated with L-asparaginase administration. *J Psychiatr Res* (1974) **10**:105–13. doi:10.1016/0022-3956(74)90030-2
45. Ubuka T, Meister A. Studies on the utilization of asparagine by mouse leukemia cells. *J Natl Cancer Inst* (1971) **46**:291–8.
46. Hubbard SC, Ivatt RJ. Synthesis and processing of asparagine-linked oligosaccharides. *Annu Rev Biochem* (1981) **50**:555–83. doi:10.1146/annurev.bi.50.070181.003011
47. Ruzzo EK, Capo-Chichi JM, Ben-Zeev B, Chitayat D, Mao H, Pappas AL, et al. Deficiency of asparagine synthetase causes congenital microcephaly and a progressive form of encephalopathy. *Neuron* (2013) **80**:429–41. doi:10.1016/j.neuron.2013.08.013
48. Leiper J, Nandi M. The therapeutic potential of targeting endogenous inhibitors of nitric oxide synthesis. *Nat Rev Drug Discov* (2011) **10**:277–91. doi:10.1038/nrd3358
49. Boger RH, Sullivan LM, Schwedhelm E, Wang TJ, Maas R, Benjamin EJ, et al. Plasma asymmetric dimethylarginine and incidence of cardiovascular disease and death in the community. *Circulation* (2009) **119**:1592–600. doi:10.1161/CIRCULATIONAHA.108.838268
50. Alderton WK, Cooper CE, Knowles RG. Nitric oxide synthases: structure, function and inhibition. *Biochem J* (2001) **357**:593–615. doi:10.1042/0264-6021:3570593
51. Feil R, Kleppisch T. NO/cGMP-dependent modulation of synaptic transmission. *Handb Exp Pharmacol* (2008) **184**:529–60. doi:10.1007/978-3-540-74805-2_16
52. Arlt S, Schulze F, Eichenlaub M, Maas R, Lehmbeck JT, Schwedhelm E, et al. Asymmetrical dimethylarginine is increased in plasma and decreased in cerebrospinal fluid of patients with Alzheimer's disease. *Dement Geriatr Cogn Disord* (2008) **26**:58–64. doi:10.1159/000144026
53. Hamel E. The cerebral circulation: function and dysfunction in Alzheimer's disease. *J Cardiovasc Pharmacol* (2014) **65**:317–24. doi:10.1097/FJC.0000000000000177
54. Hall J, Viney R, Haas M. Taking a count: the evaluation of genetic testing. *Aust N Z J Public Health* (1998) **22**:754–8. doi:10.1111/j.1467-842X.1998.tb01488.x
55. Lliffe S, Manthorpe J. The hazards of early recognition of dementia: a risk assessment. *Aging Ment Health* (2004) **8**:99–105. doi:10.1080/13607860410001649653
56. Billings PR, Kohn MA, De Cuevas M, Beckwith J, Alper JS, Natowicz MR. Discrimination as a consequence of genetic testing. *Am J Hum Genet* (1992) **50**:476–82.
57. Grosse SD, Wordsworth S, Payne K. Economic methods for valuing the outcomes of genetic testing: beyond cost-effectiveness analysis. *Genet Med* (2008) **10**:648–54. doi:10.1097/GIM.0b013e3181837217
58. Hsu JW, Willis R. Dementia risk and financial decision making by older households: the impact of information. *J Hum Cap* (2013) **2013**:45. doi:10.2139/ssrn.2339225
59. Marson DC, Sawrie SM, Snyder S, Mcinturff B, Stalvey T, Boothe A, et al. Assessing financial capacity in patients with Alzheimer disease: a conceptual model and prototype instrument. *Arch Neurol* (2000) **57**:877–84. doi:10.1001/archneur.57.6.877
60. Martin R, Griffith HR, Belue K, Harrell L, Zamrini E, Anderson B, et al. Declining financial capacity in patients with mild Alzheimer disease: a one-year longitudinal study. *Am J Geriatr Psychiatry* (2008) **16**:209–19. doi:10.1097/JGP.0b013e318157cb00
61. Triebel KL, Martin R, Griffith HR, Marceaux J, Okonkwo OC, Harrell L, et al. Declining financial capacity in mild cognitive impairment: a 1-year longitudinal study. *Neurology* (2009) **73**:928–34. doi:10.1212/WNL.0b013e3181b87971
62. Karlawish J. How are we going to live with Alzheimer's disease? *Health Aff (Millwood)* (2014) **33**:541–6. doi:10.1377/hlthaff.2014.0089
63. Hoffman D. Alzheimer's disease legislation and policy – now and in the future. *Health Aff (Millwood)* (2014) **33**:561–5. doi:10.1377/hlthaff.2013.1223
64. Guttman A, Wagner JW, Allen AL, Arras JD, Atkinson BF, Farahany NA, et al. *Presidential Commission for the Study of Bioethical Issues Report, GRAY MATTERS – Integrative Approaches for Neuroscience, Ethics, and Society.* Washington, DC: US Dept Health and Human Services (2014). http://www.bioethics.gov/sites/default/files/Gray%20Matters%20Vol%201.pdf
65. Goldman JS, Hahn SE, Catania JW, Larusse-Eckert S, Butson MB, Rumbaugh M, et al. Genetic counseling and testing for Alzheimer disease: joint practice guidelines of the American College of Medical Genetics and the National Society of Genetic Counselors. *Genet Med* (2011) **13**:597–605. doi:10.1097/GIM.0b013e31821d69b8

23

Anti-Aβ autoantibodies in amyloid-related imaging abnormalities (ARIA): candidate biomarker for immunotherapy in Alzheimer's disease and cerebral amyloid angiopathy

*Jacopo C. DiFrancesco[1,2], Martina Longoni[1,2] and Fabrizio Piazza[1,2,3]**

[1] School of Medicine, Milan Center for Neuroscience (NeuroMi), University of Milano-Bicocca, Monza, Italy, [2] The Inflammatory Cerebral Amyloid Angiopathy and Alzheimer's Disease βiomarkers (iCAβ) International Network, Monza, Italy, [3] The iCAβ-ITALY Study Group of the Italian Society for the Study of Dementia (SINdem), Monza, Italy

Edited by:
Charlotte Elisabeth Teunissen, VU University Medical Center Amsterdam, Netherlands

Reviewed by:
Darius Widera, University of Reading, UK
Ales Bartos, National Institute of Mental Health, Czech Republic

***Correspondence:**
Fabrizio Piazza, iCAβ International Network, School of Medicine, University of Milano-Bicocca, Via Cadore 48, Monza, 20900, Italy
fabrizio.piazza@unimib.it

Amyloid-related imaging abnormalities (ARIA) represent the major severe side effect of amyloid-beta (Aβ) immunotherapy for Alzheimer's disease (AD). Early biomarkers of ARIA represent an important challenge to ensure safe and beneficial effects of immunotherapies, given that different promising clinical trials in prodromal and subjects at risk for AD are underway. The recent demonstration that cerebrospinal fluid (CSF) anti-Aβ autoantibodies play a key role in the development of the ARIA-like events characterizing cerebral amyloid angiopathy-related inflammation generated great interest in the field of immunotherapy. Herein, we critically review the growing body of evidence supporting the monitoring of CSF anti-Aβ autoantibody as a promising candidate biomarker for ARIA in clinical trials.

Keywords: cerebral amyloid angiopathy related inflammation, *i*CAβ International Network, Alzheimer's disease, cerebrospinal fluid biomarker, amyloid-related imaging abnormalities, Aβ disease modifying therapies, immunotherapy, anti-amyloid antibody clinical trials

Introduction

Biomarkers for the stratification, follow-up and monitoring of the safe and effective therapeutic response of amyloid-beta (Aβ) disease-modifying therapies (DMT) represent a research priority in Alzheimer's disease (AD) (1).

Immunotherapy trials, in particular, have underlined the urgent need of safety biomarkers to avoid, or at least enable the early detection of the severe side effects of treatment termed amyloid-related imaging abnormalities (ARIA) (2). There are two types of ARIA: ARIA-E, characterized by the magnetic resonance imaging (MRI) evidence of vasogenic edema (VE) and/or sulcal effusion on fluid-attenuated inversion recovery (FLAIR), as hallmarks of inflammation at the level of the affected vessels; and ARIA-H, characterized by signal of hemosiderin deposits involving microhemorrhages (MHs) and superficial siderosis on T2*-weighted gradient echo (T2*-GRE) or susceptibility-weighted imaging (SWI), as hallmarks of cerebral amyloid angiopathy (CAA) (3) (**Figures 1A,B**).

Even if the acronym ARIA was initially referred to specifically describe the MRI abnormalities of bapineuzumab (2, 4–6), the first monoclonal antibody employed in clinical trial, the term is

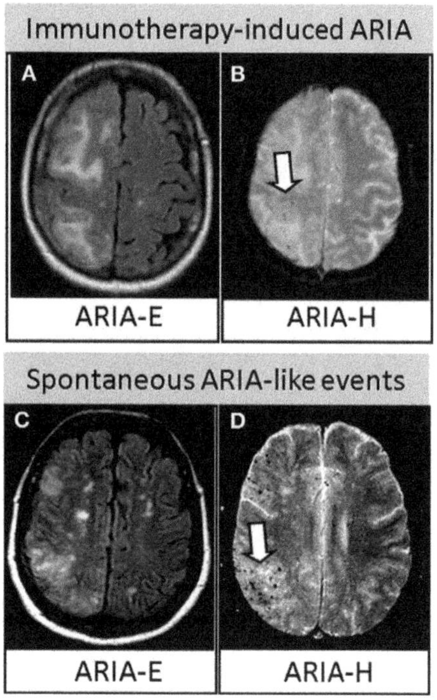

FIGURE 1 | Similarities between immunotherapy-induced ARIA and spontaneous ARIA-like events in CAA-ri. *Upper row.* Axial brain MRI revealing ARIA-E **(A)** and ARIA-H [**(B)**, arrow] in one AD patient treated with bapineuzumab. Reproduced with permission from Ref. (3). *Lower row.* Axial brain MRI revealing spontaneous ARIA-E **(C)** and ARIA-H [**(D)**, arrow] occurring in one CAA-ri patient from the "The inflammatory Cerebral Amyloid Angiopathy and Alzheimer's disease βiomarkers (*i*CAβ) International Network (20, 50)." Images **(A,C)** represent FLAIR-MRI sequences; **(B,D)** represent T2*-GRE sequences.

currently used to define the clinical–radiological side effects subsequently reported with almost all the immunotherapy strategies tested (7–12).

Today, no early biomarker able to predict the incipient occurrence of an ARIA has been already included in clinical trials. However, the current FDA guidelines for enrolling patients in studies assessing DMT require MRI evaluation, recommending to exclude patients with ≥5 MHs and with any evidence of superficial siderosis or prior parenchymal hemorrhage (3, 6). Nevertheless, MHs on MRI are relatively non-specific, reflecting a variety of pathologic conditions. MRI could thus be particularly helpful for the detection of the acute/subacute course of ARIA, but it could fail to predict patients at high risk to develop incipient occurrence of these events, both at the baseline and during the therapeutic follow-up (13–18).

The ARIA issue recently generated increasing interest after the very promising data for the Phase 1b study of aducanumab (NCT01677572) were presented at the 12th AD/PD Meeting in Nice (19) and at the Alzheimer's Association International Conference (AAIC 2015) in Washington (12). This drug demonstrated a statistically significant cognitive improvement in patients with prodromal or mild AD, together with a dose- and time-dependent reduction of deposited Aβ on amyloid-PET. Aducanumab, however, revealed an incidence of immunotherapy-related ARIA in the 55% of patients, particularly in the high-dose and *APOEε4* carriers arm, associated with a 35% of ARIA drop-outs due to the development of these side effects (19).

The recent discovery that ARIA-like events in CAA-related inflammation (CAA-ri) are mediated by increased anti-Aβ autoantibodies in the CSF, has sensibly increased the understanding of the etiological mechanisms of ARIA. CAA-ri has thus been proposed as a human spontaneous model of the drug-induced ARIA in AD (15–17).

Starting from this background, in this review we critically discuss the growing body of evidence supporting the dosage of CSF anti-Aβ autoantibody as a promising candidate biomarkers for ARIA in clinical trials (13, 15–17, 20, 21).

Immunotherapy-Induced ARIA

Trials in AD and natural history studies have suggested that the following all contribute to the development of ARIA: 1) the severity of Aβ deposition (e.g., greater in advanced stages of the disease), 2) the degree of CAA in an already impaired vasculature, 3) the *APOEε4* allele dose, and 4) the dose of drug administered.

In human clinical trials, although the mechanisms leading to ARIA are not yet fully elucidated, it is well demonstrated that increased drug dosage clearly augments the risk to develop ARIA (4, 11, 12, 19). Another interesting aspect is that *APOEε4* carriers, with higher parenchymal and vascular Aβ load, are more vulnerable to ARIA, due to the larger antibody-enhancement shift in Aβ. Consistently, the analyses of the two phase III trials of bapineuzumab showed a greater incidence of ARIA in association with the number of *APOEε4* alleles, increasing from 11.4% in *APOEε4* heterozygotes to 27.3% in *APOEε4* homozygotes. Interestingly, *APOEε4* carriers represented the well-responder group of patients, showing a dose-related reduction of CSF tau and phospho-tau and a decreased rate of Aβ accumulation on amyloid-PET after treatment with bapineuzumab (4, 6, 22), gantenerumab (11), and aducanumab (12, 19).

A retrospective revision of all MRI scans of patients included in the bapineuzumab trials identified an even larger number of ARIA cases (35%) than those previously described (17%), in line with the recent data emerged for aducanumab (55%). Particularly, ARIA-E were reported as the most common abnormalities, while nearly half of the ARIA-E positive cases also developed ARIA-H, often colocalized in the same brain regions. In addition, it has been shown that these abnormalities tended to occur early in the course of treatment, with most occurring between the first and third infusion. ARIA can present with relevant neurological signs, characterized by headache, confusion, and neuropsychiatric symptoms. Patients, however, may also experience mildly symptomatic or asymptomatic ARIA, rapidly resolving with the discontinuation of treatment (3, 4, 6, 11, 12, 19).

Of note, ARIA have always been reported to be paradoxically more represented in patients treated at the higher, but more effective, dosages of the administered therapeutic antibody (2, 4, 6–12, 19), thus dramatically increasing the interest in biomarkers for understanding, predicting, and monitoring these potential hazards (14, 15, 17).

Spontaneous ARIA-Like Events

In 2013, the discovery that the typical MRI findings of VE (ARIA-E) and multiple area of MHs and/or superficial siderosis (ARIA-H) characterizing the acute phase of CAA-ri represent a variation of drug-induced ARIA has generated great interest in the field of immunotherapy (16). Following this first evidence, several subsequent studies have clearly confirmed the clinical and radiological similarities. CAA-ri is characterized by symptomatic or mildly symptomatic acute/subacute neurological signs, mainly headache, mental confusion, psychiatric symptoms, dizziness, and focal signs. Moreover, like in AD trials, the MRI features are represented by asymmetrical and bilateral VE involving the posterior cortical/subcortical white matter, and by diffuse MHs or signs of cortical superficial siderosis (**Figures 1C,D**). Additionally, as for immunotherapy-induced ARIA, the *APOE4* genotype is overrepresented in CAA-ri patients (16, 23–30). Another interesting finding is that CAA-ri patients are typically very well responsive to immunosuppressive therapy if diagnosed and medicated promptly, rarely reporting the occurrence of successive relapses (20).

Of note, spontaneous ARIA-like events have been recently identified in prodromal (21, 31) and established AD (32), and in one case, the development of ARIA has been reported as a possible trigger for rapidly progressive dementia (21).

Interestingly, spontaneous ARIA and CAA-ri have been also described in familial forms of AD (FAD), i.e., in AβPP duplication carriers (33), in presenilin 1-associated FAD (I202F *PSEN1* mutation) (34), and in two siblings carrying the P284S *PSEN1* mutation (35). Recognition that ARIA may arise spontaneously during the course of FAD is a particular timely and important observation that further reinforces the parallelism between iatrogenic and spontaneous ARIA, given the immunotherapy trials for FAD underway.

Anti-Aβ Antibodies as Biomarker for ARIA

The lack of reliable techniques for the detection of anti-Aβ autoantibodies have so far led to contradictory results, showing a reduced (36–38), partially modified (39), unchanged (40, 41), or even increased amount in AD patients (42, 43). A possible explanation is that these studies were conducted in plasma or serum, while their CSF levels have never been clearly explored before.

The recent development of an ultra-sensitive technique able to detect the very low concentration of anti-Aβ autoantibodies in the human CSF has sensibly increased the understanding of their physio-pathological functions (16). CSF anti-Aβ autoantibodies have been demonstrated to play a key role in the etiopathogenesis of ARIA-like in CAA-ri and, today, CAA-ri is widely accepted as a human spontaneous model of the therapeutic-induced ARIA (15–17).

First, like in immunotherapy, the acute phase of CAA-ri is characterized by a specific immune reaction mediated by an increased amount of autologous CSF antibodies against the perivascular deposited Aβ typical of CAA (13, 16, 21, 44–46). Although observed in a single case study, autoantibodies have been found to be intrathecally produced and specifically increased only in CSF, while no changes has been found in the plasma, thus reflecting the immune/inflammatory mechanisms restricted to the brain (13). However, considering the less invasive procedure compared to CSF, further investigations in a larger population will be of certain interest. Second, the temporal relationship between anti-Aβ autoantibody levels and clinical and radiological improvement of CAA-ri strongly supports they are a specific trait of the VE and MHs processes (ARIA-like events) (13, 16, 21, 46). Third, like in AD-treated patients, the increased CSF level of Aβ40 and Aβ42, the decreased amyloid-PET uptake, and the higher amounts of anti-Aβ autoantibodies indicate a transient massive drainage of Aβ from the brain and vascular deposits to its soluble forms (18, 20, 31, 47). Furthermore, in line with data from passive immunization (8, 48), a reduction of both autoantibodies and neurodegenerative markers tau and P-tau in the CSF has also been demonstrated following the clinical and radiological remission of the acute phase of the disease (16, 21). Fourth, the levels of anti-Aβ autoantibodies specifically discriminate CAA-ri from sporadic CAA without inflammation, other non-CAA inflammatory and autoimmune disorders or healthy controls (13, 16, 20, 21). Fifth, anti-Aβ autoantibodies have been suggested as a possible early predictor of CAA-ri recurrence (20).

Such insights have definitively pointed out the dosage of CSF anti-Aβ autoantibodies as a very promising candidate biomarker for the diagnosis, monitoring and management of ARIA. Currently, although the validation of cut-offs for clinical diagnostic purposes is still ongoing, the dosage of CSF anti-Aβ autoantibodies in CAA-ri is already accepted as a valid support in clinical practice (49).

Future Directions in Immunotherapy Trials

The recognition that CSF anti-Aβ autoantibodies represent a valid biomarker in the diagnosis of CAA-ri paves the way for new avenues in immunotherapy of AD. Studies aiming to quantify the amount of naturally occurring anti-Aβ autoantibodies in AD patients enrolled in clinical trials should thus be taken in serious consideration (49).

The inflammatory Cerebral Amyloid Angiopathy and Alzheimer's disease βiomarkers (*i*CAβ) International Network, a World-Wide Consortium aimed to the discovery and validation of biomarkers of ARIA in the largest cohort of CAA-ri today available, represents a leading authority in the field (50).

Here is an example of the different critical information that may derive by the measurement of CSF anti-Aβ autoantibodies as promising candidate biomarker for ARIA.

Patient Engagement Biomarker

The baseline level of CSF anti-Aβ autoantibodies in AD and healthy subjects is currently unknown. A key area for future studies will be to explore the levels and time course of CSF anti-Aβ autoantibodies at the baseline (before treatment) and during immunotherapy. Of note, the high prevalence of *APOEε4* carriers and the co-localization of MHs and VE in CAA-ri (20) further strength the indication to dose anti-Aβ autoantibodies as a potential biomarker to identify those patients at higher risk of ARIA. Notably, these findings will be of direct relevance also for CAA, since the first phase I immunotherapy trial (ponezumab) for sporadic CAA has recently been launched (NCT01821118).

Drug Tailoring Biomarker

The monitoring of CSF anti-Aβ antibodies (both therapeutically administered and naturally produced) may allow personalizing treatment for a greater clinical effect, minimizing the occurrence of ARIA side effects, in order to maintain a putative "therapeutic window" for the safe clearance of vascular Aβ. This may be particularly true for patients at high risk for ARIA (*APOEε4* carriers and/or high CSF autoantibody at the baseline). This may also explain the lack of efficacy of previous immunotherapy trials compared to aducanumab. The dosage of the therapeutic antibody has often been limited due to the concerns of ARIA side-effect, leading to the exclusion of patients from the opportunity to be treated and the continuous adjustment of the therapeutic protocols.

Safety Prediction and Drug Engagement Biomarker

The identification of cut-off for ARIA-like events has been demonstrated to be a valid diagnostic biomarker in CAA-ri. The measurement of the CSF anti-Aβ antibodies titer in patients developing ARIA could allow establishing similar reference values for the prediction or, at least, the early diagnosis of these events during immunotherapy of AD. This could permit the management of treatment, e.g., reducing the dosage or delaying further infusions in patients at risk for ARIA. This could be particularly important between the second and third drug administration, since the majority of ARIA have been reported during this period (2, 4, 6, 8). Moreover, the monitoring of CSF anti-Aβ antibodies, together with the proof of reduced Aβ accumulation on amyloid-PET (11, 12, 22) and the increased level of CSF Aβ, could be proposed as an additional biomarker to monitor drug efficacy and for a better interpretation of the trial outcomes.

Biomarker for ARIA Remission at Follow-up

In the case of ARIA occurrence, an early diagnosis will allow a prompt medication, e.g., steroid administration, thus avoiding the exclusion of these patients from trials. Furthermore, the return of CSF anti-Aβ antibodies below a putative cut-off level (still to be established) could help clinicians in confirming the effective remission of ARIA, as efficiently demonstrated in CAA-ri (16).

Conclusions

In the last decade, ARIA have severely limited the development of DMT. The validation of anti-Aβ autoantibodies biomarker for the monitoring and prediction of ARIA could have critical implications to avoid the occurrence of these serious side-effects. Anti-Aβ autoantibodies may offer a unique possibility to explore the relationships between Aβ clearance and the outcomes of clinical trials, increasing the chances for developing innovative DMT.

The monitoring of CSF anti-Aβ autoantibodies could help personalized treatment. The stratification of patients based on the risk to develop ARIA could allow their allocation in the right dosage arm in order to obtain the best therapeutic window for each specific treatment and study. Of note, since we are moving to larger and longer prevention trials in prodromal and subjects at risk for AD, based on the selective enrollment of patients with positive CSF and/or amyloid-PET uptake (**Table 1**), this is a particularly timely issue that could potentially increase the risk

TABLE 1 | Use of CSF and amyloid-PET biomarkers in current immunotherapy trials of Alzheimer's disease and cerebral amyloid angiopathy (update – September 2015).

Drug	Condition	Trial phase	Biomarker use		Clinical trial government identifier
			CSF	Amyloid PET	
Solanezumab (A4 study, Expedition3, ExpeditionEXT)	Asymptomatic AD or mild to moderate AD	III	Outcome evaluation	Inclusion and outcome evaluations	NCT02008357 NCT01900665 NCT01127633
Gantenerumab	Prodromal or mild AD	III	Inclusion and outcome evaluations	Inclusion and outcome evaluations	NCT02051608 NCT01224106
Gantenerumab and Solanezumab (DIAN-TU)	Autosomal dominant AD	II III	Inclusion and outcome evaluation	Inclusion and outcome evaluation	NCT01760005
Crenezumab	Prodromal autosomal dominant AD kindred or mild to moderate AD	II	Outcome evaluations	Inclusion and outcome evaluations	NCT01998841 NCT02353598
Aducanumab (BIIB037 study, ENGAGE, EMERGE)	Prodromal or mild AD	I III	–	Inclusion and outcome evaluations	NCT01677572 NCT02484547 NCT02477800
Ponezumab	Cerebral amyloid angiopathy	II	–	–	NCT01821118
BAN2401	Early AD	II	–	Inclusion and outcome evaluations	NCT01767311

CSF, cerebrospinal fluid; AD, Alzheimer's disease.

to incur in the same side effects (ARIA) previously reported. Noteworthy, the enthusiasm for the very promising perspectives emerging for aducanumab (NCT01677572) and gantenerumab (NCT02051608 and NCT01760005) may be affected by patient complains related to the high risk of ARIA, thus reducing their feeling in the treatment. Without effective biomarkers we will have the consequence of further unacceptable delays in finding a cure for these devastating diseases.

Biomarkers for ARIA will also improve our understanding on the mechanisms of action and drug efficacy of immunotherapies, i.e., the decreased Aβ load observed on amyloid-PET (8, 11, 12, 22) and the associated positive effects on downstream markers of neurodegeneration (11, 12, 48).

Although the study of CSF and/or imaging biomarkers for ARIA is matter of current active investigation (50), as highlighted in this review, more research is obviously needed.

The validation of biomarkers for ARIA will necessarily imply a multidisciplinary approach and the more strict collaboration between pharmaceutical companies leading immunotherapy trials, clinicians, basic researchers from academy, research societies and regulatory authorities.

In the near future, the comprehension of the physiopathological mechanisms of ARIA and the discovery of early biomarkers will represent an important challenge in order to ensure safe and beneficial effects of immunotherapy (16, 17, 49). Therapeutic implications for CSF anti-Aβ autoantibodies biomarker would be of immediate application, representing a unique benefit of DMT efficacy compared to other more expensive techniques such as amyloid-PET. CSF withdrawal is in effect a common and minimally invasive diagnostic procedure widely used in clinical trials (**Table 1**). The opportunity to implement this biomarker should thus be taken in serious consideration, particularly in the suspicious of ARIA.

Author Contributions

FP contributed in the conception, design, and drafting of the work. JCD and ML contributed in the drafting and critical revision. All the Authors approved the final version of the work.

Acknowledgments

This publication was partially supported by the University of Milano-Bicocca (FAR 2015 QUOTA COMPETITIVA) and The *i*CAβ-ITALY Study Group of the Italian Society for the study of Dementia (SINdem). This work is part of the BIOMARKAPD project within the EU Joint Programme for Neurodegenerative Disease Research (JPND), and the framework of the Ivascomar project, Cluster Tecnologico Nazionale Scienze della Vita ALISEI, Italian Ministry of Research.

References

1. Lleo A, Cavedo E, Parnetti L, Vanderstichele H, Herukka SK, Andreasen N, et al. Cerebrospinal fluid biomarkers in trials for Alzheimer and Parkinson diseases. *Nat Rev Neurol* (2015) **11**:41–55. doi:10.1038/nrneurol.2014.232
2. Sperling RA, Jack CR Jr, Black SE, Frosch MP, Greenberg SM, Hyman BT, et al. Amyloid-related imaging abnormalities in amyloid-modifying therapeutic trials: recommendations from the Alzheimer's Association Research Roundtable Workgroup. *Alzheimers Dement* (2011) **7**:367–85. doi:10.1016/j.jalz.2011.05.2351
3. Barakos J, Sperling R, Salloway S, Jack C, Gass A, Fiebach JB, et al. MR imaging features of amyloid-related imaging abnormalities. *AJNR Am J Neuroradiol* (2013) **34**(10):1958–65. doi:10.3174/ajnr.A3500
4. Salloway S, Sperling R, Fox NC, Blennow K, Klunk W, Raskind M, et al. Two phase 3 trials of bapineuzumab in mild-to-moderate Alzheimer's disease. *N Engl J Med* (2014) **370**:322–33. doi:10.1056/NEJMoa1304839
5. Salloway S, Sperling R, Gilman S, Fox NC, Blennow K, Raskind M, et al. A phase 2 multiple ascending dose trial of bapineuzumab in mild to moderate Alzheimer disease. *Neurology* (2009) **73**:2061–70. doi:10.1212/WNL.0b013e3181c67808
6. Sperling R, Salloway S, Brooks DJ, Tampieri D, Barakos J, Fox NC, et al. Amyloid-related imaging abnormalities in patients with Alzheimer's disease treated with bapineuzumab: a retrospective analysis. *Lancet Neurol* (2012) **11**:241–9. doi:10.1016/S1474-4422(12)70015-7
7. Orgogozo JM, Gilman S, Dartigues JF, Laurent B, Puel M, Kirby LC, et al. Subacute meningoencephalitis in a subset of patients with AD after Abeta42 immunization. *Neurology* (2003) **61**:46–54. doi:10.1212/01.WNL.0000073623.84147.A8
8. Ostrowitzki S, Deptula D, Thurfjell L, Barkhof F, Bohrmann B, Brooks DJ, et al. Mechanism of amyloid removal in patients with Alzheimer disease treated with gantenerumab. *Arch Neurol* (2012) **69**:198–207. doi:10.1001/archneurol.2011.1538
9. Coric V, van Dyck CH, Salloway S, Andreasen N, Brody M, Richter RW, et al. Safety and tolerability of the gamma-secretase inhibitor avagacestat in a phase 2 study of mild to moderate Alzheimer disease. *Arch Neurol* (2012) **69**:1–12. doi:10.1001/archneurol.2012.2194
10. Doody RS, Thomas RG, Farlow M, Iwatsubo T, Vellas B, Joffe S, et al. Phase 3 trials of solanezumab for mild-to-moderate Alzheimer's disease. *N Engl J Med* (2014) **370**:311–21. doi:10.1056/NEJMoa1312889
11. Scheltens P. Biomarker Data from SCarlet RoAd – a Global Phase 3 Study of Gantenerumab in Patients with Prodromal AD. *The Alzheimer's Association International Conference (AAIC)* (2015). Available from: https://www.alz.org/aaic/abstracts/abstr-archives.asp
12. Sevigny J. Aducanumab (BIIB037), an Anti-Amyloid Beta Monoclonal Antibody, in Patients with Prodromal or Mild Alzheimer's Disease: Interim Results of a Randomized, Double-Blind, Placebo-Controlled, Phase 1B Study. *The Alzheimer's Association International Conference (AAIC)* (2015). Available from: https://www.alz.org/aaic/abstracts/abstr-archives.asp
13. DiFrancesco JC, Brioschi M, Brighina L, Ruffmann C, Saracchi E, Costantino G, et al. Anti-Abeta autoantibodies in the CSF of a patient with CAA-related inflammation: a case report. *Neurology* (2011) **76**:842–4. doi:10.1212/WNL.0b013e31820e773c
14. Frisoni GB. ARIA from off-key operas? *Lancet Neurol* (2012) **11**:207–8. doi:10.1016/S1474-4422(12)70021-2
15. Greenberg SM, Frosch MP. Life imitates art: anti-amyloid antibodies and inflammatory cerebral amyloid angiopathy. *Neurology* (2011) **76**:772–3. doi:10.1212/WNL.0b013e31820e7bce
16. Piazza F, Greenberg SM, Savoiardo M, Gardinetti M, Chiapparini L, Raicher I, et al. Anti-amyloid beta autoantibodies in cerebral amyloid angiopathy-related inflammation: implications for amyloid-modifying therapies. *Ann Neurol* (2013) **73**:449–58. doi:10.1002/ana.23857
17. Werring DJ, Sperling R. Inflammatory cerebral amyloid angiopathyand amyloid-modifying therapies:Variations on the same ARIA? *Ann Neurol* (2013) **73**:439–41. doi:10.1002/ana.23891
18. Yamada M. Cerebral amyloid angiopathy: emerging concepts. *J Stroke* (2015) **17**:17–30. doi:10.5853/jos.2015.17.1.17
19. BusinessWire. *Biogen Idec Presents Positive Interim Results from Phase 1B Study of Investigational Alzheimer's Disease Treatment Aducanumab (BIIB037) at 2015 AD/PD™ Conference* (2015). Available from: http://www.businesswire.com/news/home/20150320005170/en/Biogen-Idec-Presents-Positive-Interim-Results-Phase#.VS5GktysXE1

20. DiFrancesco JC, Touat M, Caulo M, Gallucci M, Garcin B, Levy R, et al. Recurrence of cerebral amyloid angiopathy-related inflammation: a report of two cases from the iCAβ International Network. *J Alzheimers Dis* (2015) **46**:1071–7. doi:10.3233/JAD-150070
21. Boncoraglio GB, Piazza F, Savoiardo M, Farina L, DiFrancesco JC, Prioni S, et al. Prodromal Alzheimer's disease presenting as cerebral amyloid angiopathy-related inflammation with spontaneous amyloid-related imaging abnormalities and high cerebrospinal fluid anti-abeta autoantibodies. *J Alzheimers Dis* (2015) **45**:363–7. doi:10.3233/JAD-142376
22. Liu E, Schmidt ME, Margolin R, Sperling R, Koeppe R, Mason NS, et al. Amyloid-beta 11C-PiB-PET imaging results from 2 randomized bapineuzumab phase 3 AD trials. *Neurology* (2015) **85**(8):692–700. doi:10.1212/WNL.0000000000001877
23. Castro Caldas A, Silva C, Albuquerque L, Pimentel J, Silva V, Ferro JM. Cerebral amyloid angiopathy associated with inflammation: report of 3 cases and systematic review. *J Stroke Cerebrovasc Dis* (2015) **24**(9):2039–48. doi:10.1016/j.jstrokecerebrovasdis.2015.04.015
24. Eng JA, Frosch MP, Choi K, Rebeck GW, Greenberg SM. Clinical manifestations of cerebral amyloid angiopathy-related inflammation. *Ann Neurol* (2004) **55**:250–6. doi:10.1002/ana.10810
25. Kinnecom C, Lev MH, Wendell L, Smith EE, Rosand J, Frosch MP, et al. Course of cerebral amyloid angiopathy-related inflammation. *Neurology* (2007) **68**:1411–6. doi:10.1212/01.wnl.0000260066.98681.2e
26. Kirshner HS, Bradshaw M. The inflammatory form of cerebral amyloid angiopathy or "cerebral amyloid angiopathy-related inflammation" (CAARI). *Curr Neurol Neurosci Rep* (2015) **15**:572. doi:10.1007/s11910-015-0572-y
27. Martucci M, Sarria S, Toledo M, Coscojuela P, Vert C, Siurana S, et al. Cerebral amyloid angiopathy-related inflammation: imaging findings and clinical outcome. *Neuroradiology* (2014) **56**:283–9. doi:10.1007/s00234-014-1330-6
28. Mendonca MD, Caetano A, Pinto M, Cruz ESV, Viana-Baptista M. Stroke-like episodes heralding a reversible encephalopathy: microbleeds as the key to the diagnosis of cerebral amyloid angiopathy-related inflammation-a case report and literature review. *J Stroke Cerebrovasc Dis* (2015) **24**(9):e245–50. doi:10.1016/j.jstrokecerebrovasdis.2015.04.042
29. Berkowitz AL, Baker JM, Miller JJ, Greenberg SM. Mystery case: cerebral amyloid angiopathy-related inflammation. *Neurology* (2014) **83**:1678–9. doi:10.1212/WNL.0000000000000930
30. Crosta F, Orlandi B, De Santis F, Passalacqua G, DiFrancesco JC, Piazza F, et al. Cerebral amyloid angiopathy-related inflammation: report of a case with very difficult therapeutic management. *Case Rep Neurol Med* (2015) **2015**:483020. doi:10.1155/2015/483020
31. Raman MR, Wiste HJ, Senjem ML, Ward CP, Jack CR Jr, Kantarci K. Spontaneous amyloid-related imaging abnormalities in a cognitively normal adult. *Neurology* (2014) **83**:1771–2. doi:10.1212/WNL.0000000000000957
32. Carlson C, Estergard W, Oh J, Suhy J, Jack CR Jr, Siemers E, et al. Prevalence of asymptomatic vasogenic edema in pretreatment Alzheimer's disease study cohorts from phase 3 trials of semagacestat and solanezumab. *Alzheimers Dement* (2011) **7**:396–401. doi:10.1016/j.jalz.2011.05.2353
33. Chamard L, Wallon D, Pijoff A, Berger E, Viennet G, Hannequin D, et al. Amyloid-related imaging abnormalities in AbetaPP duplication carriers. *J Alzheimers Dis* (2013) **37**:789–93. doi:10.3233/JAD-130629
34. Ryan NS, Lashley T, Revesz T, Dantu K, Fox NC, Morris HR. Spontaneous ARIA (amyloid-related imaging abnormalities) and cerebral amyloid angiopathy related inflammation in presenilin 1-associated familial Alzheimer's disease. *J Alzheimers Dis* (2014) **44**(4):1069–74. doi:10.3233/JAD-142325
35. Floris G, Di Stefano F, Cherchi MV, Costa G, Marrosu F, Marrosu MG. Multiple spontaneous cerebral microbleeds and leukoencephalopathy in PSEN1-associated familial Alzheimer's disease: mirror of cerebral amyloid angiopathy? *J Alzheimers Dis* (2015) **47**:535–8. doi:10.3233/JAD-150165
36. Du Y, Dodel R, Hampel H, Buerger K, Lin S, Eastwood B, et al. Reduced levels of amyloid beta-peptide antibody in Alzheimer disease. *Neurology* (2001) **57**:801–5. doi:10.1212/WNL.57.5.801
37. Song MS, Mook-Jung I, Lee HJ, Min JY, Park MH. Serum anti-amyloid-beta antibodies and Alzheimer's disease in elderly Korean patients. *J Int Med Res* (2007) **35**:301–6. doi:10.1177/147323000703500303
38. Weksler ME, Relkin N, Turkenich R, LaRusse S, Zhou L, Szabo P. Patients with Alzheimer disease have lower levels of serum anti-amyloid peptide antibodies than healthy elderly individuals. *Exp Gerontol* (2002) **37**:943–8. doi:10.1016/S0531-5565(02)00029-3
39. Conti E, Galimberti G, Tremolizzo L, Masetto A, Cereda D, Zanchi C, et al. Cholinesterase inhibitor use is associated with increased plasma levels of anti-Abeta 1-42 antibodies in Alzheimer's disease patients. *Neurosci Lett* (2010) **486**:193–6. doi:10.1016/j.neulet.2010.09.050
40. Baril L, Nicolas L, Croisile B, Crozier P, Hessler C, Sassolas A, et al. Immune response to Abeta-peptides in peripheral blood from patients with Alzheimer's disease and control subjects. *Neurosci Lett* (2004) **355**:226–30. doi:10.1016/j.neulet.2003.10.071
41. Hyman BT, Smith C, Buldyrev I, Whelan C, Brown H, Tang MX, et al. Autoantibodies to amyloid-beta and Alzheimer's disease. *Ann Neurol* (2001) **49**:808–10. doi:10.1002/ana.1061
42. Conti E, Galimberti G, Piazza F, Raggi ME, Ferrarese C. Increased soluble APPalpha, Abeta 1-42, and anti-Abeta 1-42 antibodies in plasma from down syndrome patients. *Alzheimer Dis Assoc Disord* (2010) **24**:96–100. doi:10.1097/WAD.0b013e3181aba63a
43. Nath A, Hall E, Tuzova M, Dobbs M, Jons M, Anderson C, et al. Autoantibodies to amyloid beta-peptide (Abeta) are increased in Alzheimer's disease patients and Abeta antibodies can enhance Abeta neurotoxicity: implications for disease pathogenesis and vaccine development. *Neuromolecular Med* (2003) **3**:29–39. doi:10.1385/NMM:3:1:29
44. Bogner S, Bernreuther C, Matschke J, Barrera-Ocampo A, Sepulveda-Falla D, Leypoldt F, et al. Immune activation in amyloid-beta-related angiitis correlates with decreased parenchymal amyloid-beta plaque load. *Neurodegener Dis* (2014) **13**:38–44. doi:10.1159/000352020
45. Hermann DM, Keyvani K, van de Nes J, Weimar C, Wiltfang J, Nitsch RM, et al. Brain-reactive beta-amyloid antibodies in primary CNS angiitis with cerebral amyloid angiopathy. *Neurology* (2011) **77**:503–5. doi:10.1212/WNL.0b013e318227b250
46. Kimura A, Sakurai T, Yoshikura N, Hayashi Y, Takemura M, Takahashi H, et al. Corticosteroid therapy in a patient with cerebral amyloid angiopathy-related inflammation. *J Neuroinflammation* (2013) **10**:39. doi:10.1186/1742-2094-10-39
47. Sengoku R, Matsushima S, Murakami Y, Fukuda T, Tokumaru AM, Hashimoto M, et al. (1)(1)C-PiB PET imaging of encephalopathy associated with cerebral amyloid angiopathy. *Intern Med* (2014) **53**:1997–2000. doi:10.2169/internalmedicine.53.1731
48. Blennow K, Zetterberg H, Rinne JO, Salloway S, Wei J, Black R, et al. Effect of immunotherapy with bapineuzumab on cerebrospinal fluid biomarker levels in patients with mild to moderate Alzheimer disease. *Arch Neurol* (2012) **69**:1002–10. doi:10.1001/archneurol.2012.90
49. Piazza F, Greenberg SM, Lleó A, Ferrarese C, Nitrini R, Tagliavini F, et al. Anti-Aβ Autoantibodies in CAA and AD: Different Singers for the Same ARIA? *Alzheimers Dement* (2014) **10**(4 Suppl):P221. doi:10.1016/j.jalz.2014.04.304
50. Piazza F. *The Inflammatory Cerebral Amyloid Angiopathy and Alzheimer's Disease Biomarkers International Network* (2015). Available from: https://sites.google.com/site/icabinternationalnetwork

24

Pro-apoptotic kinase levels in cerebrospinal fluid as potential future biomarkers in Alzheimer's disease

Claire Paquet**, Julien Dumurgier and Jacques Hugon

INSERM UMR-S942, Centre Mémoire de Ressources et de Recherche (CMRR) Paris Nord Ile de France, Groupe Hospitalier Lariboisière Fernand-Widal Saint-Louis, AP-HP, Université Paris Diderot, Paris, France

Edited by:
Charlotte Elisabeth Teunissen, VU University Medical Center Amsterdam, Netherlands

Reviewed by:
Jesus Avila, Centro de Biología Molecular Severo Ochoa, Spain
Andrea F. N. Rosenberger, VU University Medical Center Amsterdam, Netherlands

****Correspondence:***
Claire Paquet, INSERM UMR-S942, Centre Mémoire de Ressources et de Recherche (CMRR) Paris Nord Ile de France, Groupe Hospitalier Lariboisière Fernand-Widal Saint Louis, 200 Rue du Faubourg Saint Denis, Paris 75010, France
claire.paquet@inserm.fr

Alzheimer's disease (AD) is characterized by the accumulation of Aβ peptides, hyperphosphorylated tau proteins, and neuronal loss in the brain of affected patients. The causes of neurodegeneration in AD are not clear, but apoptosis could be one of the cell death mechanisms. According to the amyloid hypothesis, abnormal aggregation of Aβ leads to altered kinase activities inducing tau phosphorylation and neuronal degeneration. Several studies have shown that pro-apoptotic kinases could be a link between Aβ and tau anomalies. Here, we present recent evidences from AD experimental models and human studies that three pro-apoptotic kinases (double-stranded RNA kinase (PKR), glycogen synthase kinase-3β, and C-Jun terminal kinase (JNK) could be implicated in AD physiopathology. These kinases are detectable in human fluids and the analysis of their levels could be used as potential surrogate markers to evaluate cell death and clinical prognosis. In addition to current biomarkers ($A\beta_{1-42}$, tau, and phosphorylated tau), these new evaluations could bring about valuable information on potential innovative therapeutic targets to alter the clinical evolution.

Keywords: cerebrospinal fluid, pro-apoptotic kinase, PKR, GSK-3, JNK, Alzheimer's disease

Introduction

Neuropathological lesions in Alzheimer's disease (AD) include senile plaques, neurofibrillary tangles, and amyloid angiopathy leading to synaptic and neuronal degradations. Aβ is formed after the cleavage of amyloid precursor protein (APP) by β secretase (BACE1) and γ secretase (1). According to the amyloid cascade hypothesis (2), biochemical and genetic findings have suggested that Aβ accumulation can induce tau phosphorylation and aggregation, synaptic dysfunction, and neuronal alteration, responsible for clinical signs of dementia (3). The precise mechanisms of neuronal demise have not been fully elucidated; however, apoptosis has been one of the most analyzed mechanisms in previous reports. Apoptosis is a sequence of events leading to the activation of caspases and cell disintegration. It has been proposed as the predominant form of cell death in AD due to unbalanced actions between pro and anti-apoptotic proteins (4, 5). Increased expression of several pro-apoptotic kinases has been observed in AD brains and their cellular pathways could be linked to AD physiopathology (6–13).

Protein kinases represent one of the largest super families, and they are molecular switches activating and inhibiting many biological processes, such as memory, differentiation, cell division, and cell death. They belong to complex metabolisms interacting with other kinases and their dysfunctions can be associated with various diseases (14). According to Hardy's hypothesis (3), Aβ peptides can trigger protein kinases in AD participating in neuronal signaling pathways between Aβ and tau phosphorylation. Many of these kinases are also pro-apoptotic and could induce synaptic and neuronal sheddings.

Recently, reports have shown that cerebrospinal fluid (CSF) levels of $A\beta_{1-42}$, total tau (T-tau), and phosphorylated tau (ptau) were altered in AD patients and in patients with mild cognitive impairment (MCI) with higher risks to convert to AD (15). The analysis of CSF biomarkers has brought about new insights into the managing procedures of AD patients leading to new diagnostic criteria (16). The levels of these CSF biomarkers correlate with the severity of neuropathological lesions (17, 18). The use of CSF biomarkers has improved the confidence of clinicians for AD diagnosis (19) and now serves for the screening of patients in clinical trials (20). Because lumbar puncture (LP) is better known, more practiced, and well tolerated (21–24), physicians resort in CSF biomarkers more and more in clinical practice reflecting the impact on AD diagnosis (25, 26).

However, these classic CSF biomarkers are not directly predictive of the AD evolution. The need for new biomarkers remains to avoid the classification of patients by quintiles or clusters (27, 28). Furthermore, they have several pre-analytical requirements limiting the analysis to expert centers while AD patients are located everywhere in the world (29–31). Consequently, additional biomarkers are needed to predict the clinical evolution and cognitive decline, and to assess the efficiency of treatment targeting pathways of neuronal death.

This brief report will provide an overview of three pro-apoptotic protein kinases that are involved in AD physiopathology with detectable levels in biological fluids. We aim to address their place as new biomarkers reflecting the rate of neuronal death, predicting possibly the clinical evolution and requiring less pre-analytical preparations.

Pro-Apoptotic Kinases in Alzheimer's Disease

Double-Stranded RNA-Dependent Protein Kinase

Involvement of PKR in AD Pathophysiology

RNA-dependent protein kinase (PKR) is a serine/threonine pro-apoptotic kinase present in cells as non-activated. PKR plays a role in various cell functions (32) and is involved in apoptosis (33–40). Activation of PKR results from autophosphorylation on threonine residues 446 and 451 of the kinase domain (41–45). Once activated, PKR triggers several effectors and pathways leading to apoptosis including the activation of eukaryotic initiating factor 2 alpha (eiF2α), which inhibits protein synthesis. PKR participates in the activation of caspase 8, which can contribute to the conversion of procaspase 3 into caspase 3 (46, 47). More widely, PKR activates both intrinsic and extrinsic apoptotic pathways (38, 48–51). Activated and pro-apoptotic forms of PKR (pPKR) can accumulate in several neurodegenerative diseases including AD (9, 12, 52–54). In 2002, we have observed an abnormal activation of PKR in AD brains (9) and this result was confirmed by several teams (12, 52, 53). Immunohistochemical findings performed in AD brains revealed an accumulation of pPKR around senile plaques (in dystrophic neurites), in the cytoplasm of neurons especially in the hippocampus and the temporal cortex, whereas neuronal staining was more nuclear in the frontal and parietal cortex (8, 55, 56).

Using animal and cells models, we have shown that PKR is activated by Aβ peptide (8, 53, 55–61) through its activator PACT (56), and this activation plays a role in neuronal death in AD (8, 55, 56), Furthermore, we have shown that the activation of PKR (partly by Aβ) could control the levels of β-secretase (BACE1) in stressed cells. These data suggest the existence of a pathological self-sustaining loop involving PKR (1). On the other hand, we have reported a co-localization of ptau and pPKR (8). In neural cell cultures, Aβ induced the phosphorylation of PKR, glycogen synthase kinase-3β (GSK-3β), and tau. The pharmacological inhibition of PKR reduced GSK-3 activation and tau phosphorylation, suggesting that PKR could indirectly control the abnormal formation of tangles (8). Moreover, PKR has been shown to be implicated in memory (62). All these findings suggest that PKR plays a key role in the events leading to abnormal molecular signals at the origin of neurodegeneration in AD.

PKR as a New Biomarker

The analysis of PKR levels in biological fluids of AD patients was further explored. In 2006, we observed increased pPKR levels in lymphocytes from AD patients compared to controls. However, an important overlap between the two groups was found showing that this biological test was not appropriate for diagnosis (63). The CSF is in direct contact with the brain and is less influenced by peripheral factors. We have evaluated CSF PKR concentrations in AD, MCI, and control individuals. Ninety one patients were included. The levels of total PKR (T-PKR), pPKR, Aβ, T-tau, and ptau were determined by Western blots or ELISA methods. The concentrations of T-PKR and pPKR were significantly increased in AD patients and in most MCI patients compared to neurological controls. The optimal threshold for pPKR to discriminate AD patients from controls gave a sensitivity of 91.1% and a specificity of 94.3%. In the group of AD patients, concentrations of pPKR correlated with CSF levels of tau and ptau. A few AD or MCI patients with normal Aβ and tau levels had increased pPKR levels. A correct discrimination between non-AD subjects and AD patients was possible with CSF PKR evaluations (11). To understand if pPKR and ptau could be found in extracellular fluid after the induction of neural endoplasmic reticulum (ER) stress, we have carried out a study in the supernatant of stressed human neuroblastoma cells. Results have revealed an increased concentration of T-PKR, pPKR, T-tau, and ptau after cellular stress. pPKR, together with tau, are released from neural cells due to an increased membrane permeability of unknown origin or late breakdown of the apoptotic plasma membrane. The fact that especially pPKR is increased in AD CSF (317%) and much less T-PKR (38%) could suggest that mainly pPKR accumulates in affected neurons before being released in the extracellular space of AD brains (11).

In a second step, we have analyzed in the same cohort, the predictive value of CSF pPKR levels on the cognitive decline over 2 years (11, 64). Every 6 months, patients underwent neurological exams and neuropsychological assessments including a Mini Mental State Examination (MMSE) evaluation. Using a multivariate linear mixed model, our results showed that the level of CSF pPKR was associated with a more pronounced cognitive decline. In this cohort, CSF pPKR levels were the only biomarkers linked to the cognitive decline over the follow-up survey. Furthermore, although classical biomarkers are very useful to predict the clinical outcome of MCI patients, the results of biomarker levels in the two groups of amnestic MCI patients (converters and non-converters) show that PKR was the most discriminant biomarker between the two groups (64).

Glycogen Synthase Kinase-3 Protein Kinase

GSK-3β and AD Pathophysiology

Glycogen synthase kinase-3 (GSK-3) is a proline-directed serine/threonine kinase and is ubiquitously expressed with two isoforms, GSK-3α and GSK-3β (65, 66). GSK-3 has a role in many biological pathways including gene transcription, apoptosis (67), regulation of glycogen metabolism (68, 69), and microtubule stability (70, 71). GSK-3β is highly present in neurons (72) and can phosphorylate tau at 17 sites of the protein, more extensively than any other kinases (71). It is activated on two phosphorylation sites (Tyrosine 216 and Serine 9), which have opposite effects. Tyr216 phosphorylation leads to GSK-3β activation while serine 9 phosphorylation inhibits its activity (66). Evidences from several works have suggested that the involvement of GSK-3 in AD is linked to the reduction of acetylcholine synthesis (66) and to increased production of Aβ. GSK-3β can co-localize with ptau in dystrophic neurites and tangles (8, 73, 74). Enhanced GSK-3 protein levels and activity were observed in the frontal cortex and hippocampus in AD brains (8). Furthermore, in 2012, we have shown that pPKR, activated GSK-3β, and ptau proteins can be co-expressed in AD brains. In addition, PKR can modulate neuronal apoptosis and tau phosphorylation through GSK-3β activation. GSK-3 inhibition decreased tau phosphorylation without acting on PKR activation (8). It has recently been reported that a polymorphism in the GSK-3 promoter region is a risk factor for late onset AD (75). We have also shown that active Aβ immunotherapy in AD patients induced a reduction of all GSK-3β forms; active, inactive, and total (76). Overall, the inactive GSK-3β appears to be the more abundant form compared to the active form. Finally, GSK-3 is pro-apoptotic and thereby might directly contribute to neuronal death in AD (67).

GSK-3 as a Biomarker

In 2004, Hye et al. explored GSK-3 levels in circulating lymphocytes. Total GSK-3α and β and inactive GSK-3β concentrations were assessed in white blood cells in a series of 113 patients including AD, MCI, and elderly controls. The results showed increased GSK-3α (+65%) and GSK-3β (+59%) protein levels in AD and MCI compared to controls without concomitant augmentation of pGSK-3β (77).

In 2004, a decreased level of CSF GSK-3β in schizophrenic patients from a small cohort has been shown (78). The study did not evaluate activated or inactivated form of the kinase and so far no study has assessed CSF GSK-3 concentrations in AD patients.

Taking together, measurements of GSK-3 in biological fluids could be a supplemental biomarker reflecting AD pathology. Since GSK-3 is dramatically decreased in AD brains after active Aβ immunization (76), CSF GSK-3 evaluation could reflect the efficiency of this therapeutic on neuronal stress and pro-apoptotic pathways.

C-Jun N-Terminal Kinases

JNK and AD Pathophysiology

C-Jun N-terminal kinases (JNKs) are a family of serine/threonine protein kinases encoded by three genes (JNK1, JNK2, and JNK3). JNK1 and JNK2 are ubiquitous, and JNK3 is mainly expressed in the brain. JNKs are activated by phosphorylation (pJNK) through mitogen-activated protein (MAP) kinase kinase pathways induced by extracellular stimuli, such as cytokines and Aβ peptides (79). JNKs have multiple functions, including regulation of gene expression, inflammation, cell proliferation, and apoptosis (80). In the brain, while JNK1 and 2 are involved in the development, JNK3 seems principally implicated in neurodegeneration (81). Previous studies have revealed that JNKs, particularly JNK3, can control BACE1 expression levels (82), can phosphorylate APP, and enhance Aβ production (83, 84). The deletion of JNK3 has a neuroprotective effect against ischemia (85) and excitotoxicity (86, 87). Aβ-induced cell death is reduced in cultures of cortical neurons from JNK3 knockout (KO) mice, and JNKs have been implicated in experimental models of AD and Parkinson's disease. pJNK is increased in AD brains as well as upstream JNKs activators (88).

Immunohistochemical findings in AD brains have shown that the activated form of JNK (pJNK) was localized in peripheral rims of senile plaques, in neurofibrillary tangles, and granulovacuolar degenerations, as previously reported (7, 88). Neurons were modestly marked in the cytoplasm and in the nucleus in AD brains. In control brains, pJNK immunolabellings were rarely detected. The full form of JNK3 was detected, in the center and around senile plaques, as well as in the cytoplasm of neurons. Confocal imaging revealed an association between Aβ42 and JNK3 stainings in senile plaques, suggesting that JNK3 proteins may accumulate during the formation of amyloid aggregates (7). Immunochemical results revealed a significant correlation between Aβ and JNK3 levels in control and AD brains. In frontal cortex, pJNK and JNK3 could be detected in the same senile plaques. Quantification of these histological results showed an increase of JNK3 staining (+59%) and pJNK staining (+182%) in AD brains compared to control brains (7).

JNK as a CSF Biomarker

According to these results, JNK3 could be a marker of abnormal pathways in the CSF. In a recent study, CSF JNKs levels were evaluated by western blots in AD patients and neurological controls. JNK1, JNK2, and pJNK proteins were not detectable in the CSF. A significant increase of CSF JNK3 levels was found in AD patients compared to controls (+23%). Optimal cut-offs showed that the JNK3 value of 70.3 optical density units (ODU) had a sensitivity of 80% and a specificity of 73%, with an area under curve of 0.75 (7). No correlations were found between CSF JNK3 levels and age, sex, CSF levels of $A\beta_{1-42}$, T-tau, and pTau, as well as MRI evaluations using Fazekas scores (89) or Scheltens scales (90).

Patients with AD were followed for a mean period of 1.8 (±1.3) years. During the follow-up, clinicians performed 4.7 (±2.25)

MMSE tests per patient. Using linear mixed models, a longitudinal analysis using tertiles of JNK3 levels was carried out. We found that patients in the third tertile (>89 ODU) experienced a reduced and significant decline in MMSE scores over time. This association was maintained after adjusting for age, sex, educational levels, and MRI abnormalities. Comparison of the tertiles revealed that patients in the two lowest tertiles (<89 ODU) experienced a more rapid decline of MMSE scores over time than those in the upper tertile (7).

Conclusion

Apoptosis seems an important way of cellular death in AD. Several pro-apoptotic kinases are involved in the pathophysiology of AD, and the evaluations of CSF concentrations could be useful to predict the cognitive decline. In addition, since these three kinases are implicated in neuronal apoptosis, they represent new therapeutic targets that could afford neuroprotection and alter the relentless clinical evolution in AD patients.

References

1. Yan R, Vassar R. Targeting the beta secretase BACE1 for Alzheimer's disease therapy. *Lancet Neurol* (2014) **13**:319–29. doi:10.1016/S1474-4422(13)70276-X
2. Hardy JA, Higgins GA. Alzheimer's disease: the amyloid cascade hypothesis. *Science* (1992) **256**:184–5. doi:10.1126/science.1566067
3. Hardy J. The amyloid hypothesis for Alzheimer's disease: a critical reappraisal. *J Neurochem* (2009) **110**:1129–34. doi:10.1111/j.1471-4159.2009.06181.x
4. Lucassen PJ, Chung WC, Kamphorst W, Swaab DF. DNA damage distribution in the human brain as shown by in situ end labeling; area-specific differences in aging and Alzheimer disease in the absence of apoptotic morphology. *J Neuropathol Exp Neurol* (1997) **56**:887–900. doi:10.1097/00005072-199708000-00007
5. Friedlander RM. Apoptosis and caspases in neurodegenerative diseases. *N Engl J Med* (2003) **348**:1365–75. doi:10.1056/NEJMra022366
6. Checler F, Alves da Costa C. p53 in neurodegenerative diseases and brain cancers. *Pharmacol Ther* (2014) **142**:99–113. doi:10.1016/j.pharmthera.2013.11.009
7. Gourmaud S, Paquet C, Dumurgier J, Pace C, Bouras C, Gray F, et al. Increased levels of cerebrospinal fluid JNK3 associated with amyloid pathology: links to cognitive decline. *J Psychiatry Neurosci* (2015) **40**(3):151–61. doi:10.1503/jpn.140062
8. Bose A, Mouton-Liger F, Paquet C, Mazot P, Vigny M, Gray F, et al. Modulation of tau phosphorylation by the kinase PKR: implications in Alzheimer's disease. *Brain Pathol* (2011) **21**:189–200. doi:10.1111/j.1750-3639.2010.00437.x
9. Chang RC, Wong AK, Ng HK, Hugon J. Phosphorylation of eukaryotic initiation factor-2alpha (eIF2alpha) is associated with neuronal degeneration in Alzheimer's disease. *Neuroreport* (2002) **13**:2429–32. doi:10.1097/00001756-200212200-00011
10. Garcia MA, Gil J, Ventoso I, Guerra S, Domingo E, Rivas C, et al. Impact of protein kinase PKR in cell biology: from antiviral to antiproliferative action. *Microbiol Mol Biol Rev* (2006) **70**:1032–60. doi:10.1128/MMBR.00027-06
11. Mouton-Liger F, Paquet C, Dumurgier J, Lapalus P, Gray F, Laplanche JL, et al. Increased cerebrospinal fluid levels of double-stranded RNA-dependant protein kinase in Alzheimer's disease. *Biol Psychiatry* (2012) **71**:829–35. doi:10.1016/j.biopsych.2011.11.031
12. Peel AL, Bredesen DE. Activation of the cell stress kinase PKR in Alzheimer's disease and human amyloid precursor protein transgenic mice. *Neurobiol Dis* (2003) **14**:52–62. doi:10.1016/S0969-9961(03)00086-X
13. Salloway S, Sperling R, Fox NC, Blennow K, Klunk W, Raskind M, et al. Two phase 3 trials of bapineuzumab in mild-to-moderate Alzheimer's disease. *N Engl J Med* (2014) **370**:322–33. doi:10.1056/NEJMoa1304839
14. Shchemelinin I, Sefc L, Necas E. Protein kinases, their function and implication in cancer and other diseases. *Folia Biol* (2006) **52**(3):81–100.
15. Blennow K, Hampel H, Weiner M, Zetterberg H. Cerebrospinal fluid and plasma biomarkers in Alzheimer disease. *Nat Rev Neurol* (2010) **6**:131–44. doi:10.1038/nrneurol.2010.4
16. McKhann GM, Knopman DS, Chertkow H, Hyman BT, Jack CR Jr, Kawas CH, et al. The diagnosis of dementia due to Alzheimer's disease: recommendations from the national institute on aging-Alzheimer's association workgroups on diagnostic guidelines for Alzheimer's disease. *Alzheimers Dement* (2011) 7:263–9. doi:10.1016/j.jalz.2011.03.005
17. Tapiola T, Alafuzoff I, Herukka SK, Parkkinen L, Hartikainen P, Soininen H, et al. Cerebrospinal fluid {beta}-amyloid 42 and tau proteins as biomarkers of Alzheimer-type pathologic changes in the brain. *Arch Neurol* (2009) **66**:382–9. doi:10.1001/archneurol.2008.596
18. Jagust WJ, Landau SM, Shaw LM, Trojanowski JQ, Koeppe RA, Reiman EM, et al. Relationships between biomarkers in aging and dementia. *Neurology* (2009) **73**:1193–9. doi:10.1212/WNL.0b013e3181bc010c
19. Mouton-Liger F, Wallon D, Troussiere AC, Yatimi R, Dumurgier J, Magnin E, et al. Impact of cerebro-spinal fluid biomarkers of Alzheimer's disease in clinical practice: a multicentric study. *J Neurol* (2014) **261**:144–51. doi:10.1007/s00415-013-7160-3
20. Dumurgier J, Laplanche JL, Mouton-Liger F, Lapalus P, Indart S, Prevot M, et al. The screening of Alzheimer's patients with CSF biomarkers, modulates the distribution of APOE genotype: impact on clinical trials. *J Neurol* (2014) **261**:1187–95. doi:10.1007/s00415-014-7335-6
21. Paquet C, Latour F, Saulnier I, Hanon O. [Multicenter study on lumbar puncture indication, clinical practice and feasibility]. *Rev Neurol (Paris)* (2012) **168**:28–32. doi:10.1016/j.neurol.2011.08.012
22. Heitz C, Lorette A, Julian A, Roubaud C, Paquet C. [Lumbar puncture practice in case of hemorrhagic or ischemic risk: a national opinion survey]. *Rev Neurol* (2014) **170**:685–92. doi:10.1016/j.neurol.2014.05.007
23. Peskind E, Nordberg A, Darreh-Shori T, Soininen H. Safety of lumbar puncture procedures in patients with Alzheimer's disease. *Curr Alzheimer Res* (2009) **6**:290–2. doi:10.2174/156720509788486509
24. Zetterberg H, Tullhog K, Hansson O, Minthon L, Londos E, Blennow K. Low incidence of post-lumbar puncture headache in 1,089 consecutive memory clinic patients. *Eur Neurol* (2010) **63**:326–30. doi:10.1159/000311703
25. Schoonenboom NS, Reesink FE, Verwey NA, Kester MI, Teunissen CE, van de Ven PM, et al. Cerebrospinal fluid markers for differential dementia diagnosis in a large memory clinic cohort. *Neurology* (2012) **78**:47–54. doi:10.1212/WNL.0b013e31823ed0f0
26. Troussiere AC, Wallon D, Mouton-Liger F, Yatimi R, Robert P, Hugon J, et al. Who needs cerebrospinal biomarkers? A national survey in clinical practice. *J Alzheimers Dis* (2014) **40**:857–61. doi:10.3233/JAD-132672
27. Wallin AK, Blennow K, Zetterberg H, Londos E, Minthon L, Hansson O. CSF biomarkers predict a more malignant outcome in Alzheimer disease. *Neurology* (2010) **74**:1531–7. doi:10.1212/WNL.0b013e3181dd4dd8
28. Kester MI, van der Vlies AE, Blankenstein MA, Pijnenburg YA, van Elk EJ, Scheltens P, et al. CSF biomarkers predict rate of cognitive decline in Alzheimer disease. *Neurology* (2009) **73**:1353–8. doi:10.1212/WNL.0b013e3181bd8271
29. Dumurgier J, Vercruysse O, Paquet C, Bombois S, Chaulet C, Laplanche JL, et al. Intersite variability of CSF Alzheimer's disease biomarkers in clinical setting. *Alzheimers Dement* (2013) **9**:406–13. doi:10.1016/j.jalz.2012.06.006
30. Gabelle A, Dumurgier J, Vercruysse O, Paquet C, Bombois S, Laplanche JL, et al. Impact of the 2008-2012 French Alzheimer plan on the use of cerebrospinal fluid biomarkers in research memory center: the PLM study. *J Alzheimers Dis* (2013) **34**:297–305. doi:10.3233/JAD-121549
31. Lehmann S, Schraen S, Quadrio I, Paquet C, Bombois S, Delaby C, et al. Impact of harmonization of collection tubes on Alzheimer's disease diagnosis. *Alzheimers Dement* (2014) **10**(5 Suppl):S390–4.e2. doi:10.1016/j.jalz.2013.06.008
32. Proud CG. PKR: a new name and new roles. *Trends Biochem Sci* (1995) **20**:241–6. doi:10.1016/S0968-0004(00)89025-8
33. Lee SB, Esteban M. The interferon-induced double-stranded RNA-activated protein kinase induces apoptosis. *Virology* (1994) **199**:491–6. doi:10.1006/viro.1994.1151

34. Castelli JC, Hassel BA, Maran A, Paranjape J, Hewitt JA, Li XL, et al. The role of 2'-5' oligoadenylate-activated ribonuclease L in apoptosis. *Cell Death Differ* (1998) **5**:313–20. doi:10.1038/sj.cdd.4400352
35. Cotman CW, Su JH. Mechanisms of neuronal death in Alzheimer's disease. *Brain Pathol* (1996) **6**:493–506. doi:10.1111/j.1750-3639.1996.tb00878.x
36. Der SD, Yang YL, Weissmann C, Williams BR, double-stranded A. RNA-activated protein kinase-dependent pathway mediating stress-induced apoptosis. *Proc Natl Acad Sci U S A* (1997) **94**:3279–83. doi:10.1073/pnas.94.7.3279
37. Kibler KV, Shors T, Perkins KB, Zeman CC, Banaszak MP, Biesterfeldt J, et al. Double-stranded RNA is a trigger for apoptosis in vaccinia virus-infected cells. *J Virol* (1997) **71**:1992–2003.
38. Srivastava SP, Kumar KU, Kaufman RJ. Phosphorylation of eukaryotic translation initiation factor 2 mediates apoptosis in response to activation of the double-stranded RNA-dependent protein kinase. *J Biol Chem* (1998) **273**:2416–23. doi:10.1074/jbc.273.4.2416
39. Takizawa T, Ohashi K, Nakanishi Y. Possible involvement of double-stranded RNA-activated protein kinase in cell death by influenza virus infection. *J Virol* (1996) **70**:8128–32.
40. Yeung MC, Chang DL, Camantigue RE, Lau AS. Inhibitory role of the host apoptogenic gene PKR in the establishment of persistent infection by encephalomyocarditis virus in U937 cells. *Proc Natl Acad Sci U S A* (1999) **96**:11860–5. doi:10.1073/pnas.96.21.11860
41. Carpick BW, Graziano V, Schneider D, Maitra RK, Lee X, Williams BR. Characterization of the solution complex between the interferon-induced, double-stranded RNA-activated protein kinase and HIV-I trans-activating region RNA. *J Biol Chem* (1997) **272**:9510–6. doi:10.1074/jbc.272.14.9510
42. Dey M, Cao C, Dar AC, Tamura T, Ozato K, Sicheri F, et al. Mechanistic link between PKR dimerization, autophosphorylation, and eIF2alpha substrate recognition. *Cell* (2005) **122**:901–13. doi:10.1016/j.cell.2005.06.041
43. Galabru J, Hovanessian A. Autophosphorylation of the protein kinase dependent on double-stranded RNA. *J Biol Chem* (1987) **262**:15538–44.
44. Hovanessian AG. The double stranded RNA-activated protein kinase induced by interferon: dsRNA-PK. *J Interferon Res* (1989) **9**:641–7. doi:10.1089/jir.1989.9.641
45. Zhang F, Romano PR, Nagamura-Inoue T, Tian B, Dever TE, Mathews MB, et al. Binding of double-stranded RNA to protein kinase PKR is required for dimerization and promotes critical autophosphorylation events in the activation loop. *J Biol Chem* (2001) **276**:24946–58. doi:10.1074/jbc.M102108200
46. Balachandran S, Kim CN, Yeh WC, Mak TW, Bhalla K, Barber GN. Activation of the dsRNA-dependent protein kinase, PKR, induces apoptosis through FADD-mediated death signaling. *EMBO J* (1998) **17**:6888–902. doi:10.1093/emboj/17.23.6888
47. Gil J, Esteban M. The interferon-induced protein kinase (PKR), triggers apoptosis through FADD-mediated activation of caspase 8 in a manner independent of Fas and TNF-alpha receptors. *Oncogene* (2000) **19**:3665–74. doi:10.1038/sj.onc.1203710
48. Clemens MJ, Hershey JW, Hovanessian AC, Jacobs BC, Katze MG, Kaufman RJ, et al. PKR: proposed nomenclature for the RNA-dependent protein kinase induced by interferon. *J Interferon Res* (1993) **13**:241. doi:10.1089/jir.1993.13.241
49. Donze O, Deng J, Curran J, Sladek R, Picard D, Sonenberg N. The protein kinase PKR: a molecular clock that sequentially activates survival and death programs. *EMBO J* (2004) **23**:564–71. doi:10.1038/sj.emboj.7600078
50. Gil J, Alcami J, Esteban M. Induction of apoptosis by double-stranded-RNA-dependent protein kinase (PKR) involves the alpha subunit of eukaryotic translation initiation factor 2 and NF-kappaB. *Mol Cell Biol* (1999) **19**:4653–63.
51. Scheuner D, Patel R, Wang F, Lee K, Kumar K, Wu J, et al. Double-stranded RNA-dependent protein kinase phosphorylation of the alpha-subunit of eukaryotic translation initiation factor 2 mediates apoptosis. *J Biol Chem* (2006) **281**:21458–68. doi:10.1074/jbc.M603784200
52. Bando Y, Onuki R, Katayama T, Manabe T, Kudo T, Taira K, et al. Double-strand RNA dependent protein kinase (PKR) is involved in the extrastriatal degeneration in Parkinson's disease and Huntington's disease. *Neurochem Int* (2005) **46**:11–8. doi:10.1016/j.neuint.2004.07.005
53. Onuki R, Bando Y, Suyama E, Katayama T, Kawasaki H, Baba T, et al. An RNA-dependent protein kinase is involved in tunicamycin-induced apoptosis and Alzheimer's disease. *EMBO J* (2004) **23**:959–68. doi:10.1038/sj.emboj.7600049
54. Hu JH, Zhang H, Wagey R, Krieger C, Pelech SL. Protein kinase and protein phosphatase expression in amyotrophic lateral sclerosis spinal cord. *J Neurochem* (2003) **85**:432–42. doi:10.1046/j.1471-4159.2003.01670.x
55. Mouton-Liger F, Paquet C, Dumurgier J, Bouras C, Pradier L, Gray F, et al. Oxidative stress increases BACE1 protein levels through activation of the PKR-eIF2alpha pathway. *Biochim Biophys Acta* (2012) **1822**:885–96. doi:10.1016/j.bbadis.2012.01.009
56. Paquet C, Mouton-Liger F, Meurs EF, Mazot P, Bouras C, Pradier L, et al. The PKR activator PACT is induced by Abeta: involvement in Alzheimer's disease. *Brain Pathol* (2012) **22**:219–29. doi:10.1111/j.1750-3639.2011.00520.x
57. Ito M, Onuki R, Bando Y, Tohyama M, Sugiyama Y. Phosphorylated PKR contributes the induction of GRP94 under ER stress. *Biochem Biophys Res Commun* (2007) **360**:615–20. doi:10.1016/j.bbrc.2007.06.087
58. Mecha M, Torrao AS, Mestre L, Carrillo-Salinas FJ, Mechoulam R, Guaza C. Cannabidiol protects oligodendrocyte progenitor cells from inflammation-induced apoptosis by attenuating endoplasmic reticulum stress. *Cell Death Dis* (2012) **3**:e331. doi:10.1038/cddis.2012.71
59. Shimazawa M, Ito Y, Inokuchi Y, Hara H. Involvement of double-stranded RNA-dependent protein kinase in ER stress-induced retinal neuron damage. *Invest Ophthalmol Vis Sci* (2007) **48**:3729–36. doi:10.1167/iovs.06-1122
60. Singh M, Fowlkes V, Handy I, Patel CV, Patel RC. Essential role of PACT-mediated PKR activation in tunicamycin-induced apoptosis. *J Mol Biol* (2009) **385**:457–68. doi:10.1016/j.jmb.2008.10.068
61. Vaughn LS, Snee B, Patel RC. Inhibition of PKR protects against tunicamycin-induced apoptosis in neuroblastoma cells. *Gene* (2014) **536**:90–6. doi:10.1016/j.gene.2013.11.074
62. Zhu PJ, Huang W, Kalikulov D, Yoo JW, Placzek AN, Stoica L, et al. Suppression of PKR promotes network excitability and enhanced cognition by interferon-gamma-mediated disinhibition. *Cell* (2011) **147**:1384–96. doi:10.1016/j.cell.2011.11.029
63. Paccalin M, Pain-Barc S, Pluchon C, Paul C, Besson MN, Carret-Rebillat AS, et al. Activated mTOR and PKR kinases in lymphocytes correlate with memory and cognitive decline in Alzheimer's disease. *Dement Geriatr Cogn Disord* (2006) **22**:320–6. doi:10.1159/000095562
64. Dumurgier J, Mouton-Liger F, Lapalus P, Prevot M, Laplanche JL, Hugon J, et al. Cerebrospinal fluid PKR level predicts cognitive decline in Alzheimer's disease. *PLoS One* (2013) **8**:e53587. doi:10.1371/journal.pone.0053587
65. Woodgett JR. Molecular cloning and expression of glycogen synthase kinase-3/factor A. *EMBO J* (1990) **9**:2431–8.
66. Hooper C, Killick R, Lovestone S. The GSK3 hypothesis of Alzheimer's disease. *J Neurochem* (2008) **104**:1433–9. doi:10.1111/j.1471-4159.2007.05194.x
67. Beurel E, Jope RS. The paradoxical pro- and anti-apoptotic actions of GSK3 in the intrinsic and extrinsic apoptosis signaling pathways. *Prog Neurobiol* (2006) **79**:173–89. doi:10.1016/j.pneurobio.2006.07.006
68. Embi N, Rylatt DB, Cohen P. Glycogen synthase kinase-3 from rabbit skeletal muscle. Separation from cyclic-AMP-dependent protein kinase and phosphorylase kinase. *Eur J Biochem* (1980) **107**:519–27. doi:10.1111/j.1432-1033.1980.tb06059.x
69. Woodgett JR, Cohen P. Multisite phosphorylation of glycogen synthase. Molecular basis for the substrate specificity of glycogen synthase kinase-3 and casein kinase-II (glycogen synthase kinase-5). *Biochim Biophys Acta* (1984) **788**:339–47. doi:10.1016/0167-4838(84)90047-5
70. Anderton BH, Betts J, Blackstock WP, Brion JP, Chapman S, Connell J, et al. Sites of phosphorylation in tau and factors affecting their regulation. *Biochem Soc Symp* (2001) **67**:73–80.
71. Brion JP, Anderton BH, Authelet M, Dayanandan R, Leroy K, Lovestone S, et al. Neurofibrillary tangles and tau phosphorylation. *Biochem Soc Symp* (2001) **67**:81–8.
72. Leroy K, Boutajangout A, Authelet M, Woodgett JR, Anderton BH, Brion JP. The active form of glycogen synthase kinase-3beta is associated with granulovacuolar degeneration in neurons in Alzheimer's disease. *Acta Neuropathol* (2002) **103**:91–9. doi:10.1007/s004010100435
73. Pei JJ, Braak E, Braak H, Grundke-Iqbal I, Iqbal K, Winblad B, et al. Distribution of active glycogen synthase kinase 3beta (GSK-3beta) in brains staged for Alzheimer disease neurofibrillary changes. *J Neuropathol Exp Neurol* (1999) **58**:1010–9. doi:10.1097/00005072-199909000-00011
74. Elyaman W, Yardin C, Hugon J. Involvement of glycogen synthase kinase-3beta and tau phosphorylation in neuronal Golgi disassembly. *J Neurochem* (2002) **81**:870–80. doi:10.1046/j.1471-4159.2002.00838.x

75. Mateo I, Vazquez-Higuera JL, Sanchez-Juan P, Rodriguez-Rodriguez E, Infante J, Garcia-Gorostiaga I, et al. Epistasis between tau phosphorylation regulating genes (CDK5R1 and GSK-3beta) and Alzheimer's disease risk. *Acta Neurol Scand* (2009) **120**:130–3. doi:10.1111/j.1600-0404.2008.01128.x
76. Amin J, Paquet C, Baker A, Asuni AA, Love S, Holmes C, et al. Effect of Abeta immunisation on hyperphosphorylated tau: a potential role for GSK-3beta. *Neuropathol Appl Neurobiol* (2015) **41**(4):445–57. doi:10.1111/nan.12205
77. Hye A, Kerr F, Archer N, Foy C, Poppe M, Brown R, et al. Glycogen synthase kinase-3 is increased in white cells early in Alzheimer's disease. *Neurosci Lett* (2005) **373**:1–4. doi:10.1016/j.neulet.2004.10.031
78. Kozlovsky N, Regenold WT, Levine J, Rapoport A, Belmaker RH, Agam G. GSK-3beta in cerebrospinal fluid of schizophrenia patients. *J Neural Transm* (2004) **111**:1093–8. doi:10.1007/s00702-003-0127-0
79. Daher A, Laraki G, Singh M, Melendez-Pena CE, Bannwarth S, Peters AH, et al. TRBP control of PACT-induced phosphorylation of protein kinase R is reversed by stress. *Mol Cell Biol* (2009) **29**:254–65. doi:10.1128/MCB.01030-08
80. Wei W, Norton DD, Wang X, Kusiak JW. Abeta 17-42 in Alzheimer's disease activates JNK and caspase-8 leading to neuronal apoptosis. *Brain* (2002) **125**:2036–43. doi:10.1093/brain/awf205
81. Bogoyevitch MA. The isoform-specific functions of the c-Jun N-terminal Kinases (JNKs): differences revealed by gene targeting. *Bioessays* (2006) **28**:923–34. doi:10.1002/bies.20458
82. Tamagno E, Guglielmotto M, Aragno M, Borghi R, Autelli R, Giliberto L, et al. Oxidative stress activates a positive feedback between the gamma- and beta-secretase cleavages of the beta-amyloid precursor protein. *J Neurochem* (2008) **104**(3):683–95. doi:10.1111/j.1471-4159.2007.05072.x
83. Colombo A, Bastone A, Ploia C, Sclip A, Salmona M, Forloni G, et al. JNK regulates APP cleavage and degradation in a model of Alzheimer's disease. *Neurobiol Dis* (2009) **33**:518–25. doi:10.1016/j.nbd.2008.12.014
84. Yoon SO, Park DJ, Ryu JC, Ozer HG, Tep C, Shin YJ, et al. JNK3 perpetuates metabolic stress induced by Abeta peptides. *Neuron* (2012) **75**:824–37. doi:10.1016/j.neuron.2012.06.024
85. Kuan CY, Whitmarsh AJ, Yang DD, Liao G, Schloemer AJ, Dong C, et al. A critical role of neural-specific JNK3 for ischemic apoptosis. *Proc Natl Acad Sci U S A* (2003) **100**:15184–9. doi:10.1073/pnas.2336254100
86. Brecht S, Kirchhof R, Chromik A, Willesen M, Nicolaus T, Raivich G, et al. Specific pathophysiological functions of JNK isoforms in the brain. *Eur J Neurosci* (2005) **21**:363–77. doi:10.1111/j.1460-9568.2005.03857.x
87. Yang DD, Kuan CY, Whitmarsh AJ, Rincon M, Zheng TS, Davis RJ, et al. Absence of excitotoxicity-induced apoptosis in the hippocampus of mice lacking the Jnk3 gene. *Nature* (1997) **389**:865–70. doi:10.1038/38154
88. Zhu X, Raina AK, Rottkamp CA, Aliev G, Perry G, Boux H, et al. Activation and redistribution of c-jun N-terminal kinase/stress activated protein kinase in degenerating neurons in Alzheimer's disease. *J Neurochem* (2001) **76**:435–41. doi:10.1046/j.1471-4159.2001.00046.x
89. Fazekas F, Chawluk JB, Alavi A, Hurtig HI, Zimmerman RA. MR signal abnormalities at 1.5 T in Alzheimer's dementia and normal aging. *AJR Am J Roentgenol* (1987) **149**:351–6. doi:10.2214/ajr.149.2.351
90. Scheltens P, Leys D, Barkhof F, Huglo D, Weinstein HC, Vermersch P, et al. Atrophy of medial temporal lobes on MRI in "probable" Alzheimer's disease and normal ageing: diagnostic value and neuropsychological correlates. *J Neurol Neurosurg Psychiatry* (1992) **55**:967–72. doi:10.1136/jnnp.55.10.967

Permissions

All chapters in this book were first published in BADTPF, by Frontiers; hereby published with permission under the Creative Commons Attribution License or equivalent. Every chapter published in this book has been scrutinized by our experts. Their significance has been extensively debated. The topics covered herein carry significant findings which will fuel the growth of the discipline. They may even be implemented as practical applications or may be referred to as a beginning point for another development.

The contributors of this book come from diverse backgrounds, making this book a truly international effort. This book will bring forth new frontiers with its revolutionizing research information and detailed analysis of the nascent developments around the world.

We would like to thank all the contributing authors for lending their expertise to make the book truly unique. They have played a crucial role in the development of this book. Without their invaluable contributions this book wouldn't have been possible. They have made vital efforts to compile up to date information on the varied aspects of this subject to make this book a valuable addition to the collection of many professionals and students.

This book was conceptualized with the vision of imparting up-to-date information and advanced data in this field. To ensure the same, a matchless editorial board was set up. Every individual on the board went through rigorous rounds of assessment to prove their worth. After which they invested a large part of their time researching and compiling the most relevant data for our readers.

The editorial board has been involved in producing this book since its inception. They have spent rigorous hours researching and exploring the diverse topics which have resulted in the successful publishing of this book. They have passed on their knowledge of decades through this book. To expedite this challenging task, the publisher supported the team at every step. A small team of assistant editors was also appointed to further simplify the editing procedure and attain best results for the readers.

Apart from the editorial board, the designing team has also invested a significant amount of their time in understanding the subject and creating the most relevant covers. They scrutinized every image to scout for the most suitable representation of the subject and create an appropriate cover for the book.

The publishing team has been an ardent support to the editorial, designing and production team. Their endless efforts to recruit the best for this project, has resulted in the accomplishment of this book. They are a veteran in the field of academics and their pool of knowledge is as vast as their experience in printing. Their expertise and guidance has proved useful at every step. Their uncompromising quality standards have made this book an exceptional effort. Their encouragement from time to time has been an inspiration for everyone.

The publisher and the editorial board hope that this book will prove to be a valuable piece of knowledge for researchers, students, practitioners and scholars across the globe.

List of Contributors

Dilek Inekci
Nordic Bioscience, Biomarkers and Research, Herlev, Denmark
Systems Biology, Technical University of Denmark, Lyngby, Denmark

Ditte Svendsen Jonesco, Sophie Kennard, Morten Asser Karsdal and Kim Henriksen
Nordic Bioscience, Biomarkers and Research, Herlev, Denmark

Hanne Struyfs, Ellis Niemantsverdriet and Joery Goossens
Reference Center for Biological Markers of Dementia (BIODEM), Institute Born-Bunge, University of Antwerp, Antwerp, Belgium

Erik Fransen
StatUa Center for Statistics, University of Antwerp, Antwerp, Belgium

Jean-Jacques Martin
Biobank, Institute Born-Bunge, University of Antwerp, Antwerp, Belgium

Peter P. De Deyn
Reference Center for Biological Markers of Dementia (BIODEM), Institute Born-Bunge, University of Antwerp, Antwerp, Belgium
Biobank, Institute Born-Bunge, University of Antwerp, Antwerp, Belgium
Department of Neurology and Memory Clinic, Hospital Network Antwerp (ZNA) Middelheim and Hoge Beuken, Antwerp, Belgium
Department of Neurology and Alzheimer Research Center, University Medical Center Groningen (UMCG), Groningen, Netherlands

Sebastiaan Engelborghs
Reference Center for Biological Markers of Dementia (BIODEM), Institute Born-Bunge, University of Antwerp, Antwerp, Belgium
Department of Neurology and Memory Clinic, Hospital Network Antwerp (ZNA) Middelheim and Hoge Beuken, Antwerp, Belgium

Megan K. Herbert, Marijke Beenes and H. Bea Kuiperij
Department of Neurology and Parkinson Center, Donders Institute for Brain, Cognition and Behaviour, Radboud University Medical Centre, Nijmegen, Netherlands
Department of Laboratory Medicine, Radboud University Medical Centre, Nijmegen, Netherlands

Marjolein B. Aerts, Rianne A. J. Esselink and Bastiaan R. Bloem
Department of Neurology and Parkinson Center, Donders Institute for Brain, Cognition and Behaviour, Radboud University Medical Centre, Nijmegen, Netherlands
Parkinson Center, Nijmegen, Netherlands

Niklas Norgren
UmanDiagnostics, Umeå, Sweden

Marcel M. Verbeek
Department of Neurology and Parkinson Center, Donders Institute for Brain, Cognition and Behaviour, Radboud University Medical Centre, Nijmegen, Netherlands
Department of Laboratory Medicine, Radboud University Medical Centre, Nijmegen, Netherlands
Parkinson Center, Nijmegen, Netherlands

Vladimir V. Salmin and Konstantin A. Shapovalov
Department of Medical and Biological Physics, Krasnoyarsk State Medical University named after Prof. V.F. Voino-Yasenetsky, Krasnoyarsk, Russia

Yulia K. Komleva, Natalia V. Kuvacheva, Elena D. Khilazheva, Olga L. Lopatina, Elena A. Pozhilenkova and Alla B. Salmina
Department of Biochemistry, Medical, Pharmaceutical and Toxicological Chemistry, Krasnoyarsk State Medical University named after Prof. V.F. Voino-Yasenetsky, Krasnoyarsk, Russia
Research Institute of Molecular Medicine and Pathobiochemistry, Krasnoyarsk State Medical University named after Prof. V.F. Voino-Yasenetsky, Krasnoyarsk, Russia

Andrey V. Morgun
Department of Pediatrics, Krasnoyarsk State Medical University named after Prof. V.F. Voino-Yasenetsky, Krasnoyarsk, Russia

Yulia A. Uspenskaya
Research Institute of Molecular Medicine and Pathobiochemistry, Krasnoyarsk State Medical University named after Prof. V.F. Voino-Yasenetsky, Krasnoyarsk, Russia

Katja Kühbach, Maren Hülsemann, Yvonne Herrmann, Kateryna Kravchenko, Andreas Kulawik, Christina Linnartz, Luriano Peters, Kun Wang and Johannes Willbold
ICS-6 Structural Biochemistry, Forschungszentrum Jülich GmbH, Jülich, Germany

Dieter Willbold and Oliver Bannach
ICS-6 Structural Biochemistry, Forschungszentrum Jülich GmbH, Jülich, Germany
Institut für Physikalische Biologie, Heinrich-Heine-Universität Düsseldorf, Düsseldorf, Germany

Aaron Ritter and Jeffrey Cummings
Cleveland Clinic Lou Ruvo Center for Brain Health, Las Vegas, NV, USA

Dilek Inekci
Nordic Bioscience, Biomarkers and Research, Herlev, Denmark
Systems Biology, Technical University of Denmark, Lyngby, Denmark

Ditte Svendsen Jonesco, Sophie Kennard, Morten Asser Karsdal and Kim Henriksen
Nordic Bioscience, Biomarkers and Research, Herlev, Denmark

Kaj Blennow and Henrik Zetterberg
Clinical Neurochemistry Laboratory, Department of Psychiatry and Neurochemistry, Institute of Neuroscience and Physiology, The Sahlgrenska Academy at University of Gothenburg, Mölndal, Sweden

Suzanne Elizabeth Schindler and Anne M. Fagan
Department of Neurology, Knight Alzheimer's Disease Research Center, Hope Center for Neurological Disorders, Washington University School of Medicine, St. Louis, MO, USA

Megan K. Herbert and Marijke Beenes
Department of Neurology and Parkinson Center, Donders Institute for Brain, Cognition and Behaviour, Radboud University Medical Centre, Nijmegen, Netherlands
Department of Laboratory Medicine, Radboud University Medical Centre, Nijmegen, Netherlands

Marjolein B. Aerts, Rianne A. J. Esselink and Bastiaan R. Bloem
Department of Neurology and Parkinson Center, Donders Institute for Brain, Cognition and Behaviour, Radboud University Medical Centre, Nijmegen, Netherlands
Parkinson Center, Nijmegen, Netherlands

Niklas Norgren
UmanDiagnostics, Umeå, Sweden

H. Bea Kuiperij
Department of Neurology and Parkinson Center, Donders Institute for Brain, Cognition and Behaviour, Radboud University Medical Centre, Nijmegen, Netherlands
Department of Laboratory Medicine, Radboud University Medical Centre, Nijmegen, Netherlands

Marcel M. Verbeek
Department of Neurology and Parkinson Center, Donders Institute for Brain, Cognition and Behaviour, Radboud University Medical Centre, Nijmegen, Netherlands
Department of Laboratory Medicine, Radboud University Medical Centre, Nijmegen, Netherlands
Parkinson Center, Nijmegen, Netherlands

Babette L. R. Reijs
Department of Psychiatry and Neuropsychology, School for Mental Health and Neuroscience, Alzheimer Center Limburg, Maastricht University Medical Center, Maastricht, Netherlands

Charlotte E. Teunissen
Neurochemistry Laboratory and Biobank, Department of Clinical Chemistry, VU University Medical Center, Amsterdam, Netherlands

Nikolai Goncharenko and Fay Betsou
Integrated Biobank of Luxembourg, Luxembourg, Luxembourg

Kaj Blennow
Clinical Neurochemistry Laboratory, Department of Neuroscience and Physiology, Sahlgrenska University Hospital, The Sahlgrenska Academy at University of Gothenburg, Mölndal, Sweden

Inês Baldeiras
Center for Neuroscience and Cell Biology, Institute for Biomedical Imaging and Life Sciences, Faculty of Medicine, University of Coimbra, Coimbra, Portugal

Alexandre de Mendonça
Faculty of Medicine, University of Lisbon, Lisbon, Portugal

Anne-Marie Miller
Medical Gerontology, School of Medicine, Trinity College Dublin, Dublin, Ireland

José L. Molinuevo
ICN Hospital Clinic i Universitari, Institut d'Investigacions Biomèdiques August Pi i Sunyer, Barcelona, Spain

Brit Mollenhauer
Paracelsus-Elena-Klinik, Kassel, Germany
Department of Neurosurgery and Institute of Neuropathology, University Medical Center Göttingen, Göttingen, Germany

Lucilla Parnetti
Section of Neurology, Centre for Memory Disturbances, University of Perugia, Perugia, Italy

Uros Rot
Laboratory for CSF Diagnostics, Department of Neurology, University Medical Centre, Ljubljana, Slovenia

Anja Schneider
Department of Psychiatry and Psychotherapy, University Medical Center Göttingen and Translational Dementia Research Group, German Center for Neurodegenerative Diseases (DZNE), Göttingen, Germany

Anja Hviid Simonsen
Danish Dementia Research Centre, Rigshospitalet, Copenhagen University Hospital, Copenhagen, Denmark

Henrik Zetterberg
Department of Psychiatry and Neurochemistry, Institute of Neuroscience and Physiology, The Sahlgrenska Academy at the University of Gothenburg, Mölndal, Sweden
UCL Institute of Neurology, London, UK

Pieter Jelle Visser
Department of Psychiatry and Neuropsychology, School for Mental Health and Neuroscience, Alzheimer Center Limburg, Maastricht University Medical Center, Maastricht, Netherlands
Department of Neurology, Alzheimer Center, VU University Medical Center, Amsterdam, Netherlands

Maria João Leitão
Center for Neuroscience and Cell Biology (CNC), University of Coimbra, Coimbra, Portugal

Inês Baldeiras and Catarina Resende de Oliveira
Center for Neuroscience and Cell Biology (CNC), University of Coimbra, Coimbra, Portugal
Neurochemistry Laboratory, Neurology Department, Coimbra University Hospital, Coimbra, Portugal
Faculty of Medicine, University of Coimbra, Coimbra, Portugal

Sanna-Kaisa Herukka and Maria Pikkarainen
Neurology Department, Institute of Clinical Medicine, Kuopio University Hospital, University of Eastern Finland, Kuopio, Finland

Ville Leinonen
Neurosurgery of NeuroCenter, Kuopio University Hospital, Kuopio, Finland

Anja Hviid Simonsen
Danish Dementia Research Centre, Copenhagen University Hospital Rigshospitalet, Copenhagen, Denmark

Armand Perret-Liaudet
Neurobiology, Biochemistry and Molecular Biology Department, University Hospital of Lyon, Lyon, France
UMR5292, BioRan, CNRS, INSERM U1028, University of Lyon, Lyon, France
Société Française de Biologie Clinique (SFBC), Alzheimer Biomarkers Group Co-Coordination, Lyon, France

Anthony Fourier and Isabelle Quadrio
Neurobiology, Biochemistry and Molecular Biology Department, University Hospital of Lyon, Lyon, France

UMR5292, BioRan, CNRS, INSERM U1028, University of Lyon, Lyon, France

Pedro Mota Veiga
Statistics and Research - Curva de Gauss, Training and Consulting, Canas de Senhorim, Portugal

Claudia Cicognola, Davide Chiasserini and Lucilla Parnetti
Section of Neurology, Department of Medicine, Centre for Memory Disturbances, University of Perugia, Perugia, Italy

Yuhai Zhao
LSU Neuroscience Center Louisiana State University Health Science Center, New Orleans, LA, USA
Department of Cell Biology and Anatomy, LSU Neuroscience Center Louisiana State University Health Science Center, New Orleans, LA, USA

Surjyadipta Bhattacharjee
LSU Neuroscience Center Louisiana State University Health Science Center, New Orleans, LA, USA

Prerna Dua
Department of Health Information Management, Louisiana State University, Ruston, LA, USA

Peter N. Alexandrov
Russian Academy of Medical Sciences, Moscow, Russia

Camilla Steen Jensen and Anja Hviid Simonsen
Department of Neurology, Danish Dementia Research Centre, Rigshospitalet - Copenhagen University Hospital, Copenhagen, Denmark

Walter J. Lukiw
LSU Neuroscience Center Louisiana State University Health Science Center, New Orleans, LA, USA
Department of Ophthalmology, LSU Neuroscience Center Louisiana State University Health Science Center, New Orleans, LA, USA
Department of Neurology, LSU Neuroscience Center Louisiana State University Health Science Center, New Orleans, LA, USA

Steen Gregers Hasselbalch and Gunhild Waldemar
Department of Neurology, Danish Dementia Research Centre, Rigshospitalet - Copenhagen University Hospital, Copenhagen, Denmark
Department of Clinical Medicine, University of Copenhagen, Copenhagen, Denmark

Constance Delaby, Amandine Moulinier, Justine Boulanghien and Sylvain Lehmann
Laboratoire de Biochimie-Protéomique Clinique, Institute for Regenerative Medicine and Biotherapy (IRMB), CHU de Montpellier and Université Montpellier, Montpellier, France

Audrey Gabelle
Laboratoire de Biochimie-Protéomique Clinique, Institute for Regenerative Medicine and Biotherapy (IRMB), CHU de Montpellier and Université Montpellier, Montpellier, France

Centre Mémoire Ressource Recherche Languedoc Roussillon, Hôpital Gui de Chauliac, CHU de Montpellier, Montpellier, France

David Blum, Susanna Schraen-Maschke and Luc Buée
INSERM U837, CHU de Lille, Lille, France

Dany Séverac
MGXMontpellier GenomiX, Institut de Génomique Fonctionnelle, Montpellier, France

Thierry Rème
INSERM U1040, CHU de Montpellier, Montpellier, France

Ulf Andreasson and Kaj Blennow
Clinical Neurochemistry Laboratory, Institute of Neuroscience and Physiology, The Sahlgrenska Academy, University of Gothenburg, Mölndal, Sweden

Armand Perret-Liaudet
Neurobiology Laboratory, Centre for Memory Resources and Research (CMRR), Groupement Hospitalier Est (GHE), Hôpitaux de Lyon, Université Lyon, CNRS UMR5292, INSERM U1028, Lyon, France

Linda J. C. van Waalwijk van Doorn, H. Bea Kuiperij and Marcel M. Verbeek
Department of Neurology, Donders Institute for Brain, Cognition and Behaviour, Radboud University Medical Center, Nijmegen, Netherlands
Department of Laboratory Medicine, Donders Institute for Brain, Cognition and Behaviour, Radboud Alzheimer Centre, Nijmegen, Netherlands

Davide Chiasserini and Lucilla Parnetti
Laboratory of Clinical Neurochemistry, Department of Medicine, Section of Neurology, University of Perugia, Perugia, Italy

Sebastiaan Engelborghs
Reference Center for Biological Markers of Dementia (BIODEM), Institute Born-Bunge, University of Antwerp, Antwerp, Belgium
Department of Neurology and Memory Clinic, Hospital Network Antwerp (ZNA) Middelheim and Hoge Beuken, Antwerp, Belgium

Tormod Fladby
University of Oslo, Oslo, Norway
Department of Neurology, Akershus University Hospital, Lørenskog, Norway

Sermin Genc
Department of Neuroscience, Institute of Health Science, Dokuz Eylul University, Izmir, Turkey,

Niels Kruse
Department of Neuropathology, University Medical Center, Göttingen, Germany

Luka Kulic
Division of Psychiatry Research, University of Zurich, Schlieren, Switzerland

Piotr Lewczuk
Department of Psychiatry and Psychotherapy, Universitätsklinikum Erlangen, Friedrich- Alexander Universität Erlangen-Nürnberg, Erlangen, Germany

Brit Mollenhauer
Paracelsus-Elena Klinik, Kassel, Germany
Department of Neuropathology, University Medical Center Göttingen, Göttingen, Germany

Barbara Mroczko
Department of Neurodegeneration Diagnostics, Medical University of Białystok, Białystok, Poland

Eugeen Vanmechelen
ADx NeuroSciences, Ghent, Belgium

Bengt Winblad
Karolinska Institutet, Stockholm, Sweden

Henrik Zetterberg
Clinical Neurochemistry Laboratory, Institute of Neuroscience and Physiology, The Sahlgrenska Academy, University of Gothenburg, Mölndal, Sweden
Institute of Neurology, University College London, London, UK

Marleen Koel-Simmelink and Charlotte E. Teunissen
Neurochemistry Laboratory and Biobank, Department of Clinical Chemistry, Neurocampus Amsterdam, VU University Medical Center, Amsterdam, Netherlands

Aline Dorey
Center for Memory Resources and Research, Hospices Civils de Lyon, Charpennes Hospital, Lyon 1 University, Villeurbanne, France
Neurochemistry Unit, Biochemistry Department, Hospices Civils de Lyon, Groupement Hospitalier Est, Bron, France

Armand Perret-Liaudet
Center for Memory Resources and Research, Hospices Civils de Lyon, Charpennes Hospital, Lyon 1 University, Villeurbanne, France

Neurochemistry Unit, Biochemistry Department, Hospices Civils de Lyon, Groupement Hospitalier Est, Bron, France
BioRaN Team, Lyon Neuroscience Research Center, CNRS UMR 5292, INSERM U1028, Lyon 1 University, Bron, France

Yannick Tholance
Neurochemistry Unit, Biochemistry Department, Hospices Civils de Lyon, Groupement Hospitalier Est, Bron, France
WAKE Team, Lyon Neuroscience Research Center, CNRS UMR5292, INSERM U1028, Lyon 1 University, Lyon, France

Anthony Fourier and Isabelle Quadrio
Neurochemistry Unit, Biochemistry Department, Hospices Civils de Lyon, Groupement Hospitalier Est, Bron, France
BioRaN Team, Lyon Neuroscience Research Center, CNRS UMR 5292, INSERM U1028, Lyon 1 University, Bron, France

Marta del Campo, Harry A. M. Twaalfhoven and Charlotte E. Teunissen
Neurochemistry Laboratory, VU University Medical Center, Amsterdam, Netherlands
Department of Clinical Chemistry, VU University Medical Center, Amsterdam, Netherlands

Wesley Jongbloed and Marinus A. Blankenstein
Department of Clinical Chemistry, VU University Medical Center, Amsterdam, Netherlands

Robert Veerhuis
Neurochemistry Laboratory, VU University Medical Center, Amsterdam, Netherlands
Department of Psychiatry, VU University Medical Center, Amsterdam, Netherlands

Inmaculada Lopez-Font, Inmaculada Cuchillo-Ibañez, Aitana Sogorb-Esteve and Javier Sáez-Valero
Instituto de Neurociencias de Alicante, Universidad Miguel Hernández-CSIC, Sant Joan d'Alacant, Spain
Centro de Investigación Biomédica en Red sobre Enfermedades Neurodegenerativas (CIBERNED), Sant Joan d'Alacant, Spain

María-Salud García-Ayllón
Instituto de Neurociencias de Alicante, Universidad Miguel Hernández-CSIC, Sant Joan d'Alacant, Spain
Centro de Investigación Biomédica en Red sobre Enfermedades Neurodegenerativas (CIBERNED), Sant Joan d'Alacant, Spain
Unidad de Investigación, Fundación para el Fomento de la Investigación Sanitaria Biomédica de la Comunidad Valenciana (FISABIO), Hospital General Universitario de Elche, Elche, Spain

Pauline Bros
Laboratoire de Biochimie et de Protéomique Clinique - Institut de Médecine Régénérative et Biothérapies, Centre Hospitalier Universitaire de Montpellier, Montpellier, France
Laboratoire National de Métrologie et d'Essais (LNE), Paris, France

Jérôme Vialaret, Nicolas Barthelemy, Sylvain Lehmann and Christophe Hirtz
Laboratoire de Biochimie et de Protéomique Clinique - Institut de Médecine Régénérative et Biothérapies, Centre Hospitalier Universitaire de Montpellier, Montpellier, France

Vincent Delatour
Laboratoire National de Métrologie et d'Essais (LNE), Paris, France

Audrey Gabelle
Laboratoire de Biochimie et de Protéomique Clinique - Institut de Médecine Régénérative et Biothérapies, Centre Hospitalier Universitaire de Montpellier, Montpellier, France
Centre Mémoire Ressources Recherche, Centre Hospitalier Universitaire de Montpellier, Hôpital Gui de Chauliac, Université Montpellier I, Montpellier, France

Alison L. Baird, Sarah Westwood and Simon Lovestone
Department of Psychiatry, University of Oxford, Oxford, UK

Douglas Galasko
Department of Neurosciences, Shiley-Marcos Alzheimer's Disease Research Center, University of California, San Diego, La Jolla, CA, USA

Massimo S. Fiandaca
Department of Neurology, University of California Irvine, Irvine, CA, USA
Department of Neurological Surgery, University of California Irvine, Irvine, CA, USA

Xiaogang Zhong and Ming T. Tan
Department of Bioinformatics, Biostatistics and Biomathematics, Georgetown University Medical Center, Washington, DC, USA

Amrita K. Cheema
Departments of Oncology and Biochemistry, Georgetown University Medical Center, Washington, DC, USA

Michael H. Orquiza
Department of Neuroscience, Georgetown University Medical Center, Washington, DC, USA

Swathi Chidambaram
School of Medicine, Georgetown University Medical Center, Washington, DC, USA

Carole Roan Gresenz
Department of Economics, Sociology and Statistics, RAND Corporation, Arlington, VA, USA

Kevin T. FitzGerald
Pellegrino Center for Clinical Bioethics, Georgetown University Medical Center, Washington, DC, USA

Mike A. Nalls and Andrew B. Singleton
Laboratory of Neurogenetics, National Institute on Aging, National Institutes of Health, Bethesda, MD, USA

Mark Mapstone and Howard J. Federoff
Department of Neurology, University of California Irvine, Irvine, CA, USA

Jacopo C. DiFrancesco and Martina Longoni
School of Medicine, Milan Center for Neuroscience (NeuroMi), University of Milano-Bicocca, Monza, Italy
The Inflammatory Cerebral Amyloid Angiopathy and Alzheimer's Disease βiomarkers (iCAβ) International Network, Monza, Italy

Fabrizio Piazza
School of Medicine, Milan Center for Neuroscience (NeuroMi), University of Milano-Bicocca, Monza, Italy
The Inflammatory Cerebral Amyloid Angiopathy and Alzheimer's Disease βiomarkers (iCAβ) International Network, Monza, Italy
The iCAβ-ITALY Study Group of the Italian Society for the Study of Dementia (SINdem), Monza, Italy

Claire Paquet, Julien Dumurgier and Jacques Hugon
INSERM UMR-S942, Centre Mémoire de Ressources et de Recherche (CMRR) Paris Nord Ile de France, Groupe Hospitalier Lariboisière Fernand-Widal Saint-Louis, AP-HP, Université Paris Diderot, Paris, France

Index

www.ingramcontent.com/pod-product-compliance
Lightning Source LLC
LaVergne TN
LVHW060549210926
848485LV00005B/1285